Essentials of Pharmacology

Essentials of Pharmacology

Editor: Brendon Krauss

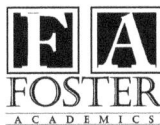

FOSTER
ACADEMICS

www.fosteracademics.com

www.fosteracademics.com

FA
FOSTER
ACADEMICS

Cataloging-in-Publication Data

Essentials of pharmacology / edited by Brendon Krauss.
    p. cm.
Includes bibliographical references and index.
ISBN 978-1-63242-510-2
1. Pharmacology. 2. Pharmacy. 3. Medical sciences. 4. Drugs. I. Krauss, Brendon.
RM300 .E87 2017
615.1--dc23

© Foster Academics, 2017

Foster Academics,
118-35 Queens Blvd., Suite 400,
Forest Hills, NY 11375, USA

ISBN 978-1-63242-510-2 (Hardback)

Printed and bound in the United States of America.

Contents

Preface

Pharmacology is the practice of designing drugs that cure or prevent disease as well as studying its effects and effectiveness. The pharmaceutical industry is ever-growing and more and more methods are being discovered to make effective drugs available. Newer medicines that are engineered in the laboratory can reduce the rehabilitation period as well as chances of relapse. This book is compiled in such a manner that it will provide in-depth knowledge about the theory and practice of pharmacology. From theories to research to practical applications, case studies related to all contemporary topics of relevance to this field have been included in this text. It will provide comprehensive knowledge to the readers. This text will be relevant to students and researchers alike in the fields of surgery, pharmacotherapy and pharmaceutical medicine.

The information shared in this book is based on empirical researches made by veterans in this field of study. The elaborative information provided in this book will help the readers further their scope of knowledge leading to advancements in this field.

Finally, I would like to thank my fellow researchers who gave constructive feedback and my family members who supported me at every step of my research.

Editor

Metformin loaded non-ionic surfactant vesicles: optimization of formulation, effect of process variables and characterization

Anchal Sankhyan and Pravin K Pawar[*]

Abstract

Background: Metformin an oral hypoglycemic has been widely used as a fist line of treatment of Type II Diabetes but in a very high dose 2–3 times a day and moreover suffers from a number of side effects like lactic acidosis, gastric discomfort, chest pain, allergic reactions being some of them. The present work was conducted with the aim of sustaining the release of metformin so as to decrease its side effects and also reduce its dosing frequency using a novel delivery system niosomes (non-ionic surfactant vesicles). Non-ionic surfactant vesicles of different surfactants were prepared using thin film hydration technique and were investigated for morphology, entrapment, in-vitro release, TEM (transmission electron microscopy) and physical stability. Optimized formulation was further studied for the effect of Surfactant concentration, DCP (Dicetyl phosphate), Surfactant: cholesterol ratio and volume of hydration. The release studies data was subjected to release kinetics models.

Results: The prepared vesicles were uniform and spherical in size. Optimized formulation MN3 entrapped the drug with 84.50±0.184 efficiency in the vesicles of the size 487.60±2.646 and showed the most sustained release of 73.89±0.126. Also it was resulted that 100 molar concentration of cholesterol and surfactant, Presence of DCP, equimolar ratio of span 60: cholesterol and 15 ml of volume of hydration were found to be optimum for miosome preparation.

Conclusions: The present work concluded metformin loaded niosomes to be effective in sustaining the drug release leading to decreased side effects and increased patient compliance.

Keywords: Anti-diabetic, Niosomes, Metformin, Dicetyl phosphate, Sustained release

Background

With the advent of therapeutics, oral delivery is the most widely used and the most convenient route of drug delivery. Despite of phenomenal advances in other dosage routes viz. injectable, inhalable, transdermal, nasal, oral delivery still remain well ahead of the pack as the preferred delivery route. Higher concentration is focused in making the oral formulations viable if it is not immediately viable, than in plumping for an alternative delivery method. The top 50 drugs selling in the world have 84% oral delivery [1]. Variety of approaches have been tried to enhance the oral bioavailability of poorly soluble drugs using the excipients with approved or GRAS (generally regarded as safe) status. Micronization by spray-drying, freeze-drying, crystallization and milling; nanosizing into nanoparticles by various techniques with high-pressure homogenization being one of most efficient; crystal engineering of polymorphs, hydrates, solvates, co-crystals, supercritical fluid and sonocrystallization; solid dispersions developed by melt-mixing, solvent evaporation, supercritical fluid and melt extrusion; solubilizing ability of cyclodextrins; solid lipid nanoparticles prepared by high-pressure homogenization and microemulsion technology and other colloidal drug delivery systems including emulsions, microemulsions, self-emulsified and self-microemulsified drug delivery systems, liposomes etc. have been widely researched for enhancement of oral bioavailability [2]. Other attempts of enhancing oral bioavailability include Solid lipid nanoparticles, mucoadhesive delivery system, lipid digestion models, Supersaturatable Formulations, nanoemulsion, nanocapsules, fast-dispersing dosage forms and pH-sensitive supramolecular assemblies [3-10].

* Correspondence: pkpawar80@yahoo.com
Chitkara College of Pharmacy, Chitkara University, Chandigarh-Patiala Highway, Rajpura, Patiala, Punjab 140401, India

Diabetes is a group of chronic carbohydrate metabolism disorders resulting from diminished or absent action of insulin by altered secretion, decreased insulin efficacy or combination of both the factors leading to hyperglycemia. Type II diabetes is the most common type counting about 90-95% of the diagnosed cases, characterized with normal or even excess of insulin levels with insulin resistance being the major cause of increased glucose levels [11]. Metformin a biguanide enhances insulin sensitivity, found to be effective in impaired glucose tolerance, obese patients and patients with cardiovascular diseases and is used as first line of drug in treatment of Type II diabetes [12].

The oral bioavailability of Metformin is 50-60% as it is BCS (Biopharmaceutical Classification System) class III drug and has site-specific absorption in the GI tract [13]. The drug has negligible plasma protein binding, relatively short half life of 1.5-4.5 hours and requires administration of 500 mg dose two or three times a day [14]. Moreover the drug suffers from serious but rare side effects of lactic acidosis with 50% mortality, chest pain, allergic reactions accompanied by high incidences of concomitant gastrointestinal symptoms such as diarrhea, abdominal discomfort, vomiting, stomachache, headache and lethargy [15]. Researchers endeavored for years to enhance the oral bioavailability, sustain the drug release for better patient compliance and reduced side effects of the most widely used oral hypoglycemic Metformin. The conventional dosage form of Metformin i.e. tablet has been modified by various approaches to get the desired results. Matrix tablets with sustained release have been prepared using hydroxypropyl methyl cellulose as a hydrophilic polymer, hydrophilic synthetic polymers and hydrophobic natural polymers and by incorporation of lipophillic waxes by melt granulation [14,16]. With the view to enhance patient compliance taste masked tablets and oro-dispersible tablets have also been formulated, also the FDA (Food and Drug Administration) has approved metformin-glipizide tablets for oral suspension, metformin-glyburide oral solution and linagliptin-metformin hydrochloride tablets [17-19]. Niosomes are non ionic surfactant vesicles having lamellar structure formed by self assembly of surfactant molecules. To improve the oral bioavailability of poorly water soluble drug like griseofulvin, the noisome (vesicular) system was developed [20]. In another report, the polysaccharide coated noisomes of propranolol HCl was developed for the oral drug delivery and studied the effect of polysaccharide cap using hydrophobic anchors on the non ionic surfactant vesicles [21]. The only novel delivery system so far utilized for the delivery of metformin is mucoadhesive ispaghula-sodium alginate beads [22]. Niosomes have been used to deliver a number of drugs and have shown pronounced benefits of enhanced bioavailability, sustained release, targeted delivery, decreased side effects, high stability, easy modification, and so on [23]. In the present investigation niosomes have been prepared to enhance oral bioavailability of class III antidiabetic drug. The nonionic surfactant vesicles have been prepared and evaluated for entrapment efficiency, in vitro drug release, particle size, zeta potential, TEM. Also the effect of various parameters viz. molar concentration and molar ratio of cholesterol and surfactant, presence of DCP and volume of hydration was studied on the various evaluated parameters. The studied system is developed for efficient treatment of Type II diabetes.

Methods

Metformin was a kind gift sample from Matrix Laboratories (Hyderabad, India). Cholesterol was supplied by Fisher Scientific (Mumbai, India). The non-ionic surfactants viz. Span 20, Span 40, Span 60, Span 80, Tween 20, Tween 80 and Brij 30 were purchased from Loba Chemie Pvt. Ltd. (Mumbai, India). Tween 60 was procured from Sisco Research Laboratories Pvt. Ltd. (Mumbai, India) and HPLC chloroform was provided by Merck Specialities Pvt. Ltd. (Mumbai, India). All the ingredients used in the procedures were of analytical grade.

Preparation of niosomes

The nano sized vesicles were prepared using Thin Film Hydration Method. The specified quantities of cholesterol, non-ionic surfactant and Dicetyl Phosphate (DCP) were completely dissolved in 10 ml HPLC chloroform contained in a clean and dry Round Bottom Flask (Table 1). The transparent solution was reduced to a thin dry film using Rotary Vaccum Evaporator (Perfit, India) at $50.00\pm2.00°C$. Metformin was dissolved in phosphate buffer pH 6.8 and the thin dry film was hydrated using this buffered drug solution. The film is allowed to hydrate for about 1 hour for the formation of niosomes [22]. Milky dispersion is prepared which is kept at 4°C for 24 hours for maturation of the formed vesicles.

Entrapment efficiency

The entrapment efficiency of the matured niosomes was determined using centrifugation method. The measured volume 5 ml of the prepared dispersion was centrifuged using cooling centrifuge (RIS-24BL, REMI India) at 6°C for 1 hour to separate the free drug from niosomes. The niosomes formed a cake floating at the top of tube and clear solvent containing the unentrapped drug remained at the bottom. The cake was resuspended in 5 ml phosphate buffer pH 6.8 and the process was repeated twice by centrifugation for 30 minutes to ensure complete removal of free drug. After suitable dilution with

Table 1 Composition (molar ratio), entrapment efficiency and particle size of metformin niosomes

Formulation code	Cholesterol	Surfactant	Dicetyl phosphate (mg)	Entrapment* efficiency (%)	Particle size* (nm)
MN1	250	Span 60 (250)	5	85.16±0.12	574.33±2.08
MN2	250	Span 60 (250)	-	87.12±0.05	636.00±2.65
MN3	100	Span 60 (100)	5	84.50±0.18	487.60±2.65
MN4	100	Span 60 (100)	-	86.51±0.15	504.66±2.52
MN5	75	Span 60 (75)	5	83.66±0.08	388.0±3.61
MN6	75	Span 60 (75)	-	84.71±0.05	496.66±3.51
MN7	250	Span 40 (250)	5	83.91±0.01	565.33±2.52
MN8	250	Span 40 (250)	-	85.07±0.08	624.67±2.08
MN9	100	Span 40 (100)	5	83.71±0.12	462.33±2.08
MN10	100	Span 40 (100)	-	84.88±0.11	496.33±1.53
MN11	75	Span 40 (75)	5	84.56±0.08	378.67±1.53
MN12	75	Span 40 (75)	-	86.63±0.02	484.67±1.53

*Mean ± SD, n = 3.

Phosphate buffer pH6.8 the clear fraction was used for the determination of free drug spectrophotometrically by UV-visible Spectrophotometer (AU-2701, Systronics, Mumbai, India) [24]. The entrapment efficiency was calculated using the formula

$$PercentEntrapmentEfficiency = \frac{InitialDrug(D_i) - Unentrappeddrug(D_u)}{InitialDrug(D_i)} X100$$

In-vitro drug release

The in-vitro drug release pattern was studied using modified USP dissolution apparatus I. Samples were placed on the dialysis membrane previously soaked overnight in phosphate buffer pH 6.8 and attached to lower end of a glass tube. The tubes were immersed in dissolution vessel containing phosphate buffer pH 6.8 maintained at 37±0.5°C. Samples were withdrawn at regular interval of time and replaced with equal amount of buffer to maintain sink condition [25]. The samples were analyzed by UV/Visible spectrophotometer (AU-2701, Systronics, Mumbai, India) for the drug release pattern. The study was continued upto 8 hours.

Particle size and zeta potential

The particle size of the non-ionic surfactant vesicles was determined by dynamic light scattering technique also known as photon correlation spectroscopy using Zetasizer Nano ZS-90 (Malvern Instruments Ltd., UK) [26]. The samples diluted suitably by filtered water (0.5 micrometer filter- Himedia) were placed in the cuvettes and the procedure was carried out at 90° angle and temperature 25°C to determine the size of the particles in the range of 0.6nm to 3 microns. The zeta potential was determined using combination of laser Doppler

velocimetry and phase analysis light scattering by Zetasizer Nano ZS-90 (Malvern Instruments Ltd.; UK). The diluted niosome dispersions were located in zeta meter cell for determination of electrophoretic mobility [27]. All the experiments were performed in triplicate.

Transmission electron microscopy

The morphology of the vesicles was examined by trammission electron microscopy (TEM). A drop of niosomal dispersion was diluted 10 times and was stratified onto a carbon-coated copper grid for 1 minute and excess was removed by filter paper. A drop of 2% phosphotungstic acid solution was stratified to stain the vesicles; excess was removed by a tip of filter paper and left to air dry. The grid was observed by transmission electron microscopy (Hitachi, H-7500) and by using imaging viewer software the images were analyzed and captured [28].

Drug release kinetic data analysis

The release data obtained from various formulations was studied further for fitness of data in different kinetic models like Zero order, First order, Higuchi and Korsmeyer-Peppas release models [29].

Physical stability testing

Physical stability of the niosomes was studied by leaching of the drug from the vesicles in the native prepared form i.e. dispersion stored under refrigeration. The optimized dispersion with the composition of cholesterol and span in 100:100 molar ratio with DCP was sealed in glass vials and stored under refrigeration temperature (2-8°C) for a period of 90 days. Samples were withdrawn at definite intervals of time and the amount of drug remaining was calculated by the method employed for entrapment efficiency determination [30].

Results

Span 20, Span 80, Tween 20, Tween 60, Tween 80 and Brij 30 did not formed thin and dry film at the round bottom flask so were not used further in the study. Thereby Span 40 and Span 60 were used for the preparation and evaluation in the study.

Morphology

The prepared niosomal solution was a homogeneous dispersion and after maturation of 24 hours was studied under the microscope for morphological evaluation. The vesicles were uniform, spherical in shape with traces of aggregation. The formulations prepared with inclusion of DCP were found to be free from aggregation.

Entrapment efficiency

The amount of drug loaded in the vesicles was determined by centrifugation method which separates the entrapped and the unentrapped drug. The percent entrapment efficiency was calculated and was found to be in the range of 83.66±0.08-87.12±0.05 (Table 1).

In-vitro release

The release pattern of the drug from the niosomes was studied using modified USP dissolution apparatus I. The formulations presented sustained release upto 8 hours with MN3 having the most sustained release of 73.89 ±0.13 at the end of 8 hours. On the basis of most sustained release and sufficient entrapment of 84.50±0.18 MN3 was selected as the optimized formulation (Figure 1) (Figure 2).

Particle size and zeta potential

The average vesicular size of niosomes of all the batches was measured in the range of 388.0±3.61-644.67±2.08 (Table 1). Also the surface charge was studied by zeta potential measurement. The niosomes were found to be stabilized by large negative values of zeta potential and the polydispersity index (PDI) was 0.123.

Transmission electron microscopy

The TEM photomicrographs clearly indicate that vesicles were uniform, unilamellar and spherical in shape. Also the positive staining showed the drug to be concentrated in the core of the vesicles with drug free bilayer (Figure 3).

Release kinetics

The study of drug release kinetics showed that in all the formulations the best fit model was found to be Korsmeyer-Peppas with 'n' smaller than 0.45 suggesting the Fickian diffusion release mechanism for the drug. Formulation MN3 showed the lowest release of 73.89±0.13 in 8 hours and had correlation coefficient (r =0.996) (Table 2).

Physical stability

The formulation investigated for physical stability studies showed the residual drug content in the niosomes to be 77.61± 0.22 at the end of three months. The results concluded that almost 99% of the drug was retained upto 1 month and at the end of the study 91.84% drug was retained by the formulation (Table 3).

Discussion

Effect of type of surfactants

The effect of non-ionic surfactant was studied on the entrapment efficiency, particle size and in-vitro release of the prepared niosomes. Span 60 and Span 40 were the two surfactants used in the study and the formulations were prepared by varying their concentrations to the same extent. Span 60 preceded Span 40 in terms of invitro release and entrapment efficiency by presenting the most sustained release in all the prepared batches and

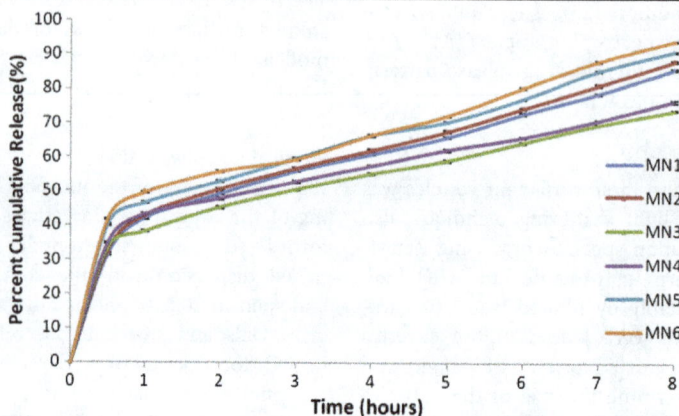

Figure 1 In vitro drug release pattern of metformin niosomes using Span 60.

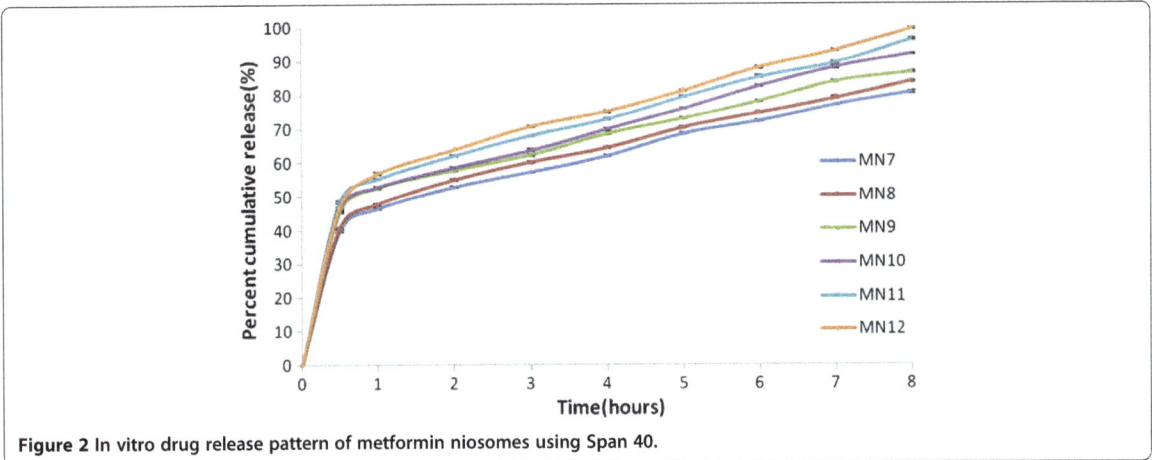

Figure 2 In vitro drug release pattern of metformin niosomes using Span 40.

higher entrapment efficiencies when compared to corresponding formulations (Figure 1) (Figure 2). Span 60 and Span 40 has the same head group and differs in the chain length of the alkyl chain which determines their performance. Span 60 having longer chain length provide more stable vesicles contributing to the higher entrapment and delayed release. Also the ordered gel state and higher phase transition temperature offered by Span 60 plays a significant role in the observed outcomes [31,32]. The size of the vesicles was slightly high in

formulations prepared by Span 60 at the same molar concentration of Span 40. This may be the repercussion of the longer alkyl chain and its stronger interactions with cholesterol molecules which resulted larger core space providing larger entrapment [33]. Decreased molar concentrations of surfactant and cholesterol reduced the entrapment of the drug and the size which may be the aftermath of the insufficient bilayer material to form a strong membrane and to encapsulate the drug efficiently. The case was not similar for the drug release an

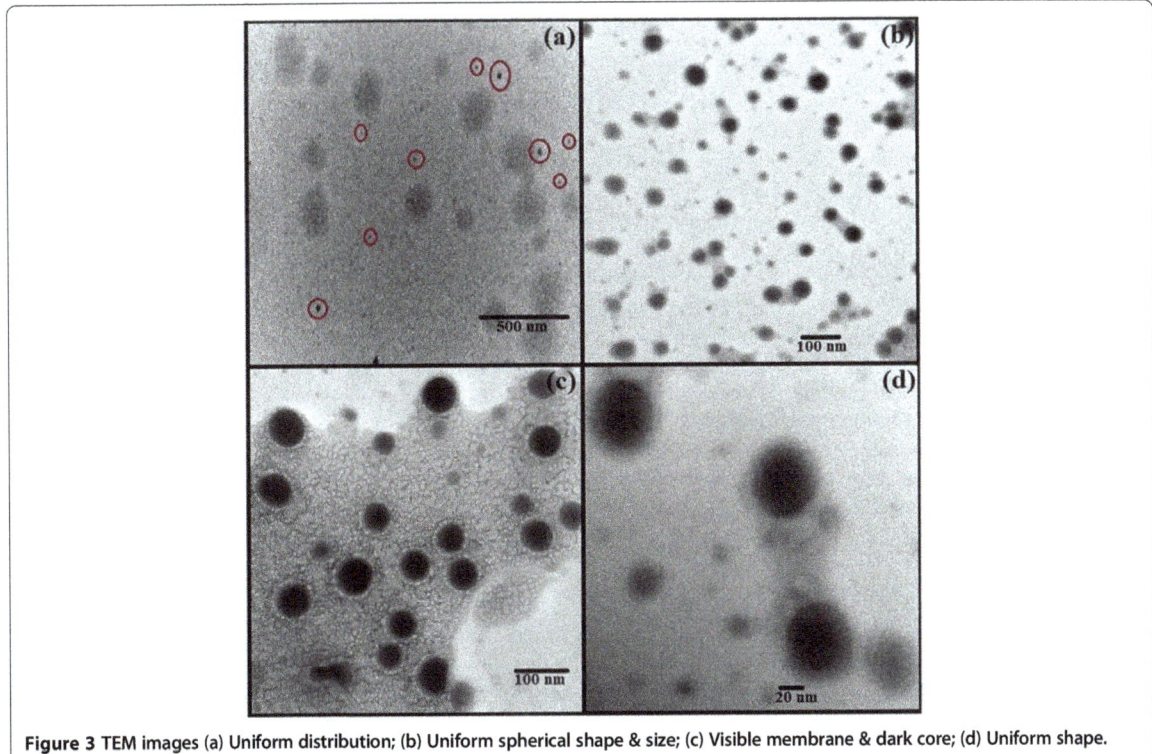

Figure 3 TEM images (a) Uniform distribution; (b) Uniform spherical shape & size; (c) Visible membrane & dark core; (d) Uniform shape.

Table 2 Drug release kinetics profile of metformin niosomes

S. NO	Formulation code	Zero order		First order		Higuchi		Korsemeyer - Peppas		
		r^2	K	r^2	K	r^2	K	r^2	K	n
1	MN1	0.851	24.00	0.566	0.137	0.973	7.98	0.993	1.620	0.267
2	MN2	0.855	24.35	0.564	0.139	0.973	7.97	0.995	1.629	0.264
3	MN3	0.809	23.66	0.541	0.135	0.953	9.75	0.996	1.580	0.261
4	MN4	0.779	25.86	0.506	0.142	0.937	11.51	0.968	1.629	0.204
5	MN5	0.824	27.81	0.511	0.150	0.954	11.07	0.975	1.660	0.252
6	MN6	0.821	28.82	0.500	0.153	0.946	11.76	0.968	1.601	0.336
7	MN7	0.760	28.96	0.474	0.151	0.927	13.51	0.992	1.664	0.203
8	MN8	0.759	29.94	0.469	0.153	0.928	13.90	0.998	1.676	0.216
9	MN9	0.734	32.70	0.440	0.160	0.909	16.13	0.960	1.714	0.184
10	MN10	0.767	32.54	0.454	0.161	0.925	15.19	0.969	1.717	0.195
11	MN11	0.754	34.53	0.440	0.165	0.920	16.47	0.991	1.739	0.198
12	MN12	0.769	34.65	0.450	0.165	0.932	15.79	0.992	1.751	0.202
13	MN13	0.812	30.27	0.487	0.156	0.943	12.70	0.957	1.692	0.214
14	MN14	0.814	23.35	0.538	0.135	0.939	9.86	0.959	1.589	0.203
15	MN15	0.793	25.36	0.509	0.141	0.929	11.30	0.952	1.624	0.190
16	MN16	0.702	37.27	0.405	0.170	0.883	19.50	0.963	1.766	0.156
17	MN17	0.820	23.06	0.546	0.134	0.948	9.46	0.988	1.579	0.223
18	MN18	0.820	24.69	0.535	0.139	0.954	9.91	0.976	1.606	0.235

*r^2=regression coefficient, K= release rate constant, n=diffusional exponent.

optimized amount was required for the controlled effect and increase or decrease in the amount of surfactant lead to early drug loss (Table 1).

Effect of DCP

Charge inducer used was also scrutinized to corroborate its effects on the characteristics of the vesicles. The negative charge induced by DCP resulted in smaller size of the vesicles leading to lower entrapment efficiency (Table 1). Charge on the surface of the bilayer cause repulsive forces which compel the vesicles to be more curved and smaller in sizes. Smaller the size smaller will be the volume enclosed in the core and smaller will be the amount of drug entrapped. DCP was also found to have an advantageous

Table 3 Stability of optimized metformin niosome formulation under refrigeration temperature (2-8°C) storage condition

Time (days)	Entrapment efficiency* (%)	Drug remaining* (%)
0	84.50±0.19	100.00±0.00
7	84.36±0.10	99.83±0.12
15	84.24±0.13	99.68±0.15
30	83.91±0.08	99.30±0.09
45	83.39±0.10	98.69±0.12
60	81.55±0.21	96.50±0.25
90	77.61±0.22	91.84±0.26

*Mean ± SD, n = 3.

impact in retarding the drug release rate which may be attributed to the stability provided by it to the membrane [34] (Figure 1) (Figure 2). DCP has reported effects of providing integrity and uniformity and preventing aggregation and fusion which have been established in the study by the maintenance of sustained release and evident reduction of aggregation in photomicrographs and visual observations [35]. Aggregation has also been lowered by sonication of the prepared dispersion clearly visible in photomicrographs of the vesicles.

Effect of surfactant: cholesterol ratio

The surfactant: cholesterol ratio used, plays a decisive determinant of the properties and the behavior of the bilayer of the niosomes. So to predict the consequences, different molar ratios of surfactants were incorporated into different batches and were investigated for the parameters of particle size, entrapment and in-vitro release. The evaluation proposed equimolar ratio to be the most apt for development of a superior delivery system providing all the required features. Surfactant is the core material for bilayer formation, but the bilayer of just the non-ionic surfactant is not strong enough to serve as host for the drug. So cholesterol having a steroidal rigid structure provides the required strength to the bilayer, despite of the fact that cholesterol itself is incapable of layer formation [36]. When the molar ratio of the surfactant was increased from 75:100 to 125:100 in context with cholesterol the entrapment enhanced to an optimum level and then declined, here the optimized ratio was equimolar i.e. 100:100. The excess of cholesterol at lower ratio tend to disrupt the regular bilayer structure leading to lower entrapment and higher drug release caused by leakage. Irregularities in the membrane structure added by the excess of cholesterol may have lead to increase in the vesicular size. With the increased ratio of the surfactant the entrapment has also improved to an optimized level as the excess of cholesterol is compensated by the added surfactant. At the molar ratio of 100:100 the surfactant and the cholesterol have the best fit arrangement in the bilayer serving to be efficient drug carrier. As the cholesterol acts as the rigidizing agent having the ability to cement the leakages, its deficiency upon increasing the ratio of the surfactant after the optimized ratio lead to the formation of leakage points resulting in lower entrapment and increased drug release [37]. The particle size has decreased with the increasing concentration of surfactant, may be due to bilayer formation with decreased cholesterol content. MN14 being the optimized formulation has highest entrapment of 84.14±0.07, with the most sustained release of 74.37±0.22 after 8 hours and the smallest particle size of all 481.33±3.06 nm (Table 4).

Effect of volume of hydration

Hydration of the thin dry film by the aqueous media is a critical step and the volume used determines the resulting features of the niosomes. The drug used being hydrophilic in nature was dissolved in the buffer and this solution was used for hydration. So the volume also altered the concentration obtained. The results showed no specific pattern of relationship between volume and the evaluated parameters. MN17 prepared using 15 ml of hydrating media served to be best fit formulation with highest entrapment and most retarded release. Any increase or decrease in volume hampered the entrapment and subsequently the release (Table 4). The possible reason for such a behavior could be stated as 15 ml providing ample space for vesicle formation. The lower volume may have lead to incomplete or distorted formation of bilayer due to excess of material and less of space. Whereas in the case of larger volume, the material have

been dispersed in large volume with large interacting area. This may have caused formation of smaller vesicles with decreased entrapment efficiency.

The in vitro release revealed prolonged delivery of the drug for about 8 hours which suffice the daily requirement in Type II diabetes treatment. The sustained release is also proven to decrease the side effects resulting from higher drug concentrations or presence of drug at the areas other than the target site [38]. Also the patient compliance is enhanced by use of niosomes with the possibility of once daily dose as compared to 2–3 doses per day. The negative zeta potential exhibit the negative charge developed on the surface causing the repulsive forces preserving the formulation from aggregation and fusion of vesicles thereby maintaining their integrity and uniformity [35]. The stability testing imply minimal drug lose from the vesicles upto 3 months at refrigeration temperature. In the light of above facts niosomes have been found to meet the requirements for successful delivery of the drug. Furthermore successful encapsulation of the drug in niosomes has also opened the doors for exploitation of other benefits presented by this novel delivery system viz. enhanced penetration, targeted delivery, reduced dose, protection from harsh environment etc.

Conclusions

The investigation conclusively supported niosomes to be an advantageous drug delivery system with high degree of entrapment and sustained release of the drug over extended period of time. The results also concluded that the studied variables have a significant impact on the entrapment and release of drug from the niosomes. Also the Molar concentration and molar ratio of cholesterol and surfactant, the charge inducer DCP and the volume of hydration used should be in optimized value and greatly influence the entrapment of drug in the vesicles and also alters the performance of niosomes. The optimized formulation (cholesterol: surfactant, 100:100 molar concentration) with DCP (5 mg) and 15 ml volume of hydration showed the most sustained release of drug and was found to be the best formulation. The careful control of all the above factors allow the production of a dosage form with sustained release capable of

Table 4 Effect of surfactant: cholesterol ratio on entrapment efficiency, particle size and in vitro drug release

Formulation code	Cholesterol:surfactant (Span 60)	Volume of hydration (ml)	Entrapment efficiency* (%)	Particle size* (nm)	In vitro drug release* (%)
MN13	100:75	15	78.84±0.09	524.33±3.06	94.18±0.50
MN14	100:100	15	84.14±0.07	481.33±3.06	74.37±0.22
MN15	100:125	15	79.27±0.04	445.33±2.08	79.03±0.10
MN16	100:100	10	66.92±0.33	490.67±2.52	94.03±0.14
MN17	100:100	15	83.37±0.09	477.33±2.08	74.60±0.33
MN18	100:100	20	79.36±0.10	455.0±2.64	78.31±0.20

*Mean ± SD, n = 3.

combating the side effects and also reducing the dosing frequency with the greater patient compliance. Suggesting metformin loaded niosomes to be an efficient drug carrier system in treatment of Type II Diabetes.

Abbreviations
DCP: Dicetyl Phosphate; TEM: Transmission Electron Microscopy.

Competing interests
The author(s) declare that they have no competing interests.

Authors' contributions
All authors have read and approved the final manuscript.

Acknowledgements
The authors are thankful to Matrix Laboratories, Hyderabad, India, for providing metformin as a kind gift sample. Authors are grateful to Dr. Madhu Chitkara, Vice chancellor, Chitkara University, Rajpura, Punjab for financial and infrastructure support for the project.

References

1. Furness G: OnDrugDelivery. [http://www.ondrugdelivery.com/publications/Oral_Drug_Delivery_07.pdf].
2. Krishnaiah YSR: Pharmaceutical technologies for enhancing oral bioavailability of poorly soluble drugs. J Bioequiv Availab 2010, 2:28–36.
3. Luo YF, Chen DW, Ren LX, Zhao XL, Qin J: Solid lipid nanoparticles for enhancing vinpocetine's oral bioavailability. J Control Release 2006, 114:53–59.
4. Schnürch AB, Guggib D, Pinter Y: Thiolated chitosans: development and in vitro evaluation of a mucoadhesive, permeation enhancing oral drug delivery system. J Control Release 2004, 94:177–186.
5. Fatouros DG, Mullertz A: In vitro lipid digestion models in design of drug delivery systems for enhancing oral bioavailability. Expert Opin Drug Metab Toxicol 2008, 4:65–76.
6. Gao P, Guyton ME, Huang T, Bauer JM, Stefanski KJ, Lu Q: Enhanced oral bioavailability of a poorly water soluble drug PNU91325 by supersaturatable formulations. Drug Dev Ind Pharm 2004, 30:221–229.
7. Vyas TK, Shahiwala A, Amiji MM: Improved oralbioavailability and brain transport of Saquinavir upon administration in novel nanoemulsion formulations. Int J Pharm 2008, 347:93–101.
8. Nassara T, Roma A, Nyskab A, Benita S: Novel double coated nanocapsules for intestinal delivery and enhanced oral bioavailability of tacrolimus, a P-gp substrate drug. J Control Release 2009, 133:77–84.
9. Sastry SV, Nyshadham JR, Fix JA: Recent technological advances in oral drug delivery – a review. Pharm Sci Technol To 2000, 3:138–145.
10. Sant VP, Smith D, Lerouxa JC: Novel pH-sensitive supramolecular assemblies for oral delivery of poorly water soluble drugs: preparation and characterization. J Control Release 2004, 97:301–312.
11. Deshpande AD, Hayes MH, Schootman M: Epidemiology of Diabetes and Diabetes-Related Complications. Phys Ther 2008, 88:1254–1264.
12. Slama G: The potential of metformin for diabetes prevention. Diabetes Metab 2003, 29:104–111.
13. Tajiri S, Kanamaru T, Yoshida K, Hosoi Y, Konno T, Yada S, Nakagami H: The Relationship between the Drug Concentration Profiles in Plasma and the Drug Doses in the Colon. Chem Pharm Bull 2010, 58:1295–1300.
14. Mandal U, Gowda V, Ghosh A, Selvan S, Solomon S, Pal TK: Formulation and Optimization of Sustained release matrix tablet of Metformin HCl 500mg using response surface methodology. Yakugaku Zasshi 2007, 127:1281–1290.
15. Brown JB, Pedula K, Barzilay J, Herson MK, Latare P: Lactic Acidosis Rates in Type 2 Diabetes. Diabetes Care 1998, 21:1659–1663.
16. Wadher KJ, Kakde RB, Umekar MJ: Formulation and Evaluation of Sustained-Release Tablets of Metformin Hydrochloride Using Hydrophilic Synthetic and Hydrophobic Natural Polymers. Indian. J Pharm Sci 2011, 73:208–215.
17. The Weinberg Group Inc.: FDA: [http://www.fda.gov/ohrms/dockets/dailys/04/may04/050404/04p-0208-cp00001-03-Attachment-02-vol1.pdf?

utm_campaign=Google2&utm_source=fdaSearch&utm_medium=website&utm_term=metformin-glipizide%20tablets%20for%20oral%20suspension&utm_content=1].
18. Lachman Consultant Services Inc.: FDA: [http://www.fda.gov/ohrms/dockets/dailys/03/Nov03/112193/03p-0534-cp00001-03-attachment-2-vol1.pdf?utm_campaign=Google2&utm_source=fdaSearch&utm_medium=website&utm_term=metformin-glyburide%20oral%20solution&utm_content=1].
19. Boehringer Ingelheim: FDA;; [http://www.accessdata.fda.gov/scripts/cder/drugsatfda/index.cfm?fuseaction=Search.DrugDetails].
20. Jadon PS, Gajbhiye V, Jadon RS, Gajbhiye KR, Ganesh N: Enhanced Oral Bioavailability of Griseofulvin via Niosomes. AAPS PharmSciTech 2009, 10:1186–1192.
21. Sihorkar V, Vyas SP: Polysaccharide coated niosomes for oral drug delivery: formulation and in vitro stability studies. Pharmazie 2000, 55:107–13.
22. Patel FM, Patel AN, Rathore KS: Release of metformin hydrochloride from ispaghula sodium alginate beads adhered cock intestinal mucosa. Int J Curr Pharmaceut Res 2011, 3:52–55.
23. Kumar GP, Rajeshwarrao P: Nonionic surfactant vesicular systems for effective drug delivery—an overview. Acta Pharmaceutica Sinica B 2011, 1:208–219.
24. Chengjiu H, David Rhodes G: Proniosomes: A Novel Drug Carrier Preparation. Int J Pharm 1999, 185:23–35.
25. Abdel-Mottaleb MMA, Lamprecht A: Standardized in vitro drug release test for colloidal drug carriers using modified USP dissolution apparatus. Drug Dev Ind Pharm 2011, 37:178–184.
26. Junyaprasert VB, Teeranachaideekul V, Supaperm T: Effect of Charged and Non-ionic Membrane Additives on Physicochemical Properties and Stability of Niosomes. AAPS PharmSciTech 2008, 9:851–859.
27. Singh G, Dwivedi H, Saraf SK, Saraf SA: Niosomal Delivery of Isoniazid - Development and Characterization. Trop J Pharm Res 2011, 10:203–210.
28. Muzzalupo R, Tavano L, Trombino S, Cassano R, Picci N, Mesa CL: Niosomes from α, ω-trioxyethylene-bis(sodium2-dodecyloxy-propylenesulfonate): Preparation and characterization. Colloids Surf B Biointerfaces 2008, 64:200–207.
29. Srinivas S, Kumar YA, Hemanth A, Anitha M: Preparation and evaluation of niosomes containing Aceclofenac. Dig J Nanomater Bios 2010, 5:249–254.
30. Shahiwala A, Misra A: Studies in topical application of niosomally entrapped nimuslide. J Pharm Pharm Sci 2002, 5:220–225.
31. Attia IA, El-Gizawy SA, Fouda MA, Donia AM: Influence of a Niosomal Formulation on the Oral Bioavailability of Acyclovir in Rabbits. AAPS PharmSciTech 2007, 8:E1–E7.
32. Hao YM, Li K: Entrapment and release difference resulting from hydrogen bonding interactions in niosome. Int J Pharm 2011, 403:245–253.
33. Manconi M, Sinico C, Valenti D, Loy G, Fadda AM: Niosomes as carriers for tretinoin. I. Preparation and properties. Int J Pharm 2002, 234:237–248.
34. Namdeo A, Jain NK: Niosomal delivery of 5-Fluorouracil. J Microencapsul 1999, 16:731–740.
35. Kandasamy R, Veintramuthu S: Formulation and Optimization of Zidovudine Niosomes. AAPS PharmSciTech 2010, 11:1119–1127.
36. Korchowiec B, Paluch M, Corvis Y, Rogalska E: A Langmuir film approach to elucidating interactions in lipid membranes: 1,2-dipalmitoyl-sn-glycero-3- phosphoethanolamine/ cholesterol/ metal cation systems. Chem Phys Lipids 2006, 144:127–136.
37. Guinedi AS, Mortada ND, Mansour S, Hathout RM: Preparation and evaluation of reverse-phase evaporation and multilamellar niosomes as ophthalmic carriers of acetazolamide. Int J Pharm 2005, 306:71–82.
38. Bayindir ZS, Yuksel N: Characterization of niosomes prepared with various nonionic surfactants for paclitaxel oral delivery. J Pharm Sci 2010, 99:2049–2060.

Preparation and radiolabeling of a lyophilized (kit) formulation of DOTA-rituximab with ^{90}Y and ^{111}In for domestic radioimmunotherapy and radioscintigraphy of Non-Hodgkin's Lymphoma

Nazila Gholipour[1*], Amir Reza Jalilian[2], Ali Khalaj[3], Fariba Johari-Daha[2], Kamal Yavari[2], Omid Sabzevari[4], Ali Reza Khanchi[2] and Mehdi Akhlaghi[5]

Abstract

Background: On the basis of results of our previous investigations on ^{90}Y-DTPA-rituximab and in order to fulfil national demands to radioimmunoconjugates for radioscintigraphy and radioimmunotherapy of Non-Hodgkin's Lymphoma (NHL), preparation and radiolabeling of a lyophilized formulation (kit) of DOTA-rituximab with ^{111}In and ^{90}Y was investigated.

Methods: ^{111}In and ^{90}Y with high radiochemical and radionuclide purity were prepared by ^{112}Cd (p,2n)^{111}In nuclear reaction and a locally developed ^{90}Sr/^{90}Y generator, respectively. DOTA-rituximab immunoconjugates were prepared by the reaction of solutions of p-SCN-Bz-DOTA and rituximab in carbonate buffer (pH = 9.5) and the number of DOTA per molecule of conjugates were determined by transchelation reaction between DOTA and arsenaso yttrium(III) complex. DOTA-rituximab immunoconjugates were labeled with ^{111}In and ^{90}Y and radioimmunoconjugates were checked for radiochemical purity by chromatography methods and for immunoreactivity by cell-binding assay using Raji cell line. The stability of radiolabeled conjugate with the approximate number of 7 DOTA molecules per one rituximab molecule which was prepared in moderate yield and showed moderate immunoreactivity, compared to two other prepared radioimmunoconjugates, was determined at different time intervals and against EDTA and human serum by chromatography methods and reducing SDS-polyacrylamide gel electrophoresis, respectively. The biodistribution of the selected radioimmunoconjugate in rats was determined by measurement of the radioactivity of different organs after sacrificing the animals by ether asphyxiation.

Results: The radioimmunoconjugate with approximate DOTA/rituximab molar ratio of 7 showed stability after 24 h at room temperature, after 96 h at 4°C, as the lyophilized formulation after six months storage and against EDTA and human serum. This radioimmunoconjugate had a biodistribution profile similar to that of ^{90}Y-ibritumomab, which is approved by FDA for radioimmunotherapy of NHL, and showed low brain and lung uptakes and low yttrium deposition into bone.

Conclusion: Findings of this study suggest that further investigations may result in a lyophilized (kit) formulation of DOTA-rituximab which could be easily radiolabeled with ^{90}Y and ^{111}In in order to be used for radioimmunotherapy and radioscintigraphy of B-cell lymphoma in Iran.

Keywords: Rituximab, ^{90}Y, ^{111}In, Lymphoma-B, Biodistribution, Radioimmunotherapy

* Correspondence: gholipour@razi.tums.ac.ir
[1]Department of Radiopharmacy, Faculty of Pharmacy, Tehran University of Medical Sciences, P.O. Box: 14155–6451, Tehran, Iran
Full list of author information is available at the end of the article

Introduction

Non-Hodgkin's Lymphoma (NHL) also known as B and T cell lymphoma is a form of blood cancer originating in lymphatic system. Many investigations for treatment of NHL have been based on the development of antibody against CD-20 antigens which are expressed on the surface of B-cells [1]. Results of these investigations have led to drugs such as rituximab [2,3], a chimeric antibody for immunotherapy of CD20-positive low-grade NHL, and ibritumomab and tositumomab derived from immortalized mouse cells for the treatment of follicular lymphoma [4]. Since NHL is multifocal and radiosensitive [1,5,6], anti-CD20 monoclonal antibodies (mAbs) labeled with [111]In (^{111}In-ibritumomab) for imaging, [90]Y ([90]Y- ibritumomab, Zevalin) for therapy and [131]I (^{131}I-tositumomab, Bexxar) for imaging and therapy have been approved for use in patients with NHL [4,7,8]. It has been shown that the response rate of NHL in radioimmunotherapy (RIT) with ^{90}Y-ibritumomab tiuxetan compared to rituximab immunotherapy is higher and unlike chemotherapy is not associated with severe mucositis, hair loss, or persistent nausea [1,5,8-10].

Radiolabeled Murine antibodies compared to those of humanized chimeric antibodies have shorter *in vivo* half-lives [1,5] and as a result lower toxicities due to non-specific body irradiation. However these antibodies as foreign proteins may induce immunologic and anaphylactic reactions [11] in patients because of development of human anti murine antibody (HAMA) response and have not been approved for re-injection or retreatment [5,7,12]. Consequently, considerable investigations have been carried out for the preparation of radioimmunoconjugates from rituximab, a chimeric antibody which induce distinctly less antibody responses and preparation of rituximab labeled with [90]Y [13,14], [111]In [15], [153]Sm [16], [177]Lu [17-19], [64]Cu [20], [149] Tb, [213]Bi, [227]Th and [225]Ac [11], through an additionally attached chelating agents such as different chemical forms of DTPA or DOTA [21,22] onto antibody, have been described. Due to high costs of commercially available radiolabeled anti CD20 monoclonal antibodies and on the basis of results of our previous investigations on ^{90}Y-DTPA-rituximab [14], where an unexpected high lung uptake was observed, and in the search for a radioimmunoconjugate of higher efficiency and lower toxicity, preparation of DOTA-rituximab which compared to DTPA-rituximab has higher stability appeared of interest. The aim of the present study was to develop a lyophilized formulation of DOTA-rituximab that could be labeled with ^{111}In and ^{90}Y in order to fulfil national demands to radioimmunoconjugates for radioscintigraphy and radioimmunotherapy of Non-Hodgkin's Lymphoma (NHL). While preparation of ^{90}Y-DOTA-rituximab has been reported [13], but characteristics, stability at different time intervals and different temperatures and biodistribution of the prepared radioimmunoconjugate have not been explained in details. This manuscript describes the synthesis, purification, and chemical characterization of a lyophilized (kit) DOTA-rituximab conjugate for labeling with ^{90}Y and ^{111}In and the radiochemical purity, in-vitro stability and biodistribution of the resulting radioimmunoconjugates.

Materials and methods

Materials

p-SCN-Bz-DOTA with %94 purity was obtained from Macrocyclics Inc. (NJ, USA). Rituximab (Reditux) was a pharmaceutical sample purchased from Cinnagen Co. (Tehran, Iran). Radio-TLC scanning was performed using a Bioscan AR-2000 radio TLC scanner instrument (Bioscan, Paris, France). A high purity germanium (HPGe) detector coupled with a Canberra™ (model GC1020-7500SL) multichannel analyzer and a dose calibrator ISOMED 1010 (Dresden, Germany) were used for counting radioactivity of organs of rats in biodistribution study. Analytical HPLC was performed by Shimadzu LC-10AT, armed with flow scintillation analyzer (Packard-150 TR) and UV-visible (Shimadzu) equipped with Whatman Partisphere C-18 column 250×4.6 mm, (Whatman Co. NJ, USA). Animal studies were performed in accordance with the United Kingdom Biological Council's Guidelines on the Use of Living Animals in Scientific Investigations, 2nd Edn. which was approved by Animal Ethics Committee of the Deputy of Research of Nuclear Science and Technology Research Institute (NSTRI) of Iran.

Preparation and quality control of ^{111}In-InCl₃

[111]In-InCl^3 solution was produced by [112]Cd (p,2n)[111]In nuclear reaction using a 30 MeV cyclotron in Agricultural, Medical and Industrial Research School (AMIRS) and purified by cation exchange chromatography on Dowex 50×8 resin. Gamma spectroscopy of the final sample was carried out by counting in an HPGe detector. Differential-pulsed anodic stripping polarography was used to ensure that the amount of cadmium, indium and copper ions in the sample are not higher than those of internationally accepted limits. The ^{111}In-InCl₃ solution was evaporated. The residue was dissolved in ultra-pure water and filtered under sterile condition. The radiochemical purity of the final ^{111}In solution was checked in 10 mM DTPA (pH = 5.0) solution (R_f of free [111]In^{3+} = 0.8) [15,23].

Preparation and quality control of ^{90}Y-YCl₃

^{90}Y-YCl₃ solution was prepared at Nuclear Science and Technology and Research Institute of Atomic Energy Organization of Iran by ion exchange chromatography technique through elution from an in-house made ^{90}Sr/^{90}Y generator which was developed for research purposes.

The radionuclidic purity of the solution for the presence of other radionuclides was tested by beta spectroscopy using liquid scintillation counter (LSC). The radiochemical purity of $^{90}YCl_3$ was checked by radio-TLC using 10 mM DTPA (pH = 5.0) solution (R_f of free $^{90}Y^{3+}$ = 0.8) [24].

Preparation of DOTA-rituximab immunoconjugates

DOTA-rituximab immunoconjugates were prepared according to the reported method [18] with only slight modifications. Briefly, one milliliter of rituximab solution (10 mg/ml) was freed from excipients first by ultrafiltration using Vivaspin-2 filter (30 kDa, Sartorius AG, 2 × 10 min at 2.684 g) and then by washing three times with carbonate buffer (1 ml, 0.2 M Na_2CO_3, pH = 9.5). The antibody was then removed from the upper part of filter using 3.5 ml of carbonate buffer (0.2 M Na_2CO_3, pH = 9.5). The final concentration of rituximab was determined by a biophotometer (Eppendorf) at OD = 280 nm and found to be 2.73 mg/ml. The structural integrity of the antibody was confirmed by reducing SDS-PAGE electrophoresis [13]. 1.1 ml aliquots of resulting rituximab (3 mg, 2×10^{-5} mmol/1.1 ml) solution in three sterile and pyrigen-free vials were treated with the solution of p-SCN-Bz-DOTA in carbonate buffer (0.2 M, pH = 9.5) in molar ratios of 5 (0.073 mg, 10^{-4} mmol), 15(0.22 mg, 3×10^{-4} mmol), and 25 (0.36 mg, 5×10^{-4} mmol), respectively. The solutions were gently mixed for 20 times by pipetting up and down and then incubated at room temperature for 24 h. The coupling reactions were terminated and unreacted p-SCN-Bz-DOTA were removed by adjustment of the pH of solutions to 7.0 using ammonium acetate buffer (0.25 M, pH = 5.5), followed by ultrafiltration and then washing three times with ammonium acetate buffer (0.25 M, pH = 5.5). The immunoconjugates were then removed from upper part of filters with 1 ml aliquots of ammonium acetate buffer (0.25 M, pH = 5.5). The concentration of the antibody in final immunoconjugate solutions were measured by a biophotometer and found to be around 2.84 mg/ml. The antibody solutions were dispensed in sterile vials at a quantity of 0.3 mg per vials and treated with 30 µl aliquots of mannitol solution (mannitol Ph Eur, 80 mg/ml in ultrapure water). Finally, the formulated immunoconjugate antibody solutions were freeze dried to obtain white pellets which were stored at −18°C.

Determination of the number of DOTA molecules per one rituximab molecule in DOTA-rituximab immunoconjugates

The DOTA to rituximab ratios were determined on the basis of a transchelation between DOTA and arsenaso yttrium (III) complex from a standard curve for absorbance of arsenaso yttrium (III) complex at 652 nm which was constructed for a series of solutions containing 8.1 µM AAIII, 3.9 µM Y(III) and different concentrations of p-SCN-Bz-DOTA (0–20 µM) in 0.15 M ammonium acetate buffer (pH = 7) [25].

Determination of the stability of the lyophilized (Kit) DOTA-rituximab immunoconjugates

Stability and degradation of the lyophilized DOTA-rituximab immunoconjugate kit (with selected DOTA: antibody ratio) was checked by integrity test using reducing SDS-polyacrylamide gel electrophoresis (reducing SDS-PAGE) at frequent monthly intervals (for 6 months) according to the method of Laemmli [26].

Radiolabeling and quality control of the radiolabeled immunoconjugates

Typically, 510 MBq of $^{111}InCl_3$ solution in 0.2 M HCl in conical vials were dried under a flow of nitrogen and residues were dissolved in 1500 µl of ammonium acetate buffer (pH = 5.5). 500 µl aliquots of ammonium acetate buffer were added to the vials containing lyophilized immunoconjugates (three different DOTA: antibody ratios) and the vials were mixed using pipetting up and down (10-20×) to dissolve immunoconjugates. Then 500 µl (170 MBq) aliquots of ^{111}In solution were added to vials and after mixing gently for 5 min by up and down pipetting, mixtures were incubated at 37°C for 1–2 h.

The radiochemical purity of the products was determined by ITLC on Whatman No.2, using 10 mM DTPA as mobile phase and HPLC on a C-18 column using a gradient system as a reported routine method in this laboratory [27]. To increase the radiochemical purity, the radioimmunoconjugates were purified by chromatography using PD-10 columns (GE healthcare) and ammonium acetate buffer (pH = 7.0) as eluting solvent. The final solutions were then passed through 0.22 micron biological filters for stability and biodistribution studies. Radiolabeling of the immunoconjugates with ^{90}Y and quality control of the resulting radioimmunoconjugate were carried out by the same method which was described for the preparation and quality control of ^{111}In-DOTA-rituximab.

Determination of the Immunoreactivity of radioimmunoconjugates

The immunoreactivity of radioimmunoconjugates were determined by the use of the cell-binding assay on Raji cell line, using 5 sequential dilutions of 10^6-10^7 cells in exponential growth (microscopic determination generally indicated >90% viability). A known amount (6 ng) of antibody labeled with 2.54 MBq of ^{111}In and ^{90}Y, was incubated with cells in 200 µl of phosphate-buffered saline (0.15 molar NaCl and 0.01 molar phosphate buffer, pH = 7.0) containing 5% fetal calf serum and NaN_3

(0.02% w/v) for 2 h at 37°C. Nonspecific binding, generally less than 3%, was assessed by competition with 100 μg of unlabeled antibody and results were used for determination of specific binding which were analyzed at maximal observed binding on 10^7 cells by extrapolating to infinite antigen excess according to the reported method [28]. The Student T-test for paired samples was used for statistical comparison of results.

Determination of the stability of radiolabeled DOTA-rituximab against EDTA

A 0.1 ml aliquot of the radiolabeled product with approximate number of 7 molecules of DOTA per rituximab molecule was mixed with 0.1 ml of ethylenediaminetetraacetic acid (30 mM, pH = 7.4) and allowed to incubate for 4 h at room temperature. The radiochemical purity of incubated solution was evaluated by radio-TLC [15].

Determination of the stability of radiolabeled DOTA-rituximab in the presence of human serum

^{111}In- and ^{90}Y-DOTA-rituximab mixtures were incubated in freshly prepared human serum for 12 h at 37°C. Radiolabeling stability was assessed by size exclusion chromatography on a Sepharose column (1 × 30 cm) and using phosphate buffer solution as eluent at a flow rate of 0.5 ml/min. To obtain elution chromatogram, the incubated mixture was applied on the column and 1 ml fractions were collected and their radioactivities were determined. To calibrate the column, the control samples including free ^{111}In and ^{90}Y, radiolabeled human serum albumin and radiolabeled DOTA-rituximab were separately applied to the column for retention volume determination [15,16].

Radiolabeling efficiency of the lyophilized (Kit) DOTA-rituximab conjugates

The radiolabeling efficiency of the lyophilized DOTA-rituximab immunoconjugate (kit) was investigated by monthly radiolabeling with ^{111}In and ^{90}Y and ITLC analysis [15].

Determination of the stability of the lyophilized (kit) radioimmunoconjugates

For evaluation of the stability of radiolabeled DOTA-rituximab, the radiochemical purities of samples of the final solution after storage at 4°C for 4 days and at 25°C for 24 h were determined by radio-TLC analysis [15]. Integrity of radiolabeled DOTA-rituximab was checked by reducing SDS-polyacrylamide gel electrophoresis [26].

Determination of biodistribution of ^{111}In-DOTA-rituximab and ^{90}Y-DOTA-rituximab in rats

Male rates weighing 250-300 g were randomly divided into four groups. The first and second groups were

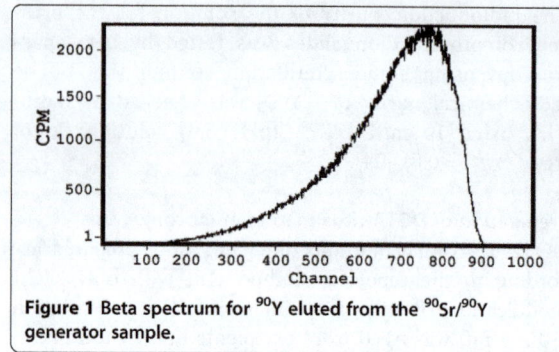

Figure 1 Beta spectrum for ^{90}Y eluted from the ^{90}Sr/^{90}Y generator sample.

administrated intravenously 0.3 mCi/kg aliquots of ^{111}In-Rituximab and ^{90}Y-rituximab solutions, respectively. The third and fourth groups were administered intravenously 250 mg/m^2 of unlabeled rituximab, 2 hours before injection 0.3 mci/kg aliquots of ^{111}In-Rituximab and ^{90}Y-rituximab, to block CD-20 positive binding sites on the B-cells in the circulation and spleen [9]. The animals were sacrificed by ether asphyxiation at the exact time intervals, and the distribution of radioactivity, represented as percent of injected dose per gram (%ID/g), was determined by measurement of radioactivity of samples from different organs using a beta-scintillator detector for ^{90}Y samples and an HPGe detector for counting the area under the curve of the 171 keV peak for ^{111}In [15,16].

Results

Preparation and quality control of radionuclides

^{111}In as ^{111}InCl$_3$ solution with a specific activity of higher than1.55 GBq/μg indium at time of calibration was obtained by a non-carrier-added method. Quality control of the radionuclidic [15] showed the presence of 171 and 245 keV gamma energies, originating from ^{111}In

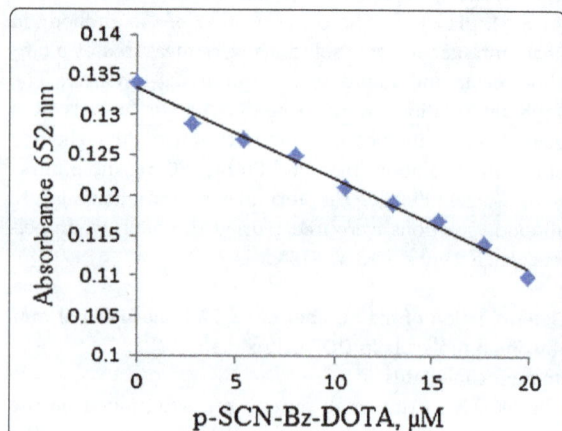

Figure 2 The relationship between the absorbance of the complex and the molarities of p-SCN-Bz-DOTA at 652 nm.

Table 1 The approximate number of DOTA molecules per rituximab molecule, radiolabeling yields, specific activity and radioimmunoreactivity of the prepared immunoconjugates and radioimmunoconjugates

Rituximab: DOTA molar ratio	Approximate number of DOTA per rituximab	Radiolabeling yield for ^{111}In (%)[a]	Radiolabeling yield for ^{90}Y (%)[a]	Specific activity (MBq/mg)[b]	
				^{111}In	^{90}Y
1:5	4	55.3	49.5	358	312
1:15	7	84	78	463	431
1:25	9	92	84	514	455

[a]Labeling conditions; 0.3 mg of immunoconjugate, 170 MBq of radioisotope, ammonium acetate buffer pH = 5.5, 37°C.
[b]Specific activity is calculated based on measured antibody concentration (UV) and radioactivity (dose calibrator).

and a purity of higher than %99. The concentrations of cadmium (from target material) and copper (from target support) were 0.1 ppm which was below the internationally accepted levels and the radiochemical purity of ^{111}In-InCl$_3$ was higher than %98.

^{90}Y was obtained from the natural decay of its parent, ^{90}Sr (t$_{1/2}$, 29 y) by an in house designed ^{90}Sr/^{90}Y generator which was developed for the research purpose. ^{90}Sr was the only radionuclide impurity resulting from the production process and in all the yttrium (^{90}Y) chloride solutions eluted from the generator the ^{90}Sr/^{90}Y ratio was ≤ 10^{-5}. Figure 1 shows beta spectrum for Y-90 eluted from the ^{90}Sr/^{90}Y generator [24].

Determination of the number of DOTA molecules per one rituximab molecule in DOTA-rituximab conjugates

Figure 2 shows dependency of absorbance of arsenaso yttrium (III) complex at 652 nm on molarities of p-SCN-Bz-DOTA which was determined by arsenazo spectrophotometric method [25]. The solid line represents linear relationship between the absorbance, A$_{652nm}$ and the concentration of 0–20 μM of p-SCN-Bz-DOTA. The approximate numbers of chelating group per rituximab molecule for immunoconjugates which were obtained by using different molar ratios of reactants are presented in Table 1.

Radiolabeling and quality control of the immunoconjugates

The yields for radiolabeling of immunoconjugates are presented in Table 1. In radio-TLC experiments, the best eluent system for free ^{90}Y and ^{111}In detection was 10 mM DTPA aqueous solution (R$_f$ of 0.8). Due to the size and charge of the protein (≈150,000 D), radiolabeled DOTA-rituximab remained at the sample origin but radiolabeled DOTA showed high R$_f$ values. Figure 3 shows the radiochromatograms of free ^{90}Y and ^{90}Y-rituximab. Free ^{111}In and ^{111}In-rituximab pair showed similar radiochromatograms.

Figure 4 shows HPLC chromatograms of free ^{111}In, ^{111}In-P-SCN-Bz-DOTA and ^{111}In-rituximab. Both free indium and radiolabeled DOTA eluted rapidly but ^{111}In-DOTA-rituximab was eluted at 14.8 min. ^{90}Y, ^{90}Y-P-

SCN-Bz-DOTA and ^{90}Y-DOTA-rituximab showed similar radiochromatograms.

Results for the immunoreactivity of radioimmunoconjugates

The average immunoreactivity for radioimmunoconjugates with approximate DOTA/rituximab ratios of 4, 7 and 9 were %91.4, %72.8 and %47.3, respectively.

Results for the stability of radioimmunoconjugate against EDTA and human serum

Table 2 represents radiochemical stability of radioimmunoconjugates which were checked by radio-TLC analysis at 4°C after 4 days and at 25°C after 24 h. There was a decrease of about 1-2% in radiochemical purity of radioimmunoconjugates in the presence of EDTA, indicating of their stabilities [15].

^{111}In- and ^{90}Y-DOTA-rituximab were also stable in the presence of the fresh human serum. Analysis of

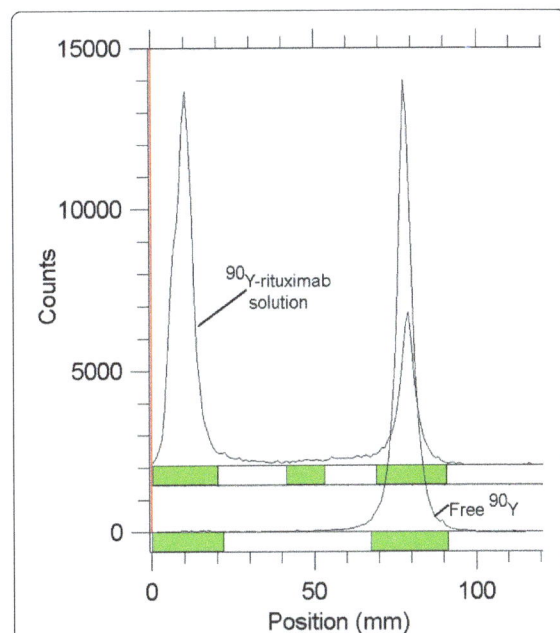

Figure 3 Radio-TLC chromatograms of ^{90}YCl$_3$ solution and ^{90}Y-DOTA-rituximab solution.

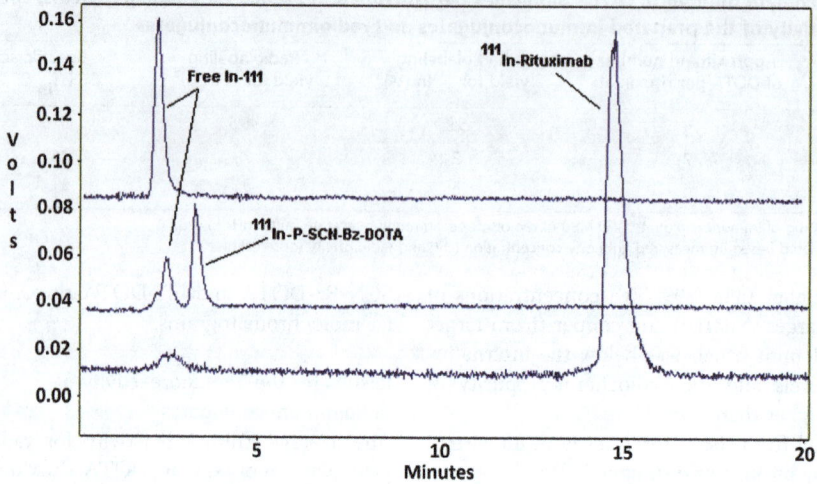

Figure 4 HPLC chromatograms of free ^{111}In, ^{111}In-DOTA and ^{111}In-rituximab.

aliquots of the samples after 24 h incubation by size exclusion chromatography showed that %96-98 of the radioactivity was associated with the radiolabeled DOTA-rituximab [13,14].

As it is shown in Figure 5, the reducing SDS-PAGE patterns for rituximab, DOTA-rituximab and ^{90}Y-DOTA-rituximab immunoconjugates were similar. Interestingly, the reducing SDS-PAGE results compared with a result for a commercially available rituximab sample showed no clear indication for antibody degradation. Similar results were obtained for monthly integrity tests on stored DOTA-rituximab immunoconjugate kits. The efficiencies of indium-111 radiolabeling of DOTA-rituximab kit (DOTA/antibody ratio = 7), measured monthly for six months, were 85.2 ± 3.1, 84.3 ± 1.7, 86.4 ± 2.8, 83.7 ± 3.4, 85.8 ± 1.9 and 84.8 ± 3.3, respectively. Reliable efficiencies also were observed for radioimmunoconjugate obtained by radiolabeling of DOTA-rituximab kit (DOTA/antibody ratio = 7) with [90]yttrium.

Table 2 In vitro stability of ^{111}In-DOTA-rituximab

Incubation time (h)	Radiochemical purity (%)[a]	
	25°C	4°C
0	96.4 ± 1.7	96.4 ± 1.7
6	96.1 ± 2.1	96.3 ± 1.4
12	95.7 ± 2.3	94.5 ± 2.7
24	96.6 ± 1.2	95.9 ± 1.4
48	ND[b]	94.8 ± 2.6
72	ND	95.7 ± 1.5
96	ND	96.3 ± 1.3

[a]For each time point, n = 3.
[b]Not Determined.

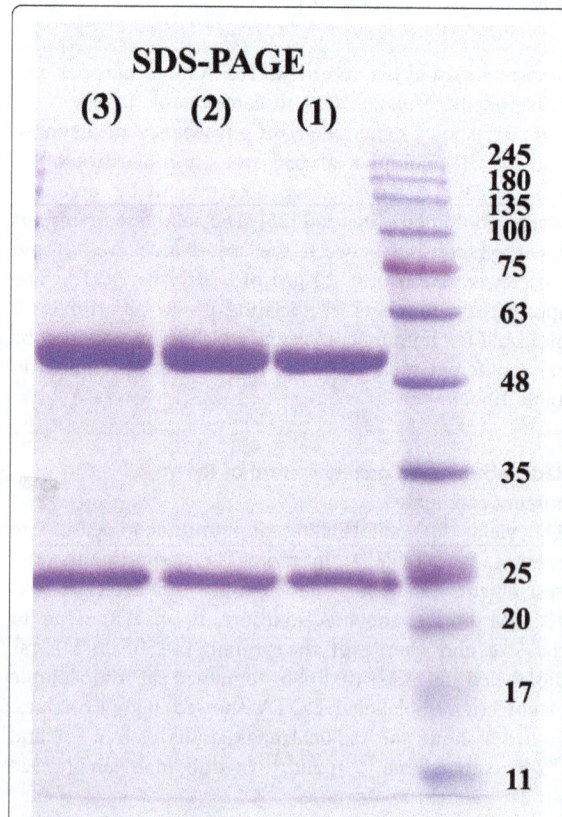

Figure 5 Reducing SDS-PAGE lane patterns for rituximab (1), DOTA-rituximab conjugate (2) and ^{90}Y-DOTA-rituximab conjugate (3).

Results for the biodistribution study

Figure 6 shows the biodistribution profiles of ^{111}In-DOTA-rituximab and ^{90}Y-DOTA-rituximab in male rats (first and second groups) which were determined by measurement of the radioactivities of the weighted samples of rat organs. Both groups showed similar biodistribution profiles. Over time, the liver and spleen uptakes were increased by reduction in the radioactivity of blood circulation. In the case of pre-injection of 250 mg/m^2 of unlabeled rituximab (third and fourth groups), a faster clearance of radioactivity from blood circulation in comparison with first and second groups was observed. Figure 7 shows the biodistribution of ^{111}In-DOTA-rituximab and ^{90}Y-DOTA-rituximab after pre-injection of unlabeled rituximab. In these two groups, also biodistribution profiles were approximately similar. Lungs uptakes in groups 3 and 4 were lower compared to groups 1 and 2. Brain and bone showed very low uptake in all groups.

Discussion

In this study preparation of a lyophilized (kit) formulation for radiolabeling of DOTA-rituximab with ^{90}Y for radioimmunotherapy of B cells lymphoma and with ^{111}In for radioimmunoscintigraphy as well as estimation of administered dose of ^{90}Y-DOTA-rituximab was investigated. [111]In was prepared by [112]Cd (p,2n)[111]In nuclear reaction and ^{90}Y was prepared by ^{90}Sr/^{90}Y generator which was developed locally for research purpose.

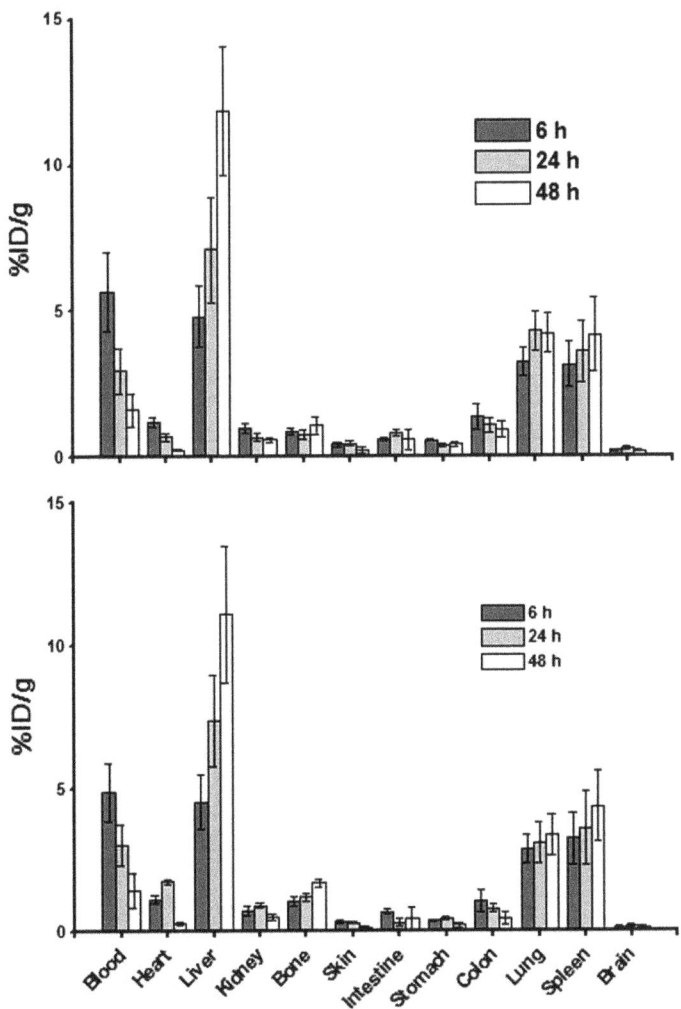

Figure 6 Percentage of injected dose per gram (%ID/g) of ^{111}In-DOTA-Rituximab (up) and ^{90}Y-DOTA-rituximab (down) with approximate DOTA/rituximab molar ratio of 7 in rat organs.

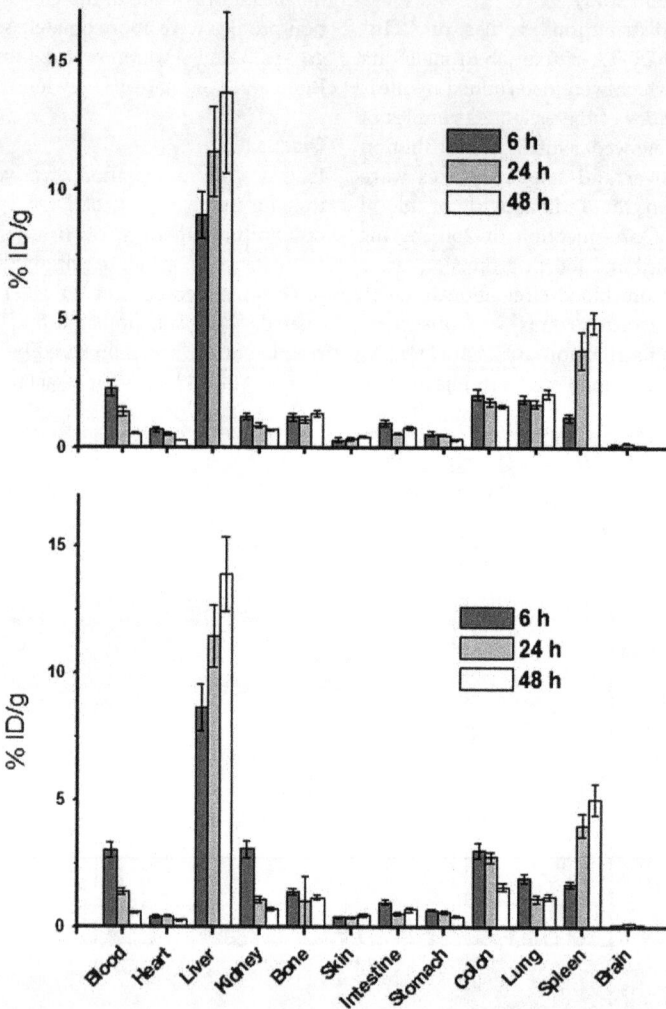

Figure 7 Percentage of injected dose per gram (ID/g%) of ^{90}Y-DOTA-rituximab (up) and ^{111}In-DOTA-rituximab (down) with approximate DOTA/rituximab molar ratio of 7 in rat organs in rat organs, 250 mg/m^2 of unlabeled rituximab was injected 2 h before injection of radioimmunoconjugates.

DOTA-rituximab immunoconjugates with approximate number of 4, 7 and 9 molecules of DOTA per one rituximab molecule were obtained by incubation of excess 5, 15 and 25 folds of p-SCN-benzyl-DOTA with rituximab using 0.2 M sodium carbonate buffer of pH = 9.5. DOTA-rituximab conjugates were successfully radiolabeled with ^{111}In and ^{90}Y, and the radiolabeling yields and efficiencies of radioimmunoconjugates which increased by increase in of DOTA/antibody molar ratios are reported in Table 1.

The immunoreactivity of radioimmunoconjugates compared to commercially available rituximab determined by Lindmo method [28] on Raji cells decreased by increase in DOTA/rituximab molar ratios and the average immunoreactivity for approximate molar ratios of 4, 7 and 9

were %91.4, %72.8 and %47.3, respectively. These findings suggest that increase in molar ratio of DOTA/antibody results to nonspecific conjugation of DOTA to antibody from antigen binding sites [29].

Due to the importance of both immunoreactivity and specific activity of radioimmunoconjugate and their oppositional behavior toward increasing the number of DOTA molecules per one antibody molecule, the immunoconjugate with approximate DOTA/antibody ratio of 7, with moderate immunoreactivity and specific activity, was selected for stability and bio-distribution studies. The selected radioimmunoconjugate showed stability when it was determined after 24 h at room temperature, after 96 h at 4°C, and after six months as lyophilized formulation. The selected radioimmunoconjugate was also stable to either EDTA or serum challenge for the duration of either experiment.

In agreement with results of studies on biodistribution of other labeled antibodies such as [90]Y- ibritumomab, ^{131}I-tositumomab and ^{177}Lu-Anti CD-20 [9,11,17,30], in this study after administration of ^{111}In-DOTA-rituximab and ^{90}Y-DOTA-rituximab with approximate DOTA/rituximab molar ratio of 7 in male rats the activity of blood circulation declined slowly and the activity of liver, spleen and other reticulloendothelial organs increased gradually. In the cases that rats were pre-treated with unlabeled rituximab the clearance of the radioactivity from the blood circulation was faster and the initial uptake of the activity in spleen was lower which could be attributed to blockade of CD-20 positive binding sites on B-cells in blood circulation and spleen [9]. The selected radioimmunoconjugate of this study also similar to ^{90}Y-ibritumomab did not have any significant brain uptake and compared to ^{90}Y-DTPA-rituximab of our previous investigation [14] showed significantly lower lung accumulation and ^{90}Y deposition in the bone which may be explained by possible cross-linking or cyclization of antibody with cyclic DTPA dianhydride [31] and lower stability of DTPA conjugates compared with DOTA conjugates.

Conclusion

Results of this study showed that radiolabeling of the lyophilized formulation (kit) of DOTA-rituximab having approximate DOTA/rituximab molar ratio of 7 with ^{90}Y and [90]In results in radioimmunoconjugates with moderate radioimmunoreactivity, and good stability and biodistribution profile. These findings suggest that further investigations may result in a kit formulation which could be easily radiolabeled with ^{111}In and ^{90}Y and to be used for radioimmunotherapy and radioscintigraphy of B cells lymphoma in Iran.

Abbreviations
DOTA: 1,4,7,10-tetraazacyclododecane-1,4,7,10-tetraacetic acid; p-SCN-Bz-DOTA: p-benzyl isothiocyanate-1,4,7,10-tetraazacyclododecane-1,4,7,10-tetraacetic acid; NHL: Non-Hodgkin's lymphoma; TLC: Thin layer chromatography; HPLC: High pressure liquid chromatography; SDS-PAGE: Sodium dodecyl sulfate-polyacrylamide gel electrophoresis.

Competing interests
The authors declare that they have no competing interests.

Authors' contributions
NG: Study design, preparing and radiolabeling of immunoconjugate, biodistribution studies and preparing of the manuscript. ARJ: Collaboration in study design, preparing of ^{111}In and the manuscript. AK: Collaboration in study design and preparing of the manuscript. FJD: Participation in radiolabeling of immunoconjugates. KY: Participation in the immunoreactivity studies. OS: Participation in the immunoreactivity studies. ARK: Participation in the preparation of yttrium-90. MA: Collaboration in study design, Participation in the preparation of the manuscript. All authors read and approved the final manuscript.

Acknowledgements
The authors wish to thank Dr. Mirzai for participating in the ^{111}In preparation and Mr. Mojarrabie Tabrizi and Mr. Salimi for participating in the ^{90}Y preparation and measurements and Mr. S. Daneshvari for participatation in the conducting animal studies and finally Mr. Naserian for participating in the integrity tests.

Author details
[1]Department of Radiopharmacy, Faculty of Pharmacy, Tehran University of Medical Sciences, P.O. Box: 14155–6451, Tehran, Iran. [2]Radiation Application Research School, Nuclear Science and Technology Research Institute, P.O. Box: 14395–836, Tehran, Iran. [3]Department of Medicinal Chemistry, Faculty of Pharmacy, Tehran University of Medical Sciences, P.O. Box: 14155–6451, Tehran, Iran. [4]Depatment of Toxicology and Pharmacology, School of Pharmacy, Tehran University of Medical Sciences, P.O. Box: 14176–14411, Tehran, Iran. [5]Research Center for Nuclear Medicine, Tehran University of Medical Sciences, P.O. Box: 14117–13137, Tehran, Iran.

References
1. Dillman RO: Radioimmunotherapy of B-cell lymphoma with radiolabeled anti-CD20 monoclonal antibodies. Clin Exp Med 2006, 6:1–12.
2. McLaughlin P, Grillo-López AJ, Link BK, Levy R, Czuczman MS, Williams ME, Heyman MR, Bence-Bruckler I, White CA, Cabanillas F, Jain V, Ho AD, Lister J, Wey K, Shen D, Dallaire BK: Rituximab chimeric anti-CD20 monoclonal antibody therapy for relapsed indolent lymphoma: half of patients respond to a four-dose treatment program. J Clin Oncol 1998, 16:2825–2833.
3. Hainsworth JD, Burris HA, Morrissey LH, Litchy S, Scullin DC Jr, Bearden JD 3rd, Richards P, Greco FA: Rituximab monoclonal antibody as initial systemic therapy for patients with low-grade non-Hodgkin lymphoma. Blood 2000, 95:3052–3056.
4. Macklis RM, Pohlman B: Radioimmunotherapy for non-Hodgkin's lymphoma: a review for radiation oncologists. Int J Radiat Oncol Biol Phys 2006, 66:833–841.
5. Leahy MF, Seymour JF, Hicks RJ, Turner JH: Multicenter phase II clinical study of iodine-131-rituximab radioimmunotherapy in relapsed or refractory indolent non-Hodgkin's lymphoma. J Clin Oncol 2006, 24:4418–4425.
6. Skvortsova I, Popper BA, Skvortsov S, Saurer M, Auer T, Moser R, Kamleitner H, Zwierzina H, Lukas P: Pretreatment with rituximab enhances radiosensitivity of non-Hodgkin's lymphoma cells. J Radiat Res 2005, 46:241–248.
7. Jacobs SA: Yttrium ibritumomab tiuxetan in the treatment of non-Hodgkin's lymphoma: current status and future prospects. Biologics 2007, 1:215–227.
8. Tennvall J, Fischer M, Bischof Delaloye A, Bombardieri E, Bodei L, Giammarile F, Lassmann M, Oyen W, Brans B, Therapy Committee, EANM; Oncology Committee, EANM; Dosimetry Committee, EANM: EANM procedure guideline for radio-immunotherapy for B-cell lymphoma with ^{90}Y-radiolabeled ibritumomab tiuxetan (Zevalin). Eur J Nucl Med Mol Imaging 2007, 34:616–622.
9. Chamarthy MR, Williams SC, Moadel RM: Radioimmunotherapy of non-Hodgkin's lymphoma: from the 'magic bullets' to 'radioactive magic bullets'. Yale J Biol Med 2011, 84:391–407.
10. DeNardo GL: Treatment of Non-Hodgkin's Lymphoma (NHL) with radiolabeled antibodies (mAbs). Semin Nucl Med 2005, 35:202–211.
11. Antonescu C, Bischof Delaloye A, Kosinski M, Monnin P, Schaffland AO, Ketterer N, Grannavel C, Kovacsovics T, Verdun FR, Buchegger F: Repeated injections of 131I-rituximab show patient-specific stable biodistribution and tissue kinetics. Eur J Nucl Med Mol Imaging 2005, 32:943–951.
12. Kaminski MS, Radford JA, Gregory SA, Leonard JP, Knox SJ, Kroll S, Wahl RL: Re-treatment with I-131 tositumomab in patients with non-Hodgkin's lymphoma who had previously responded to I-131 tositumomab. J Clin Oncol 2005, 23:7985–7993.
13. Vaes M, Bron D, Vugts DJ, Paesmans M, Meuleman N, Ghanem GE, Guiot T, Vanderlinden B, Thielemans K, Van Dongen G, Flamen P, Muylle K: Safety and efficacy of radioimmunotherapy with [90]Yttrium-rituximab in patients with relapsed CD20+ B cell lymphoma: a feasibility study. J Cancer Sci Ther 2012, 4:394–400.

14. Gholipour N, Vakili A, Radfar E, Jalilian AR, Bahrami-Samani A, Shirvani-Arani S, Ghannadi-Maragheh M: Optimization of 90 Y-antiCD20 preparation for radioimmunotherapy. *J Can Res Ther* 2013, 9:199–204.

15. Jalilian AR, Sardari D, Kia L, Rowshanfarzad P, Garousi J, Akhlaghi M, Shanehsazzadeh S, Mirzaii M: Preparation, quality control and biodistribution studies of two [^{111}In]-Rituximab immunoconjugates. *Sci Pharm* 2008, 76:151–170.

16. Bahrami-Samani A, Ghannadi-Maragheh M, Jalilian AR, Yousefnia H, Garousi J, Moradkhani S: Development of [153]Sm-DTPA-rituximab for radioimmunotherapy. *Nukleonika* 2009, 54:271–277.

17. Audicio PF, Castellano G, Tassano MR, Rezzano ME, Fernandez M, Riva E, Robles A, Cabral P, Balter H, Oliver P: [^{177}Lu]DOTA-anti-CD20: labeling and pre-clinical studies. *Appl Radiat Isot* 2011, 69:924–928.

18. Forrer F, Chen J, Fani M, Powell P, Lohri A, Müller-Brand J, Moldenhauer G, Maecke HR: In vitro characterization of (177)Lu-radiolabeled chimeric anti-CD20 monoclonal antibody and a preliminary dosimetry study. *Eur J Nucl Med Mol Imaging* 2009, 36:1443–1452.

19. Yousefnia H, Radfar E, Jalilian AR, Bahrami-Samani A, Shirvani-Arani S, Arbabi A, Ghannadi-Maragheh M: Development of ^{177}Lu-DOTA-anti-CD20 for radioimmunotherapy. *J Radioanal Nucl Chem* 2011, 287:199–209.

20. Jalilian AR, Mirsadeghi L, Yari-kamrani Y, Rowshanfarzad P, Kamali-dehghan M, Sabet M: Development of [^{64}Cu]-DOTA-anti-CD20 for targeted therapy. *J Radioanal Nucl Chem* 2007, 274:563–568.

21. De León-Rodríguez LM, Kovacs Z: The synthesis and chelation chemistry of DOTA-peptide conjugates. *Bioconjug Chem* 2008, 19:391–402.

22. Chappell LL, Ma D, Milenic DE, Garmestani K, Venditto V, Beitzel MP: Synthesis and evaluation of novel bifunctional chelating agents based on 1,4,7,10-tetraazacyclododecane-N, N′, N″, N‴-tetraacetic acid for radiolabeling proteins. *Nucl Med Biol* 2003, 30:581–595.

23. Sadeghpour H, Jalilian AR, Akhlaghi M, Kamali-dehghan M, Mirzaii M: Preparation and biodistribution of [^{111}In]- rHu Epo for erythropoietin receptor imaging. *J Radioanal Nucl Chem* 2008, 278:117–122.

24. Vakili A, Jalilian AR, Yavari K, Shirvani-Arani S, Khanchi AR, Bahrami-Samani A, Salimi B, Khorrami-Moghadam AR: Preparation and quality control and biodistribution studies of [^{90}Y]-DOTA-cetuximab for radioimmunotherapy. *J Radioanal Nucl Chem* 2013, 296:1287–1294.

25. Dadachova E, Chappell LL, Brechbiel MW: Spectrophotometric method for determination of bifunctional macrocyclic ligands in macrocyclic ligand-protein conjugates. *Nucl Med Biol* 1999, 26:977–982.

26. Laemmli UK: Cleavage of structural proteins during the assembly of the head of bacteriophage T4. *Nature* 1970, 227:680–685.

27. Jalilian AR, Akhlaghi M: HPLC analysis of radiogallium labeled proteins using a two solvent system. *J Liq Chromatogr Related Technol* 2013, 36:731–739.

28. Lindmo T, Boven E, Cuttitta F, Fedorko J, Bunn PA Jr: Determination of the immunoreactive fraction of radiolabeled monoclonal antibodies by linear extrapolation to binding at infinite antigen excess. *J Immunol Methods* 1984, 72:77–89.

29. Flieger D, Renoth S, Beier I, Sauerbruch T, Schmidt-Wolf I: Mechanism of cytotoxicity induced by chimeric mouse human monoclonal antibody IDEC-C2B8 in CD20-expressing lymphoma cell lines. *Cell Immunol* 2000, 204:55–63.

30. Perk LR, Visser OJ, Stigter-van Walsum M, Vosjan MJ, Visser GW, Zijlstra JM, Huijgens PC, van Dongen GA: Preparation and evaluation of (89)Zr-Zevalin for monitoring of (90)Y-Zevalin biodistribution with positron emission tomography. *Eur J Nucl Med Mol Imaging* 2006, 33:1337–1345.

31. Liu S: Bifunctional coupling agents for radiolabeling of biomolecules and target-specific delivery of metallic radionuclides. *Adv Drug Delivery Rev* 2008, 60:1347–1370.

3

The effect of piperine on midazolam plasma concentration in healthy volunteers, a research on the CYP3A-involving metabolism

Mohammad Mahdi Rezaee[1], Sohrab Kazemi[1,3], Mohammad Taghi Kazemi[1], Saeed Gharooee[1], Elham Yazdani[1], Hoda Gharooee[1], Mohammad Reza Shiran[2] and Ali Akbar Moghadamnia[1,3*]

Abstract

Some studies showed that piperine (the alkaloid of *piper nigrum*) can change the activities of microsomal enzymes. Midazolam concentration is applied as a probe to determine the CYP3A enzyme activity. This study was done to determine piperine pretreatment role on midazolam plasma concentration.

Twenty healthy volunteers (14 men and 6 women) received oral dose of piperine (15 mg) or placebo for three days as pretreatment and midazolam (10 mg) on fourth day of study and the blood samples were taken at 0.5, 2.5 and 5 h after midazolam administration. The midazolam plasma levels were assayed using HPLC method (C18 analytical column, 75:25 methanol:water as mobile phase, UV detector at 242 nm wavelength and diazepam as internal standard). Data were fit in a "one-compartment PK model" using *P-Pharm 1.5* software and analyzed under statistical tests. The mean ±SD of the age and body mass index were 24.3 ± 1.83 years (range: 21–28 years) and 23.46± 2.85, respectively. The duration of sedation in piperine receiving group was greater that the placebo group (188±59 *vs.* 102±43 min, p<0.0001). Half-life and clearance of midazolam were higher in piperine pretreatment group compared to placebo [1.88±0.03 *vs.* 1.71± 0.04 h (p<0.0001) and 33.62 ± 0.4 *vs.* 37.09 ± 1.07 ml/min (p<0.0001), respectively]. According to the results, piperine can significantly increases half-life and decreases clearance of midazolam compared to placebo. It is suggested that piperine can demonstrate those effects by inhibition CYP3A4 enzyme activity in liver microsomal system.

Keywords: Piperine, Midazolam, CYP3A, Clearance, Half-life, Microsomal hepatic metabolism, HPLC

Introduction

Some specific substances of food products and additives can manipulate drugs disposition and fate in body through mechanisms that make changes their plasma concentration [1-3]. These changes will exert as inducers or inhibitors of hepatic microsomal enzymes or transporters [1,3-5]. Black pepper (piper nigrum) has been used widely throughout the world. It has been shown that pepper can change metabolism of some drugs in those that take foods containing high pepper [6]. Piperine is an isolated alkaloid of black pepper [7] that belongs to capsaicin like family

[8]. Animal studies have previously demonstrated that piperine inhibits several enzymatic pathways involving P450, as well as phase II metabolism [9,10].

Grilled meat using wood charcoal, smoked meats, foods containing cruciferous vegetables, and some medicinal plants can induce several microsomal and transporter enzymes and decrease plasma concentration of xenobiotics, such as cyclosporine A and anti-HIV protease inhibitors [11]. Other drugs, such as verapamil induces CYP3A4 and increases transport of p-glycoproteine precursor [11]. On the other hand, some foods such as grape fruit can increase plasma concentration of felodipine, nitrondipine, secoanavir and cyclosporine A by inhibiting of CYP3A [12,13]. It has been suggested that pretreatment piperine in mice, may result in increasing plasma concentration of theophylline [9,14]. This similar effect of piperine on plasma level of theophylline, rifampine, phenytoin and

* Correspondence: moghadamnia@yahoo.com
[1]Department of Pharmacology, Babol University of Medical Sciences, Babol, Iran
[3]Cellular and Molecular Biology Research Centre, Babol University of Medical Sciences, Babol, Iran
Full list of author information is available at the end of the article

propranolol has been observed in human studies [15]. It has been reported that administration of 1 g of black pepper as a single dose, may increase time-concentration area under the curve (AUC) of phenytoin more than two times compared to placebo.

CYP3A enzymes are the most important enzymatic group that involve in drug metabolism. More than 50% of microsomal enzymes are made up of CYP3A and about 60% of drugs used in treatment (e.g. calcium channel blockers, corticosteroids, sex hormones, macrolide antibiotics, benzodiazepines and immunosuppressant drug cyclosporine) are metabolized by CYP3A [16]. Plasma concentration of some drugs such as midazolam and caffeine can serve as a probe of the enzyme activity [17,18]. Midazolam is a short acting sedative bezodiazepins that is mainly metabolized by CYP3A4 [7]. Determination of plasma concentration of midazolam can help to assess the activity level of CYP3A4 [6].

Based on the mentioned effect of piperine and the important role of CYP3A in drug metabolism, this study was designed to investigate the effect of three days pretreatment of low dose piperine on midazolam plasma concentration in healthy volunteers.

Materials and methods

This study has been approved by ethics committee of Babol University of Medical Sciences (Babol, Iran) and recorded in IRCT (Iranian registry of clinical trials) data bank with registration number:IRCT201203129271N1. All healthy volunteers were given information of the aims of the study, methods and possible outcomes of the treatment so that they could understand the main objective of the investigation. All selected participants signed a written informative consent form and then they were entered into the study. Although, neither midazolam nor piperine have serious side effects at lower doses, all participants were allowed to leave the study at any time of the follow up when they developed considerable complications.

Type of study

This was a cross-over controlled study on two groups (n=10) of healthy volunteers. A one-month period was considered as wash out time between two trials. Based on previous reports in 100 healthy volunteers of Mazandaran province (Northern Iran) to find out the CYP3A activity and recorded moderate activity in this sample size of the population [17,18], all participants were selected from Babol, one of the big cities of the province. After providing adequate information to the subjects, eligible healthy volunteers will be enrolled in the study. Inclusion criteria: being healthy; age ranging 18 to 35; normal diet; not receiving microsomal enzyme inhibitor or inducer agents for at least 7 days before the study; not using black pepper for at least 7 days before the study. Exclusion criteria: age

being below 18 and above 35; smocking; pregnancy; metabolic disorders; high pepper diet, receiving enzyme inhibitors or inducers.

Drugs & chemicals

Midazolam (Exir Lorestan, Iran), EDTA (Sigma Chemical Co. USA), piperine (Merck, Germany), n-hexan, HPLC grade methanol, isoamyl alcohol and HCl (Merck, Germany) and deionized water were used. Standard form of midazolam and diazepam as base (used as internal standard) were prepared from Dr. Abidi Pharmaceuitical Company (Tehran, Iran).

Devices

Centrifuge (Clements 2000, Australia) and HPLC [(Knauer, Germany); column Eurospher 100–5 C18 of silica gel, dimension: 250 × 4.6 mm with pre-column, UV detector, EZchrom Elite software] were used.

Steps

All participants received adequate description about the setting, treatment schedule and outcome of drug administration. Then they recorded their personal information including age, sex, height, weight, general health situation, and history of drug use, food sensitivity, smoking, occupation, education and consent to the study in a special form.

Drug administration and sampling

Healthy volunteers regardless of gender were randomly divided into two control and piperine receiving groups (n=20 per group). The subject received placebo or piperine (1 capsule 15 mg of piperine daily for 3 days before midazolam) and midazolam (10 mg as an oral single dose) on fourth day of the study. Total period of the study is 4 days. Blood samples (maximum 10 ml) were taken at 0.5, 2.5 and 5 hour after midazolam administration. After a month as a wash out period, the treatment program was exchanged between placebo and piperine groups and all steps were done as same as the previous.

Blood samples preparation

Blood samples were transferred into labeled tubes containing Ca-EDTA and shake gently to mix Ca-EDTA with blood for preventing of coagulation.The samples were centrifuged at 3500 ×g for 15 min and supernatant plasma layer transferred into a blank tube. Until the assay of midazolam or diazepam concentration, the plasma samples were kept at −20°C.

HPLC assay

For measurement of the drugs concentration, plasma samples were removed from the freezer condition and left in the laboratory to convert from frozen into a liquid sample. Then 0.5 ml of thawed plasma sample was transferred into a capped falcon tube. In the next step, 100 micl of 1 M NaOH and 100 micl isoamyl alcohol were added. After a gently shaking, 4.5 ml of n-hexan was added and shake for 1 minute. The final solutions were centrifuged at 300 ×g for 5 min. After this step, 4.2 ml of supernatant was drawn and transferred into a plastic tube and 100 miclof 0.05 M HCl was added to the solution and centrifuged similar as the previous. Then the supernatant (organic layer) was discarded and the remaining was directly injected into the HPLC.

HPLC analysis

The separation was carried out at ambient temperature using a single-column isocratic reverse-phase method. The mobile phase consisted of 75% methanol and 25% water. Flow rate was set at 0.8 ml/min. The extracts were detected by UV detector at 242 nm wavelength. Twenty micl of the aqueous layer of final extract was injected into the HPLC using a Hamilton's syringe. The injection was repeated 3 times for each sample. Peaks area and height were considered for midazolam and diazepam detection and used for calculation of the drugs concentration in the final plasma extract.

Standard preparations

A working solution containing 10 micg of midazolam in 1 mL of mobile phase was prepared. Six standard solutions of different concentrations of midazolam (20, 50, 75, 100, 150 and 200 ng/ml) were prepared. Then 20 micl of 25 ng/ml of diazepam solution as internal standard as added to each standard concentration of midazolam.

Data handling and analysis

Data were analyzed in two steps. The first; personal information of the participants and data of drugs assay were handled using Excel software. Calibration curves were plotted based on peak area and/or height ratio of midazolam to diazepam.

The slope, intercept and R^2 coefficient were calculated. Coefficient variation (CV) for this analysis was 3.8%.

The second; pharmacokinetic (PK) parameters such as absorption rate constant (Ka), clearance, half-life and volume of distribution of midazolam in the placebo and piperine groups were calculated based on assumed one-compartment kinetics using *P-Pharm* software.

Based on non-parametric distribution, data of three concentrations by time were analyzed using Friedman test. Wilcoxon U-test was used for the results of clearance, volume of distribution and half-life of midazolam in piperine group compared to placebo. The difference of the PK parameters between two groups was considered statistically significant at $p < 0.05$.

Table 1 Comparison of the mean (±SD) of onset and duration of sedative effect and frequency of sedation and amnesia following midazolam administration in placebo and piperine pretreatment groups (n=20)

	Onset of drug effect (min)	End of drug effect (min)	Sedation	Amnesia
Placebo	11.25 (±4.5)	102 (±43)	16	4
Piperine	11.75 (±4.9)	188 (±59)	20	**7**
p value	NS*	0.0001	NS	NS

*NS: non-significant.

Results

The age range of the participants was from 21 to 28 year (24.3±1.83). Six subjects were female and 14 were male (mean±SD of age: males: 25±1.26, females: 22.66±1.86). All participants were healthy volunteer and selected from Mazandaran province. The subjects' weight ranged from 49 to 101 kg (68.05±2.85). Their average (±SD) BMI was 23.46 (±2.85).

Clinical features

All the subjects experienced sedation and mild hypnosis following midazolam administration. This situation was transient and they've got improvement during next 4 hours after administration of midazolam. In some subjects, severe sedation and dizziness were observed in placebo and piperine groups (30% and 55%, respectively). The mean duration of the sedation in piperine receiving group was greater than placebo (188±59 *vs.* 102±43 min, p<0.0001) (Table 1).

Duration of midazolam sedative effect in piperine pretreatment group in the females was greater than the males when compared to placebo (p=0.027 and p<0.001) (Figure 1). Seven subjects of piperine group showed predominant amnesia but only 4 subjects were amnesic in placebo group. One subject of piperine group showed

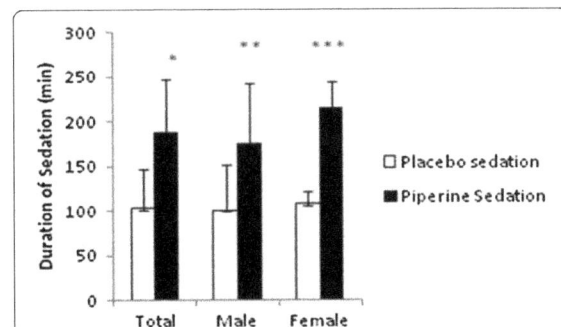

Figure 1 Comparison of duration of sedation (min) after midazolam (10 mg, p.o.) in placebo and piperine pretreatment (15 mg p.o. in three sequential days before midazolam) groups. Total data and data by sex are shown for 20 subjects. Sedation in piperine pretreatment group is greater than placebo group (*p<0.001, **p<0.01, ***p<0.0001).

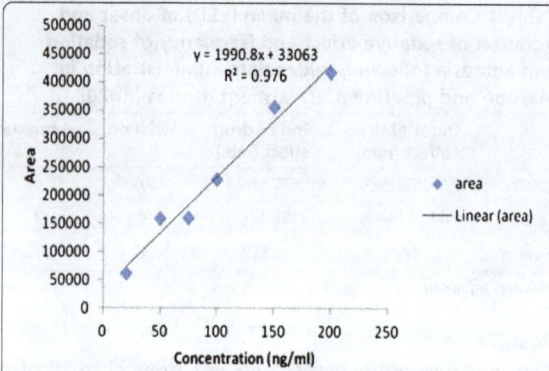

Figure 2 Peak area ratios (midazolam/diazepam)-concentration curve of six different concentrations (ng/ml) of midazolam containing equal diazepam (25 ng/ml) as internal standard.

hiccup when receiving midazolam that was disappeared during first hours after drug administration. The supine position was recommended for participants suffering from severe dizziness and possible hypotension.

Standard curve

Six concentrations (20, 50, 75, 100, 150 and 200 ng/ml) as standard solution of midazolam were prepared. Equal volume of diazepam solution (25 ng/ml) as internal standard was spiked on each concentration of midazolam. Based on peak area ratios of different concentration of midazolam on diazepam, the standard curve was obtained (Figure 2). The linearity (R^2) constant and the line equation are shown in the Figure 2.

The chromatograms of standard midazolam (50 ng/ml) and diazepam (25 ng/ml) are shown in Figure 3. Diazepam was used as internal standard.

The comparison of primary data of drug concentrations showed a significant different between placebo and piperine pretreatment groups at 2.5 and 5 hours after midazolam (p=0.015 and p=0.002, respectively). Analysis of intra-group variation of concentration by time showed a significant profile (p=0.03). There was no significant difference in AUC_{0-5} of placebo compared to piperine pretreatment group (411.1± 235.4 *vs.* 495, 9 ± 273, respectively).Pharmacokinetics parameters were estimated in an assumed one-compartment model using *P-Pharm* software. For comparing final estimation, non-parametric paired Wilcoxon U-test was applied.

All PK parameters except of Vd, in piperine pretreated subjects has demonstrated a significant difference compared to placebo (p<000.1). Half-life of midazolam in piperine pretreatment group is considerably greater than in placebo (Table 2). For this reason, it could be said that piperine may decrease metabolism of midazolam.

After modeling with input of initial data assumption (Cl= 40 ml/min, Vd=80 L, Ka=1, F=1), concentration-time curves were plotted. Individual Bayesian fits of concentration (ng/ml) of midazolam by time (h) profile placebo and piperine pretreatment are shown in Figure 4.

The population plasma midazolam concentrations time curves in placebo (A) and piperine (B) treatment groups are shown in Figure 4. Based on the figure (A), one subject showed an out of range concentration at the time of 2.5 h. It is considered that the maximum concentration in placebo group occurred at 1.5 h after midazolam administration.

Discussion

This investigation showed 3 days piperine pretreatment can significant increase elimination half-life (t1/2) and decrease clearance of midazolam when compared to control. Our results can demonstrate a possible relation between midazolam concentration and CYP3A activity.

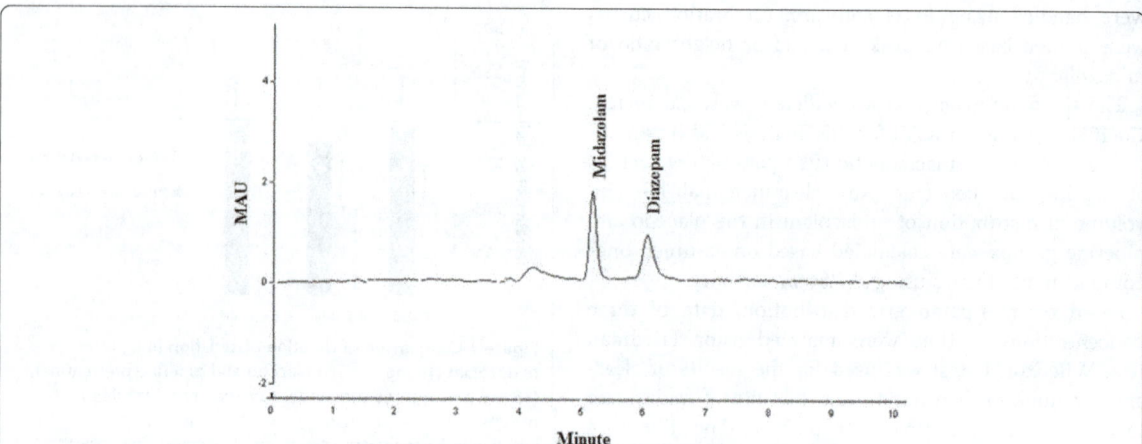

Figure 3 Chromatograms of midazolam standard concentration (50 ng/ml) and diazepam (25 ng/ml).

Table 2 Comparison of pharmacokinetics (PK) data of midazolam in placebo and piperine pretreatment groups

Group	Clearance	Volume	Kel†	T1/2‡
Placebo (n=20)				
Mean	37.09	91.44	0.41	1.71*
Min	34.27	87.63	0.390	1.63
Max	38.48	93.03	0.42	1.78
S.D.	1.07	1.54	0.01	0.04
Fold	1.12	1.06	1.1	1.1
C.V.	2.89	1.69	2.62	2.61
Piperine (n=20)				
Mean	33.62	91.43	0.37	1.88
Min	32.63	84.45	0.35	1.86
Max	34.02	92.35	0.37	1.96
S.D.	0.4	1.7	0.01	0.03
Fold	1.04	1.09	1.05	1.05
C.V.	1.2	1.86	1.29	1.33

†Elimination rate constant.
‡Half- life.
*$p < 0.0001$ (with piperine group).

This enzyme has an important role in microsomal drug metabolisms. Thirty percent of cytochrome P450 enzymes of liver are made of CY3A4 [19]. It has been estimated that CYP3A4 is responsible for 50 percent of the metabolism of all drugs that being eliminated via hepatic microsomal enzymatic system [20,21]. In addition to having an active role in hepatic metabolism of drugs, CYP3A4 is sufficiently active in the small intestine [22,23]. CYP3A4 is active in the metabolism of lipophilic substrates such as fentanyl, alfentanil, oxycodone, and methadone [24-28]. CYP3A4 inhibitors that have been well studied include: azole antifungal agents and a number of the macrolide antibodies [29]. There are clinically important examples such as midazolam, alprozolam, atorvastatin, simvastatin, felodipine, nifedipine, and cyclosporine that are affected by this system [29]. Among the CYP3A substrates, midazolam has been introduced as a predominant substrate of CYP3A4 and CYP3A5 [29]. The metabolism of intravenous midazolam can reflect to the rate of hepatic CYP3A activity but when it is administered by mouth, the metabolism can demonstrate both liver and enteral origin of CYP3A [22,23]. Any changes in CYP3A enzymatic pathway, may affect midazolam metabolism. CYP3A activity can be affected by different factors such as genetics, nutritional, environmental, and hormonal and disease conditions. These variations in CYP3A activity may create some problems in dosing of the drugs those are metabolized by this enzymatic system. These variations may increase drug interaction episodes and cause side effects to the patients. More than 50% of drugs that are eliminated by liver microsomal enzymes are metabolized by CYP3A system [20,21].

In the present study piperine the main alkaloid of black pepper [7], could significantly prolong life time of midazolam in body. This may increase the pharmacologic activity and can induce and prolong sedative-hypnotic properties of the drug. These effects of piperine may be the result of inhibition of CYP3A4 activity. Previous animal studies have demonstrated that piperine inhibits several CYP450 mediated pathways [30]. Piperine is a selective non-competitive inhibitor of CYP3A but has lower activity on the other microsomal enzymes. It can inhibit activity UDP-glucuronosyl transferase as well [31,32]. Pretreatment of piperine in mice induced higher plasma levels of theophylline, rifampin, phenytoin and propranolol and Q10-CoA compared to control [33,34]. Such an effect has been reported in a previous clinical study [15]. It has been reported that a single dose of 1 g of black pepper can increase the AUC (area under the curve of plasma concentration-time) of phenytoin [14]. In the present study piperine was given in low dose and seems that in this dose, it can change important PK parameters such as clearance and t/12 of midazolam. It

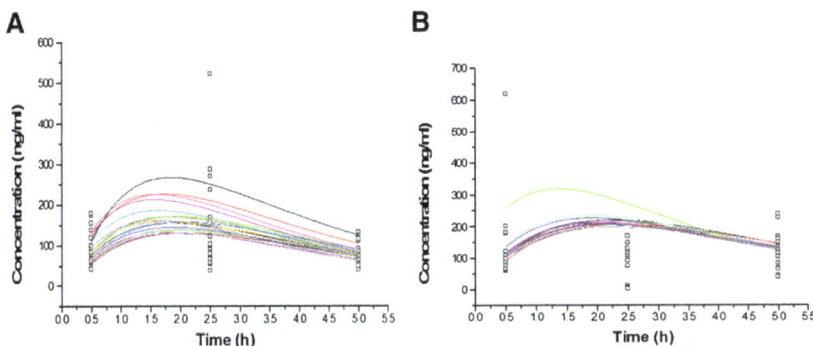

Figure 4 Bayesian predicted (thin line) and observed (symbols) plasma midazolam concentrations in placebo (A) and piperine (B) receiving groups. Note the different scales of concentrations in the figures.

means that piperine's direct effect on midazolam elimination is not assumed and it can increase the half-life of midazolam via inhibition of its hepatic microsomal elimination. This may increase duration and severity of side effects of subject drugs (substrate of CYP3A) following their elevated plasma levels. As we already showed the midazolam side effects in piperine pretreated subjects were considerable compared to placebo. The inhibition or induction of enteral CYP3A4 and p-glycoprotein can mediate considerable drug interactions. These of interactions may be due to a considerable variation in drug action from no effect to toxic effect of drugs [35-38].

The genes of CYP3A4 and p-glycoprotein are expressed in enterocytes and the bioavailability of many drugs such as cyclosporine A, midazolam, verapamil, HIV protease inhibitors and digoxin could be affected by the enzyme and transporter [11,36,38-40]. Metabolism of midazolam when prescribed intravenously shows the activity of hepatic CYP3A, but when it is prescribed orally, it can show the activity of both hepatic and intestinal CYP3A [41,42]. After oxidative metabolism, midazolam changes into one of its main metabolites, hydroxide midazolam, in liver, and is mediated in an exceptional rout by CYP3A isoforms [43,44]. Piperine inhibits p-glycoprotein and CYP3A activity. Since, these proteins become expressed in enterocytes and hepatocytes; they have an effective role in first-pass metabolism of subject drugs. Piperine content of nutritional regimen can change the levels of p-glycoprotein and CYP3A substrates in blood when those administered by mouth [45]. However more researches are needed to prove intestinal or hepatic effects of piperine, especially to justify their mechanism in the present study. In this investigation duration of sedation and possible hypnosis action of midazolam in females was longer than the males. This may be to the result from higher plasma level of midazolam after piperine pretreatment in female subjects. Perhaps, it is concluded that sex may be an important factor to obtaining plasma concentration of midazolam. This may be due to higher activity of CYP3A4 in female at normal condition compared to male [46-49]. In a previous phenotyping study by the authors, similar results by sex variability on CYP3A activity has been reported [17]. For this reason more clinical effects are expected in females if the enzyme becomes inhibited.

Conclusion

Individual PK variations can significantly determine CYP3A activity in general population. This may predispose patients to demonstrate unexpected drug manifestations compared to normal subjects. According to the present investigation, piperine may inhibit CYP3A4 activity and increase the level of midazolam as a substrate of the enzyme.

Competing interests
The authors declared that they have no competing interests.

Authors' contributions
MMR: data collection and executive affairs; SK: laboratory works and review literature searching; MTK: lab tests and data collection; SGh: HPLC model setting; EY and HGh: data collection; MRS: study design and modeling; AAM: study design, to register study in IRCT, data handling and statistical analysis, manuscript writing and correction. All authors read and approved the final manuscript.

Acknowledgements
Authors wish with to give their special thanks to Dr. Amin Rostami, professor of the University of Manchester (UK) for his co-operation to hand *P-Pharm* software, Dr. Roueini, professor of Tehran University of Medical Sciences and Dr. Abidi Pharmaceutical Company for their co-operation to kindly provide standards midazolam and diazepam and Mrs. Hashemi and Dr. Aliasghar Sefidgar for their technical efforts and finally all the participants. This investigation (*project No: 8827910*) has been financially supported by Research Affairs division of Babol University of Medical Sciences.

Author details
[1]Department of Pharmacology, Babol University of Medical Sciences, Babol, Iran. [2]Department of Pharmacology, Mazandaran University of Medical Sciences, Sari, Iran. [3]Cellular and Molecular Biology Research Centre, Babol University of Medical Sciences, Babol, Iran.

References
1. Evans AM: **Influence of dietary components on the gastrointestinal metabolism and transport of drugs.** *Ther Drug Monit* 2000, **22:**131–136.
2. Wilkinson GR: **The effects of diet, aging and disease-states on presystemic elimination and oral drug bioavailability in humans.** *Adv Drug Deliv Rev* 1997, **27:**129–159.
3. Walter-Sack I, Klotz U: **Influence of diet and nutritional status on drug metabolism.** *Clin Pharmacokinet* 1996, **31:**47–64.
4. Ayrton A, Morgan P: **Role of transport proteins in drug absorption, distribution and excretion.** *Xenobiotica* 2001, **31:**469–497.
5. Wilkinson GR: **Cytochrome P4503A (CYP3A) metabolism: prediction of in vivo activity in humans.** *J Pharmacokinet Biopharm* 1996, **24:**475–490.
6. Lauterburg BH, Velez ME: **Glutathione deficiency in alcoholics: risk factor for paracetamol hepatotoxicity.** *Gut* 1988, **29:**1153–1157.
7. Durgaprasad S, Pai CG, Vasanthkumar, Alvres JF, Namitha S: **A pilot study of the antioxidant effect of curcumin in tropical pancreatitis.** *Indian J Med Res* 2005, **122:**315–318.
8. Kapelyukh Y, Paine MJ, Marechal JD, Sutcliffe MJ, Wolf CR, Roberts GC: **Multiple substrate binding by cytochrome P450 3A4: estimation of the number of bound substrate molecules.** *Drug Metab Dispos* 2008, **36:**2136–2144.
9. Atal CK, Zutshi U, Rao PG: **Scientific evidence on the role of Ayurvedic herbals on bioavailability of drugs.** *J Ethnopharmacol* 1981, **4:**229–232.
10. Singh J, Dubey RK, Atal CK: **Piperine-mediated inhibition of glucuronidation activity in isolated epithelial cells of the guinea-pig small intestine: evidence that piperine lowers the endogenous UDP-glucuronic acid content.** *J Pharmacol Exp Ther* 1986, **236:**488–493.
11. Darbar D, Fromm MF, Dell'Orto S, Kim RB, Kroemer HK, Eichelbaum M, Roden DM: **Modulation by dietary salt of verapamil disposition in humans.** *Circulation* 1998, **98:**2702–2708.
12. Bailey DG, Malcolm J, Arnold O, Spence JD: **Grapefruit juice-drug interactions.** *Br J Clin Pharmacol* 1998, **46:**101–110.
13. Kane GC, Lipsky JJ: **Drug-grapefruit juice interactions.** *Mayo Clin Proc* 2000, **75:**933–942.
14. Velpandian T, Jasuja R, Bhardwaj RK, Jaiswal J, Gupta SK: **Piperine in food: interference in the pharmacokinetics of phenytoin.** *Eur J Drug Metab Pharmacokinet* 2001, **26:**241–247.
15. Zutshi RK, Singh R, Zutshi U, Johri RK, Atal CK: **Influence of piperine on rifampicin blood levels in patients of pulmonary tuberculosis.** *J Assoc Physicians India* 1985, **33:**223–224.

16. Kreek MJ, Garfield JW, Gutjahr CL, Giusti LM: Rifampin-induced methadone withdrawal. *N Engl J Med* 1976, **294**:1104–1106.

17. Shiran MR, Gharooee Ahangar S, Rostamkolaee S, Sefidgar SAA, Baradaran M, Hashemi M, Baleghi M, *et al*: Phenotyping of CYP3A by oral midazolam in healthy mazandarani volunteers. *J Babol Univ Med SCI* 2011, **13**:19–25.

18. Rostamkolaee S, Gharooee Ahangar S, Kazemi M, Shiran MR, Moghadamnia AA: Determination of CYP1A1 phenotype in a sample of healthy volunteers. *J Babol Univ Med SCI* 2011, **14**:25–32.

19. Shimada T, Yamazaki H, Mimura M, Inui Y, Guengerich FP: Interindividual variations in human liver cytochrome P-450 enzymes involved in the oxidation of drugs, carcinogens and toxic chemicals: studies with liver microsomes of 30 Japanese and 30 Caucasians. *J Pharmacol Exp Ther* 1994, **270**:414–423.

20. Johnson WW: Cytochrome P450 inactivation by pharmaceuticals and phytochemicals: therapeutic relevance. *Drug Metab Rev* 2008, **40**:101–147.

21. Guengerich FP: Mechanisms of cytochrome P450 substrate oxidation: MiniReview. *J Biochem Mol Toxicol* 2007, **21**:163–168.

22. Kato M: Intestinal first-pass metabolism of CYP3A4 substrates. *Drug Metab Pharmacokinet* 2008, **23**:87–94.

23. Paine MF, Hart HL, Ludington SS, Haining RL, Rettie AE, Zeldin DC: The human intestinal cytochrome P450 "pie". *Drug Metab Dispos* 2006, **34**:880–886.

24. Feierman DE, Lasker JM: Metabolism of fentanyl, a synthetic opioid analgesic, by human liver microsomes. Role of CYP3A4. *Drug Metab Dispos* 1996, **24**:932–939.

25. Ferrari A, Coccia CP, Bertolini A, Sternieri E: Methadone–metabolism, pharmacokinetics and interactions. *Pharmacol Res* 2004, **50**:551–559.

26. Lalovic B, Phillips B, Risler LL, Howald W, Shen DD: Quantitative contribution of CYP2D6 and CYP3A to oxycodone metabolism in human liver and intestinal microsomes. *Drug Metab Dispos* 2004, **32**:447–454.

27. Klees TM, Sheffels P, Dale O, Kharasch ED: Metabolism of alfentanil by cytochrome p4503a (cyp3a) enzymes. *Drug Metab Dispos* 2005, **33**:303–311.

28. Trescot AM, Datta S, Lee M, Hansen H: Opioid pharmacology. *Pain Physician* 2008, **11**:S133–S153.

29. Pelkonen O, Turpeinen M, Hakkola J, Honkakoski P, Hukkanen J, Raunio H: Inhibition and induction of human cytochrome P450 enzymes: current status. *Arch Toxicol* 2008, **82**:667–715.

30. Volak LP, Ghirmai S, Cashman JR, Court MH: Curcuminoids inhibit multiple human cytochromes P450, UDP-glucuronosyltransferase, and sulfotransferase enzymes, whereas piperine is a relatively selective CYP3A4 inhibitor. *Drug Metab Dispos* 2008, **36**:1594–1605.

31. Atal CK, Dubey RK, Singh J: Biochemical basis of enhanced drug bioavailability by piperine: evidence that piperine is a potent inhibitor of drug metabolism. *J Pharmacol Exp Ther* 1985, **232**:258–262.

32. Reen RK, Singh J: In vitro and in vivo inhibition of pulmonary cytochrome P450 activities by piperine, a major ingredient of piper species. *Indian J Exp Biol* 1991, **29**:568–573.

33. Bano G, Raina RK, Zutshi U, Bedi KL, Johri RK, Sharma SC: Effect of piperine on bioavailability and pharmacokinetics of propranolol and theophylline in healthy volunteers. *Eur J Clin Pharmacol* 1991, **41**:615–617.

34. Pattanaik S, Hota D, Prabhakar S, Kharbanda P, Pandhi P: Effect of piperine on the steady-state pharmacokinetics of phenytoin in patients with epilepsy. *Phytother Res* 2006, **20**:683–686.

35. Fromm MF, Kim RB, Stein CM, Wilkinson GR, Roden DM: Inhibition of P-glycoprotein-mediated drug transport: a unifying mechanism to explain the interaction between digoxin and quinidine [seecomments]. *Circulation* 1999, **99**:552–557.

36. Greiner B, Eichelbaum M, Fritz P, Kreichgauer HP, von Richter O, Zundler J, Kroemer HK: The role of intestinal P-glycoprotein in the interaction of digoxin and rifampin. *J Clin Invest* 1999, **104**:147–153.

37. Thummel KE, O'Shea D, Paine MF, Shen DD, Kunze KL, Perkins JD, Wilkinson GR: Oral first-pass elimination of midazolam involves both gastrointestinal and hepatic CYP3A-mediated metabolism. *Clin Pharmacol Ther* 1996, **59**:491–502.

38. Westphal K, Weinbrenner A, Zschiesche M, Franke G, Knoke M, Oertel R, Fritz P, *et al*: Induction of P-glycoprotein by rifampin increases intestinal secretion of talinolol in human beings: a new type of drug/drug interaction. *Clin Pharmacol Ther* 2000, **68**:345–355.

39. Fromm MF, Busse D, Kroemer HK, Eichelbaum M: Differential induction of prehepatic and hepatic metabolism of verapamil by rifampin. *Hepatology* 1996, **24**:796–801.

40. Kim RB, Fromm MF, Wandel C, Leake B, Wood AJ, Roden DM, Wilkinson GR: The drug transporter P-glycoprotein limits oral absorption and brain entry of HIV-1 protease inhibitors. *J Clin Invest* 1998, **101**:289–294.

41. Paine MF, Shen DD, Kunze KL, Perkins JD, Marsh CL, McVicar JP, Barr DM, *et al*: First-pass metabolism of midazolam by the human intestine. *Clin Pharmacol Ther* 1996, **60**:14–24.

42. Wandel C, Bocker RH, Bohrer H, de Vries JX, Hofmann W, Walter K, Kleingeist B, *et al*: Relationship between hepatic cytochrome P450 3A content and activity and the disposition of midazolam administered orally. *Drug Metab Dispos* 1998, **26**:110–114.

43. Kronbach T, Mathys D, Umeno M, Gonzalez FJ, Meyer UA: Oxidation of midazolam and triazolam by human liver cytochrome P450IIIA4. *Mol Pharmacol* 1989, **36**:89–96.

44. Ghosal A, Satoh H, Thomas PE, Bush E, Moore D: Inhibition and kinetics of cytochrome P4503A activity in microsomes from rat, human, and cdna-expressed human cytochrome P450. *Drug Metab Dispos* 1996, **24**:940–947.

45. Bhardwaj RK, Glaeser H, Becquemont L, Klotz U, Gupta SK, Fromm MF: Piperine, a major constituent of black pepper, inhibits human P-glycoprotein and CYP3A4. *J Pharmacol Exp Ther* 2002, **302**:645–650.

46. Gleiter CH, Gundert-Remy U: Gender differences in pharmacokinetics. *Eur J Drug Metab Pharmacokinet* 1996, **21**:123–128.

47. Miao J, Jin Y, Marunde RL, Kim S, Quinney S, Radovich M, Li L, *et al*: Association of genotypes of the CYP3A cluster with midazolam disposition in vivo. *Pharmacogenomics J* 2009, **9**:319–326.

48. Tanaka E: Gender-related differences in pharmacokinetics and their clinical significance. *J Clin Pharm Ther* 1999, **24**:339–346.

49. Harris RZ, Benet LZ, Schwartz JB: Gender effects in pharmacokinetics and pharmacodynamics. *Drugs* 1995, **50**:222–239.

4

Bioactive Terpenoids and Flavonoids from *Daucus littoralis* Smith subsp. *hyrcanicus* Rech.f, an Endemic Species of Iran

Fatemeh Yousefbeyk[1†], Ahmad Reza Gohari[1†], Zeinabsadat Hashemighahderijani[2†], Sayed Nasser Ostad[2†], Mohamad Hossein Salehi Sourmaghi[2], Mohsen Amini[3], Fereshteh Golfakhrabadi[1], Hossein Jamalifar[4] and Gholamreza Amin[1*†]

Abstract

Background: *Daucus littoralis* Smith subsp. *hyrcanicus* Rech.f. (Apiaceae) is an endemic species in northern parts of Iran where it is commonly named Caspian carrot. The fruits have been used as condiment.

Methods: In a series of *in vitro* assays, antioxidant (DPPH and FRAP assays), cytotoxic and antimicrobial activities of different extracts of roots and fruits were evaluated for the first time. The separation and purification of the compounds were carried out on the most potent extracts using various chromatographic methods and identified by spectroscopic data (^{1}H and ^{13}C NMR).

Results: The results showed that among the extracts only fruit methanol extract (FME) has significant antioxidant activity ($IC_{50} = 145.93$ μg.ml^{-1} in DPPH assay and 358 ± 0.02 mmol FeII/g dry extract in FRAP assay). The radical scavenging activity of FME at 400 μg.ml^{-1} was comparable with α-tocopherol (40 μg.ml^{-1}) and with BHA (100 μg.ml^{-1}) ($p > 0.05$). FME did not show any toxicity against cancerous and normal cell lines. Fruit ethyl acetate extract (FEE) had cytotoxic activity against breast carcinoma and hepatocellular carcinoma cells (IC_{50} 168.4 and 185 μg.ml^{-1}, respectively), while it did not possess antioxidant activity in comparison with α-tocopherol and BHA as standard compounds. Ethyl acetate and methanol extract of fruits showed antimicrobial activity against *Staphylococcus aureus* (MIC: 3.75 mg.ml^{-1}) and *Candida albicans* (MIC: 15.6 and 7.8 mg.ml^{-1}, respectively). Four terpenoids were isolated form FEE including: β-sitosterol (1), stigmasterol (2), caryophyllene oxide (3), β-amyrin (4). Also, three flavonoids namely quercetin 3-O-β-glucoside (5), quercetin 3-O-β-galactoside (6) and luteolin (7) were isolated from FME.

Conclusion: This study showed that FEE and FME of *D. littoralis* Smith subsp. *hyrcanicus* Rech.f. had the highest biological activities which may be correlated with *in vitro* cytotoxic, antimicrobial and antioxidant activities of terpenoids and flavonoids components of the extracts.

Keywords: *Daucus littoralis* Smith subsp. *hyrcanicus* Rech.f, Antioxidant, Cytotoxic activity, Antimicrobial

Background

Daucus littoralis Smith subsp. *hyrcanicus* Rech.f. (Umbelliferae or Apiaceae) is an endemic species which is distributed in north of Iran (Mazandaran and Guilan provinces). It is an annual or perennial herb growing up to 3 to 10 cm high on the sandy dunes of Caspian Sea coasts where the

* Correspondence: amin@tums.ac.ir
†Equal contributors
[1]Department of Pharmacognosy, Faculty of Pharmacy and Medicinal Plants Research Centre, Tehran University of Medical Sciences, Tehran 14155-6451, Iran
Full list of author information is available at the end of the article

fruits have been used as condiment by the rural population [1]. The fruits of the related species, *D. carota*, have been used in Traditional Chinese Medicine (TCM) as a remedy for the treatment of ancylostomiasis, dropsy, chronic kidney diseases and bladder afflictions [2]. A wide range of pharmacologic properties such as antibacterial, antifungal, anthelmintic, hepatoprotective and cytotoxic activities have been reported on *D. carota* [2]. Phytochemical studies indicated the presence of sesquiterpenes, chromones, flavonoids, coumarins and anthocyanins from *D. carota* [2], sesquiterpene lactone [3] and phenylpropanoid triesters [4] from *D. glaber* (Forssk.) Thell. Recently we reported the composition and antimicrobial activity of the essential oil from leaves and stems, fruits, flowers and roots of *D. littoralis* Smith subsp. *hyrcanicus* Rech.f. [5]. No data on the phytochemistry and biological activity have been published for this species. In this study, we investigated the antioxidant, antimicrobial and cytotoxic activities of different extracts from roots and fruits of this plant. Also the isolation and structure elucidation of active compounds from most active extracts are reported.

Methods
General procedures
^{1}H and ^{13}C-NMR spectra was acquired using a Bruker Avance TM500 DRX (500 MHz for ^{1}H and 125 MHz for ^{13}C) spectrometer with tetramethylsilane as an internal standard, and chemical shifts are given in δ (ppm). Column chromatography was performed using silica gel (70–230, 230–400 mesh) (Merck, Germany) and Sephadex LH$_{20}$ (Fluka,Switzerland). Silica gel 60 F254 precoated plates (Merck, Germany) were used for TLC. The spots were detected by spraying anisaldehyde-H$_2$SO$_4$ (Sigma-Aldrich Chemie, Germany) reagent followed by heating. HPLC separations were carried out on a Knauer system (Smart line system, Germany) connected to a photodiode array detector. All the solvents, standards and reagents were obtained from Merck (Germany).

Plant material
The plant was collected from Bandar-e-Anzaly sea coast, province of Guilan, north of Iran, during the fruiting stage in June 2012. A voucher specimen of plant (6734-TEH) was deposited in Herbarium of Department of Pharmacognosy, Faculty of Pharmacy, Tehran University of Medical Sciences, Tehran, Iran.

Extraction and Isolation
The roots and fruits of plant (1 kg, each) were powdered and extracted successively with ethyl acetate, methanol and methanol–water (1:1), at room temperature. The fruit ethyl acetate extract (FEE) (88 g) was subjected to silica gel column chromatography (CC) with CHCl$_3$: AcOEt (9: 1) as eluent to give ten fractions (A-J). The fraction H (5 g) was submitted to silica gel CC with hexane: AcOEt (8: 2) to obtain 20 fractions (Ha- Ht). The fractions Hm and Hr result compounds 1 and 2 (5 and 5.3 mg). The fraction Hc (300 mg) was subjected to CC with hexane: AcOEt (9: 1) to give three fractions (Hc$_1$-Hc$_3$). Compound 3 (5.9 mg) was obtained from the fraction Hc$_3$ (25 mg) by silica gel CC and hexane: CHCl$_3$: AcOEt (18: 1: 1) as mobile phase.

The fraction Hd (500 mg) was chromatographed on Sephadex LH$_{20}$ with CHCl$_3$: MeOH (3:7) to obtain nine fractions (Hd$_1$-Hd$_9$). Fraction Hd$_9$ (30 mg) was subjected

to normal phase semi-HPLC a Eurospher column (250 × 18 mm i.d.) and a PDF detector (λ: 210 nm).The initial eluted ratio was adjusted with 95: 5 (hexane: AcOEt) and delivered to the column for 20 min (flow-rate: 3 ml. min^{-1}). Then the eluted ratio was changed to 85:15 (hexane: AcOEt) until 50 min. The program was continued with the same ratio of solvents for next 20 min (70 min after starting point). The compound 4 (5.5 mg) was purified with this method.

The FME was dissolved in distilled water and after filtration; the aqueous solution was extracted with petroleum ether three times. The water soluble phase was evaporated to dryness and then extracted with n-BuOH for three times. The butanolic extract (8 g) was subjected to column chromatography on Sephadex LH$_{20}$ with MeOH to obtain 7 fractions (B$_1$-B$_7$). Fraction B$_6$ was submitted to reversed phase semi- HPLC including a Eurospher (column 250 × 20 mm i.d.) and a PDA detector (λ: 310 nm). Mobile phase including 40:60 (H$_2$O: MeOH) was delivered at flow rate 3 ml.min^{-1} to give compounds 5 and 6 (5.5 and 5 mg respectively).

For purification of fraction B$_7$, a gradient reversed phase semi-HPLC was used with the same column, flow rate and detection condition. The eluted ratio was adjusted with 65:35 (H$_2$O: MeOH) as starting ratio and delivered to the column for 50 min and then was changed to 9:11 (H$_2$O: MeOH) until 70 min. Chromatography was continued with the same ratio of mobile phase for next 100 min (170 min after starting point) to give compound 7 (6.5 mg).

Antimicrobial activity of extracts
Antimicrobial activity of different extracts were tested against a Gram-positive (*Staphylococcus aureus* ATCC 6538), two Gram-negatives (*Escherichia coli* ATCC 8739 and *Pseudomonas aeruginosa* ATCC 9027) and a fungal strain (*Candida albicans* ATCC 1023). Minimum inhibitory concentration (MIC) of the extracts was determined by broth micro dilution method using 96 U-shaped wells plates [6]. A stock solution of 300 mg.ml^{-1} from each extract was prepared in DMSO. Then two-fold serial dilution of the stock solution of each extract (100 µl) was prepared by using Mueller Hinton Broth (MHB) and Sabourad Dextrose Broth (SDB) (100 µl, each) in ten wells. The stock microbial suspension with twofold test inoculum was prepared in MHB and SDB from a 24-h old culture. Then aliquot of 100 µl of twofold test strain inoculum was added to each well to reach the final inoculum size of 5 × 10^5 cfu.ml^{-1} [7]. The minimum bactericidal concentration (MBC) was determined by quantitative subculture of 100 µl from each clear well onto Mueller Hinton Agar (MHA) and Sabourad Dextrose Agar (SDA) plates. Plates were incubated at 37°C and 20-25°C for bacterial and fungal strains, for 48 h, respectively. The MBC

is defined as the lowest concentration of extracts that results in more than 99.9% killing of the bacteria being tested [7].

Antioxidant activity

DPPH radical-scavenging activity assay

The antioxidant activity of extracts were measured by the DPPH (2, 2′-diphenyl-1-picrylhydrazyl) free radical scavenging method based on an established protocol [8]. Sample solutions (1 ml) in methanol at different concentration were added to DPPH methanol solution (2 ml, 40 µg.ml^{-1}). The mixtures were incubated at room temperature for 30 min and the absorbance was measured at 517 nm. Vitamin E and butyl hydroxyanisole (BHA) were used as positive controls. IC$_{50}$ values (indicate the concentration of the test samples providing 50% radical scavenging) were calculated from graph-plotted scavenging percentage against extract concentration.

Ferric reducing antioxidant potential (FRAP scavenging) assay:

The FRAP assay was done according to the method described by Benzie and Strain [9,10]. Briefly, the FRAP reagent contained 5 ml of a (10 mmol.l^{-1}) TPTZ (2, 4, 6- tripyridyl- s- triazine) solution in 40 mmol.l^{-1} HCl plus 5 ml of (20 mmol.l^{-1}) FeCl$_3$ and 50 ml of (0.3 mmol.l^{-1}) acetate buffer, pH 3.6 and was prepared freshly. Aliquots of extract (50 µl) were mixed with FRAP reagent (1.5 ml), incubated at 37°C, for 10 min, and then the absorbance was measured at 593 nm. For construction of calibration curve, five concentrations of FeSO$_4$ .7H$_2$O (125, 250, 500, 750, 1000 mmol.l^{-1}) were used. The antioxidant activities were expressed as the concentration of antioxidants having a reducing ability equivalent for 1 mmol.l^{-1} FeSO$_4$ [11].

Measurement of total phenolic contents

Total phenolics were determined colorimetrically by the Folin-Ciocalteu method as described by Miliauskas, et al. [12]. The prepared extracts (1 ml) were mixed with 5 ml of Folin-Ciocalteu reagent (previously diluted tenfold with distilled water) and allowed to stand at room temperature for 10 min. A 4 ml sodium bicarbonate solution (75 g.l^{-1}) was added to the mixture. After 30 min at room temperature, absorbance was measured at 765 nm using a UV spectrophotometer (Pharmacia Biotech). Total phenolics were quantified by calibration curve obtained from measuring the absorbance of a known concentration of gallic acid (GA) standard (20–200 mg.l^{-1}). The concentrations are expressed as milligrams of gallic acid equivalents (GA) per g dry extract [11].

Cell cultures and cytotoxicity assay

Three cancerous cell lines HT29 (colon carcinoma), HepG2 (hepatocellular carcinoma), MCF7 (breast ductal carcinoma) and a normal cell line NIH-3T3 (Swiss mouse embryo fibroblast) were purchased from the Pasteur Institute, Tehran, Iran. The cells were maintained in RPMI 1640, supplemented with 10% fetal bovine serum, 0.28 units.ml^{-1} insulin, 100 µg.ml^{-1} streptomycin, 100 units.ml^{-1} penicillin, and 0.3 mg.ml^{-1} glutamine. The cells were grown at 37°C in a humidified atmosphere of 5% CO$_2$. The cytotoxicity of different extracts was assayed using the MTT cytotoxicity assay. The cells (1×10^4) were plated in 100 µl of medium/well in 96-well plates (NUNC, Denmark). After 48 hours incubation at 37°C, in 5% CO$_2$, and a humidified atmosphere, the different extracts were added to the cells of different concentrations (800, 400, 200, 100, 50, 25, 12.5 and 6, 25 µg.ml^{-1}). Methotrexate (positive control) and extracts were incubated at 37°C, in 5% CO$_2$, humidified atmosphere, for 48 hours. After 48 hours, 25 µl of 5 mg.ml^{-1} MTT (dissolved in PBS) was added per well. After three hours of incubation, the MTT solution was removed and the cells were washed twice with 100 µl of PBS. One hundred and fifty microliters of DMSO was added per well, to solubilize the formazan crystals. The optical densities of the wells were then measured at 570 nm (690 nm reference wavelength). By referring to the control (medium with DMSO), the cell survival was assessed [13]. The median growth inhibitory concentration (IC$_{50}$ values) was obtained from the IC$_{50}$ of dose response curve in the Sigma Plot 12 software. Each data is the mean value of three independent experiments and presented as mean ± SD.

Results and discussion

In the present study extracts from roots and fruits of D. littoralis Smith subsp. hyrcanicus Rech.f. were investigated for bioactivity, the first time. Among the tested extracts, fruits methanol extract (FME) and fruit ethyl acetate extract (FEE) showed highest bioactive properties. As shown in Table 1, FME had the highest content of total phenol (99.1 ± 0.08 mg gallic acid equivalent/g dry extract) and the highest antioxidant activity in the DPPH assay (IC$_{50}$ = 145.93 µg.ml^{-1}) and in FRAP assay (358 ± 0.02 mmol FeII/g dry extract). Radical scavenging activity of FME at 400 µg.ml^{-1} was comparable with α-tocopherol (40 µg.ml^{-1}) and BHA (100 µg.ml^{-1}) ($p > 0.05$). Other extracts did not have any antioxidant activity in comparison with α-tocopherol and BHA. Other extracts did not have any significant antioxidant activities.

The results of antimicrobial assays are shown in Table 2. Among the extracts, only FME exhibited antimicrobial activity against all four microorganisms. FME showed better antimicrobial activity against S. aureus

Table 1 Antioxidant activity and total phenolic content of different extracts from fruits and roots of *D. littoralis* subsp. *hyrcanicus*

	DPPH	FRAP	Total phenol contents
	(μg.ml^{-1})	(mmol FeII/g dry extract)	(mg GAE/g dry extract)
FEE	789.74	44.6 ± 0.2	25.13 ± 0.06
FME	145.93	358 ± 0.02	99.1 ± 0.08
FMWE	172.3	306 ± 0.08	41.35 ± 0.04
REE	>1000	78 ± 0.01	36.06 ± 0.01
RME	467.2	258 ± 0.30	32.12 ± 0.03
RMWE	269.75	214 ± 0.20	27.79 ± 0.01
Vitamin E	14.12	313 ± 0.01	-
BHA	7.8	880 ± 0.06	-

Key to extracts employed: FEE: Fruts Ethyl acetate Extract; FME: Fruits Methanol Extract; FMWE: Fruits Methanol–water Extract; REE: Roots Ethyl acetate Extract; RME: Roots Methanol Extract; RMWE: Roots Methanol–water Extract.

(MIC: 3.75 and MBC: 7.5 mg.ml^{-1}), whereas it showed weak activity towards Gram negative bacteria.

Antiproliferative activity was determined in HepG2, MCF7, HT-29, and NIH-3T3 cells, shown in Table 3. Only FEE and root ethyl acetate extract (REE) showed toxicity on cancerous cell lines. FEE showed higher cytotoxicity on HepG2 and MCF7 (IC$_{50}$ 185.01 ± 2.1 and 168 ± 1.5 μg.ml^{-1}, respectively) than REE.

The FEE and FME were used for isolation and purification of main components with different chromatography methods. From FEE four terpenoids including β-sitosterol (1), stigmasterol (2) caryophyllene oxide (3) and β-amyrin (4) were isolated. Three flavonoids including: quercetin 3-O-β-glucoside (5), quercetin 3-O-β-galactoside (6) and luteolin (7) were isolated from FME (Figure 1). Compounds 1–7 were identified by comparison of their

spectroscopic data (^{1}H-NMR, ^{13}C-NMR) with those in the literature and authentic compounds from our laboratory [14-16]. Spectroscopic data of compounds 1-7 are provided in Additional file 1.

β-Amyrin is a pentacyclic triterpene with anti-inflammatory, antimicrobial, antifungal, antiviral and cytotoxic properties [17]. β-Amyrin isolated from MeOH extracts of *Byrsonima crassifolia* showed moderate antimicrobial activity against *S. aureus* and *C. albicans* (MIC: 0.5 and 1.02 mg.ml^{-1}, respectively) [18]. The better activity of FEE against *S. aureus* and *C. albicans* seems to be due to the presence of β-amyrin. β-Sitosterol and stigmasterol are two of the most prevalent phytostrols in the plant kingdom [19]. *In vivo* investigation showed that oral consumption of stigmasterol inhibits the absorption of sterols and cholesterol from the intestinal tract and suppress the biosynthesis of cholesterol and bile acids in rats [19]. β-Sitosterol modulates the production of inflammatory cytokines, and reduces prostate enlargement [20]. It showed cytotoxic activity against colon carcinoma (COLO 320 DM), breast cancer and Bowes cell lines [21]. β-Caryophyllene oxide has shown cytotoxic activity against HepG2, AGS (human lung cancer cells), HeLa (human cervical adenocarcinoma cells), SNU-1 (human gastric cancer cell) and SNU-16 (human stomach cancer), with IC$_{50}$ values of 3.95, 12.6, 13.55, 16.79, and 27.39 μM, respectively [22]. The cytotoxic activity of FEE against MCF7 and HepG2 seems to be due to the presence of β-sitosterol, β-amyrin and β-caryophyllene oxide.

In general, phenolic compounds possess antibacterial and antifungal properties [23]. Among them, flavonoids are well known for their antibacterial, antifungal, antiviral, antioxidant, anti-inflammatory activities [24]. The antioxidant activity of flavonoids is due to their capability as radical scavengers [25]. Many medicinal plants containing flavonoids have been reported for their antibacterial activity [23]. The high amount of total phenols

Table 2 Minimum inhibitory concentration (MIC) and minimum bactericidal concentration (MBC) of deferent extract of fruits and roots of *D. littoralis* subsp. *hyrcanicus*

Microorganisms	*Staphylococcus aureus*		*Escherichia coli*		*Pseudomonas aeruginosa*		*Candida albicans*	
	MIC	MBC	MIC	MBC	MIC	MBC	MIC	MBC
FEE	3.7	7.5	-	-	-	-	15.6	15.6
FME	3.7	7.5	>100	>100	62.5	>100	7.8	15.6
FMWE	-	-	-	-	-	-	-	-
REE	-	-	-	-	-	-	-	-
RME	>100	>100	-	-	-	-	-	-
RMWE	>100	>100	-	-	-	-	-	-

Note: MIC and MBC were determined by broth micro dilution method and expressed in mg.ml^{-1}(W/V); Key to extracts employed: FEE: Fruits Ethyl acetate Extract; FME: Fruits Methanol Extract; FMWE: Fruits Methanol–water Extract; REE: Roots Ethyl acetate Extract; RME: Roots Methanol Extract; RMWE: Roots Methanol–water Extract.

Table 3 Cytotoxic activity of different extracts of fruits and roots *D. littoralis* subsp. *hyrcanicus* using MTT assay

	HepG2	MCF7	HT-29	NIH-3T3
FEE	185.01 ± 2.1	168.41 ± 1.5	412.8 ± 1.3	149.48 ± 1.1
FME	- [a]	-	-	-
FMWE	-	-	-	-
REE	219.58 ± 1.1	279.68 ± 2.6	351.26 ± 3.2	155.34 ± 1.3
RME	935.34 ± 2.4	-	-	-
RMWE	-	-	-	-
Methotrexate	-	0.16 ± 0.09	0.23 ± 0.02	0.24 ± 0.01

Notes: Results are expressed as IC_{50} values (µg.m.l⁻¹), [a] inactive ($IC_{50} > 1000$); Key to cell Lines employed: HepG2(Hepatocellular carcinoma); MCF7 (breast carcinoma); HT29 (colon carcinoma); NIH-3T3 (Swiss embryo fibroblast). Key to extracts employed: FEE: Fruts Ethyl acetate Extract; FME: Fruits Methanol Extract; FMWE: Fruits Methanol–water Extract; REE: Roots Ethyl acetate Extract; RME: Roots Methanol Extract; RMWE: Roots Methanol–water Extract.

and in particular quercetin 3-O-β-glucoside, quercetin 3-O-β-galactoside and luteolin are responsible for better antibacterial activity of FME.

Conclusion

In this study, a screening of different extracts of *D. littoralis* Smith subsp. *hyrcanicus* Rech.f. was carried out for the first time. The presence of β-sitosterol, β-amyrin and β -caryophyllene oxide explained the cytotoxic activity of FEE in breast carcinoma and hepatocellular carcinoma cell lines. The high amount of phenolic compounds and flavonoids was responsible for the antioxidant and antimicrobial activity of FME. Based on these observations, FEE and FME can be good candidates for further *in vivo* biological studies and phytochemical investigations.

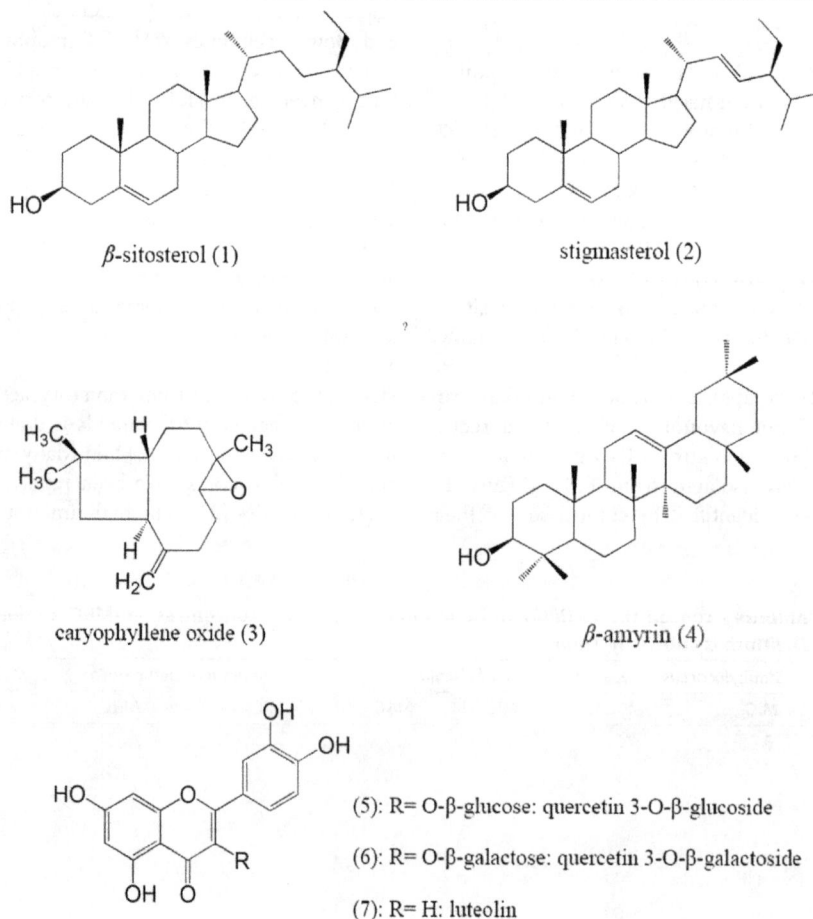

Figure 1 Structures of compounds 1-7 isolated form *D. littoralis* Smith subsp. *hyrcanicus* Rech.f including β-sitosterol (1), stigmasterol (2), caryophyllene oxide (3), β-amyrin (4), quercetin 3-O-β-glucoside (5), quercetin 3-O-β-galactoside (6) and luteolin (7).

Additional file

Additional file 1: Spectroscopic data of compounds 1-7 isolated from *D. littoralis* Smith subsp. *hyrcanicus* Rech.f.:

Competing interests

No conflict of interest has been declared.

Authors' contributions

FY performed plant preparation, extraction, isolation, identification of plant substances, evaluated antimicrobial activity of extracts, advised on antioxidant and total phenol content method and drafted the manuscript. AR-G advised on separation of plant substances and identification of compounds. ZH carried out antioxidant assays, total phenol content and cytotoxic activity of the extracts. SN-O advised on cytotoxic activity of extract by MTT assay. MH-SS conceived the study and edited the manuscript. MA advised on NMR techniques of isolated compounds. FG contributed in antimicrobial assay and edited the manuscript. HJ advised antimicrobial activity of extracts. GR-A did the botanical studies and identified scientific name of the Plant, conceived the study and edited the manuscript. All authors read and approved the final manuscript.

Acknowledgements

This investigation granted by research chancellor of Tehran University of Medical Sciences. The authors are grateful to Dr. Mohsen Amin (Faculty of Pharmacy, Tehran University of Medical Sciences) for proof reading and revising the manuscript. Also we acknowledge Mr Amir Yousefbeyk for his assistance in collecting plants.

Author details

[1]Department of Pharmacognosy, Faculty of Pharmacy and Medicinal Plants Research Centre, Tehran University of Medical Sciences, Tehran 14155-6451, Iran. [2]Department of Toxicology, Pharmacology and Nanotechnology Research Centre, Tehran University of Medical Sciences, Tehran 14155-6451, Iran. [3]Department of Medicinal Chemistry, Faculty of Pharmacy, Tehran University of Medical Sciences, Tehran 14155-6451, Iran. [4]Department of Drug and Food Control, Faculty of Pharmacy and Pharmaceutical Quality Assurance Research Centre, Tehran University of Medical Sciences, Tehran 14155-6451, Iran.

References

1. Mozafarian V: *Flora of Iran. (Umbelliferae) volume 162*. Tehran: Research Institute of Forests and Rangelands; 2007.
2. Fu HW, Zhang L, Yi T, Chen RN, Wang X, Tian JK: **Two New guaiane-type sesquiterpene glycosides from the fruits of *Daucus carota* L.** *Chem Pharm Bull* 2010, **58**:125–128.
3. Sallam AA, Hitotsuyanagi Y, Mansour ESS, Ahmed AF, Gedara S, Fukaya H, Takeya K: **Sesquiterpene Lactones from *Daucus glaber*.** *Helv Chim Acta* 2010, **93**:48–57.
4. Sallam AA, Hitotsuyanagi Y, Mansour ESS, Ahmed AF, Gedara S, Fukaya H, Takeya K: **Phenylpropanoid triesters from *Daucus glaber*.** *Phytochem Lett* 2009, **2**:188–191.
5. Yousefbeyk F, Gohari AR, Salehi Sourmaghi MH, Amini M, Jamalifar H, Golfakhrabadi F, Ramezani N, Amin GH: **Chemical composition and antimicrobial activity of essential oils from different parts of *Daucus littoralis* Smith subsp. *hyrcanicus*.** *Rech J Essent Oil Bear.* in press.
6. NCCLS: *Methods for Dilution Antimicrobial Susceptibility Tests for Bacteria that Grow Aerobically. Approved Standard M7-A7*. Pennsylvania: Wayne; 2006.
7. Vazirian M, Taheri Kashani S, Shams Ardekani M, Khanavi M: **Antimicrobial activity of lemongrass (*Cymbopogon citratus (DC) Stapf.*) essential oil against food-borne pathogens added to cream filled cakes and pastries.** *J Essent Oil Res* 2010, **24**:579–582.
8. Yassa N, Razavi-Beni H, Hadjiakhoondi A: **Free radical scavenging and lipid peroxidation activity of the Shahani black grape.** *Pak J Biol Sci* 2008, **11**:1–4.
9. Benzie IF, Strain JJ: **The ferric reducing ability of plasma (FRAP) as ameasure of "antioxidant power": the FRAP assay.** *Anal Biochem* 1996, **239**:70–76.
10. Moradi-Afrapoli F, Asghari B, Saeidnia S, Ajani Y, Mirjani M, Malmir M, Dolatabadi Bazaz R, Hadjiakhoondi A, Salehi P, Hamburger M, Yassa N: **vitro α-glucosidase inhibitory activity of phenolic constituents from aerial parts of *Polygonum hyrcanicum*.** *Daru* 2012, **20**:37–41.
11. Sadati N, Khanavi M, Mahrokh A, Nabavi S, Sohrabipour J, Hadjiakhoondi A: **Comparison of Antioxidant Activity and Total Phenolic Contents of some Persian Gulf Marine Algae.** *J Med Plants* 2011, **10**:73–79.
12. Miliauskas G, Venskutonis P, Beek T: **Screening of radical cavenging activiy of some medicinal and aromatic plant extract.** *Food Chem* 2004, **85**:231–237.
13. Momtaz S, Lall N, Hussein A, Ostad S, Abdollahi M: **Investigation of the possible biological activities of a poisonous South African plant; Hyaenanche globosa (Euphorbiaceae).** *Phacog Mag* 2010, **6**:34–41.
14. Goad LJ, Akihisa T: *Analysis of sterols*. London: Blackie Academic & Professional; 1997.
15. Gohari AR, Hadjiakhoondi A, Sadat-Ebrahimi S, Saeidnia S, Shafiee A: **Cytotoxic triterpenoids from *Satureja macrantha* C.A. Mey.** *Daru* 2005, **13**:177–181.
16. Agrawal P: *Carbon-13 NMR of Flavonoids*. New York: Elsevier; 1989.
17. Hernández Vázquez L, Palazon J, Navarro-Ocana A: *The pentacyclic triterpenes a, β amyrins: A review of sources and biological activities. Phytochemicals - A Gglobal perspective of their role in nutrition and health*. InTech. Crotia: In Tech Europ; 2012.
18. Rivero-Cruz JF, Sánchez-Nieto S, Benítez G, Casimiro X, Ibarra-Alvarado C, Rojas-Molina A, Rivero-Cruz B: **Antibacterial compounds isolated from *Byrsonima crassifolia*.** *Rev Latinoamer Quím* 2009, **37**:155–163.
19. Saeidnia S, Permeh P, Gohari A, Mashinchian-Moradi A: **Gracilariopsis persica from Persian Gulf Contains Bioactive Sterols.** *Iranian J Pharmal Res* 2012, **11**:845–849.
20. Paniagua-Perez R, Madrigal-Bujaidar E, Reyes-Cadena S, Molina-Jaso D, Perez Gallaga J, Silva-Miranda A, Velazcoet O, Hernandezal N, Chamorro G: **Genotoxic and cytotoxic studies of beta-sitosterol and pteropodine in mouse.** *J Biomed Biotechnol* 2005, **3**:242–2473.
21. Baskar AA, Ignacimuthu S, Paulraj GM, Numair KSA: **Potential of β-Sitosterol in experimental colon cancer model - an In vitro and In vivo study.** *BMC Complement Altern Med* 2010, **10**:24–34.
22. Jun NJ, Mosaddik A, Moon JY, Jang KC, Lee DS, Ahn KS, Cho SK: **Cytotoxic activity of β-Caryophyllene oxide isolated from Jeju Guava (*Psidium cattleianum* Sabine) Leaf Rec.** *Nat Prod* 2011, **5**:242–246.
23. Martini N, Katerere D, Eloff J: **Biological activity of five antibacterial flavonoids from *Combretum erythrophyllum* (Combretaceae).** *J Ethnopharmacol* 2004, **93**:207–212.
24. Cushnie TT, Lamb AJ: **Antimicrobial activity of flavonoids.** *Int J Antimicrob Ag* 2005, **26**:343–356.
25. Saeidnia S, Abdollahi M: **Who plays dual role in cancerous and normal cells? Natural antioxidants or free radicals or cell environment.** *Int J Phamacol* 2012, **8**:711–712.

5

Antidepressant effects of crocin and its effects on transcript and protein levels of CREB, BDNF, and VGF in rat hippocampus

Faezeh Vahdati Hassani[1], Vahideh Naseri[1], Bibi Marjan Razavi[2], Soghra Mehri[3], Khalil Abnous[4] and Hossein Hosseinzadeh[3*]

Abstract

Background: Antidepressants have been shown to affect levels of brain-derived neurotrophic factor (BDNF) and VGF (non-acronymic) whose transcriptions are dependent on cAMP response element binding protein (CREB) in long term treatment. The aim of this study was to verify the subacute antidepressant effects of crocin, an active constituent of saffron (*Crocus sativus* L.), and its effects on CREB, BDNF, and VGF proteins, transcript levels and amount of active, phosphorylated CREB (P-CREB) protein in rat hippocampus.

Methods: Crocin (12.5, 25, and 50 mg/kg), imipramine (10 mg/kg; positive control) and saline (1 mL/kg; neutral control) were administered intraperitoneally (IP) to male Wistar rats for 21 days. The antidepressant effects were studied using the forced swimming test (FST) on day 21 after injection. Protein expression and transcript levels of genes in the rat hippocampus were evaluated using western blot and quantitative reverse transcription-polymerase chain reaction (qRT-PCR), respectively.

Results: Crocin significantly reduced the immobility time in the FST. Western blot analysis showed that 25 and 50 mg/kg of crocin increased the levels of CREB and BDNF significantly and dose dependently. All doses of crocin increased the VGF levels in a dose-dependent manner. Levels of p-CREB increased significantly by 50 mg/kg dose of crocin. Only 12.5 mg/kg crocin could significantly increase the transcript levels of BDNF. No changes in CREB and VGF transcript levels were observed in all groups.

Conclusions: These results suggest that crocin has antidepressant-like action by increasing CREB, BDNF and VGF levels in hippocampus.

Keywords: Crocin, Antidepressant, Forced swimming test, qRT-PCR, Western blot

Background

Depression, a serious and prevalent mental disorder, has been predicted to be one of 10 leading causes of disabilities that affects up to 21% of world population by 2020 [1]. Due to side effects including inability to drive a car, dry mouth, constipation, and sexual dysfunction, the majority of patients have low compliance and refuse to take synthetic antidepressants in appropriate doses [2,3]. Thus, there is a need for more tolerable and less toxic

agents such as natural plant products which are important sources of new antidepressant drugs [4,5]. Contrary to what is expected, existing antidepressant drug treatments which based on the monoamine hypothesis are just effective in almost one-third of depressed patients. Moreover, clinical manifestations take 3–4 weeks to start; although changes in synaptic monoamine levels occur within hours. This delay in clinical efficacy may be due to neurobiological adaptive mechanisms in hippocampus including alterations in synaptic plasticity and neurogenesis which require synthesis of new proteins [6-10]. CREB (cAMP response element binding protein) is a transcription factor upregulated and phosphorylated by chronic antidepressant treatment. Phosphorylation

* Correspondence: Hosseinzadehh@mums.ac.ir
[3]Pharmaceutical Research Center, Department of Pharmacodynamics and Toxicology, School of Pharmacy, Mashhad University of Medical Sciences, Mashhad, Iran
Full list of author information is available at the end of the article

promotes the association of CREB with CREB-binding protein, a co-activator protein that plays role in assembly of an active transcription complex, enabling target gene expression [11]. VGF (non-acronymic) and BDNF (brain-derived neurotrophic factor) whose transcriptions are dependent on CREB, involved in depressive disorders. VGF is a neuropeptide which enhances hippocampal synaptic plasticity and has roles in energy balance and regulation of homeostasis. It also acts as antidepressant-like agent in the forced swimming test (FST) behavioral model of depression [7]. BDNF, widely expressed in mammalian brain, has been implicated in survival of neurons during hippocampal development, neural regeneration, synaptic transmission, synaptic plasticity, and neurogenesis [12].

Crocus sativus L. (Iridaceae) stigma commonly known as saffron is widely cultivated in Iran and is used in modern and traditional medicines. In addition, results of different studies on pharmacological properties of saffron and its constituents, crocetin, crocin and safranal, are similar to findings as described by Avicenna. Crocin (crocetin digentiobiose ester), a unique water-soluble carotenoid, is one of the pharmacological active constituent of saffron [13,14]. Extensive studies has evaluated saffron extracts and crocin for their pharmacological benefits such as anti-tumor and cytotoxic [15-19], antioxidant [20], antinociceptive and anti-inflammatory [21,22], aphrodisiac [23], antitussive [24], cardioprotective and hypotensive [25-27] activities. Their various effects on central nervous system including improvement of spatial cognitive abilities [28,29], anti-anxiety action [30], reducing morphine withdrawal, morphine-induced conditioned place preference, and dependence [31,32], and anticonvulsant activities [33] were also investigated. The antidepressant effects of different extracts of stigmas, petals, and corms of *C. sativus* L. and their active constituents were evaluated in acute preclinical studies and shown to be significantly more beneficial than placebo [34-37]. In the present study, we first investigated the antidepressant effects of crocin in rats using the FST; then, the protein and transcript levels of CREB, BDNF, and VGF in rat hippocampus were measured in order to understand the underlying molecular mechanism of antidepressant effects of crocin.

Methods

Animals

Adult male Wistar Albino rats, weighing 250–300 g, were provided by Animal House, School of Pharmacy, Mashhad University of Medical Sciences, Iran. Four rats were housed in standard plastic cages in the colony room under 12-h light/dark cycle, $22 \pm 2°C$ and 40-50% humidity conditions. Animals had free access to food and water before and during the study. This study was approved by the ethical committee (No:88587) of Mashhad University of Medical Sciences.

Chemicals

High Pure RNA Tissue Kit (#12033674001, Roche, Germany) was used for RNA extraction and EXPRESS One-Step SYBR® GreenER™ SuperMix Kit (#11780-200, Invitrogen, USA) for qRT-PCR. Bio-Rad Protein Assay Kit (#500-0002, Bio-Rad, USA) to determine protein contents. Imipramine hydrochloride obtained from Marham Daru, Iran. Tris–HCl, (ethylenediaminetetraacetic acid) EDTA, Sodium fluoride (NaF), sodium orthovanadate (Na_3VO_4), β-glycerol phosphate, sodium deoxycholate (NaDC), complete protease inhibitor cocktail (P8340), phenylmethylsulfonyl fluoride (PMSF), Sodium dodecyl sulfate (SDS), 2-mercaptoethanol (2-ME), Bromophenol blue (BPB), glycerol, and Tris Buffered Saline with Tween® 20 (TBST), and Tween® 20 purchased from Sigma-Aldrich, Germany.

Crocin extraction

Crocin was extracted and purified as previously described by Hadizadeh and colleagues [38]. Ten g saffron stigmas powders were suspended in 25 mL ethanol 80% (0°C) and vortexed for 2 min. After that, the suspension was centrifuged at 4000 rpm for 10 min and the supernatant was separated. This step was repeated 6 times by addition of 25 mL ethanol 80%. The resulting extract was kept in a sealed thick walled glass container at –5°C for 24 days in darkness. The formed crystals were separated from the solution and washed with acetone to remove remaining water. The obtained crystals were then dissolved in 120 mL ethanol 80% and kept at –5°C for 20 extra days. The purity of total crocin was more than 97% and the amount of obtained crocin from the initial stigmas powder was 10%. The purity of crocin crystals was determined using UV-visible spectrophotometery and HPLC [38].

Treatments

Thirty rats were randomly divided into 5 different treatment groups (n = 6). Different doses of crocin (12.5, 25, and 50 mg/kg) [28,39] were administered intraperitoneally (IP) for 21 days. Neutral and positive control groups received (IP) 1 mL/kg saline and 10 mg/kg imipramine, respectively [40,41]. Crocin and imipramine were dissolved in saline right before injections. All treatments were injected in a volume of 1 mL/kg. After 21 days of treatment, rats were examined in the FST one hour after the final injections. Then, all treated rats were killed by decapitation. Hippocampi were separated immediately and frozen in liquid nitrogen and stored at –80°C until use.

Forced swimming test (FST)

The FST was conducted between 10:00 and 14:00 hours. The test involved two individual sections (2 days) using a cylindrical tank made of glass, 80 cm tall, 30 cm in diameter, and filled with water (23-25°C) to a depth of 40 cm in which rats could not touch the bottom of the tank. On the 1st day (pretest), rats placed individually in the tank for 15 min and then they were removed from the water and placed in cages equipped with warmers. Tanks were cleaned and filled with fresh water between experiments. Twenty four hours after the pretest, rats were retested for 6 min under the same condition. The retest observations were recorded using a Panasonic digital camcorder (Model NO. NV-DS65EN). During the last 4 min of the retest, immobility (no additional activity other than those movements necessary to keep the rat head off the water) times were scored by an observer unaware of the treatment groups [42,43].

Tissue collection

Rats (n = 6) immediately were sacrificed by decapitation after the FST under stress free conditions. Each decapitation performed in a room isolated from other rodents. The animal head was positioned completely in the opening of the guillotine and guillotine lever was quickly depressed. After that, Brain was removed, dissected on ice in 3–4 min following decapitation. The brain was cut in half using a midline incision and the midbrain was gently removed. The hippocampus is delineated by a large vessel running along its length. Hippocampi were isolated; tissue at each end of them was cut, washed by saline, rapidly frozen in liquid nitrogen and stored at −80°C for subsequent processing.

Protein extraction

To prepare samples for western blotting, tissues were homogenized in the homogenization buffer containing Tris–HCl 50 mM (pH: 7.4), 2 mM EDTA, 10 mM NaF, 1 mM Na_3VO_4, 10 mM β-glycerol phosphate, 0.2% w/v NaDC, 1 mM PMSF, and complete protease inhibitor cocktail using polytron homogenizer (POLYTRON® PT 10–35, Kinematica, Switzerland) in ice. After centrifugation at $10000 \times g$ for 15 min at 4°C, Supernatants were collected on ice and protein contents were determined using Bio-Rad Protein Assay Kit and all concentrations were adjusted to 10 mg/mL. Equal volumes of SDS sample buffer containing 4% w/v SDS, 10% v/v 2-ME, 100 mM Tris-base, 0.2% w/v BPB, and 20% v/v glycerol were added to the samples and incubated in boiling water for 5 min. Blue homogenates were stored at −80°C until use.

Western blot

Immuno blotting analysis performed on the prepared samples to assess the levels of CREB, p-CREB, BDNF, and VGF. Briefly, samples containing equivalent amounts of 50 µg of total protein were loaded to SDS-PAGE gel and then transferred to PVDF membrane by electrophoresis. Blots were blocked with 5% non-fat dry milk in TBST for 3 h at room temperature. After blocking, blots were probed with specific primary antibodies: rabbit monoclonal anti-serum against CREB (#9197, Cell Signaling, USA), mouse monoclonal anti-serum against p-CREB (Ser133) (#9196, Cell Signaling, USA), rabbit polyclonal anti-serum against BDNF (#ab46176, Abcam, USA) and VGF (#ab74140, Abcam, USA), and mouse and rabbit monoclonal anti-serums against β-actin (# 3700 and # 4970, Cell Signaling, USA) at 1:1000 dilutions for 2 h at room temperature. Membranes were washed 3 times with 0.1% Tween® 20 and TBST. Then, blots were incubated with antimouse and rabbit horse radish peroxidase labeled IgG (#7076 and #7074, Cell Signaling, USA) as secondary antibodies at 1:3000 dilutions for 1 h at room temperature. Finally, protein bands were visualized using an enhanced chemiluminescence reagent (Pierce ECL western blotting substrate) and Alliance Gel-doc (Alliance 4.7 Gel doc, UVtec UK). UV Tec software (UK) was used to semi quantify protein bands intensities. All blots were normalized against intensities of corresponding β-actin protein bands.

RNA extraction

Total RNAs were extracted from rat hippocampi using High Pure RNA Tissue Kit according to the manufacturer's instructions. The quantity and quality of the isolated RNAs were assessed using NanoDrop 2000 UV–vis spectrophotometer (Thermo Scientific, USA).

Quantitative RT-PCR

QRT-PCR was performed to analyze transcript levels of CREB, BDNF, and VGF using EXPRESS One-Step SYBR® GreenER™ SuperMix Kit for one-step qRT-PCR according to the manufacturer's instructions and a StepOne™ Real-Time PCR System (ABI, USA). Data were analyzed using the $\Delta\Delta Ct$ method [44].

The following real-time PCR protocol was used for all genes: activation of reverse transcriptase and cDNA synthesis (5 min @ 50°C), PCR activation (2 min @ 95°C), 40 cycles of denaturation (15 s @ 95°C) and annealing/extension (1 min @ 60°C). At the end of the PCR, a melting curve analysis was performed by gradually increasing the temperature from 60 to 95°C with a heating rate of 0.3°C/s.

Primers for the selected genes were designed using Beacon designer 7.8 (Biosoft, USA) and their specificity was confirmed by BLAST (http://www.ncbi.nlm.nih.gov/tools/primer-blast/). β-actin was used as endogenous control gene. Primers were purchased from Metabion international AG, Germany (Table 1).

Table 1 Primers used for qRT-PCR

Gene			Amplicon length (bp)
VGF	Forward	5'-GATGACGACGACGAAGAC-3'	100
	Reverse	5'-CGATGATGCTGACCACAT-3'	
β-actin	Forward	5'GGGAAATCGTGCGTGACATT-3'	76
	Reverse	5'- GCGGCAGTGGCCATCTC-3'	
CREB	Forward	5'-CCAAACTAGCAGTGGGCAGT-3'	140
	Reverse	5'- GAATGGTAGTACCCGGCTGA-3'	
BDNF	Forward	5'-TCTACGAGACCAAGTGTAATCC-3'	152
	Reverse	5'- TATGAACCGCCAGCCAAT-3'	

Statistical analysis

Data were analyzed using GraphPad InStat version 3.00 (GraphPad Software, San Diego, California, USA) with One-way Analysis of Variance (ANOVA) followed by Tukey post-hoc test and plotted in GraphPad Prism version 3.00 (GraphPad Software, San Diego California USA). All data presented as mean ± Standard error of the mean (S.E.M). P values less than 0.05 were considered to be statistically significant.

Results

Forced swimming test

As shown in Figure 1, subacute administration of crocin (12.5 and 50 mg/kg: $**p < 0.01$; 25 mg/kg: $*p < 0.05$) and imipramine (10 mg/kg, $**p < 0.01$) significantly reduced the immobility time as compared with neutral control group that received saline. All doses of crocin could reduce the immobility time, but not in a dose dependent manner.

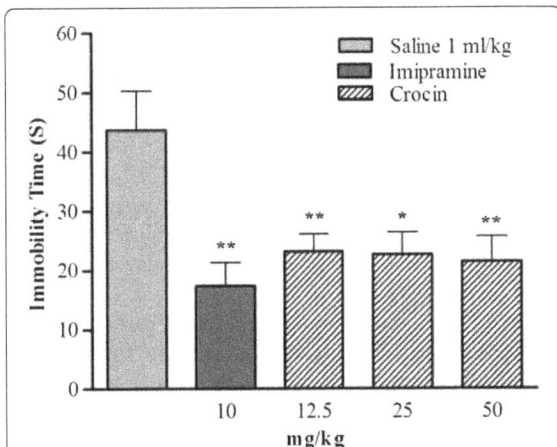

Figure 1 Effects of the subacute administration of crocin and imipramine on immobility time of rats subjected to the forced swimming test. The data are expressed as mean ± S.E.M; n = 6. All groups were compared to neutral control group (saline) according to ANOVA followed by Tukey post-hoc test: $*p < 0.05$, $**p < 0.01$.

Western blot assay

Effects of the subacute treatment with crocin (12.5, 25, and 50 mg/kg, IP) on the CREB, p-CREB, BDNF, and VGF protein expression in the hippocampus are shown in Figure 2. Statistical analysis indicated a significant and dose-dependent effect of treatment with crocin on the CREB expression as compared with control: 25 mg/kg (37.80%, $*p < 0.05$) and 50 mg/kg (55.6%, $***p < 0.001$). Effect of imipramine on the CREB level was higher than that of in crocin treated groups (Figure 2A). Crocin at a dose of 12.5 mg/kg showed no appreciable effect on the CREB expression as compared with saline group. Treatment with high dose of crocin (50 mg/kg) significantly increased the expression of p-CREB (43.52%, $**p < 0.01$) as shown in Figure 2B. As shown in Figure 2C, there were 41.63% ($**p < 0.01$) and 67.79% ($***p < 0.001$) increase in the levels of BDNF after treatment with 25 and 50 mg/kg crocin as compared with control, respectively. Treatment with 12.5 mg/kg crocin could not significantly change the BDNF protein level. The effect of 50 mg/kg crocin on the level of BDNF was similar to 10 mg/kg imipramine ($***p < 0.001$ vs. saline). Crocin at all doses, compared to saline, could significantly and dose dependently increase the VGF levels in a dose-dependent manner: 12.5 mg/kg (32.95%, $p < 0.05$), 25 mg/kg (54.35%, $p < 0.001$), and 50 mg/kg (80.54%, $p < 0.001$). Crocin at doses of 25 and 50 mg/kg could increase the VGF levels similar to that of imipramine ($***p < 0.001$ vs. saline, Figure 2D).

Quantitative RT-PCR

Figure 3 illustrates the effects of the subacute treatment with crocin (12.5, 25, and 50 mg/kg, IP) and imipramine (10 mg/kg, IP) on the CREB, BDNF and VGF transcript levels in rat hippocampi. The lowest dose of crocin (12.5 mg/kg) could significantly increase the BDNF transcript levels in the hippocampus ($*p < 0.05$) as compared with saline group. No significant changes were observed in the transcript levels of CREB and VGF in different experimental groups.

Discussion

In the present study we demonstrated that subacute administration of crocin in all doses (12.5, 25, and 50 mg/kg) decreased the immobility time of rats in the forced swimming test (FST), however this effect was not in a dose-dependent manner. Subacute treatment with 10 mg/kg imipramine as positive control also decreased the immobility time. In order to understand the molecular mechanism of crocin-induced subacute antidepressant effects in the hippocampus, the protein and transcript levels of anti-depressant related genes were studied. Our data showed that crocin increased the protein levels of CREB, p-CREB, BDNF, and VGF in the

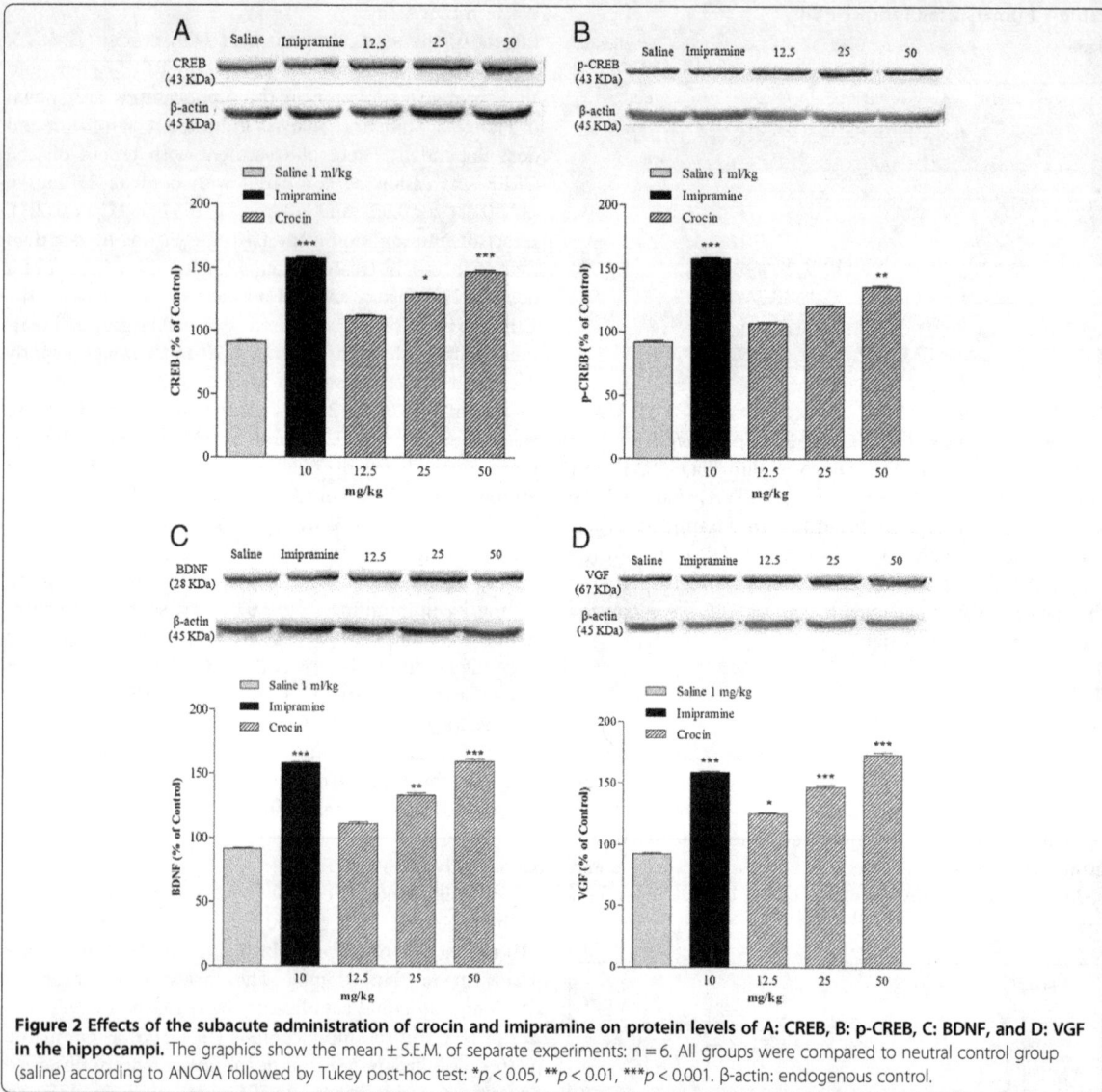

Figure 2 **Effects of the subacute administration of crocin and imipramine on protein levels of A: CREB, B: p-CREB, C: BDNF, and D: VGF in the hippocampi.** The graphics show the mean ± S.E.M. of separate experiments: n = 6. All groups were compared to neutral control group (saline) according to ANOVA followed by Tukey post-hoc test: $*p < 0.05$, $**p < 0.01$, $***p < 0.001$. β-actin: endogenous control.

hippocampus. Treatment with 12.5 mg/kg crocin significantly increased in BDNF transcript level.

In late 1970s, FST was accepted as a beneficial model to predict the antidepressant effects of drugs on animal [42]. The antidepressant effects of different saffron extracts and crocin in acute administration in mice and rats have already been reported in previous studies using the FST. Furthermore, in the open field activity test, crocin did not show a significant effect on total locomotion [34-37]. The studies have been reported that acute and chronic administration of imipramine (10 mg/kg) significantly reduced the immobility time and confirmed its antidepressant effects [40,41]. In our study, imipramine (10 mg/kg) like previous reports decreased the

immobility time as compared with neutral control group. The administration of crocin in different doses also reduced the immobility time, similar to that of imipramine. Therefore, our results suggest that crocin has antidepressant effects in subacute treatment.

Hippocampus is a region in the brain that plays a central role in processing of emotions and controlling of behavior in response to fear and anxiety [45]. Preclinical and Clinical studies have shown that the hippocampus is affected by stress. Death and atrophy of hippocampal neurons have been reported in rats exposed to stress and high levels of glucocorticoids [46]. The reduction of hippocampus size in patients with recurrent depression and posttraumatic stress disorder has been observed

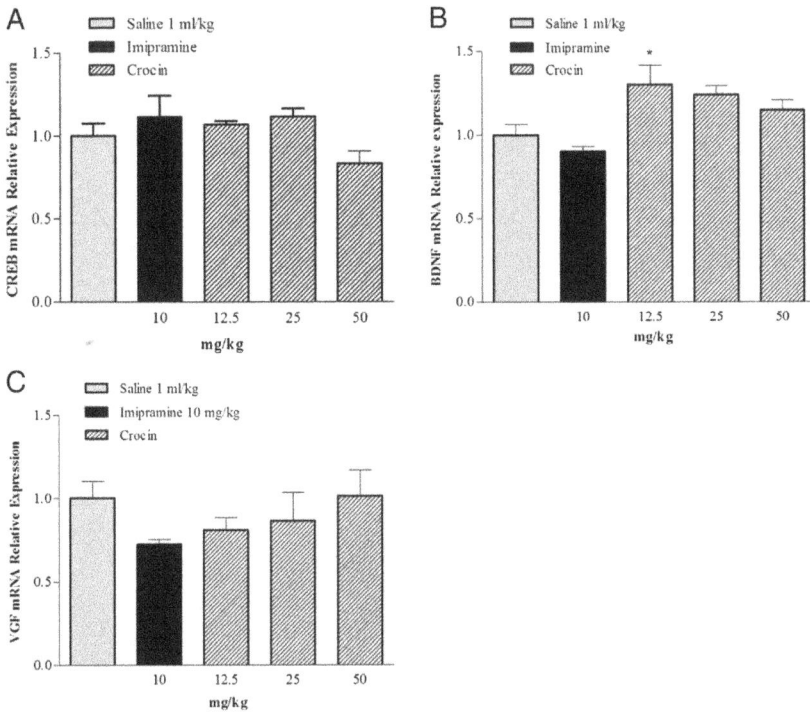

Figure 3 Effects of the subacute administration of crocin and imipramine on transcript levels of A: CREB, B: BDNF, and C: VGF. Data are expressed as mean ± S.E.M; n = 4. All groups were compared to neutral control group (saline) according to ANOVA followed by Tukey post-hoc test: *$p < 0.05$.

[47-49]. It is well established that structural and functional modifications of hippocampus are associated with antidepressant treatments. These changes include alterations in synaptic plasticity, neurogenesis, and synaptogenesis and most likely require the transcription and protein expression of new molecules such as CREB, BDNF and VGF [7].

Chronic treatment with antidepressants enhances, activates and induces the phosphorylation of CREB that produces antidepressant behavioral response in rodents and human [7,11,50,51]. Various antidepressants have shown different effects on CREB protein and mRNA levels. For example, 21 days administration of several different types of antidepressant drugs including fluoxetine (a serotonin (5-HT) selective reuptake inhibitor), desipramine (a selective norepinephrine (NE) reuptake inhibitor), imipramine (a nonselective 5-HT and NE reuptake inhibitor, 15 mg/kg), and tranylcypromine (a monoamine oxidase inhibitor) significantly increased levels of CREB mRNA in rat hippocampus and only fluoxetine significantly increased CREB protein levels [11,51]. Conversely, similar doses and time course of administration showed that neither desmethylimipramine nor fluoxetine could increase CREB protein levels;

however, both could increase CREB phosphorylation, but only in the frontal cortex and not in the hippocampus [11]. In addition, it was shown that imipramine at dose of 20 mg/kg could only increase CREB protein levels in prefrontal cortex but not in hippocampus [52]. The administration of fluoxetine and reboxetine (a NE reuptake inhibitor) for 14 days at a dose of 10 mg/kg resulted in increased levels of CREB mRNA in the hippocampus, but desipramine at the same dose did not have significant effect on CREB mRNA level [50]. In transgenic mice model of depression imipramine (10 mg/kg) increased CREB mRNA levels only in the cortex, whereas fluoxetine (10 mg/kg) could increase the levels of CREB mRNA in the cortex and the hippocampus [53]. The results of the present study showed that crocin administration could increase the CREB protein levels in the hippocampus dose dependently. P-CREB significantly increased only with 50 mg/kg of crocin. Desmethylimipramine and fluoxetine has been reported to increase CREB phosphorylation in other region of the brains like cortex [11]. In our study, no significant changes in CREB mRNA levels were observed in hippocampus. Therefore, crocin-induced changes in CREB and p-CREB protein and CREB mRNA levels may be involved in other brain regions such as cortex similar to previous reports [11,53]. However more supportive data are necessary to confirm this hypothesis.

BDNF structurally belongs to the neurotrophin family that plays an important role in regulation of neuronal differentiation including neurotransmitter content and neuronal survival [54]. Recent studies have shown that after treatment with antidepressants, levels of BDNF significantly increased in plasma [55,56]. It was evidenced that use of imipramine as a nonselective 5-HT and NE reuptake inhibitor at doses of 10 and 20 mg/kg was effective to increase BDNF protein levels in both prefrontal cortex and hippocampus [52]. It has been shown that longer treatment with citalopram (a serotonergic agent) could significantly increase the level of BDNF transcript [57]. In addition, both acute and chronic use of norepinephrine re-uptake inhibitors (desipramine and maprotiline) had no effect on BDNF mRNA levels, while serotonergic antidepressants (fluoxetine and paroxetine) altered BDNF gene expression, but not in acute administration [58]. In the current study, subacute treatment with crocin in a dose-dependent manner increased the BDNF protein levels compared to the neutral control treatment group. Crocin could significantly increase the BDNF transcript level as compared to saline group. Due to the result of present and past studies, the effect of crocin on BDNF expression levels is similar to serotonergic drugs.

VGF is a neuropeptide that has been shown to be involved in maintaining energy balance, mediating hippocampal synaptic plasticity, and antidepressant responses [7,59]. In several animal models of depression local application of VGF into the midbrain or hippocampus produced antidepressant responses [60]. Due to the different studies, VGF gene is an important target for BDNF and serotonin. This agent besides exercise may activate intracellular pathways that may lead to the VGF expression [59]. Antidepressants do not show the same effects on VGF gene expression. Although Hunsberger and colleagues reported that VGF expression was not affected by different classes of antidepressants [61], there are some reports that show fluoxetine and paroxetine, but not imipramine and desipramine could increase the VGF expression [60]. Our results showed that transcript levels of VGF were not increased following administration of different doses of crocin, however, VGF protein expression significantly and dose-dependently elevated after treatment with crocin.

Conclusions

In conclusion, our study showed that subacute administration of crocin has antidepressant effects in rats. Crocin administration significantly increased the CREB, p-CREB, BDNF, and VGF protein expressions in rat hippocampus.

Competing interests
The authors declare that they have no competing interests.

Authors' contributions
HH and KA designed the study. SM and BMR were the supervisors. FVH and VN participated in doing the experiments. FVH draft the manuscript. All authors read and approved the final manuscript.

Acknowledgments
This research was supported by Vice Chancellor of Research, Mashhad University of Medical Sciences. The results described in this paper are part of a Pharm. D. thesis.

Author details
[1]School of Pharmacy, Mashhad University of Medical Sciences, Mashhad, Iran. [2]Targeted Drug Delivery Research Centre, Department of Pharmacodynamics and Toxicology, School of Pharmacy, Mashhad University of Medical Sciences, Mashhad, Iran. [3]Pharmaceutical Research Center, Department of Pharmacodynamics and Toxicology, School of Pharmacy, Mashhad University of Medical Sciences, Mashhad, Iran. [4]Pharmaceutical Research Center, Department of Medicinal Chemistry and Department of Biotechnology, Mashhad University of Medical Sciences, Mashhad, Iran.

References
1. Murray CJ, Lopez AD: Alternative projections of mortality and disability by cause 1990–2020: global burden of disease study. *Lancet* 1997, 349:1498–1504.
2. Demyttenaere K: Compliance during treatment with antidepressants. *J Affect Disord* 1997, 43:27–39.
3. Blackwell B: Antidepressant drugs: side effects and compliance. *J Clin Psychiatry* 1982, 43:14–21.
4. Schulz V: Safety of St John's Wort extract compared to synthetic antidepressants. *Phytomedicine* 2006, 13:199–204.
5. Modaghegh MH, Shahabian M, Esmaeili HA, Rajbai O, Hosseinzadeh H: Safety evaluation of saffron (Crocus sativus) tablets in healthy volunteers. *Phytomedicine* 2008, 15:1032–1037.
6. Schechter LE, Ring RH, Beyer CE, Hughes ZA, Khawaja X, Malberg JE, Rosenzweig-Lipson S: Innovative approaches for the development of antidepressant drugs: current and future strategies. *NeuroRx* 2005, 2:590–611.
7. Thakker-Varia S, Alder J: Neuropeptides in depression: role of VGF. *Behav Brain Res* 2009, 197:262–278.
8. Dranovsky A, Hen R: Hippocampal neurogenesis: regulation by stress and antidepressants. *Biol Psychiatry* 2006, 59:1136–1143.
9. Castren E: Is mood chemistry? *Nat Rev Neurosci* 2005, 6:241–246.
10. Adell A, Castro E, Celada P, Bortolozzi A, Pazos A, Artigas F: Strategies for producing faster acting antidepressants. *Drug Discov Today* 2005, 10:578–585.
11. Blendy JA: The role of CREB in depression and antidepressant treatment. *Biol Psychiatry* 2006, 59:1144–1150.
12. Yu H, Chen ZY: The role of BDNF in depression on the basis of its location in the neural circuitry. *Acta Pharmacol Sin* 2011, 32:3–11.
13. Hosseinzadeh H, Nassiri-Asl M: Avicenna's (Ibn Sina) the Canon of Medicine and Saffron (Crocus sativus): a review. *Phytother Res* 2013, 27:475–483.
14. Rezaee R, Hosseinzadeh H: Safranal: from an aromatic natural product to a rewarding pharmacological agent. *Iran J Basic Med Sci* 2013, 16:12–26.
15. Behravan J, Hosseinzadeh H, Rastgoo A, Hessani M: Evaluation of the cytotoxic activity of crocin and safranal using potato disc and brine shrimp assays. *Physiol Pharmacol* 2010, 13:397–403.
16. Garcia-Olmo DC, Riese HH, Escribano J, Ontanon J, Fernandez JA, Atienzar M, Garcia-Olmo D: Effects of long-term treatment of colon adenocarcinoma with crocin, a carotenoid from saffron (Crocus sativus L.): an experimental study in the rat. *Nutr Cancer* 1999, 35:120–126.
17. Hosseinzadeh H, Behravan J, Ramezani M, Ajgan K: Anti-tumor and cytotoxic evaluation of Crocus sativus L. stigma and petal extracts

using brine shrimp and potato disc assays. *J Med Plants* 2005, **4**:59–65.

18. Rastgoo M, Hosseinzadeh H, Alavizadeh H, Abbasi A, Ayati Z, Jaafari MR: Antitumor Activity of PEGylated Nanoliposomes Containing Crocin in Mice Bearing C26 Colon Carcinoma. *Planta medica* 2013, **79**:447–451.

19. Salomi MJ, Nair SC, Panikkar KR: Inhibitory effects of Nigella sativa and saffron (Crocus sativus) on chemical carcinogenesis in mice. *Nutr Cancer* 1991, **16**:67–72.

20. Hosseinzadeh H, Shamsaie F, Mehri S: Antioxidant activity of aqueous and ethanolic extracts of Crocus sativus L. stigma and its bioactive constituents, crocin and safranal. *Pharmacogn Mag* 2009, **5**:419–424.

21. Amin B, Hosseinzadeh H: Evaluation of aqueous and ethanolic extracts of saffron, *Crocus sativus* L., and its constituents, safranal and crocin in allodynia and hyperalgesia induced by chronic constriction injury model of neuropathic pain in rats. *Fitoterapia* 2012, **83**:888–895.

22. Hosseinzadeh H, Younesi HM: Antinociceptive and anti-inflammatory effects of Crocus sativus L. stigma and petal extracts in mice. *BMC Pharmacol* 2002, **2**:7.

23. Hosseinzadeh H, Ziaee T, Sadeghi A: The effect of saffron, Crocus sativus stigma, extract and its constituents, safranal and crocin on sexual behaviors in normal male rats. *Phytomedicine* 2008, **15**:491–495.

24. Hosseinzadeh H, Ghenaati J: Evaluation of the antitussive effect of stigma and petals of saffron (Crocus sativus) and its components, safranal and crocin in guinea pigs. *Fitoterapia* 2006, **77**:446–448.

25. Imenshahidi M, Hosseinzadeh H, Javadpour Y: Hypotensive effect of aqueous saffron extract (Crocus sativus L.) and its constituents, safranal and crocin, in normotensive and hypertensive rats. *Phytother Res* 2010, **24**:990–994.

26. Mehdizadeh R, Parizadeh MR, Khooei A-R, Mehri S, Hosseinzadeh H: Cardioprotective Effect of Saffron Extract and Safranal in Isoproterenol-Induced Myocardial Infarction in Wistar Rats. *Iran J Basic Med Sci* 2013, **16**:56–63.

27. Razavi M, Hosseinzadeh H, Abnous K: Sadat Motamedahariaty V, Imenshahidi M: Crocin Restores Hypotensive Effect of Subchronic Administration of Diazinon in Rats. *Iran J Basic Med Sci* 2012, **16**:64–72.

28. Hosseinzadeh H, Sadeghnia HR, Ghaeni FA, Motamedshariaty VS, Mohajeri SA: Effects of saffron (Crocus sativus L.) and its active constituent, crocin, on recognition and spatial memory after chronic cerebral hypoperfusion in rats. *Phytother Res* 2012, **26**:381–386.

29. Hosseinzadeh H, Ziaei T: Effects of Crocus sativus stigma extract and its constituents, crocin and safranal, on intact memory and scopolamine-induced learning deficits in rats performing the Morris water maze task. *J Med Plants* 2006, **5**:40–50.

30. Hosseinzadeh H, Noraei NB: Anxiolytic and hypnotic effect of Crocus sativus aqueous extract and its constituents, crocin and safranal, in mice. *Phytother Res* 2009, **23**:768–774.

31. Hosseinzadeh H, Jahanian Z: Effect of Crocus sativus L. (saffron) stigma and its constituents, crocin and safranal, on morphine withdrawal syndrome in mice. *Phytother Res* 2010, **24**:726–730.

32. Imenshahidi M, Zafari H, Hosseinzadeh H: Effects of crocin on the acquisition and reinstatement of morphine-induced conditioned place preference in mice. *Pharmacologyonline* 2011, **1**:1007–1013.

33. Hosseinzadeh H, Talebzadeh F: Anticonvulsant evaluation of safranal and crocin from Crocus sativus in mice. *Fitoterapia* 2005, **76**:722–724.

34. Hosseinzadeh H, Karimi G, Niapoor M: Antidepressant effects of Crocus sativus stigma extracts and its constituents, crocin and safranal, in mice. *J Med Plants* 2004, **3**:48–58.

35. Hosseinzadeh H, Motamedshariaty V, Hadizadeh F: Antidepressant effect of kaempferol, a constituent of saffron (Crocus sativus) petal, in mice and rats. *Pharmacologyonline* 2007, **2**:367–370.

36. Karimi GR, Hosseinzadeh H, Khaleghpanah P: Study of antidepressant effect of aqueous and ethanolic extract of Crocus sativus in mice. *Iran J Basic Med Sci* 2001, **4**:11–15.

37. Wang Y, Han T, Zhu Y, Zheng CJ, Ming QL, Rahman K, Qin LP: Antidepressant properties of bioactive fractions from the extract of Crocus sativus L. *J Nat Med* 2010, **64**:24–30.

38. Hadizadeh F, Mohajeri SA, Seifi M: Extraction and purification of crocin from saffron stigmas employing a simple and efficient crystallization method. *Pak J Biol Sci* 2010, **13**:691–698.

39. Pitsikas N, Sakellaridis N: Crocus sativus L. extracts antagonize memory impairments in different behavioural tasks in the rat. *Behav Brain Res* 2006, **173**:112–115.

40. Fortunato JJ, Reus GZ, Kirsch TR, Stringari RB, Fries GR, Kapczinski F, Hallak JE, Zuardi AW, Crippa JA, Quevedo J: Chronic administration of harmine elicits antidepressant-like effects and increases BDNF levels in rat hippocampus. *J Neural Transm* 2010, **117**:1131–1137.

41. Nakamura K, Tanaka Y: Antidepressant-like effects of aniracetam in aged rats and its mode of action. *Psychopharmacology (Berl)* 2001, **158**:205–212.

42. Porsolt RD, Le Pichon M, Jalfre M: Depression: a new animal model sensitive to antidepressant treatments. *Nature* 1977, **266**:730–732.

43. Detke MJ: Rickels M, Lucki I: Active behaviors in the rat forced swimming test differentially produced by serotonergic and noradrenergic antidepressants. *Psychopharmacology (Berl)* 1995, **121**:66–72.

44. Livak KJ, Schmittgen TD: Analysis of relative gene expression data using real-time quantitative PCR and the 2(−Delta Delta C(T)) Method. *Methods* 2001, **25**:402–408.

45. Yee BK, Zhu SW, Mohammed AH, Feldon J: Levels of neurotrophic factors in the hippocampus and amygdala correlate with anxiety- and fear-related behaviour in C57BL6 mice. *J Neural Transm* 2007, **114**:431–444.

46. Smith MA, Makino S, Kvetnansky R, Post RM: Stress and glucocorticoids affect the expression of brain-derived neurotrophic factor and neurotrophin-3 mRNAs in the hippocampus. *J Neurosci* 1995, **15**:1768–1777.

47. Videbech P, Ravnkilde B: Hippocampal volume and depression: a meta-analysis of MRI studies. *Am J Psychiatry* 2004, **161**:1957–1966.

48. Sheline YI, Wang PW, Gado MH, Csernansky JG, Vannier MW: Hippocampal atrophy in recurrent major depression. *Proc Natl Acad Sci U S A* 1996, **93**:3908–3913.

49. Bremner JD, Narayan M, Anderson ER, Staib LH, Miller HL, Charney DS: Hippocampal volume reduction in major depression. *Am J Psychiatry* 2000, **157**:115–118.

50. Tiraboschi E, Tardito D, Kasahara J, Moraschi S, Pruneri P, Gennarelli M, Racagni G, Popoli M: Selective phosphorylation of nuclear CREB by fluoxetine is linked to activation of CaM kinase IV and MAP kinase cascades. *Neuropsychopharmacology* 2004, **29**:1831–1840.

51. Nibuya M, Nestler EJ, Duman RS: Chronic antidepressant administration increases the expression of cAMP response element binding protein (CREB) in rat hippocampus. *J Neurosci* 1996, **16**:2365–2372.

52. Reus GZ, Stringari RB, Ribeiro KF, Ferraro AK, Vitto MF, Cesconetto P, Souza CT, Quevedo J: Ketamine plus imipramine treatment induces antidepressant-like behavior and increases CREB and BDNF protein levels and PKA and PKC phosphorylation in rat brain. *Behav Brain Res* 2011, **221**:166–171.

53. Blom JM, Tascedda F, Carra S, Ferraguti C, Barden N, Brunello N: Altered regulation of CREB by chronic antidepressant administration in the brain of transgenic mice with impaired glucocorticoid receptor function. *Neuropsychopharmacology* 2002, **26**:605–614.

54. Davies AM: The role of neurotrophins in the developing nervous system. *J Neurobiol* 1994, **25**:1334–1348.

55. Aydemir O, Deveci A, Taneli F: The effect of chronic antidepressant treatment on serum brain-derived neurotrophic factor levels in depressed patients: a preliminary study. *Prog Neuropsychopharmacol Biol Psychiatry* 2005, **29**:261–265.

56. Gervasoni N, Aubry JM, Bondolfi G, Osiek C, Schwald M, Bertschy G, Karege F: Partial normalization of serum brain-derived neurotrophic factor in remitted patients after a major depressive episode. *Neuropsychobiology* 2005, **51**:234–238.

57. Russo-Neustadt AA, Alejandre H, Garcia C, Ivy AS, Chen MJ: Hippocampal brain-derived neurotrophic factor expression following treatment with reboxetine, citalopram, and physical exercise. *Neuropsychopharmacology* 2004, **29**:2189–2199.

58. Coppell AL, Pei Q, Zetterstrom TS: Bi-phasic change in BDNF gene expression following antidepressant drug treatment. *Neuropharmacology* 2003, **44**:903–910.

59. Malberg JE, Monteggia LM: VGF, a new player in antidepressant action? *Sci Signal* 2008, **1**:pe19.

60. Allaman I, Fiumelli H, Magistretti PJ, Martin JL: **Fluoxetine regulates the expression of neurotrophic/growth factors and glucose metabolism in astrocytes.** *Psychopharmacology (Berl)* 2011, **216:**75–84.

61. Hunsberger JG, Newton SS, Bennett AH, Duman CH, Russell DS, Salton SR, Duman RS: **Antidepressant actions of the exercise-regulated gene VGF.** *Nat Med* 2007, **13:**1476–1482.

5,6-Dimethoxybenzofuran-3-one derivatives: a novel series of dual Acetylcholinesterase/ Butyrylcholinesterase inhibitors bearing benzyl pyridinium moiety

Hamid Nadri[1], Morteza Pirali-Hamedani[2], Alireza Moradi[1], Amirhossein Sakhteman[1], Alireza Vahidi[3], Vahid Sheibani[4], Ali Asadipour[4], Nouraddin Hosseinzadeh[5], Mohammad Abdollahi[2], Abbas Shafiee[2] and Alireza Foroumadi[4,5*]

Abstract

Background: Several studies have been focused on design and synthesis of multi-target anti Alzheimer compounds. Utilizing of the dual Acetylcholinesterase/Butyrylcholinesterase inhibitors has gained more interest to treat the Alzheimer's disease. As a part of a research program to find a novel drug for treating Alzheimer disease, we have previously reported 6-alkoxybenzofuranone derivatives as potent acetylcholinesterase inhibitors. In continuation of our work, we would like to report the synthesis of 5,6-dimethoxy benzofuranone derivatives bearing a benzyl pyridinium moiety as dual Acetylcholinesterase/Butyrylcholinesterase inhibitors.

Methods: The synthesis of target compounds was carried out using a conventional method. Bayer-Villiger oxidation of 3,4-dimethoxybenzaldehyde furnished 3,4-dimethoxyphenol. The reaction of 3,4-dimethoxyphenol with chloroacetonitrile followed by treatment with HCl solution and then ring closure yielded the 5,6-dimethoxy benzofuranone. Condensation of the later compound with pyridine-4-carboxaldehyde and subsequent reaction with different benzyl halides afforded target compounds. The biological activity was measured using standard Ellman's method. Docking studies were performed to get better insight into interaction of compounds with receptor.

Results: The in vitro anti acetylcholinesterase/butyrylcholinesterase activity of compounds revealed that, all of the target compounds have good inhibitory activity against both Acetylcholinesterase/Butyrylcholinesterase enzymes in which compound 5b (IC50 = 52 ± 6.38nM) was the most active compound against acetylcholinesterase. The same binding mode and interactions were observed for the reference drug donepezil and compound 5b in docking study.

Conclusions: In this study, we presented a new series of benzofuranone-based derivatives having pyridinium moiety as potent dual acting Acetylcholinesterase/Butyrylcholinesterase inhibitors.

* Correspondence: aforoumadi@yahoo.com
[4]Neuroscience Research Center, Kerman University of Medical Sciences, Kerman, Iran
[5]Drug design & Development Research Center, Tehran University of Medical Sciences, Tehran, Iran
Full list of author information is available at the end of the article

Introduction

Alzheimer's disease (AD) is a progressive and age-dependent neurodegenerative brain disorder that leads to dementia, cognitive impairment, and memory loss [1,2]. The main cause of Alzheimer's disease etiology is not completely known however, many diverse factors such as hippocampal acetylcholine (Ach) decrease, β-amyloid (Aβ) aggregation and τ-protein deposits seem to play significant roles in initiation and progression of the disease [3-5]. Based on these findings three hypotheses was established: cholinergic, β-amyloid and tau hypothesis.

Regarding cholinergic hypothesis one of the most useful approaches for improving AD's symptoms is to design new agents that raise the acetylcholine in the cholinergic system [6]. Acetylcholinesterase (AChE) is responsible for hydrolysis of acetylcholine in the synaptic cleft, therefore; employing the AChE inhibitors could be a helpful strategy to increase the level of acetylcholine in the damaged cholinergic neurons [7]. Several compounds have been previously synthesized as AChE inhibitors and successfully used to treat AD, such as Donepezil, Galantamine and Rivastigmine (Figure 1) [8].

Moreover, it has been demonstrated that the inhibition of AChE may lead to an increase in Butyrylcholinesterase (BuChE) activity in the hippocampus that causes hydrolysis of AChE by a new way. Therefore, the maintenance of AChE/BuChE activity ratio in the hippocampus as seen in the healthy brain, could improve the signs and symptoms of AD [9]. As a result, design and synthesis of dual AChE/BuChE inhibitors should be considered to find more potent agents against AD [10].

In an earlier report, we have presented the preparation and evaluation of some new (Z)-1-benzyl-4-((6-alkoxy-3-oxobenzofuran-2(3H)-ylidene) methyl)pyridinium (Figure 2) as AChE inhibitors [11]. Most of these compounds proved to be potent AChE inhibitors in vitro, among which compounds bearing methoxy group on position 6 of benzofuran ring showed the most activity. Furthermore, it was reported that 5,6-dimethoxy benzofuranone structure is important to show more affinity toward the enzyme in some aurone-based AChE inhibitors [12,13]. Following these reasons and in pursuit of our previous study a series of new 5,6-dimethoxy benzofuran derivatives were designed, synthesized and evaluated for AChE/BuChE inhibitory activities. In this study, we decided to investigate the possible increase in the enzyme inhibitory activity by replacing the less hydrophilic 6-alkoxy benzofuranone scaffold with a more polar 5,6-dimethoxy benzofuranone motif. The final compounds have been tested for their ability to inhibit both AChE and BuChE using Ellman's method [14].

Materials and methods

Chemistry

All chemicals were obtained from Merck AG, Aldrich and Acros Chemicals. Thin layer chromatography (TLC) was carried out on Merck pre-coated silica gel F254 plates with various mobile phase systems, to check reaction progress and product mixtures. The Separating column chromatography and flash chromatography were done with silica gel (70-230 mesh). The ^{1}H nuclear magnetic resonance (NMR) spectra were recorded in DMSO-d_6 and/or CDCl$_3$ on a Bruker FT-500 MHz spectrometer with tetramethylsilane (TMS) as the internal standard. Coupling constants were reported in Hertz (Hz) and chemical shifts are given as δ value (ppm) relative to TMS as internal standard. To express spin multiplicities, s (singlet), d (doublet), t (triplet), q (quartet), dd (double doublet) and m (multiplet) were used. Mass spectra were obtained at 70 eV in a Finigan TSQ-70 spectrometer. Infrared (IR) spectra were determined using

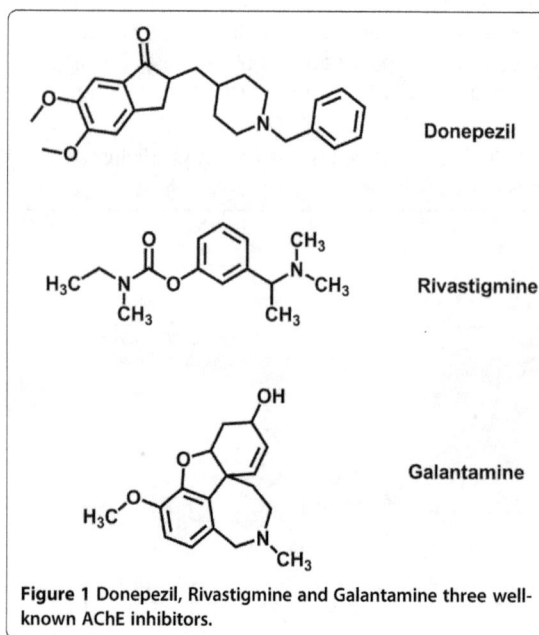

Figure 1 Donepezil, Rivastigmine and Galantamine three well-known AChE inhibitors.

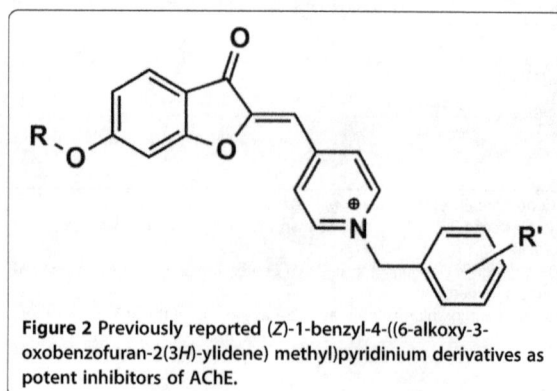

Figure 2 Previously reported (Z)-1-benzyl-4-((6-alkoxy-3-oxobenzofuran-2(3H)-ylidene) methyl)pyridinium derivatives as potent inhibitors of AChE.

a Nicolet FT-IR Magna 550 spectrophotometer. All melting points were determined using Kofler hot stage apparatus and are uncorrected.Elemental microanalyses were done on a Perkin–Elmer 240-C apparatus for C, H, and N. For better understanding of spectral data, the general structure and atom numbering of final compounds are depicted in Figure 3.

Synthesis of 3,4-dimethoxyphenol (1)

A mixture of m-chloro-peroxybenzoic acid (m-CPBA) (7 g, 32.5 mmol) in the dry dichloromethane (DCM) (40 ml) was prepared at 0°C and vigorously stirred. Then a solution of 3,4-dimethoxybenzaldehyde (5 g, 30 mmol) in the dry DCM (10 ml) was added dropwise during 1 hour. The resulting mixture was kept at room temperature and then refluxed for 16 hours. After cooling, the mixture was washed with aqueous solution of saturated sodium hydrogen carbonate (3×20 ml) followed by washing with sodium thiosulfate 10% (25 ml) to neutralize excess amount of m-CPBA. The solvent was then evaporated under reduced pressure and the resulting crude material was dissolved in methanol. The solution was stirred for 4 - hours with excess amount of sodium hydroxide 10% solution at room temperature. The pH of solution was adjusted to 1 using HCl 6 N solution. The solution was then extracted with DCM (3×25 ml) washed with brine and dried using anhydrous Na_2SO_4. The solvent was removed to yield brown syrup, which was purified with column chromatography using petroleum ether and ethyl acetate (1:1) as eluent to give compound 1. White brown solid, m. p. 74–78°C, 84% yield [15].

Synthesis of 2-chloro-1-(2-hydroxy-4,5-dimethoxyphenyl) ethanone (2)

To a mixture of 3,4-dimethoxyphenol (1) (4.93 g, 32 mmol) and chloroacetonitrile (2.4 g, 32 mmol) in dry ether (150 ml) was added anhydrous $ZnCl_2$ (1.44 g, 10.6 mmol). The mixture was cooled to 0°C and HCl gas was bubbled

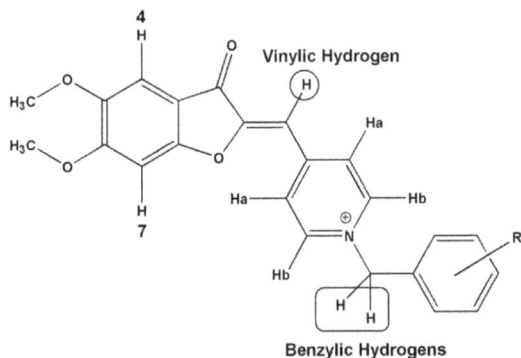

Figure 3 General structure and atom numbering of final compounds.

through the reaction for 2.5 hours. The mixture was left in the room temperature overnight and then cooled to 0°C. The precipitated iminium was filtered off and washed three times with ether. The imine was dissolved in 160 ml of 1 N HCl and refluxed for 90 min. The resulting mixture was extracted with DCM (3×100 ml) and the solvent was removed under reduced pressure to give 2.88 g white brown solid 40% yield (no further purification was needed).

Synthesis of 5,6-dimethoxybenzofuran-3(2H)-one (3)

The crude extract of 2-chloro-1-(2-hydroxy-4,5-dimethoxyphenyl)ethanone (2) (1.15 g, 5 mmol) was dissolved in 10 ml ethanol and then refluxed for 10 min under argon. Sodium acetate trihydrate (700 mg) was added thereto and refluxed for 10 min again. The resulting mixture was cooled immediately and then filtered off. The solvent was evaporated and compound 3 was yielded by re-crystallization from ethanol. White needle crystals, m.p. 163–165, 470 mg, 48%. IR v_{max}/cm^{-1} (KBr) : 1708 (C = O), ^{1}H NMR (CDCl$_3$, 80 MHz), 7.02 (s, 1H, H$_{4\text{-aromatic}}$) 6.59 (s, 1H, H$_{7\text{-aromatic}}$) 4.61 (s, 2H, H$_{2\text{-aliphatic}}$) 3.97 (s, 3H, -OCH$_3$) 3.87 (s, 3H, -OCH$_3$), EI-MS m/z (%) 194 (M$^+$, 100), 165 (45), 135 (88), 34 (57).

Synthesis of (Z)-5,6-dimethoxy-2-(pyridin-4-ylmethylene) benzofuran-3(2H)-one (4)

5,6-dimethoxybenzofuran-3(2H)-one 3 (388 mg, 2 mmol), pyridine-4-carbaldehyde (308 mg, 2.88 mmol) and PTSA (548 mg, 3.18 mmol) were suspended in the dry toluene (25 ml) and refluxed using Dean-Stark apparatus for 2 - hours. After cooling the resulting mixture, the precipitated solid was filtered off. The wet solid was suspended in aqueous 10% NaHCO$_3$ solution (50 ml) and stirred for 60 - minutes at room temperature. The filtered resulting solid was washed with water (50 ml) and then air dried. The crude solid was purified by re-crystallization from acetonitrile to yield compound 4. 400 mg, 70% yield, m.p. 265–268°C, IR v_{max}/cm^{-1} (KBr) : 1705 (C = O), 1635 (C = C alkene), ^{1}H NMR (CDCl$_3$, 80 MHz), 8.69 (dd, 2H, H$_{a\text{-pyridine}}$, $J = 4.5$ Hz, $J = 2$ Hz), 7.70 (dd, 2H, H$_{b\text{-pyridine}}$, $J = 5$ Hz, $J = 1.5$ Hz), 7.17 (s, 1H, H$_4$), 6.83 (s, 1H, H$_7$), 6.69 (s, 1H, H$_{vinylic}$), 4.03 (s, 3H, -OCH$_3$), 3.91 (s, 3H, -OCH$_3$), EI-MS m/z (%) 284 ((M$^+$ + 1), 100), 224 (90), 33 (65).

General procedure for the synthesis of 1-benzyl-4-((5,6-dimethoxy-3-oxobenzofuran-2(3H)-ylidene)methyl) pyridinium halide derivatives (5a-g)

(Z)-5,6-Dimethoxy-2-(pyridin-4-ylmethylene) benzofuran-3(2H)-one (4) (1 equiv.), was suspended in 7 ml dry acetonitrile and heated under reflux condition. Afterwards different substituted benzyl halides (1.2 equiv.) were added thereto. The mixture was refluxed for 2–3 hours followed by cooling to room temperature. After that the solvent was evaporated and 15 ml n-hexane was added to the residue. The resulting mixture was filtered off and the precipitated crystals were separated, washed with n-hexane and dried. Flash chromatography of the crystals using the chloroform-methanol (99–1) as the mobile phase, furnished the final compounds 5a-g.

(Z)-1-Benzyl-4-((5,6-dimethoxy-3-oxobenzofuran-2(3H)-ylidene) methyl) pyridinium bromide (5a)

Starting from (Z)-5,6-dimethoxy-2-(pyridin-4-ylmethylene) benzofuran-3(2H)-one (1 mmol, 0.283 g) and benzyl bromide (1.2 mmol, 0.205 g), compound 5a was obtained, quantitative yield, mp over 300°C, IR ν_{max}/cm^{-1} (KBr) : 1689 (C = O), 1607 (C = C alkene), ^{1}H NMR (DMSO-d$_6$, 500 MHz), 9.20 (d, 2H, H$_{a-Pyridine}$, J = 6.7 Hz), 8.51 (d, 2H, H$_{b-pyridine}$, J = 6.7 Hz), 7.55-7.46 (m, 5H, H$_{phenyl}$), 7.27 (s, 1H, H$_{4-benzofuranone}$), 7.25 (s, 1H, H$_{7-benzofuranone}$), 7.04 (s, 1H, H$_{vinylic}$), 5.85 (s, 2H, H$_{benzylic}$), 3.98 (s, 3H, -OCH$_3$), 3.83(s, 3H, -OCH$_3$), EI-MS m/z (%) 283 (10), 91 (100), 77 (15), 43 (38), Anal. Calcd.for C$_{23}$H$_{20}$BrNO$_4$: C, 60.81; H, 4.44; N, 3.08 Found: C, 60.68; H, 4.72; N, 3.24.

(Z)-1-(4-Fluorobenzyl)-4-((5,6-dimethoxy-3-oxobenzofuran-2 (3H)-ylidene) methyl) pyridinium bromide (5b)

Starting from (Z)-5,6-dimethoxy-2-(pyridin-4-ylmethylene) benzofuran-3(2H)-one (1 mmol, 0.283 g) and 4-fluoro-benzyl bromide (1.2 mmol, 0.226 g), compound 5b was obtained, quantitative yield, mp 276–279°C, IR ν_{max}/cm^{-1} (KBr) : 1687 (C = O), 1608 (C = C alkene), ^{1}H NMR (DMSO-d$_6$, 500 MHz), 9.22 (d, 2H, H$_{a-pyridine}$, J = 6.7 Hz), 8.52 (d, 2H, H$_{b-pyridine}$, J = 6.75 Hz), 7.67-7.64 (m, 2H, H$_{phenyl}$), 7.32-7.28 (m, 2H, H$_{phenyl}$), 7.25 (s, 1H, H$_{4-benzofuranone}$), 7.23 (s, 1H, H$_{7-benzofuranone}$), 7.04 (s, 1H, H$_{vinylic}$), 5.86 (s, 2H, H$_{benzylic}$), 3.97 (s, 3H, -OCH$_3$), 3.82(s, 3H, -OCH$_3$), EI-MS m/z (%) 283 (12), 109 (100), 95 (18), 43 (40), Anal. Calcd.for C$_{23}$H$_{19}$BrFNO$_4$: C, 58.49; H, 4.05; N, 2.97 Found: C, 58.85; H, 4.17; N, 2.74.

(Z)-1-(3-Methylbenzyl)-4-((5,6-dimethoxy-3-oxobenzofuran-2 (3H)-ylidene) methyl) pyridinium chloride (5c)

Starting from (Z)-5,6-dimethoxy-2-(pyridin-4-ylmethylene) benzofuran-3(2H)-one (1 mmol, 0.283 g) and 3-methyl-benzyl chloride (1.2 mmol, 0.169 g), compound 5c was obtained, quantitative yield, mp 293–295°C, IR ν_{max}/cm^{-1} (KBr) : 1694 (C = O), 1605 (C = C alkene), ^{1}H NMR (DMSO-d$_6$, 500 MHz), 9.25 (d, 2H, H$_{a-pyridine}$, J = 6.4 Hz), 8.51 (d, 2H, H$_{b-pyridine}$, J = 6.45 Hz), 7.48-7.41 (m, 3H, H$_{phenyl}$), 7.33 (s, 1H, H$_{phenyl}$), 7.26 (s, 1H, H$_{4-benzofuranone}$), 7.24 (s, 1H, H$_{7-benzofuranone}$), 7.03 (s, 1H, H$_{vinylic}$), 5.83 (s, 2H, H$_{benzylic}$), 3.94 (s, 3H, –OCH$_3$), 3.80 (s, 3H, –OCH$_3$), 2.3 (s, 3H, H –CH$_{3phenyl}$), EI-MS m/z (%) 283 (12), 105

(100), 91 (16), 43 (38), Anal. Calcd.for C$_{24}$H$_{22}$ClNO$_4$: C, 68.00; H, 5.23; N, 3.30 Found: C, 68.34; H, 5.05; N, 3.42.

(Z)-1-(2-Fluorobenzyl)-4-((5,6-dimethoxy-3-oxobenzofuran-2 (3H)-ylidene) methyl) pyridinium chloride (5d)

Starting from (Z)-5,6-dimethoxy-2-(pyridin-4-ylmethylene) benzofuran-3(2H)-one (1 mmol, 0.283 g) and 2-fluorobenzyl chloride (1.2 mmol, 0.173 g), compound 5d was obtained, quantitative yield, mp over 300°C, IR ν_{max}/cm^{-1} (KBr) : 1701 (C = O), 1608 (C = C alkene), ^{1}H NMR (DMSO-d$_6$, 500 MHz), 9.19 (d, 2H, H$_{a-pyridine}$, J = 5.8 Hz), 8.53 (d, 2H, H$_{b-pyridine}$, J = 5.95 Hz), 7.65-7.62 (m, 1H, H$_{phenyl}$), 7.54-7.52 (m, 1H, H$_{phenyl}$), 7.34-7.31 (m, 2H, H$_{phenyl}$), 7.26 (s, 1H, H$_{4-benzofuranone}$), 7.23 (s, 1H, H$_{7-benzofuranone}$), 7.05 (s, 1H, H$_{vinylic}$), 5.94 (s, 2H, H$_{benzylic}$), 3.95 (s, 3H, –OCH$_3$), 3.80 (s, 3H, –OCH$_3$), EI-MS m/z (%) 283 (16), 109 (100), 95 (18), 43 (35), Anal. Calcd.for C$_{24}$H$_{22}$ClNO$_4$: C, 68.00; H, 5.23; N, 3.30 Found: C, 68.12; H, 5.32; N, 3.37.

(Z)-1-(3-Fluorobenzyl)-4-((5,6-dimethoxy-3-oxobenzofuran-2 (3H)-ylidene) methyl) pyridinium chloride (5e)

Starting from (Z)-5,6-dimethoxy-2-(pyridin-4-ylmethylene) benzofuran-3(2H)-one (1 mmol, 0.283 g) and 3-fluorobenzyl chloride (1.2 mmol, 0.173 g), compound 5e was obtained, quantitative yield, mp 291–294°C, IR ν_{max}/cm^{-1} (KBr) : 1690 (C = O), 1611 (C = C alkene), ^{1}H NMR (DMSO-d$_6$, 500 MHz), 9.29 (d, 2H, H$_{a-pyridine}$, J = 6 Hz), 8.52 (d, 2H, H$_{b-pyridine}$, J = 6.2 Hz), 7.51-7.50 (m, 2H, H$_{phenyl}$), 7.43-7.41 (m, 1H, H$_{phenyl}$), 7.30-7.27 (m, 1H, H$_{phenyl}$), 7.26 (s, 1H, H$_{4-benzofuranone}$), 7.23 (s, 1H, H$_{7-benzofuranone}$), 7.04 (s, 1H, H$_{vinylic}$), 5.9 (s, 2H, H$_{benzylic}$), 3.95 (s, 3H, –OCH$_3$), 3.8 (s, 3H, –OCH$_3$), EI-MS m/z (%) EI-MS m/z (%) 283 (19), 109 (100), 95 (15), 43 (32), Anal.Calcd.for C$_{23}$H$_{19}$ClFNO$_4$: C, 64.57; H, 4.48; N, 3.27 Found: C, 64.72; H, 4.23; N, 3.16.

(Z)-1-(2-Methylbenzyl)-4-((5,6-dimethoxy-3-oxobenzofuran-2 (3H)-ylidene) methyl) pyridinium chloride (5f)

Starting from (Z)-5,6-dimethoxy-2-(pyridin-4-ylmethylene) benzofuran-3(2H)-one (1 mmol, 0.283 g) and 2-methyl-benzyl chloride (1.2 mmol, 0.169 g), compound 5f was obtained, quantitative yield, mp 287–290°C, IR ν_{max}/cm^{-1} (KBr) : 1692 (C = O), 1607(C = C alkene), ^{1}H NMR (DMSO-d$_6$, 500 MHz), 9.08 (d, 2H, H$_{a-pyridine}$, J = 6.85 Hz), 8.52 (d, 2H, H$_{b-pyridine}$, J = 6.8 Hz), 7.81- 7.78 (m, 1H, H$_{phenyl}$), 7.45-7.38 (m, 1H, H$_{phenyl}$), 7.32-7.30 (m, 2H, H$_{phenyl}$), 7.29 (s, 1H, H$_{4-benzofuranone}$), 7.24 (s, 1H, H$_{7-benzofuranone}$), 6.99 (s, 1H, H$_{vinylic}$), 5.88 (s, 2H, H$_{benzylic}$), 3.99 (s, 3H, –OCH$_3$), 3.84 (s, 3H, –OCH$_3$), 2.35 (s, 3H, H CH$_{3phenyl}$) EI-MS m/z (%) 283 (21), 105 (100), 91 (18), 43 (40), Anal. Calcd.for C$_{24}$H$_{22}$ClNO$_4$: C, 68.00; H, 5.23; N, 3.30 Found: C, 68.26; H, 5.15; N, 3.25.

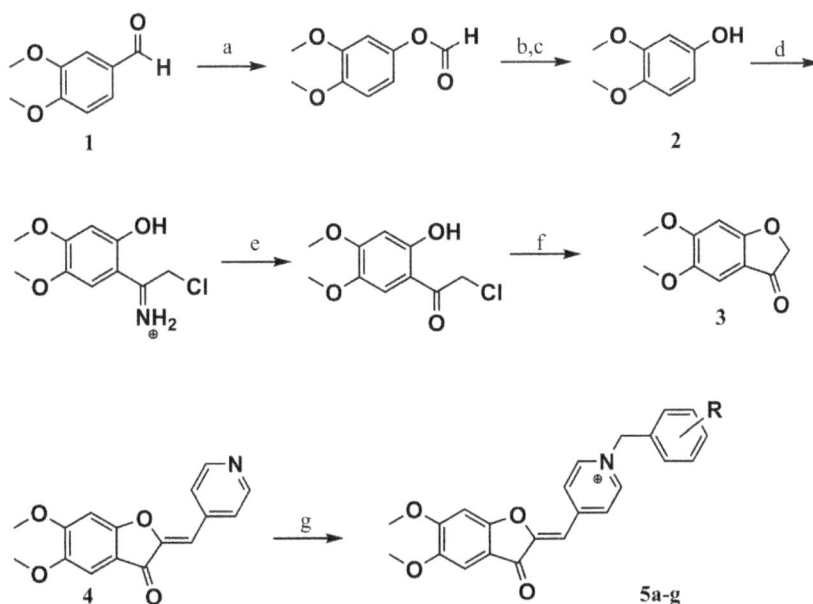

Scheme 1 Synthetic routes to final compounds 5a-g (a) *m*-CPBA, CH2Cl2, reflux 16 hrs; (b) NaOH 10%, r.t., stir., 4 hrs; (c) HCl 6 N; (d) ClCH2CN, HCl gas, ZnCl2, 0°C, 2.5 hrs, stir.; (e) HCl 1 N, reflux, 90 min; (f) Sodium acetate trihydrate, ethanol, reflux, 10 min; (g) Pyridine-4-carboxaldehyde, PTSA, toluene, reflux; (h) Substituted benzyl halide, CH3CN, reflux.

(Z)-1-(4-Methylbenzyl)-4-((5,6-dimethoxy-3-oxobenzofuran-2 (3H)-ylidene) methyl) pyridinium chloride (5g)

Starting from (Z)-5,6-dimethoxy-2-(pyridin-4-ylmethylene) benzofuran-3(2H)-one (1 mmol, 0.283 g) and 4-methylbenzyl chloride (1.2 mmol, 0.169 g), compound 5g was obtained, quantitative yield, mp 294–297°C, IR v_{max}/cm^{-1} (KBr) : 1690 (C = O), 1606 (C = C alkene), ^{1}H NMR (DMSO-d$_6$, 500 MHz), 9.24 (d, 2H, H$_{a-pyridine}$, $J = 6.4$ Hz), 8.49 (d, 2H, H$_{b-pyridine}$, $J = 6.5$ Hz), 7.47 (d, 2H, $J = 6.3$ Hz, H$_{phenyl}$), 7.26 (d, 2H, $J = 6.4$ Hz, H$_{phenyl}$), 7.20 (s, 1H, H$_{4-benzofuranone}$), 7.17 (s, 1H, H$_{7-benzofuranone}$), 6.96 (s, 1H, H$_{vinylic}$), 5.80 (s, 2H, H$_{benzylic}$), 3.95 (s, 3H, –OCH$_3$), 380 (s, 3H, –OCH$_3$), 2.28 (s, 3H, H –CH$_{3phenyl}$), EI-MS *m/z* (%) 283 (17), 105 (100), 91 (22), 43 (31), Anal. Calcd.for C$_{24}$H$_{22}$ClNO$_4$: C, 68.00; H, 5.23; N, 3.30 Found: C, 67.76; H, 5.38; N, 3.19.

Biological activity

AChE (AChE, E.C. 3.1.1.7, Type V-S, lyophilized powder, from *electric eel*, 1000 unit), Cholinesterase from equine serum were purchased from Sigma–Aldrich (Steinheim, Germany). DTNB (5, 5′-Dithiobis-(2-nitrobenzoic acid)), KH$_2$PO$_4$, K$_2$HPO$_4$, KOH, NaHCO$_3$, BTChI (butyrylthiocholine iodide) and ATChI (acetylthiocholine iodide) were obtained from Fluka (Buchs, Switzerland). To afford an assay concentration range (10^{-4} to 10^{-9} M), the tested compounds were dissolved in a mixture of 20 ml distilled water and 5 ml methanol followed by dilution in 0.1 M KH$_2$PO$_4$/K$_2$HPO$_4$ buffer (pH 8.0) to obtain final concentration.

The colorimetric Ellman's method was applied to evaluate anti AChE/BuChE activity of tested compounds. The solutions temperature was adjusted to 25°C prior to use. Five different concentrations of each compound were tested to obtain 20% to 80% inhibition of AChE and/or BuChE activity. The assay medium contained 3 ml of 0.1 M phosphate buffer pH 8.0, 100 μl of 0.01 M 5, 5′-dithio-bis(2-nitrobenzoic acid), 100 μl of 2.5 unit/mL enzyme solution (AChE, E.C. 3.1.1.7, Type V-S, lyophilized powder, from *electric eel* or BuChE from equine serum).

Then 100 μl of each tested compounds, were added to the assay medium and pre-incubated at 25°C for 15 min followed by adding 20 μl of substrate (acetylthiocholine iodide or butyrylthiocholine iodide). After that the rate of absorbance change was measured at 412 nm for 2 minutes. The blank reading solution was used to justify non-enzymatic hydrolysis of substrate during the assay. The blank solution contained 3 ml buffer, 200 μl water, 100 μl DTNB and 20 μl substrate. As a reference, an identical solution of the enzyme without the inhibitor is processed following the same protocol. The rate of the substrate enzymatic hydrolysis was calculated, and % inhibition of the tested compounds was calculated. Each concentration was evaluated in triplicate, and the

Table 1 AChE/BuChE inhibitory activity of compounds 5a-g compared with Donepezil hydrochloride (IC$_{50}$ = Mean ± SD)

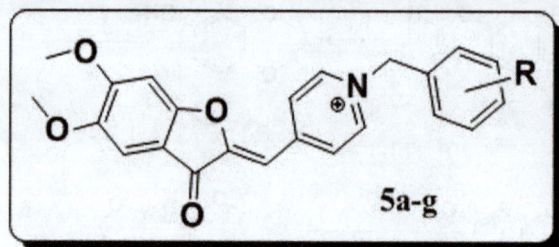

Compounds	R	AChE (IC$_{50}$ ± SD)[a] (nM)	BuChE (IC$_{50}$ ± SD)[a] (nM)	Selectivity for AChE[b] (S.I)
5a	H	86 ± 10.94	1400 ± 85	16.27
5b	2-F	52 ± 6.38	1620 ± 73	31.15
5c	3-F	115 ± 15.56	740 ± 23	6.43
5d	4-F	74 ± 11.32	960 ± 41	12.97
5e	2-CH$_3$	262 ± 27.49	3620 ± 84	13.81
5f	3-CH$_3$	208 ± 31.72	5310 ± 115	25.52
5g	4-CH$_3$	514 ± 29.53	7600 ± 260	14.78
Donepezil hydrochloride	-	31 ± 5.12	5400 ± 95	174.19

[a] Data are means ± standard deviation of three independent experiments.
[b] Selectivity Index (S.I): IC$_{50}$ BuChE/ IC$_{50}$ AChE.

IC$_{50}$ values were determined from inhibition curves (% of inhibition versus log inhibitor's concentration) graphically. Kapková et al. reported more details of the procedure [16,17].

Docking study

Docking simulation studies were done using Autodock Vina 1.1.1 [18]. For this purpose, the pdb structure of acetylcholinesterase (1EVE) was retrieved from the

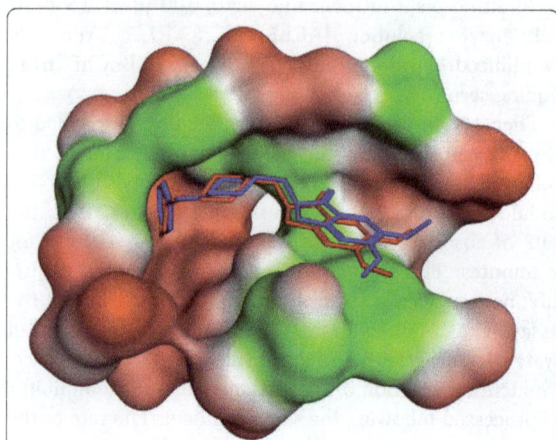

Figure 4 The superposition of the docked Donepezil (blue) and reference Donepezil (red) into the active site of the AChE.

Brookhaven protein database (RCSB)(http://www.rcsb.org) as a complex bound with inhibitor Donepezil. Subsequently, all water molecules and the co-crystallized ligand were removed from the pdb structure. Afterward the polar hydrogens were added to the receptor and pdbqt format of the receptor was created using Autodock Tools 1.5.4 [19]. The ligand coordinates were generated using Marvine-Sketch 5.8.3, 2012, ChemAxon (http://www.chemaxon.com). Then the structures were converted to pdbqt using Open babel 2.3.1 [20]. The docking site was defined by establishing a box at geometrical center of the native ligand present in the above mentioned PDB structure with the dimensions of 40, 40, and 40. The exhaustiveness parameter was set to 80 and the box center was set to the dimensions of x = 2.023, y = 63.295, z = 67.062. Finally, the lowest energy conformations between the AChE and inhibitor were selected for analyzing the interactions. The results were visualized using Chimera 1.6 [21].

Results and discussion
Chemistry

The target compounds (5a-g) were synthesized as illustrated in Scheme 1. The convenient Baeyer–Villiger oxidation of 3,4-dimethoxybenzaldehyde furnished 3,4-dimethoxyphenol (1) in a good yield [15]. Reaction of 3,4-dimethoxyphenol (1) with chloroacetonitrile using ZnCl$_2$ as Lewis acid yielded 2-chloro-1-(2-hydroxy-4,5-dimethoxyphenyl)ethane iminium as a key intermediate.

chloride or bromide derivatives were refluxed with compound (4) in dry acetonitrile to obtain final compounds (5a-g).

Biological activity

The new series of 5,6-dimethoxybenzofuranone derivatives bearing the benzyl pyridinium moiety was evaluated for AChE/BuChE activity using slightly modified Ellman's protocol.

The type and position of substituents on benzyl moiety could alter the electronic and steric properties of the phenyl ring. Therefore, the affinity of the target compounds toward the enzyme could be modified by changing the substituent on benzyl moiety.

The anti AChE/BuChE activity data of the target compounds were summarized in Table 1.

According to the data, all of the synthesized compounds have shown considerable anti AChE/BuChE activity however, did not reach the inhibition level of the reference compound (Donepezil hydrochloride IC$_{50}$ = 31 ± 5.12 nM).

As already shown in our previous study, the substitution on phenyl ring with small electron withdrawing group such as fluorine atom makes the compounds more active rather than their unsubstituted counterparts. In an opposite way the methyl phenyl substituted compounds proved to be less active than the unsubstituted compounds. In this study using the identical substitution on the ring, the anti cholinesterase activity of 5,6-dimethoxy-benzofuranone derivatives has changed in the same way. Regardless of the substitution on phenyl ring, the activity of more

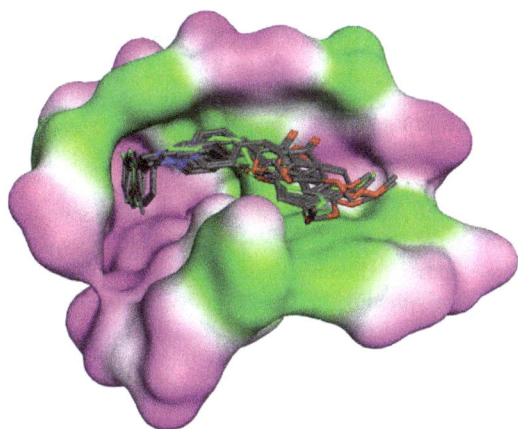

Figure 5 The superposition of best docked poses of all target compounds (colored by element) as well as Donepezil (green) into the gorge of AChE.

Afterwards, 2-chloro-1-(2-hydroxy-4,5-dimethoxyphenyl) ethanone (2) was prepared followed by treatment of iminium intermediate using hydrochloric acid. Intermolecular cyclization of compound (2) using sodium acetate resulted in formation of 5,6-dimethoxy-benzofuran-3(2H)-one (3) [22]. Condensation of 5,6-dimethoxybenzofuran-3(2H)-one (3) with 4-formyl pyridine in the presence of PTSA gave (Z)-5,6-dimethoxy-2-(pyridin-4-ylmethylene) benzofuran-3(2H)-one (4). As previously reported, the configuration of exocyclic formed double bond was assigned as Z (cis) isomer [11]. Appropriate benzyl

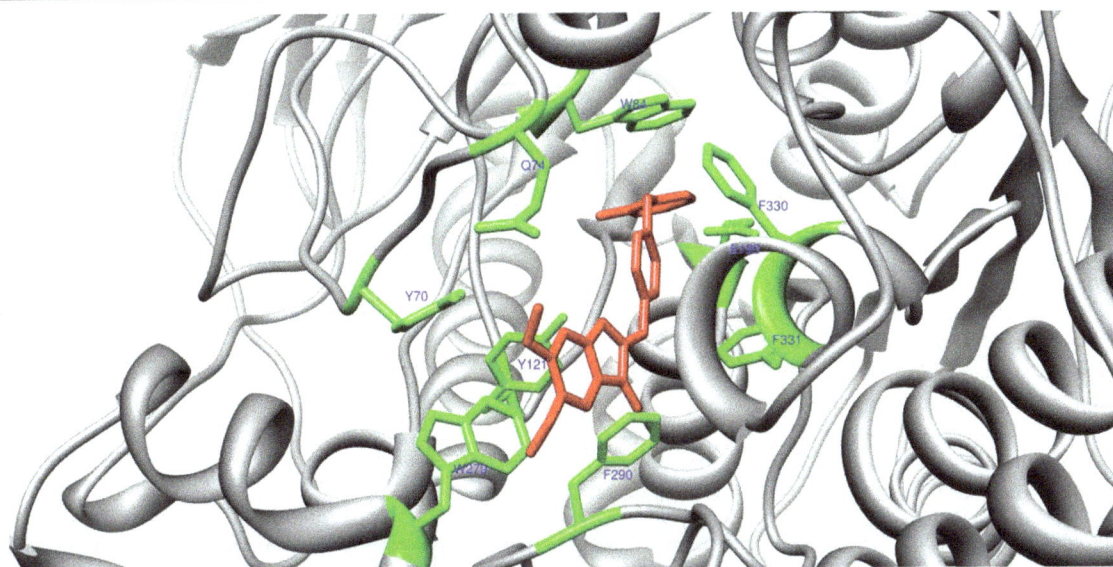

Figure 6 The interacting mode of the most active compound 5b with the active site of AChE.

polar 5,6-dimethoxybenzofuranone derivatives were slightly diminished, compared to 6-alkoxy benzofuranone derivatives that were previously reported [11].

As anticipated, the compound 5b ($IC_{50} = 52 \pm 6.38$ nM) containing 2-F substituent exhibited the highest inhibitory activity toward the enzyme. However, its activity was less than its counterparts bearing 6-methoxy ($IC_{50} = 10 \pm 6.87$ nM), 6-ethoxy ($IC_{50} = 32 \pm 7.75$ nM) and 6-propoxy ($IC_{50} = 50 \pm 9.86$) on benzofuranone.

Similarly, the 3 and 4-flouro phenyl compounds have shown lower activity in respect to corresponding 6-alkoxy benzofuranone series.

According to Table 1, changing the *ortho* position of fluorine to either *meta* or *para* decreased the activity as in compound (5c) with significantly diminished activity ($IC_{50} = 115 \pm 15.56$).

Accordingly, methyl substituted compounds have exhibited the order of activity as follow: 5f > 5e > 5g. Insertion of methyl group on phenyl ring in any position reduced the activity in comparison with unsubstituted compound (5a).

In an accord to these findings, it was concluded that substitution on position 3 with F and position 4 with – CH_3 was not tolerated.

Docking simulation study

In order to investigate the binding mode for interaction of the target compounds with AChE, docking studies were performed. First the co-crystallized ligand was docked back into the binding site of the enzyme and superposed with the native ligand (Figure 4).

Being satisfied with the reasonable RMSD between the docked and native ligands (RMSD = 0.78 Å), the docking protocol was verified for further docking studies of the target compounds. The best docked poses of the synthesized compounds on the target were superposed and showed to be similarly docked in the gorge of AChE. As shown in Figure 5, this pattern of orientation resembled very much to that observed for donepezil.

In order to figure out the binding mode for interaction of the compounds, the most active compound (5b) was subjected to further analysis. As depicted in Figure 6, the 5,6-dimethoxybenzofuranone fragment of the ligand was well accommodated in the PAS (Peripheral Anionic Site) through a π–π stacking of the phenyl ring of benzofuranone and indole moiety of Trp279. This interaction was reinforced by a hydrogen bonding between the 6-methoxy of 5b and the hydroxyl group of Tyr70. In addition, the benzyl pyridinium part of the ligand was oriented towards the anionic site (AS) composed by Phe330, Trp84 and Glu199. The interactions responsible for stabilization of bezyl pyridinium in the active site included two π–π stacking and a π-cation interaction. The π-cation interaction was formed between Phe330 and the quaternary

nitrogen of pyridine ring. Regarding the two π–π interactions, one was between 2-flouro substituted phenyl ring and Trp84 and the other between pyridine ring and Phe330. The same binding mode and interactions were also observed for the reference drug (Donepzil) [23].

Conclusions

In this study, we presented new benzofuranone-based derivatives of the pyridinium type. The inhibitory activity of new synthesized compounds were tested toward AChE using slightly modified Ellman's method and compared to those of other derivatives of this class synthesized earlier by our research group. Regarding the biological data, it was revealed that all tested compounds inhibited the AChE in nanomolar range concentration, in which compound 5b, was the most potent compound against AChE. Furthermore a same binding mode and interactions was observed for the reference drug Donepzil and compound 5b in docking study.

In conclusion, 5,6-dimethoxybenzofurane derivatives containing methylbenzyl substituent on pyridine ring demonstrated to be more potent than their corresponding 6-ethoxy and 6-propoxy benzofuranone derivatives [11].

Competing interests
The authors declare that they have no competing interests.

Authors' contributions
HN participated in the synthesis of compounds and performing biological assay. AF, Ash, AA and MP contributed in design of compounds, supervision of synthetic part, elucidation of the target compounds structure and manuscript preparation. AM, AS and AV performed the docking study and participated in manuscript preparation. NH partook in synthetic section. The biological assay part is supervised by VS and MA. All authors read and approved the final manuscript.

Acknowledgements
Molecular graphics and analyses were performed with the UCSF Chimera package. Chimera is developed by the 25 Resource for Biocomputing, Visualization, and Informatics at the University of California, San Francisco.

Author details
[1]Department of Medicinal Chemistry, Faculty of Pharmacy and Neurobiomedical Research Center, Shahid Sadoughi University of Medical Sciences, Yazd 8915173143, Iran. [2]Faculty of Pharmacy and Pharmaceutical Sciences Research Center, Tehran University of Medical Sciences, Tehran, Iran. [3]Herbal Medicine Center, Shahid Sadoughi University of Medical Sciences, Yazd 8915173143, Iran. [4]Neuroscience Research Center, Kerman University of Medical Sciences, Kerman, Iran. [5]Drug design & Development Research Center, Tehran University of Medical Sciences, Tehran, Iran.

References
1. Kung HF, Lee CW, Zhuang ZP, Kung MP, Hou C, Plossl K: **Novel stilbenes as probes for amyloid plaques.** *J Am Chem Soc* 2001, **123**:12740–12741.
2. Forstl H, Kurz A: **Clinical features of Alzheimer's disease.** *Eur Arch Psychiatry Clin Neurosci* 1999, **249**:288–290.
3. Fernandez-Bachiller MI, Perez C, Campillo NE, Paez JA, Gonzalez-Munoz GC, Usan P, Garcia-Palomero E, Lopez MG, Villarroya M, Garcia AG, Martinez A, Rodriguez-Franco MI: **Tacrine-melatonin hybrids as multifunctional agents for Alzheimer's disease, with cholinergic, antioxidant, and neuroprotective properties.** *ChemMedChem* 2009, **4**:828–841.

4. Yankner BA, Dawes LR, Fisher S, Villa-Komaroff L, Oster-Granite ML, Neve RL: Neurotoxicity of a fragment of the amyloid precursor associated with Alzheimer's disease. *Science* 1989, **245**:417–420.

5. Masters CL, Simms G, Weinman NA, Multhaup G, McDonald BL, Beyreuther K: Amyloid plaque core protein in Alzheimer's disease and Down syndrome. *Proc Natl Acad Sci U S A* 1985, **82**:4245–4249.

6. Bartus RT, Dean RL III, Beer B, Lippa AS: The cholinergic hypothesis of geriatric memory dysfunction. *Science* 1982, **217**:408–414.

7. Richman DP, Agius MA: Treatment of autoimmune myasthenia gravis. *Neurology* 2003, **61**:1652–1661.

8. Repantis D, Laisney O, Heuser I: Acetylcholinesterase inhibitors and memantine for neuroenhancement in healthy individuals: a systematic review. *Pharmacol Res* 2010, **61**:473–481.

9. Karlsson D, Fallarero A, Brunhofer G, Mayer C, Prakash O, Mohan CG, Vuorela P, Erker T: The exploration of thienothiazines as selective butyrylcholinesterase inhibitors. *Eur J Pharm Sci* 2012, **47**:190–205.

10. Musial A, Bajda M, Malawska B: Recent developments in cholinesterases inhibitors for Alzheimer's disease treatment. *Curr Med Chem* 2007, **14**:2654–2679.

11. Nadri H, Pirali-Hamedani M, Shekarchi M, Abdollahi M, Sheibani V, Amanlou M, Shafiee A, Foroumadi A: Design, synthesis and anticholinesterase activity of a novel series of 1-benzyl-4-((6-alkoxy-3-oxobenzofuran-2(3H)-ylidene) methyl) pyridinium derivatives. *Bioorg Med Chem* 2010, **18**:6360–6366.

12. Sheng R, Lin X, Zhang J, Chol KS, Huang W, Yang B, He Q, Hu Y: Design, synthesis and evaluation of flavonoid derivatives as potent AChE inhibitors. *Bioorg Med Chem* 2009, **17**:6692–6698.

13. Sheng R, Xu Y, Hu C, Zhang J, Lin X, Li J, Yang B, He Q, Hu Y: Design, synthesis and AChE inhibitory activity of indanone and aurone derivatives. *Eur J Med Chem* 2009, **44**:7–17.

14. Ellman GL, Courtney KD, Andres V Jr, Feather-Stone RM: A new and rapid colorimetric determination of acetylcholinesterase activity. *Biochem Pharmacol* 1961, **7**:88–95.

15. Li CC, Xie ZX, Zhang YD, Chen JH, Yang Z: Total synthesis of wedelolactone. *J Org Chem* 2003, **68**:8500–8504.

16. Kapkova P, Alptuzun V, Frey P, Erciyas E, Holzgrabe U: Search for dual function inhibitors for Alzheimer's disease: synthesis and biological activity of acetylcholinesterase inhibitors of pyridinium-type and their Abeta fibril formation inhibition capacity. *Bioorg Med Chem* 2006, **14**:472–478.

17. Alptuzun V, Kapkova P, Baumann K, Erciyas E, Holzgrabe U: Synthesis and biological activity of pyridinium-type acetylcholinesterase inhibitors. *J Pharm Pharmacol* 2003, **55**:1397–1404.

18. Trott O, Olson AJ: AutoDock Vina: improving the speed and accuracy of docking with a new scoring function, efficient optimization, and multithreading. *J Comput Chem* 2010, **31**:455–461.

19. Sanner MF: Python: a programming language for software integration and development. *J Mol Graph Model* 1999, **17**:57–61.

20. O'Boyle NM, Banck M, James CA, Morley C, Vandermeersch T, Hutchison GR: Open Babel: an open chemical toolbox. *J Cheminform* 2011, **3**:33.

21. Pettersen EF, Goddard TD, Huang CC, Couch GS, Greenblatt DM, Meng EC, Ferrin TE: UCSF Chimera–a visualization system for exploratory research and analysis. *J Comput Chem* 2004, **25**:1605–1612.

22. Lee CY, Chew EH, Go ML: Functionalized aurones as inducers of NAD(P)H: quinone oxidoreductase 1 that activate AhR/XRE and Nrf2/ARE signaling pathways: synthesis, evaluation and SAR. *Eur J Med Chem* 2010, **45**:2957–2971.

23. Sugimoto H, Iimura Y, Yamanishi Y, Yamatsu K: Synthesis and structure-activity relationships of acetylcholinesterase inhibitors: 1-benzyl-4-[(5,6-dimethoxy-1-oxoindan-2-yl)methyl]piperidine hydrochloride and related compounds. *J Med Chem* 1995, **38**:4821–4829.

7

Cost analysis of pharmaceutical care provided to HIV-infected patients

Renata Cavalcanti Carnevale[1], Caroline de Godoi Rezende Costa Molino[1], Marília Berlofa Visacri[1*], Priscila Gava Mazzola[1] and Patricia Moriel[1,2]

Abstract

Background: Studies have shown that pharmaceutical care can result in favorable clinical outcomes in human immunodeficiency virus (HIV)-infected patients, however, few studies have assessed the economic impact. The objective of this study was to evaluate the clinical and economic impact of pharmaceutical care of HIV-infected patients.

Methods: A controlled ambispective study was conducted in Brazil from January 2009 to June 2012. Patients were allocated to either intervention or control group. The control group was followed according to standard care while the intervention group was also followed by a pharmacist at each physician appointment for one year. Effectiveness outcomes included CD4+ count, viral load, absence of co-infections and optimal immune response, and economic outcomes included expenses of physician and pharmaceutical appointments, laboratory tests, procedures, and hospitalizations, at six months and one year.

Results: Intervention and control groups included 51 patients each. We observed significant decreases in total pharmacotherapy problems during the study. At six months, the intervention group contained higher percentages of patients without co-infections and of patients with CD4+ >500 cells/mm^3. None of the differences between intervention and control group considering clinical outcomes and costs were statistically significant. However, at one year, the intervention group showed higher percentage of better clinical outcomes and generated lower spending (not to procedures). An additional health care system daily investment of US$1.45, 1.09, 2.13, 4.35, 1.09, and 0.87 would be required for each additional outcome of viral load <50 copies/ml, absence of co-infection, CD4+ >200, 350, and 500 cells/mm^3, and optimal immune response, respectively.

Conclusion: This work demonstrated that pharmaceutical care of HIV-infected patients, for a one-year period, was able to decrease the number of pharmacotherapy problems. However, the clinical outcomes and the costs did not have statistical difference but showed higher percentage of better clinical outcomes and lower costs for some items.

Keywords: Pharmacoeconomics, Pharmaceutical care, HIV-infected patients

* Correspondence: mariberlofa@gmail.com
[1]Department of Clinical Pathology, Faculty of Medical Sciences (FCM), University of Campinas (UNICAMP), Alexander Fleming, 105, 13083-881 Campinas, SP, Brazil
Full list of author information is available at the end of the article

Introduction

Since 1996, Brazil has had a public health system program that provides free antiretroviral therapy, laboratory tests, and procedures to HIV-infected patients. This program has been internationally recognized as a major initiative against HIV [1]. However, this program alone does not guarantee safety and effectiveness of treatment because HIV treatment requires long-term therapy. Treatment of HIV includes a large number of drugs and drug interactions, and requires careful monitoring of therapy, with the goal of decreasing viral resistance and drug-related problems [1-3].

Studies have investigated the effects of pharmaceutical care on the rational use of drugs in HIV-infected patients [4-6]. March et al. demonstrated that HIV-infected patients followed by a clinical pharmacist show significant improvements in CD4+ levels and viral load and a decrease in toxic effects related to treatment [7]. This reduction in toxicity improves the quality of life and treatment adherence of the patients [8]. In addition, a systematic analysis (including data from January 1980 to June 2011) revealed that providing pharmaceutical care to HIV-infected patients was associated with statistically significant improvements in treatment adherence and had a positive impact on viral suppression [9].

Despite the variety of pharmaceutical care studies conducted with HIV-infected patients, remarkably few include an economic analysis. There is a need to go beyond the investigation of clinical outcomes generated by pharmaceutical care. Studies that include the economic impact of pharmaceutical care are necessary to justify the implementation or expansion of pharmaceutical care services [10].

In addition to the lack of economic studies on pharmaceutical care conducted with HIV-infected patients, another limitation is that, even though the studies available demonstrate that pharmaceutical care practice can contribute to the reductions of costs, they focus only on the costs associated with drugs, physician appointments, and hospitalizations. The available literature does not present studies regarding the impact of pharmaceutical care on the costs associated with laboratory tests and procedures [9,11-13]. Moreover, the majority of pharmacoeconomic studies present many methodological limitations, such as the lack of a control group and non-inclusion of costs associated with pharmacist appointments [14]. Thus, it has become imperative to conduct well-designed studies in the area of pharmaceutical care in order to obtain a clearer comprehension of its economic impact [14]. Well-designed studies investigating economic impact should be encouraged because they enable the rationalization of resources in health care, where the available resources are limited [15].

This study was designed to perform a pharmacoeconomic analysis of the impact of pharmaceutical care on HIV-infected patients over a one-year period by measuring both clinical and health care system economic outcomes.

Methods

This was a one-year, ambispective, controlled study, with a systematic sample by quota controls, paired according to random characteristics. A retrospective chart review and a prospective pharmaceutical care follow-up were conducted. The study was conducted at a hospital in the state of São Paulo, Brazil. The Hospital Ethics Committee approved the research, and informed consent was obtained from all patients.

The inclusion criteria for the study were as follows: outpatients diagnosed with HIV/AIDS (Human Immunodeficiency Virus/Acquired Immunodeficiency Syndrome), aged between 18 and 60 years, having body mass index (BMI) lower than 30 kg/m^2, and receiving antiretroviral therapy (ART). Obese patients were not included because they present higher incidences of hyperlipidemia, hypertension, and insulin resistance, and because some HIV/AIDS medications such as protease inhibitors can cause weight gain and fat accumulation, it would not be possible to determine whether the weight gain was related to the medication or to the background disease in such patients [16-19]. Patients who were unable to return for later appointments/exams, who refused to participate, who have psychiatric disease (that unable them to follow the medical appointments schedule and the pharmacist interventions), and those who were pregnant were excluded. Patients were enrolled in the study from January 2009 to June 2011 and were assigned in a 1:1 ratio to either intervention or control group by the clinical pharmacy team. Control group patients were matched to intervention group patients according to gender and baseline CD4+ count.

For one year, the intervention group was followed by the clinical pharmacy staff, composed of two pharmacists trained by the hospital clinical pharmacy team regarding HIV/AIDS and pharmaceutical care, after routine medical appointments at the hospital, using a method developed and adapted to the reality of the hospital, based on the Pharmacist's Workup of Drug Therapy (PWDT) method [20]. The control group was not followed by the clinical pharmacy team, and its data were collected through review of medical charts encompassing the same period.

Initial and final pharmacotherapy problems were accounted for and classified as necessity, effectiveness, safety, or therapy compliance pharmacotherapy problems only for the intervention group [21]. The clinical pharmacy team performed written and verbal pharmacist interventions with the intervention group, which were accounted for and classified as pharmacist-patient or pharmacist-physician interventions and as resolutive pharmacotherapy problems, preventive pharmacotherapy problems, quality of life, or referral to other medical specialties interventions. The classifications used for pharmacotherapy problems and pharmacist interventions are in accordance with those used in another publication by the authors [22].

The five effectiveness outcomes were as follows: CD4+ count higher than 200 cells/mm^3, 350 cells/mm^3, and 500 cells/mm^3; viral load lower than 50 copies/ml; and absence of co-infections. The co-infections considered by the study were as follows: bacterial co-infections (urinary infection, shigellosis, infected sebaceous cysts, cellulitis, pneumonia, and hordeolums), viral co-infections (cytomegalovirus, influenza, *Herpes zoster*, *Herpes simplex*, human papillomavirus, viral conjunctivitis, and warts), parasitic co-infection (microsporidiosis, isosporiasis, coccidiosis, and neurocryptococcosis), and fungal co-infections (oral moniliasis, onychomycosis, and tinea pedis). Effectiveness outcomes were measured at six months and one year of study and were obtained through medical chart review for both groups. Additionally, using a decision tree model, we established the number of patients from both groups that achieved, after one year of study, an optimal immune response as characterized by viral load <50 copies/ml, absence of co-infection, and CD4+>500 cells/mm^3.

For cost analysis, we identified the number of appointments (medical/nursing/nutrition/physical therapy/speech therapy/dental), laboratory tests, procedures, and hospitalizations per patient in the first six months, the last six months, and in one year, for both groups, through review of their medical charts. For the intervention group, we also included the cost of the pharmacist appointment. The DATASUS database [23] provided the monetary values for all these items. Values were quoted in US dollars ($).

Cost analysis was performed for the one-year period, considering both the effectiveness and the costs of appointments, laboratory tests, procedures, hospitalizations, total cost, and total cost without procedures.

Statistical analysis of the results was performed by SAS System for Windows (Statistical Analysis System, version 9.2). For baseline characteristics analysis, chi-square, Fisher's exact, and Mann–Whitney tests were performed. For co-infection, CD4+ and viral load analysis and generalized estimating tests were performed. For costs analysis, ANOVA for repeated measures, with a transformation by positions, was performed. The significance level was set at 5% (P ≤0.050).

Results

The study screened 140 HIV-infected patients being treated at the hospital on an outpatient basis. Thirty-eight patients were excluded: two were pregnant; nine interrupted the treatment at the hospital; eight were transferred from the hospital; and nineteen had not returned for the second pharmaceutical appointment in the first six months of the study (Figure 1). Finally, 51 patients each were allocated to intervention and control groups. A medical chart review provided the demographic data and initial information for both study groups (Table 1). The two study groups had similar baseline characteristics, indicating homogeneity.

There were a total of 230 pharmaceutical appointments (143 in the initial six months and 87 in the final six months). During these appointments, 219 pharmacist interventions were performed. Among them, 185 (84.5%) were pharmacist-patient interventions and 34 (15.5%) were pharmacist-physician interventions; 116 (53.0%) were preventive interventions, 55 (25.1%) were resolutive interventions, 42 (19.2%) were quality of life interventions, and six (2.7%) were referral to other medical specialties

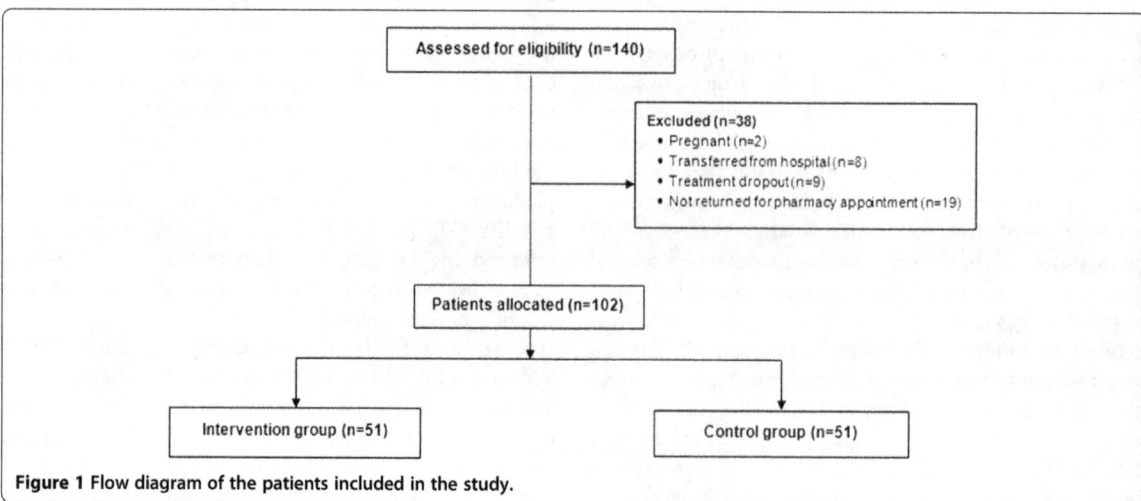

Figure 1 Flow diagram of the patients included in the study.

Table 1 Baseline characteristics of intervention group and control group

Characteristics	Control group N=51	Intervention group N=51	P value
Age (Mean [SD], years)	40.5 [9.2]	41.3 [8.8]	0.580ᵃ
Men - % (n)	66.7 (34)	66.7 (34)	1.000ᵇ
Ethnicity - % (n)			0.830ᵇ
Caucasian	70.6 (36)	68.6 (35)	
Black/ african descent	29.4 (15)	31.4 (16)	
HIV Diagnosis(Mean [SD], years)	7.5 [5.6]	8.3 [6.4]	0.690ᵃ
HIV Treatment Duration (Mean [SD], years)	5.7 [4.2]	6.5 [5.5]	0.780ᵃ
Number of tablets/day (Mean [SD])	9.3 [4.4]	10.1 [4.2]	0.250ᵃ
ART changes during the first 4 weeks of the study - % (n)	9.8 (5)	7.8 (4)	1.000ᶜ
CD4 + (Mean [SD], cells/mm³)	304.0 [277.1]	310.4 [302.0]	0.980ᵃ
CD4 + >200 cells/mm³ % (n)	56.9 (29)	54.9 (28)	0.840ᵇ
CD4 + >350 cells/mm³ % (n)	31.4 (16)	33.3 (17)	0.830ᵇ
CD4 + >500 cells/mm³ % (n)	15.7 (8)	17.7 (9)	0.800ᵇ
Viral load <50 copies/ml % (n)	60.8 (31)	64.8 (33)	0.190ᵇ
Number of Comorbidities (Mean [SD])	2.5 [1.6]	2.8 [2.1]	0.730ᵃ
Type of comorbidities % (n)			
Hepatitis C	23.5 (12)	21.6 (11)	0.630ᵇ
Tobaccoism	15.8 (8)	11.8 (6)	0.570ᵇ
Neurotoxoplasmosis	9.8 (5)	9.8 (5)	0.510ᵇ
Hypertriglyceridemia	3.9 (2)	9.8 (5)	0.440ᶜ
Pulmonary tuberculosis	13.7 (7)	3.9 (2)	0.160ᶜ
ART regimen % (n)			0.800ᵇ
TDF+3TC+EFV	17.6 (9)	21.6 (11)	
AZT+3TC+EFV	15.7 (8)	21.6 (11)	
AZT+3TC+LPV/r	9.8 (5)	7.8 (4)	
TDF+3TC+LPV/r	11.8 (6)	11.8 (6)	
Others	45.1 (23)	37.2 (19)	
Substance abuse % (n)			0.418ᵇ
Alcohol	19.6 (10)	29.4 (15)	
Tobacco	27.4 (14)	33.3 (17)	
Illicit drugs	13.73 (7)	7.8 (4)	

Note: ᵃMann-Whitney test; ᵇChi-square test;ᶜFisher's exact test.
Abbreviations: ART, antiretroviral therapy; AZT, zidovudine; CD4+, lymphocyte T CD4+; EFV, efavirenz; LPV/r, lopinavir/ritonavir; n, absolute number of patients; SD, standard deviation; TDF, tenofovir; 3TC, lamivudine.

interventions. We also observed significant decreases in total pharmacotherapy problems (from 248 to 145; 41.5%, P <0.001), necessity problems (from 55 to 26; 52.7%, P <0.001), and safety problems (from 161 to 96; 40.4%, P <0.001). A decrease in the other pharmacotherapy problems was also detected; however, it was not statistically

significant: effectiveness problems (from 12 to 11; 8.4%, P =1.0000) and compliance problems (from 20 to 12; 40.0%, P =0.760).

Regarding clinical outcomes, in the initial six months, the intervention group contained higher percentages of patients without co-infections and of patients with CD4+ >500 cells/mm³. At one year, the intervention group showed higher percentage of better clinical outcomes: absence of co-infection, viral load <50 copies/ml, CD4+ >200 cells/mm³, CD4+ >350 cells/mm³, and CD4+ >500 cells/mm³ (Table 2). However, none of these differences was statistically significant. In addition, by using the decision tree model to establish the number of patients from each study group that achieved an optimal immune response (Figure 2), it was possible to infer that pharmaceutical care improves a patient's immune response.

At six months, the intervention group presented with two bacterial, five viral, and two fungal co-infections and, at one year, presented with two bacterial, one viral, two parasitic, and one fungal co-infections. At six months, the control group presented with five bacterial, three viral, two parasitic, and one fungal co-infections, and at one year, presented with one bacterial, five viral, and three parasitic co-infections.

At one year of study, the intervention group spent less per day on appointments, laboratory tests, and hospitalizations, but spent more on procedures and in total than the control group. Moreover, only the intervention group spent on pharmaceutical appointments. Compared with the control group, the intervention group annually generated savings per patient of $3.20 associated with appointments, $23.19 with laboratory tests, and $5.94 with hospitalizations. The intervention group also generated additional annual costs per patient of $50.60 associated with procedures, $12.88 with pharmaceutical appointments, and $31.13 with total costs (Table 3). However, the difference in costs between the groups was not statistically significant. The stark contrast in the costs associated with procedures was caused by two hip surgeries performed on patients from the intervention group, which together added $1,916.09 to the total expenses. This amount corresponds to 48.0% of the total spent on procedures in the first six months of the study ($3,991.04). Excluding the costs of these procedures from the total costs, the results demonstrate that compared with the control group, the intervention group would have spent $19.40 less per patient per year (Table 3).

Cost analysis identified the additional costs associated with procedures and total costs required to achieve each of the clinical outcomes outlined in the study (Table 4). Moreover, we found that, for each $1.00 spent on pharmaceutical care, there was a loss of $1.42 per day. However, when the costs associated with procedures were excluded

Table 2 Co-infection, viral load and CD4+ at baseline, 6 months, and at one year of study

	Control Group N=51			Intervention Group N=51			P value[a]
	Basal % (n)	6 months % (n)	1 year % (n)	Basal % (n)	6 months % (n)	1 year % (n)	
Absence of co-infection	/	72.6 (37)	56.9 (29)	/	76.5 (39)	64.7 (33)	0.092
Viral load <50 copies/ml	60.8 (31)	76.5 (39)	68.6 (35)	64.8 (33)	58.8 (30)	74.5 (38)	0.869
CD4+>200 cells/mm^3	56.9 (29)	68.6 (35)	74.5 (38)	54.9 (28)	70.8 (34)	78.4 (40)	0.793
CD4+>350 cells/mm^3	31.4 (16)	37.3 (19)	49.0 (25)	33.3 (17)	37.5 (18)	51.0 (26)	0.977
CD4+>500 cells/mm^3	15.7 (8)	17.7 (9)	19.6 (10)	17.7 (9)	20.8 (10)	27.5 (14)	0.599

Note: [a]Statistical significance value - Generalized estimating equations (GEE) test.
Abbreviation: CD4+, lymphocyte T CD4+.

from final costs, for each $1.00 spent on pharmaceutical care, there was a benefit of $2.51 per day. No relationship could be identified between the total daily costs generated by the patients and the reductions of pharmacotherapy problems (P =0.292; correlation R =0.15039; Spearman correlation coefficient test), or between the total costs and the number of pharmacist interventions (P =0.706; correlation R = −0.05412; Spearman correlation coefficient test).

Discussion

Pharmaceutical interventions were mostly of the pharmacist-patient type, which prevented therapy compliance errors (i.e., the patients needed clarifications regarding the use of medication, especially regarding dosage, drug interactions, and adherence). This type of intervention can help increase patient adherence to therapy. Hirsch et al. demonstrated in a cohort study with 2,234 patients that patients undergoing pharmaceutical care had greater adherence to antiretroviral therapy than patients not undergoing pharmaceutical care [6].

The decreases observed for all pharmacotherapy problem types are consistent with the literature. Studies have shown that pharmacist interventions can effectively identify, prevent, and solve pharmacotherapeutic problems [24,25]. Problems relating to safety were the most frequently encountered in our study. Other researchers have also identified a high frequency of issues related to inappropriate dosage and safety [5,26-29]. Carcelero et al. demonstrated that the most frequent issues with hospitalized HIV-infected patients are caused by combinations of contraindicated or not recommended drugs and by dosage errors, which happen in approximately one in five patients [5].

During one year of study, compared to the control group, the intervention group showed higher percentage of clinical outcomes, however there was no statistical difference. The better clinical response is associated with slower disease progression and a lower risk of complications, opportunistic infections, and co-infections [1,30-32]. We speculate that owing to these better clinical outcomes,

the intervention group needed less hospitalization, laboratory tests, and medical appointments than the control group did.

Even though the difference in costs between the groups was not statistically significant, we can expect to see an overall, long-term cost analysis for the intervention group due its better clinical outcomes than the control group.

The lower costs associated with appointments and hospitalizations generated by the intervention group, compared with those of the control group, are consistent with the literature. Horberg et al. [13] and McPherson-Baker et al. [33] showed that the pharmacist's presence may decrease the number of appointments and, therefore, the costs for HIV-infected patients. A systematic review that included 32 articles pertaining to the impact of pharmaceutical care on HIV-infected patients showed that pharmaceutical care is associated with cost savings because it decreases the number of physician appointments, hospitalizations, and emergency visits [9]. A study in China found that total hospitalization costs in a group undergoing pharmaceutical care were significantly lower than those in a control group ($1,442.3 [684.9] vs. $1,729.6 [773.7], P <0.001) [34]. Furthermore, a Taiwanese study showed that the replacement of intravenous levofloxacin with its oral form, performed by a pharmacist, decreased hospital stays from 27.2 to 16.1 days (P =0.001), thereby lowering hospital costs [35]. Nevertheless, we found no studies in the literature that described the impact that pharmaceutical care has on the costs associated with laboratory tests and procedures.

In this study, an economic analysis that correlates the effectiveness and the costs of pharmacotherapy demonstrated that pharmaceutical care is dominant (less expensive and more effective), when we consider the effectiveness outcomes and the costs associated with appointments, laboratory tests, and hospitalizations. However, the intervention group generated higher costs associated with procedures and total costs than those of the control group. Furthermore, this study demonstrates

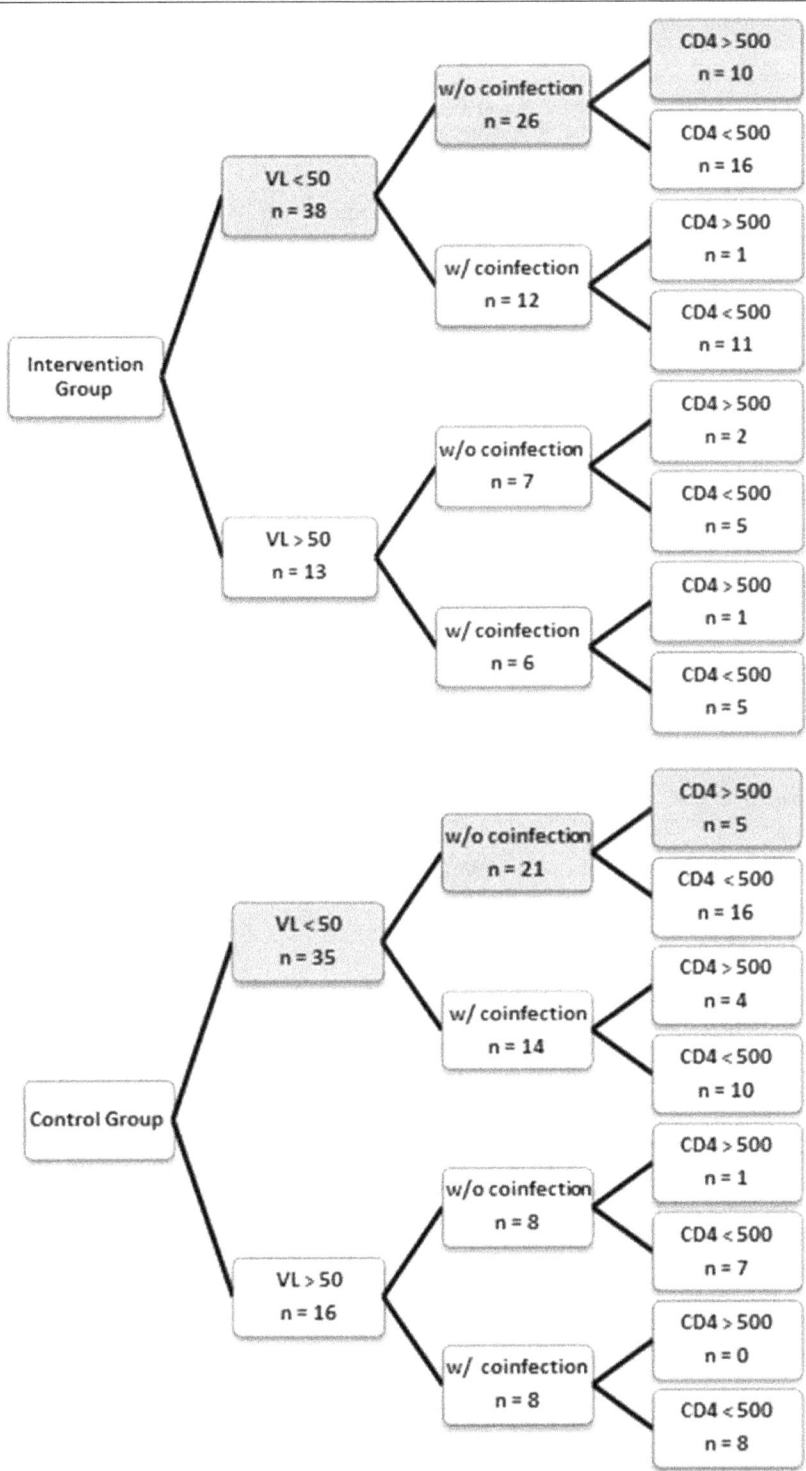

Figure 2 Optimal response immune for control and intervention groups. Abbreviation: CD4, CD4+ lymphocites; VL, viral load; w/o, without; w/, with.

Table 3 Study length of time and total daily costs (US$) for control and intervention groups

Study period	Control Group N=51			Intervention Group N=51		
	6 m (i)	6 m (f)	Final	6 m (i)	6 m (f)	Final
Length of time (mean [SD], days)	180.2[41.8]	190.5[6.4]	370.7[41.3]	196.8[29.3]	190.2[56.4]	387.0[39.8][a]
Appointments						
Total cost (US$) /day	8.65	6.49	**7.53**	8.01	6.12	**7.08**
Individual mean [SD] (US$)	0.17[0.08]	0.13[0.09]	**0.15[0.07]**	0.16[0.09]	0.12[0.08]	**0.14[0.07]**
Laboratory tests						
Total cost (US$) /day	38.07	25.35	**31.48**	33.33	22.96	**28.24**
Individual mean [SD] (US$)	0.75[0.74]	0.50[0.46]	**0.62[0.43]**	0.65[0.61]	0.45[0.43]	**0.55[0.44]**
Procedures						
Total cost (US$) /day	3.75	4.81	**4.29**	20.28	2.11	**11.36**
Individual mean [SD] (US$)	0.07[0.22]	0.09[0.21]	**0.08[0.17]**	0.40[1.11]	0.04[0.09]	**0.22[0.57]**
Hospitalization						
Total cost (US$) /day	2.62	2.53	**2.57**	2.30	1.17	**1.74**
Individual mean [SD] (US$)	0.05[0.30]	0.05[0.18]	**0.05[0.17]**	0.05[0.13]	0.02[0.10]	**0.03[0.09]**
Pharmacist						
Total cost (US$) /day	0.0	0.0	**0.0**	2.20	1.39	**1.80**
Individual mean [SD] (US$)	NA	NA	**NA**	0.05[0.02]	0.03[0.02]	**0.04[0.02]**
Total						
Final cost/day (US$)	53.09	39.18	**45.88**	66.13	33.74	**50.23**
Individual mean [SD] (US$)	1.04[0.99]	0.77[0.70]	**0.90[0.60]**	1.30[1.33]	0.66[0.55]	**1.00[0.81]**
Total excluding procedures						
Final cost/day (US$)	49.34	34.36	**41.58**	45.84	31.63	**38.87**
Individual mean [SD] (US$)	0.97[0.94]	0.67[0.63]	**0.82[0.56]**	0.90[0.71]	0.62[0.05]	**0.77[0.53]**

Note: [a] ANOVA results for repeated measures with a transformation by positions (P=0.057).
Abbreviations: 6m (i), initial 6 months; 6m (f), final 6 months; SD, Standard deviation.
Obs. The cost is the sum of the daily costs for all patients.

the importance of considering the costs associated with procedures. Here, if costs of procedures were disregarded when calculating the daily costs, the total costs of the intervention group would have been lower than those of the control group.

Table 4 Incremental Cost Effectiveness Ratio analysis per day for procedures and total costs (US$)

For each additional outcome of:	ICER (US $/day)	ICER (US$/day)
	Procedures	Total Cost (with procedures)
Viral load <50 copies/ml	2.36	1.45
Absence of co-infection	1.77	1.09
CD4+>200 cells/mm³	3.53	2.18
CD4+>350 cells/mm³	7.07	4.35
CD4+>500 cells/mm³	1.77	1.09
Optimal immune response	1.41	0.87

Abbreviation: ICER, Incremental Cost Effectiveness Ratio.

Cost analysis identified a negative relationship when considering total cost, which contradicts the literature. According to Brennan et al., a $1.00 investment in pharmaceutical care showed a $3.00 return [36]. A meta-analysis demonstrated that 85% of the studies describe positive economic impacts of pharmaceutical care and concluded that the median benefit:cost ratio was 4.68:1 [10]. However, it should be noted that costs associated with laboratory tests and procedures were not included in these studies. In our study, by disregarding the procedures cost, the relationship becomes positive (2.51:1). Inclusion of costs associated with laboratory tests and procedures explains why this study showed different results than the results from the literature, and these differences clarify the need for well-designed studies that include the costs associated with procedures and laboratory tests, for a better understanding of the relationships among pharmaceutical care, HIV-infected patients, and the economy.

Limitations

This study has some limitations. There was no randomization of patients; the pharmacy staff was not blinded; pharmacotherapy problems were not verified for the control group (it was considered unethical to identify pharmacotherapy problems without providing any intervention); and the biggest limitation was our inability to retrieve the costs associated with the use of drugs, due to lack of information in the patient's medical charts. Several studies have analyzed the costs associated with the use of drugs [9,11-13,37] because they make a significant contribution to health care costs, especially in the context of hospital care, which represents 15%–25% of total health care costs. In a study conducted at the Maine Medical Center to guide the use of antibiotics, the pharmacist performed 74 interventions, which reduced the costs associated with antibiotics use, especially by replacing parenteral with oral formulations, generating savings of approximately $400.00 per patient and decreasing the length of hospital stay [38]. Therefore, with more comprehensive patient data, important additional savings regarding the use of drugs to treat co-infections could have been verified, since the intervention group had fewer co-infections than the control group did. For example, tuberculosis is common co-infection among HIV-infected patients and its treatment consists of a combination of rifampicin, isoniazid, and pyrazinamide [32], generating a cost of $316.56 per patient [39].

Conclusion

Our study presents important information about the impact that pharmaceutical care of HIV-infected patients can have on costs associated with procedure and laboratory tests. This information could not be found elsewhere in the literature, which indicates the need for well-designed and more complete studies.

This work demonstrated that pharmaceutical care of HIV-infected patients, for a one-year period, was able to decrease the number of pharmacotherapy problems. In addition, the intervention group presented higher percentage of better clinical outcomes and lower costs associated with appointments, laboratory tests, and hospitalizations than control group, however, there was no statistical difference; and, conversely, higher total costs and costs associated with procedures than those of the control group (no statistical significance). Additional pharmacoeconomic studies focused on pharmaceutical care are necessary to achieve a more comprehensive and reliable analysis.

Competing interests
The authors declare that they have no competing interests.

Authors' contributions
RCC, CGRCM, PGM and PM were responsible for concept and design. RCC and CGRCM collected data. RCC, CGRCM, PGM and PM interpreted data. RCC, MBV and PM were involved in the writing of manuscript. MBV and PM revised the manuscript. All authors read and approved the final manuscript.

Acknowledgments
The researchers would like to thank the hospital medical staff for their support and collaboration during the research, and Coordination for the Improvement of Higher Level Personnel (CAPES) and State of São Paulo Research Foundation (FAPESP) for financial support.

Author details
[1]Department of Clinical Pathology, Faculty of Medical Sciences (FCM), University of Campinas (UNICAMP), Alexander Fleming, 105, 13083-881 Campinas, SP, Brazil. [2]Faculty of Pharmaceutical Sciences (FCF), University of Campinas (UNICAMP), Sérgio Buarque de Holanda, 25, 13083-859 Campinas, SP, Brazil.

References
1. Brazil, Ministry of Health, Secretária de Vigilância em Saúde, Programa Nacional de DST e Aids: Recomendações para Terapia Anti–retroviral em Adultos Infectados pelo HIV 2008 [http://www.ensp.fiocruz.br/portal-ensp/judicializacao/pdfs/491.pdf]
2. Dipiro J, Talbert R, Yees G, Matzke G, Wells B, Posey L: Pharmacotherapy: A Pathophysiologic Approach. 6th edition. Rio de Janeiro: Mcgraw Hill Companie; 2007.
3. Okie S: Fighting HIV-Lessons from Brazil. N Engl J Med 2006, 354:1977–1981.
4. Ma A, Chen DM, Chau FM, Saberi P: Improving adherence and clinical outcomes through an HIV pharmacist's interventions. AIDS Care 2010, 22:1189–1194.
5. Carcelero E, Tuset M, Martin M, De Lazzari E, Codina C, Miró J, Gatell J: Evaluation of antiretroviral-related errors and interventions by the clinical pharmacist in hospitalized HIV-infected patients. HIV Med 2011, 12:494–499.
6. Hirsch J, Gonzales M, Rosenquist A, Miller T, Gilmer T, Best B: Antiretroviral therapy adherence, medication use, and health care costs during 3 years of a community pharmacy medication therapy management program for Medi-Cal beneficiaries with HIV/AIDS. J Manag Care Pharm 2011, 17:213–223.
7. March K, Mak MM, Louie SG: Effects of pharmacists' interventions on patient outcomes in an HIV primary care clinic. Am J Heal Syst Pharm 2007, 64:2574–2578.
8. Mocroft A, Youle M, Moore A, Sabin CA, Madge S, Lepri AC, Tyrer M, Chaloner C, Wilson D, Loveday C, Johnson MA, Phillips AN: Reasons for modification and discontinuation of antiretrovirals: results from a single treatment centre. AIDS 2001, 15:185–194.
9. Saberi P, Dong BJ, Johnson MO, Greenblatt RM, Cocohoba JM: The impact of HIV clinical pharmacists on HIV treatment outcomes: a systematic review. Patient Prefer Adherence 2012, 6:297–322.
10. Schumock GT, Butler MG, Meek PD, Vermeulen LC, Arondekar BV, Bauman JL: Evidence of the economic benefit of clinical pharmacy services: 1996–2000. Pharmacotherapy 2003, 23:113–132.
11. Bozek PS, Perdue BE, Bar-Din M, Weidle PJ: Effect of pharmacist interventions on medication use and cost in hospitalized patients with or without HIV infection. Am J Health Syst Pharm 1998, 55:1151–1155.
12. Engles-Horton LL, Skowronski C, Mostashari F, Altice FL: Clinical guidelines and pharmacist intervention program for HIV-infected patients requiring granulocyte colony-stimulating factor therapy. Pharmacotherapy 1999, 19:356–362.
13. Horberg M, Hurley L, Silverberg M, Kinsman C, Quesenberry C: Effect of clinical pharmacists on utilization of and clinical response to antiretroviral therapy. J Acquir Immune Defic Syndr 2007, 44:531–539.
14. De Rijdt T, Willems L, Simoens S: Economic effects of clinical pharmacy interventions: a literature review. Am J Health Syst Pharm 2008, 65:1161–1172.
15. Areda CA, Bonizio RC, Freitas O: Pharmacoeconomy : an indispensable tool for the rationalization of health costs. Braz J Pharm Sci 2011, 47:231–240.

16. Bavinger C, Bendavid E, Niehaus K, Olshen RA, Olkin I, Sundaram V, Wein N, Holodniy M, Hou N, Owens DK, Desai M: Risk of cardiovascular disease from antiretroviral therapy for HIV : a systematic review. PLoS One 2013, 8:e59551.

17. Dube MP: Disorders of glucose metabolism in patients infected with human immunodeficiency virus. Clin Infect Dis 2000, 31:1467–1475.

18. Friis-Møller N, Sabin CA, Data Collection on Adverse Events of Anti-HIV Drugs (DAD) Study Group, Weber R, D'Arminio Monforte A, El-Sadr WM, Reiss P, Thiébaut R, Morfeldt L, De Wit S, Pradier C, Calvo G, Law MG, Kirk O, Phillips AN, Lundgren JD: Combination antiretroviral therapy and the risk of myocardial infarction. N Engl J Med 2003, 349:1993–2003.

19. Crum-Cianflone N, Roediger MP, Eberly L, Headd M, Marconi V, Ganesan A, Weintrob A, Barthel RV, Fraser S, Infectious Disease Clinical Research Program HIV Working Group, Agan BK: Increasing rates of obesity among HIV-infected persons during the HIV epidemic. PLoS One 2010, 5:e10106.

20. Strand LM, Cipolle RJ, Morley PC: Documenting the clinical pharmacists activities: back to basics. Drug Intell Clin Pharm 1988, 22:63–67.

21. University of Minnesota College of Pharmacy. Pharmacy workup notes [http://www.pharmacy.umn.edu/medmanagenotes/]

22. Molino CGRC, Carnevale RC, Rodrigues AT, Visacri MB, Moriel P, Mazzola PG: Impact of pharmacist interventions on drug-related problems and laboratory markers in outpatients with human immunodeficiency virus infection. Ther Clin Risk Manag 2014, 10:631–639.

23. DATASUS: SGTAP - Sistema de Gerenciamento da Tabela de Procedimentos, Medicamentos e OPM do SUS [http://sigtap.datasus.gov.br/tabela-unificada/app/sec/inicio.jsp].

24. Ruiz I, Olry A, López MA, Prada JL, Causse M: Prospective, randomized, two-arm controlled study to evaluate two interventions to improve adherence to antiretroviral therapy in Spain. Enferm Infecc Microbiol Clin 2010, 28:409–415.

25. Martin S, Wolters P, Calabrese S, Toledo-Tamula MA, Wood LV, Roby G, Elliott-DeSorbo DK: The antiretroviral regimen complexity index. A novel method of quantifying regimen complexity. J Acquir Immune Defic Syndr 2007, 45:535–544.

26. Mok S, Minson Q: Drug-related problems in hospitalized patients with HIV infection. Am J Health Syst Pharm 2008, 65:55–59.

27. Rastegar D, Knight A, Monolakis J: Antiretroviral medication errors among hospitalized patients with HIV infection. Clin Infect Dis 2006, 43:933–938.

28. Pastakia S, Corbett A, Raasch R, Napravnik S, Correll T: Frequency of HIV-related medication errors and associated risk factors in hospitalized patients. Ann Pharmacother 2008, 42:491–497.

29. Misson J, Clark W, Kendall M: Therapeutic advances: protease inhibitors for the treatment of HIV-1 infection. J Clin Pharm Ther 1997, 22:109–117.

30. Osterberg L, Blaschke T: Adherence to medication. N Engl J Med 2005, 353:487–497.

31. Langford SE, Ananworanich J, Cooper DA: Predictors of disease progression in HIV infection : a review. Aids Res Ther 2007, 4:1–14.

32. Brazil, Ministry of Health, Secretaria de Vigilancia em Saúde, Departamento de DST Aids e Hepatites Virais: Boletim Epidemiológico - AIDS e DST. 2012 [http://www.aids.gov.br/sites/default/files/anexos/publicacao/2011/50652/boletim_aids_2011_final_m_pdf_26659.pdf]

33. McPherson-Baker S, Malow RM, Penedo F, Jones DL, Schneiderman N, Klimas NG: Enhancing adherence to combination antiretroviral therapy in non-adherent HIV-positive men. AIDS Care 2000, 12:399–404.

34. Shen J, Sun Q, Zhou X, Wei Y, Qi Y, Zhu J, Yan T: Pharmacist interventions on antibiotic use in inpatients with respiratory tract infections in a Chinese hospital. Int J Clin Pharm 2011, 33(6):929–933.

35. Yen Y-H, Chen H-Y, Wuan-Jin L, Lin Y-M, Shen WC, Cheng K-J: Clinical and economic impact of a pharmacist-managed i.v.-to-p.o. conversion service for levofloxacin in Taiwan. Int J Clin Pharmacol Ther 2012, 50:136–141.

36. Brennan TA, Dollear TJ, Hu M, Matlin OS, Shrank WH, Choudhry NK, Grambley W: An integrated pharmacy-based program improved medication prescription and adherence rates in diabetes patients. Health Aff (Millwood) 2012, 31:120–129.

37. Lee AJ, Boro MS, Knapp KK, Meier JL, Korman NE: Clinical and economic outcomes of pharmacist recommendations in a Veterans Affairs medical center. Am J Health Syst Pharm 2002, 59:2070–2077.

38. Janknegt R, Meer JWM van der: Sequential therapy with intravenous and oral cephalosporins. J Antimicrob Chemother 1994, 33:169–177.

39. Brazilian Health Surveillance Agency (ANVISA): Preços máximos de medicamentos por princípio ativo para compras públicas – monodrogas/ preços fábrica (PF) e preço máximo de venda ao governo (PMVG) [http://portal.anvisa.gov.br/wps/wcm/connect/de29e2004baf729293c5dbbc0f9d5b29/LISTA_CONFORMIDADE_GOV_2012-06-19.pdf?MOD=AJPERES. Accessed July 12, 2014].

8

Genome expression analysis by suppression subtractive hybridization identified overexpression of Humanin, a target gene in gastric cancer chemoresistance

Negar Mottaghi-Dastjerdi[1,2], Mohammad Soltany-Rezaee-Rad[1,2], Zargham Sepehrizadeh[1], Gholamreza Roshandel[3], Farzaneh Ebrahimifard[4] and Neda Setayesh[1*]

Abstract

Background: In cancer cells, apoptosis is an important mechanism that influences the outcome of chemotherapy and the development of chemoresistance. To find the genes involved in chemoresistance and the development of gastric cancer, we used the suppression subtractive hybridization method to identify the genes that are overexpressed in gastric cancer tissues compared to normal gastric tissues.

Results: In the suppression subtractive hybridization library we constructed, the most highly overexpressed genes were humanin isoforms. Humanin is a recently identified endogenous peptide that has anti-apoptotic activity and has been selected for further study due to its potential role in the chemoresistance of gastric cancer. Upregulation of humanin isoforms was also observed in clinical samples by using quantitative real-time PCR. Among the studied isoforms, humanin isoform 3, with an expression level of 4.166 ± 1.44 fold, was the most overexpressed isoform in GC.

Conclusions: The overexpression of humanin in gastric cancer suggests a role for chemoresistance and provides new insight into the biology of gastric cancer. We propose that humanin isoforms are novel targets for combating chemoresistance in gastric cancer.

Keywords: Apoptosis, Chemoresistance, Gastric cancer, Suppression subtractive hybridization, Humanin

Background

Gastric cancer (GC) is the fourth most common type of malignancy and the second leading cause of cancer mortality, which has increased in developing countries [1,2]. Different genetic and epigenetic alterations are involved in the development of GC which include alterations in oncogenes (*c-erbB2*), tumor suppressor genes (*p53*), DNA repair genes (*hMLH1*), cell cycle regulators (*cyclin E*), and signaling molecules (*TGFB1/2*) [3,4]. Identification of the molecular mechanisms that contribute to the pathogenesis of GC could help us find targets for early diagnosis, classification, and treatment of it [2]. Although some gene alterations have been identified in GC, the fundamental

molecular mechanisms leading to it need to be elucidated [5-7]. Finding the genes that are differentially expressed in GC is one of the best approaches in establishing new biomarkers and therapeutic targets. In addition, these studies could improve our knowledge about molecular biology and carcinogenesis of GC.

Chemotherapy has been an important treatment for gastrointestinal cancers [2], although its success rate is limited due to chemoresistance (e.g. resistance to cisplatin, 5-fluorouracil, mitomycin C or doxorubicin). It is widely accepted that the apoptotic capacity of cancer cells is critical in determining its response to chemotherapeutic agents. The anti-apoptotic nature of cancer cells becomes a mechanism in its chemoresistance, and allows the tumor to survive [8,9]. In addition cell survival processes have an important role in chemoresistance; autophagy has been identified in chemoresistance and is

* Correspondence: nsetayesh@tums.ac.ir
[1]Department of Pharmaceutical Biotechnology and Pharmaceutical Biotechnology Research Center, School of Pharmacy, Tehran University of Medical Sciences, Tehran 1417614411, Iran
Full list of author information is available at the end of the article

known as a survival factor for tumor cells in the early stages of carcinogenesis. Autophagy is increased by the level of stress but the resulting event varies which could either lead to survival by inhibition of autophagy or to an apoptotic cell death [10]. Many high throughput studies have documented the genes alterations in GC [3,4], although they failed to encompass a complete view of their molecular pathogenesis and chemoresistance. Along with these studies, towards establishing more data about the genes alterations in GC, our research used suppression subtractive hybridization (SSH), a high throughput gene expression analysis method: this requires no prior knowledge about gene selection. The SSH is a method of selective amplification of differentially expressed sequences, which overcomes the technical drawbacks of traditional subtraction methods. Some of the advantages of the SSH method include minute amounts of required initial mRNA, elimination of the need for physical separation of single- and double-stranded molecules, equalization of the abundance of mRNA sequences within the target population and suitable for detection of rare transcripts [11].

In our study, among the identified genes from the constructed SSH library, we found four isoforms of Humanin (HN, HN1 [EMBL: CR612552, GenBank: AC131055, Swiss-Prot: P0CJ68], HN3 [EMBL: AL109955, GenBank: AL135939, Swiss-Prot: P0CJ70], HN6 [EMBL: AC231380, GenBank: AC231380, Swiss-Prot: P0CJ73], and HN10 [EMBL: AL158819, GenBank: AL158819, Swiss-Prot: P0CJ77]) as the overexpressed genes in GC. While it has been demonstrated that Humanin (HN) bears an endogenous synthesis source [12], the precise origin of its gene (or genes) is not specified [13]. HN is a recently identified endogenous peptide that protects cells against cytotoxicity and suppresses apoptosis caused by various stimuli, e.g., serum deprivation, UV irradiation, or staurosporine [13]. The cytoprotective effects of HN seems to be through various mechanisms including its antiapoptotic, metabolic (improvement of the mitochondrial bioactivity) and anti-inflammatory effects [14]. Furthermore, considering the antiapoptotic effects of HN through its binding to Bax, a Bcl-2 family pro-apoptotic protein [15], HN could mask pro-apoptotic effects of chemotherapy agents.

We provide new information about genes associated with the development of GC, particularly those involved in the chemoresistance of cancer cells: this can have a significant influence on treatment for this type of cancer that could be considered as a target in drug discovery in combating chemoresistance in gastric cancer, which typically has a poor prognosis.

Methods
Tissue sample preparation
In establishing the main SSH library, both normal and tumor gastric tissues were collected from a 64-year-old

male patient during surgery. A pathologist dissected the target tissues under the microscope with special care for minimal contamination of nonepithelial cells, and RNA*later*® (Ambion, Austin, TX, USA) was used to stabilize the RNA during storage. Hematoxylin–eosin (H&E) staining was done on the tissue to determine the tumor type and its degree of invasion.

In order to check the expression of the differentially expressed genes by quantitative real-time PCR (qRT-PCR), ten clinical tissue samples (five tumor and five normal samples) were collected from patients with endoscopy: all samples were obtained prior to chemotherapy. The consent form of The Biologic Sampling Ethics Committee, Tehran University of Medical Sciences (TUMS) was received from each patient before surgery or endoscopy.

Total RNA extraction
Total RNA was extracted from tissues with the TriPure Isolation Reagent (Roche Applied Science, Indianapolis, IN, USA). Its concentration and purity were analyzed using the Biophotometer (Eppendorf, Hamburg, GY), and its integrity was visually checked with 1% denatured agarose gel.

mRNA isolation
Isolation of mRNA was done with the DynaBead® mRNA Isolation Kit (Dynal, Lake Success, NY, USA). Briefly, the appropriate amount of DynaBeads oligo (dT)$_{25}$ was equilibrated with 100 µl of binding buffer (100 mM Tris–HCl, 500 mM LiCl, 10 mM EDTA, 1% LiDS, and 5 mM DTT). Diluted total RNA and equilibrated DynaBeads were then mixed and incubated for 5 min at 37°C in a shaking incubator. The beads were washed twice using 200 µl of washing buffer (10 mM Tris–HCl, 0.15 M LiCl, and 1 mM of EDTA). 10 µl of elution buffer was added to the DynaBeads and incubated for 2 min at 67°C. The DynaBeads were placed on the magnet, and the eluted mRNA in supernatant was then isolated. The purified mRNA was checked with 1% denatured agarose gel.

Suppression subtractive hybridization (SSH)
Using the SSH method, the subtracted library can be created from one sample pair (including cancerous and normal tissues) in both forward and reverse directions, while the expression of the achieved genes are checked in clinical tissue samples with analysis methods that included qRT-PCR [16]. In this study, SSH was carried out with the PCR-Select™ cDNA Subtraction Kit (Clontech, Palo Alto, CA, USA) according to the manufacturer's protocol. In summary, first- and second-strand cDNA were synthesized using 2 µg mRNA from the gastric cancerous (tester) and normal (driver) tissues, and digested with *Rsa* I. For the reverse subtraction, the tester was used as driver, and the driver was used as

tester. Tester cDNA was subdivided into two portions, and special adaptors were added to each. After two hybridizations between the tester and driver (towards eliminating non-altered genes in the two samples), the remaining differentially expressed sequences were amplified with two PCR rounds using *Pwo* enzyme to reduce any background products and to enrich the differentially expressed sequences. For identification of the differentially overexpressed genes, the constructed library (products of the secondary PCR step of SSH) was then cloned and sequenced as the following steps.

Cloning and confirmation of the positive clones

The secondary PCR product of the SSH method was purified with the PCR Product Purification Kit (Roche Applied Sciences, Indianapolis, IN, USA), cloned into pUC19 plasmid vectors and transformed into *Escherichia coli* NovaBlue competent cells (Novagen, Madison, WI, USA). Randomly selected positive colonies were first confirmed with a colony PCR, using N1 and N2R primers (Table 1). Plasmids from the confirmed positive clones were isolated by the High Pure Plasmid Isolation Kit (Roche Applied Sciences, Indianapolis, IN, USA) and used in single direction DNA sequencing with the BigDye Terminator Version 3.1 Sequencing Kit and a 3730xl Automated Sequencer (Applied Biosystems, Foster City, CA, USA). To identify these sequences, similarity searches were carried out with BLAST (http://blast.ncbi.nlm.nih.gov/Blast.cgi).

Analysis of the subtraction efficiency

Real-time PCR was used to estimate the efficiency of subtraction by comparing the abundance of a non-differentially expressed gene (a housekeeping gene: beta actin) before and after subtraction. Reactions were prepared by adding 10 µl of SYBR Premix Ex Taq (Takara, Kusatsu, Japan), 1 µl of the sample, 0.8 µl of the primers (10 µM), 0.4 µl of ROX dye and DEPC-treated water to a final volume of 20 µl. The thermal program for the reaction cycles was 10 min at 95°C, followed by 40 cycles of 30 sec at 95°C, and 1 min at 60°C. Melting curve analysis was done by increasing the temperature from 65°C to 95°C in 0.1°C/sec increments for each fluorescence acquisition, using the Step-One-Plus Apparatus (Applied Biosystems, Foster City, CA, USA). Relative expression of the beta actin gene in the subtracted and non-subtracted samples was used in the calculation of subtraction efficiency.

Quantitative real-time PCR (qRT-PCR)

Quantitative expression analysis was performed with real-time PCR (Applied Biosystems, Foster City, CA, USA) for the SSH-identified HN isoforms. Primer design was done with PrimerSelect, Version 7.1.0 (DNAstar, Madison, WI, USA) and synthesized by the TAG Company (TAG Copenhagen, Copenhagen, Denmark) (Table 1). The qRT-PCR was run with SYBR Premix Ex Taq (Takara, Kusatsu, Japan) in a final volume of 20 µl, containing 2X master mix 10 µl, each with forward and reverse primers (10 µM) 1 µl, ROX dye II 0.4 µl, and cDNA 2 µl.

The PCR thermocycle program was set at 95°C for 10 min followed by 40 cycles of 95°C for 30 sec, 62°C for 30 sec. Melt curve analysis followed the PCR step and increased the temperature from 65°C to 95°C, with 0.1°C/sec increments in each fluorescence reading.

Statistical analysis

The relative gene expression of HN isoforms in tumor and normal tissues was analyzed using the Livak method [17]. The statistical significance was set at $P < 0.05$.

Results

Histological examination

Histological results indicated that the tumor was a moderately differentiated, mucin-producing type of gastric adenocarcinoma, located in the prepyloric area. Local

Table 1 Designed primers sequences used to quantify gene expression by real-time PCR

Primer name	Accession number	Length	Sequence (5′ to 3′)	Annealing temp	Location	Product size
HN1-F	NM_001190452.1	20	CGCAGGCCCTAAACTACCAG	61°C	1091-1110	206 bp
HN1-R	NM_001190452.1	20	TGCTACTGTCGATGTGGACC		1277-1296	
HN3-F	NM_001190472.1	20	GGTGATAGCTGGCTGGCTTA	59°C	180-199	164 bp
HN3-R	NM_001190472.1	20	ATTAGTGGCTGCTTTTGGGC		324-343	
HN6-F	NM_001190487.1	20	TTTACCCAGGCGCAGTGGAC	62°C	60-79	247 bp
HN6-R	NM_001190487.1	22	GGCTCAGTAGGCTTATCACCAC		285-306	
HN10-F	NM_001190708.1	23	CGAGAAGACCCTATGTATGGAGC	61°C	603-625	137 bp
HN10-R	NM_001190708.1	20	AGGTTGCTCGGAGGTTGAAT		720-739	
N1	Based Ligated Adaptor	22	TCGAGCGGCCGCCCGGGCAGGT	68°C		
N2-R	Based Ligated Adaptor	20	AGCGTGGTCGCGGCCGAGGT			
ACTB-F	NM_001101.3	21	ATGGCCACGGCTGCTTCCAGC	60°C	763-783	322 bp
ACTB-R	NM_001101.3	21	CAGGAGGAGCAATGATCTTGA		1064-1084	

invasion to the lymph node was observed in two of the six pre-gastric lymph nodes (Figure 1).

Suppression subtractive hybridization (SSH)

Cloning of the two subtracted libraries (forward and reverse), ranged from 100–800 base pairs in size (Figure 2A), resulted in 120 clones. Among the overexpressed genes from the forward library, three clones had sequences, which were identical to four isoforms of HN; HN1, HN3, HN6, and HN10. They were selected for qRT-PCR analysis due to their probable role in the chemoresistance of GC cells.

Subtraction efficiency

Real-time PCR analysis demonstrated that beta actin has an 8.9-fold reduction in the subtracted library, compared with the non-subtracted library (Figure 2B). This resulting reduction verified the accuracy of the applied method in finding differentially expressed genes in GC.

Quantitative real-time PCR (qRT-PCR)

To confirm the results obtained from the constructed SSH library, relative gene expression of HN isoforms was checked in some endoscopic tissue samples. The results showed overexpression of HN isoforms in clinical tissue samples (Figure 3). These results confirmed the efficiency of the SSH library, which also indicated that these isoforms were significantly overexpressed in GC. Between the studied isoforms, HN3 with an expression level of 4.166 ± 1.44 fold was the most overexpressed isoform in GC.

Discussion

This study focused on the overexpressed genes associated with gastric adenocarcinoma as the most prevalent and life-threatening type of cancer in Iran [18]. Chemoresistance of tumor cells is a therapeutic defeat that affects treatment outcomes with cancer [19]. Development of resistance is a common occurrence in GC, with apoptosis considered to be one of the major mechanisms in tumorigenesis and chemoresistance of cells [9,19].

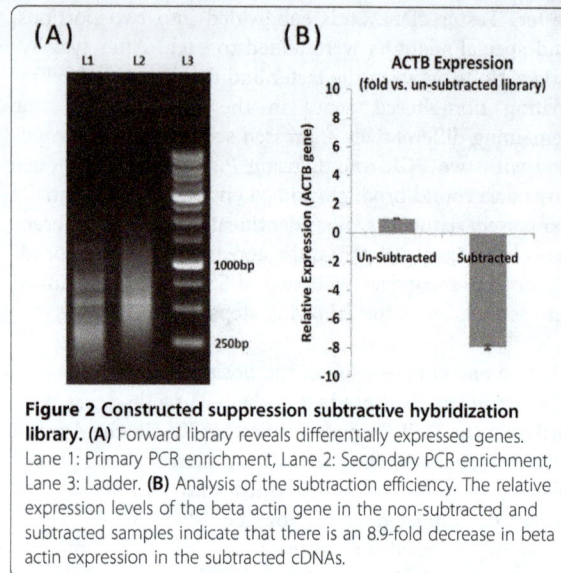

Figure 2 Constructed suppression subtractive hybridization library. (A) Forward library reveals differentially expressed genes. Lane 1: Primary PCR enrichment, Lane 2: Secondary PCR enrichment, Lane 3: Ladder. **(B)** Analysis of the subtraction efficiency. The relative expression levels of the beta actin gene in the non-subtracted and subtracted samples indicate that there is an 8.9-fold decrease in beta actin expression in the subtracted cDNAs.

Two important mechanisms involved in this resistance are the loss of pro-apoptotic signals and the gain of anti-apoptotic mechanisms [20].

Using SSH in this study, HN isoforms, the anti-apoptotic endogenous peptides with a potential role in the chemoresistance of GC cells were identified. Furthermore, upregulation of identified HN isoforms were confirmed using qRT-PCR. The importance of this study is the specific isoforms of HN identified as the overexpressed genes in GC (HN isoforms 1, 3, 6 and 10). Due to the high similarities between HN isoforms and lack of isoform-specific antibodies, detection of HN isoforms at the protein level by western blotting or IHC was not provided in this study.

Our study identified the HN gene as an overexpressed gene in GC. It is a newly discovered 24-amino acid peptide; with 75 bases in an open reading frame and 950 bases downstream of the 5′ end of the HN cDNA (HN cDNA is 99% similar to mitochondrial DNA) [21,22].

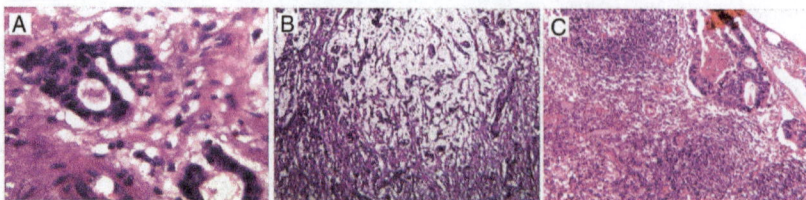

Figure 1 Histological features of the resected gastric cancerous tissue stained by H&E to determine the cancer type and metastasis. (A) Tubular structure formation, which characterizes these cancerous cells as an adenocarcinoma tumor type. **(B)** Mucin producing type of GC could be determined by the white matrix surrounded the cancerous cells. **(C)** Cross-sectional analysis of a pre-gastric lymph node. The tubular formation of the gastric adenocarcinoma cells and lymph node follicles could be observed.

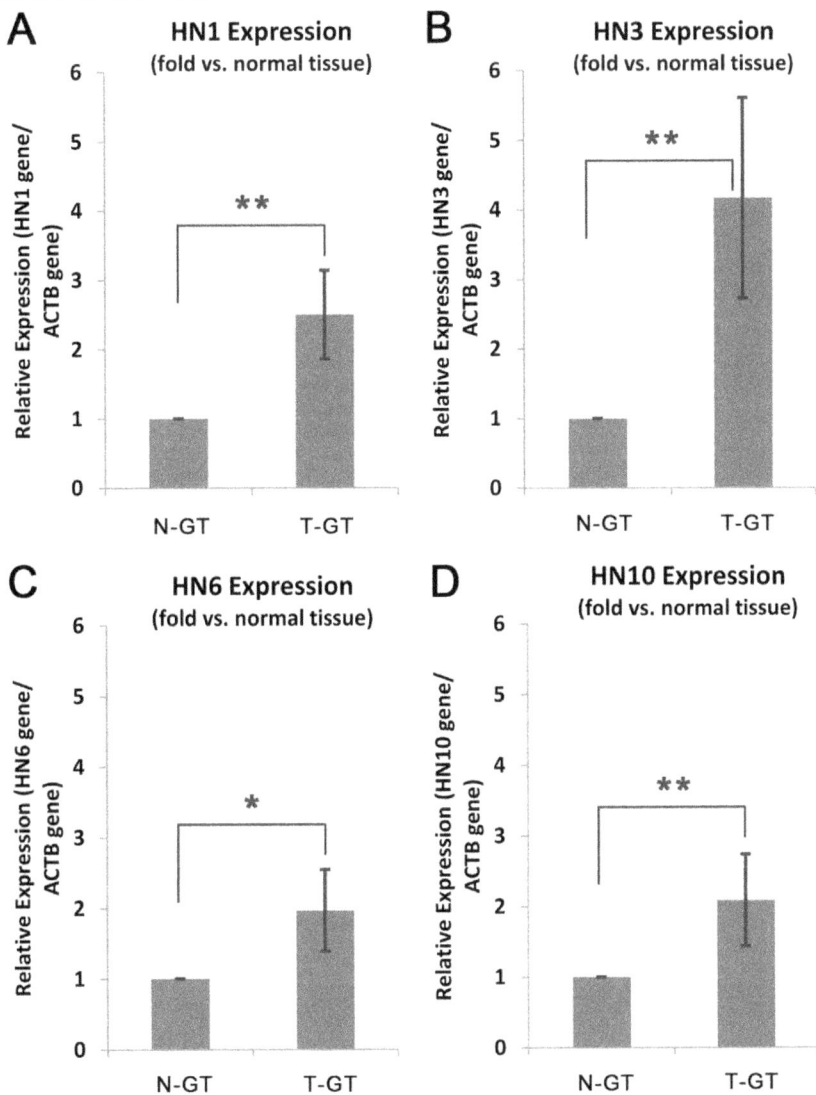

Figure 3 Relative gene expression analysis of HN isoforms in normal and tumor tissue samples, using qRT-PCR. **(A)** HN1 isoform. **(B)** HN3 isoform. **(C)** HN6 isoform. **(D)** HN10 isoform. N-GT: normal gastric tissue, T-GT: tumor gastric tissue. Whiskers represent the STDEV of expression in samples (n = 10). *P < 0.05, **P < 0.01.

Recently, studies have shown that HN is specifically bound to BAX, tBID, and BimEL and executes its anti-apoptotic activity through selective attachment to BAX and translocation inhibition of BAX to the mitochondria [15,23,24]. There have been many *in vitro* studies demonstrating the protective characteristic of HN in different cell types [25-29]. The results suggest that HN could increase the energy produced by mitochondria [30]. Furthermore, HN could similarly increase the ATP- vs. pyrovate-biogenesis, which leads to the assumption that HN may have an important role in mitochondrial dysfunction-related diseases, including cancer [23,30,31]. HN overexpression in GC

could be related to stress in a microenvironment of cancer cells (e.g., nutrient deprivation) that triggers apoptosis [24]. Cancer cells, along with the upregulation of the HN gene as an anti-apoptotic factor, combated apoptosis in them. In addition, nutrient deprivation and continuous cell division demanded additional energy resources. In this way, HN as a function of ATP production in cancer cells could diminish metabolic stresses.

Our results showed that HN3, with a 4.166 ± 1.44 -fold increase in GC tissues, is the dominant isoform. HN isoforms have a unique coding sequence for the HN peptide. Various isoforms in the HN gene with different 5′-UTR and 3′-UTR might have probable roles in the stability of its peptide. Peptides with the highest stability, with increased residence time in cancer cells, could also have more influence in tumorigenesis and chemoresistance [32].

Our results suggest that upregulation of HN in GC could be an important molecular event in its tumorigenesis. Given its anti-apoptotic activity in cancer cells, it could be one of the fundamental mechanisms in chemoresistance of GC cells: upregulation of HN alleviates metabolic stresses by ATP production which could have an important role in the early stages of tumorigenesis. HN can potentially serve as a new biomarker in the diagnosis of GC since it is present in blood circulation. To date, HN was not considered a key gene in the chemoresistance of tumor cells; future studies that target HN in gastric chemoresistance cells may have a valuable impact on the therapeutic modality used for this cancer.

Conclusions

In conclusion, using the SSH method, the overexpression of HN 1, 3, 6, and 10 isoforms were identified for the first time in gastric cancer cells. Considering the fundamental role of anti-apoptosis in the chemoresistance of cancer cells and the high expression level of HN in GC, further studies are needed to evaluate the role of HN isoforms and chemoresistance. In addition, since overexpression of HN isoforms could lead to chemoresistance in GC this gene could be a candidate in drug discovery investigations for targeting chemoresistance in this cancer.

Competing interests
All authors declare that they have no competing interests.

Authors' contributions
NMD carried out the construction of suppression subtractive hybridization and helped to draft the manuscript. MSRR carried out the qRT-PCR analysis. NS participated in study design and helped to draft the manuscript. GR participated in collecting endoscopic normal and tumor tissues. FE participated in resection of SSH pair samples (tumor and normal tissues) by surgery. ZS conceived of the study, and participated in its design and coordination and helped to draft the manuscript. All authors read and approved the final manuscript.

Acknowledgment
This study was supported by Grant No. 1192 from the Research Council of the Tehran University of Medical Sciences.

Author details
[1]Department of Pharmaceutical Biotechnology and Pharmaceutical Biotechnology Research Center, School of Pharmacy, Tehran University of Medical Sciences, Tehran 1417614411, Iran. [2]Pharmaceutical Sciences Research Center, Sari School of Pharmacy, Mazandaran University of Medical Sciences, Sari, Iran. [3]Golestan Research Center of Gastroenterology and Hepatology, Golestan University of Medical Sciences, Golestan, Iran. [4]Department of General Surgery, School of Medicine, Shahid Beheshti University of Medical Sciences, Tehran, Iran.

References
1. Bray F, Ren JS, Masuyer E, Ferlay J: Global estimates of cancer prevalence for 27 sites in the adult population in 2008. *Int J Cancer* 2013, **132**(5):1133–1145.
2. Layke JC, Lopez PP: Gastric cancer: diagnosis and treatment options. *Am Fam Physician* 2004, **69**(5):1133.
3. Yamashita K, Sakuramoto S, Watanabe M: Genomic and epigenetic profiles of gastric cancer: potential diagnostic and therapeutic applications. *Surg Today* 2011, **41**(1):24–38.
4. Nagini S: Carcinoma of the stomach: a review of epidemiology, pathogenesis, molecular genetics and chemoprevention. *World J Gastrointest Oncol* 2012, **4**(7):156.
5. Hussein NR: Helicobacter pylori and gastric cancer in the Middle East: a new enigma? *WJG* 2010, **16**(26):3226.
6. Wu CW, Chen GD, Fann CSJ, Lee AFY, Chi CW, Liu JM, Weier U, Chen JY: Clinical implications of chromosomal abnormalities in gastric adenocarcinomas. *Genes Chromosom Cancer* 2002, **35**(3):219–231.
7. Hou Q, Wu YH, Grabsch H, Zhu Y, Leong SH, Ganesan K, Cross D, Tan LK, Tao J, Gopalakrishnan V: Integrative genomics identifies RAB23 as an invasion mediator gene in diffuse-type gastric cancer. *Cancer Res* 2008, **68**(12):4623–4630.
8. Wilson T, Longley D, Johnston P: Chemoresistance in solid tumours. *Ann Oncol* 2006, **17**(suppl 10):315–324.
9. Oki E, Baba H, Tokunaga E, Nakamura T, Ueda N, Futatsugi M, Mashino K, Yamamoto M, Ikebe M, Kakeji Y, Maehara Y: Akt phosphorylation associates with LOH of PTEN and leads to chemoresistance for gastric cancer. *Int J Cancer* 2005, **117**(3):376–380.
10. Tyson JJ, Baumann WT, Chen C, Verdugo A, Tavassoly I, Wang Y, Weiner LM, Clarke R: Dynamic modelling of oestrogen signalling and cell fate in breast cancer cells. *Nat Rev Cancer* 2011, **11**(7):523–532.
11. Diatchenko L, Lau Y, Campbell AP, Chenchik A, Moqadam F, Huang B, Lukyanov S, Lukyanov K, Gurskaya N, Sverdlov ED: Suppression subtractive hybridization: a method for generating differentially regulated or tissue-specific cDNA probes and libraries. *Proc Natl Acad Sci* 1996, **93**(12):6025–6030.
12. Tajima H, Niikura T, Hashimoto Y, Ito Y, Kita Y, Terashita K, Yamazaki K, Koto A, Aiso S, Nishimoto I: Evidence for in vivo production of Humanin peptide, a neuroprotective factor against Alzheimer's disease-related insults. *Neurosci Lett* 2002, **324**(3):227–231.
13. Bodzioch M, Lapicka-Bodzioch K, Zapala B, Kamysz W, Kiec-Wilk B, Dembinska-Kiec A: Evidence for potential functionality of nuclearly-encoded humanin isoforms. *Genomics* 2009, **94**(4):247–256.
14. Zapala B, Kaczynski L, Kiec-Wilk B, Staszel T, Knapp A, Thoresen GH, Wybranska I, Dembinska-Kiec A: Humanins, the neuroprotective and cytoprotective peptides with antiapoptotic and anti-inflammatory properties. *Pharmacol Rep* 2010, **62**(5):767–777.
15. Guo B, Zhai D, Cabezas E, Welsh K, Nouraini S, Satterthwait AC, Reed JC: Humanin peptide suppresses apoptosis by interfering with Bax activation. *Nature* 2003, **423**(6938):456–461.
16. Diatchenko L, Lukyanov S, Lau Y-FC, Siebert PD: [20] Suppression subtractive hybridization: a versatile method for identifying differentially expressed genes. *Methods Enzymol* 1999, **303**:349–380.
17. Livak KJ, Schmittgen TD: Analysis of relative gene expression data using real-time quantitative PCR and the $2^{-\Delta\Delta C_T}$ Method. *Methods* 2001, **25**(4):402–408.
18. Malekzadeh R, Derakhshan MH, Malekzadeh Z: Gastric cancer in Iran: epidemiology and risk factors. *Arch Iran Med* 2009, **12**(6):576–583.
19. Hajra KM, Tan L, Liu JR: Defective apoptosis underlies chemoresistance in ovarian cancer. In *Ovarian Cancer. Volume 622*. Edited by Coukos G, Berchuck A, Ozols R. New York: Springer; 2008:197–208.
20. Reuter S, Eifes S, Dicato M, Aggarwal BB, Diederich M: Modulation of anti-apoptotic and survival pathways by curcumin as a strategy to induce apoptosis in cancer cells. *Biochem Pharmacol* 2008, **76**(11):1340–1351.
21. Lee C, Yen K, Cohen P: Humanin: a harbinger of mitochondrial-derived peptides? *Trends Endocrinol Metab* 2013.
22. Nishimoto I, Matsuoka M, Niikura T: Unravelling the role of Humanin. *Trends Mol Med* 2004, **10**(3):102–105.

23. Yen K, Lee C, Mehta H, Cohen P: The emerging role of the mitochondrial-derived peptide humanin in stress resistance. *J Mol Endocrinol* 2013, **50**(1):R11–R19.

24. Kariya S, Takahashi N, Ooba N, Kawahara M, Nakayama H, Ueno S: **Humanin inhibits cell death of serum-deprived PC12h cells.** *Neuroreport* 2002, **13**(6):903–907.

25. Hashimoto Y, Ito Y, Niikura T, Shao Z, Hata M, Oyama F, Nishimoto I: **Mechanisms of neuroprotection by a novel rescue factor humanin from Swedish mutant amyloid precursor protein.** *Biochem Biophys Res Commun* 2001, **283**(2):460–468.

26. Hashimoto Y, Niikura T, Chiba T, Tsukamoto E, Kadowaki H, Nishitoh H, Yamagishi Y, Ishizaka M, Yamada M, Nawa M: **The cytoplasmic domain of Alzheimer's amyloid-β protein precursor causes sustained apoptosis signal-regulating kinase 1/c-Jun NH2-terminal kinase-mediated neurotoxic signal via dimerization.** *J Pharmacol Exp Ther* 2003, **306**(3):889–902.

27. Ikonen M, Liu B, Hashimoto Y, Ma L, Lee K-W, Niikura T, Nishimoto I, Cohen P: **Interaction between the Alzheimer's survival peptide humanin and insulin-like growth factor-binding protein 3 regulates cell survival and apoptosis.** *Proc Natl Acad Sci* 2003, **100**(22):13042–13047.

28. Jung SS, Van Nostrand WE: **Humanin rescues human cerebrovascular smooth muscle cells from Aβ-induced toxicity.** *J Neurochem* 2003, **84**(2):266–272.

29. Wang D, Li H, Yuan H, Zheng M, Bai C, Chen L: **Humanin delays apoptosis in K562 cells by downregulation of P38 MAP kinase.** *Apoptosis* 2005, **10**(5):963–971.

30. Kariya S, Takahashi N, Hirano M, Ueno S: **Humanin improves impaired metabolic activity and prolongs survival of serum-deprived human lymphocytes.** *Mol Cell Biochem* 2003, **254**(1–2):83–89.

31. Kariya S, Hirano M, Furiya Y, Ueno S: **Effect of humanin on decreased ATP levels of human lymphocytes harboring A3243G mutant mitochondrial DNA.** *Neuropeptides* 2005, **39**(2):97–101.

32. Audic Y, Hartley RS: **Post-transcriptional regulation in cancer.** *Biol Cell* 2004, **96**(7):479–498.

9

Development of MY-DRG casemix pharmacy service weights in UKM Medical Centre in Malaysia

Saad Ahmed Ali Jadoo[1,2*], Syed Mohamed Aljunid[2], Amrizal Muhammad Nur[2], Zafar Ahmed[2] and Dexter Van Dort[3]

Abstract

Background: The service weight is among several issues and challenges in the implementation of case-mix in developing countries, including Malaysia. The aim of this study is to develop the Malaysian Diagnosis Related Group (MY-DRG) case-mix pharmacy service weight in University Kebangsaan Malaysia-Medical Center (UKMMC) by identifying the actual cost of pharmacy services by MY-DRG groups in the hospital.

Methods: All patients admitted to UKMMC in 2011 were recruited in this study. Combination of Step-down and Bottom-up costing methodology has been used in this study. The drug and supplies cost; the cost of staff; the overhead cost; and the equipment cost make up the four components of pharmacy. Direct costing approach has been employed to calculate Drugs and supplies cost from electronic-prescription system; and the inpatient pharmacy staff cost, while the overhead cost and the pharmacy equipments cost have been calculated indirectly from MY-DRG data base. The total pharmacy cost was obtained by summing the four pharmacy components' cost per each MY-DRG. The Pharmacy service weight of a MY-DRG was estimated by dividing the average pharmacy cost of the investigated MY-DRG on the average of a specified MY-DRG (which usually the average pharmacy cost of all MY-DRGs).

Results: Drugs and supplies were the main component (86.0%) of pharmacy cost compared o overhead cost centers (7.3%), staff cost (6.5%) and pharmacy equipments (0.2%) respectively. Out of 789 inpatient MY-DRGs case-mix groups, 450 (57.0%) groups were utilized by the UKMMC. Pharmacy service weight has been calculated for each of these 450 MY-DRGs groups. MY-DRG case-mix group of Lymphoma & Chronic Leukemia group with severity level three (C-4-11-III) has the highest pharmacy service weight of 11.8 equivalents to average pharmacy cost of RM 5383.90. While the MY-DRG case-mix group for Circumcision with severity level one (V-1-15-I) has the lowest pharmacy service weight of 0.04 equivalents to average pharmacy cost of RM 17.83.

Conclusion: A mixed approach which is based partly on top-down and partly on bottom up costing methodology has been recruited to develop MY-DRG case-mix pharmacy service weight for 450 groups utilized by the UKMMC in 2011.

Keywords: Diagnosis related groups, Pharmacy, Service weight, Malaysia

Background

Drug costs constitute the majority of health system pharmacy budgets and continue to increase faster than other health care expenditures [1]. It is accounting for more than 15.2% of total health expenditure in the world in 2000 [2] and almost a fifth of all health spending on average across OECD countries [3]. In 2006, Pharmaceutical spending ranges from a mean of (19.7% to 30.4%) in the high-income countries and the low-income countries respectively as a share of total health expenditure [4]. However, one third of the world population lacks reliable access to essential drugs [2].

Falkenberg and Tomson [5] indicated that "around 50% of all medicines worldwide are prescribed, dispensed, or sold inappropriately". These inefficient and ineffective uses of medicines make it continuously a target for cost control, management evaluation and policy regulation [1,6].

* Correspondence: drsaadalezzi@gemail.com
[1]United Nations University-International Institute for Global Health (UNU-IIGH), Kuala Lumpur, Malaysia
[2]International Centre for Case-Mix and Clinical Coding (ITCC), University Kebangsaan Malaysia Medical Centre, Jalan Yaacob Latiff, 56000 Cheras, Kuala Lumpur, Malaysia
Full list of author information is available at the end of the article

The development of Diagnosis Related group (DRG) in 1960s as a system comparing resource utilization across groups of patients with the same principal diagnosis greatly facilitated pharmacoeconomic evaluation [7]. The major determinant of pharmacy expenditure in any health institution is the patient complexity, so for a more effective drug costs control, methods for case mix adjustment should be considered [8].

Today more than 40 countries worldwide implemented case-mix system for various purposes and in varying levels [9,10]. The importance of the Case mix and associated cost weights is directly proportional with the increasing demand for the development of new hospital funding methodologies in many countries. The integrity of both the case-mix grouper algorithm employed and the associated relative cost weights has a direct impact on the integrity of these new funding methodologies. While, the calculation of cost weights and the development of a case-mix grouper depends on the availability of patient level case cost [11,12].

Cost is the resources spent to generate the benefits. Resources may be in the form of money, time, labour or other resources used to produce a product such as health services. However, the calculation of actual costs is not easy issue and commonly it is based on best estimates and averages across the hospital system. It was noted that during the implementation of case-mix based payment systems the attention was focused on the coding and generation of accurate and comprehensive DRG activity data. This interest is mainly because the methodologies analyzing activity patterns are well established and standards for DRG classification and coding are well documented, as well as the accurate patient's records that have been properly coded into grouper make the case-mix data quite acceptable for the purpose of defining hospital production. Thus, the costing of hospital services including the pharmacy is often neglected unintentionally. The price is different to cost, but without the understanding of costs, pricing is not possible. If prices are difficult to set, then payment models that fairly pay for what hospitals produce cannot be formulated [13,14].

UKMMC is one of the leading hospitals in Malaysia that implemented the case-mix system in 2002, as an appropriated provider payment mechanism, in line with continues national health reform process towards the provision of equitable and efficient health services [15]. "Cost weights or the relative weights are an important component of prospective payment system, since they provide the variation in payment levels that reflect the relative resources required for visits within each classification group" [16]. Cost weight was among several issues and challenges that faced the implementation of casemix in Malaysia [17]. This study aimed to develop the

pharmacy service weights in UKMMC by identifying the pharmacy services and the actual cost of care.

Methodology
Study background
This was a retrospective study with data collected from inpatients pharmacy electronic prescription and the Case-Mix database of University Kebangsaan Malaysia Medical Center (UKMMC) of year 2011. UKMMC was formed as a result of the amalgamation of the Faculty of Medicine and Hospital of University Kebangsaan Malaysia (HUKM) in early 2008. The Centre provides a broad range of teaching and tertiary referral services in over 1050 licensed inpatient beds, supported by extensive outpatient services, in addition to the primary emergency reception centre for the south eastern suburbs of Kuala Lumpur, the capital city of Malaysia. In 2011, there were 384, 496 outpatient and 35, 303 inpatient occasions of services reported in this hospital (i.e. number of admissions or number of admitted patients). The total budget of the UKMMC was in excess of 473 million Malaysian Ringgit (USD 150 million) with a 3453 total number of staff and covered area of 90203.00 (m2). Currently the UKMMC consists of a hospital, Faculty of Medicine, Institute of Medical Molecular Research (UMBI) and affiliated with UKM for teaching undergraduate and post graduate medical students [18,19].

Profile of UKMMC pharmacy
The UKMMC pharmacy is in charge of pharmacy services for all in and outpatients of UKMMC. The total pharmacy budget (drugs and supplies only) of 2011 was in excess of RM 89,870,771 equivalent to USD 28,466,240 (Exchange Rate of 27th August 2014) with a 123 total number of staff and covering area of 2187 (m2). The UKMMC pharmacy office allocated almost 16% (RM 13, 880, 484.98) of the annual pharmacy drugs and supplies budget to inpatient services and recruiting only 16% (20 persons) of the total staff to manage and distribute inpatient services [19].

Sample size and study period
The study used information on the pharmacy costs of all patients admitted to UKMMC from 1st January to 31st December 2011, comprising the 35, 303 separations. The average length of stay (ALOS) of these patients was 5.5 days, representing 193,824 days of patient care [19].

DRG assignment
In this study, over 20,192 inpatient electronic-prescriptions with ALOS of 6.6 days were assigned a DRG. There were 633 DRGs identified in the study, 10.3% of which had only 1 case and 28.9% had less than 5 cases. DRG O-6-12-I, Vaginal Delivery with other Procedure Excluding Sterilization

&/Or Dilation & Curettage (3.75%), was the highest volume DRG identified in this study. The range of length of stay varied from 1 to 69 days, and the highest proportion of patients (16.4%) and (20.6%) separated on the second and third day after admission respectively.

Data issues
The following steps have been done to develop the MY-DRG case-mix pharmacy service weight in UKMMC by identifying the actual cost of pharmacy services by MY-DRG groups in the hospital.

Step one: identifying the pharmacy component
In order to estimate the total costs of a particular health service, it is important to identify all the relevant costs and those who bear these costs [20]. In this study the pharmacy component has been identified to include four main contributors:

- The drugs and supplies cost.
- The cost of in-patient pharmacy staff.
- The overhead cost centres allocation.
- The pharmacy equipment cost.

Step two: calculation of the total pharmacy cost
A mixed approach which is based partly on top-down (step-down) and partly on bottom up or activity based (ABC) costing methodology has been recruited in order to calculate the pharmacy cost per patient or episodes [15,21]. The required data (retrospective data) for ABC approach were the all inpatient e-prescriptions and the total number of the inpatient pharmacy staff for year 2011 in UKMMC. While the data needed for top down costing were the total of hospital expenditures, total number of hospital staff, total hospital floor area and total number of inpatients for year 2011, in UKMMC.

a. Top down costing:
    The main purpose of this step is to determine the pharmacy use of the indirect (overhead) cost centers. Normally starts (at the top) with total expenditures and then divides these by a measure of total output (e.g. patient visits, days or admissions) to give an "average" cost per patient per visit, per day or per admission [22,23]. The top-down approach is cheaper and faster than a bottom up approach because of less data intensive and fewer research skills needed and data can be collected from routine resources [15].

The pharmacy use of the overhead cost centers and allocation factors
The overhead cost centers included in this study are the administration, maintenance, utility, cleaning services, security, general store and consumable, information technology (IT) centre, library, tax and insurance, rent, The central sterile services department (CSSD), telephone and fax centers. Data on the annual total cost for each center has been collected from the financial department of UKMMC. Table 1 shows the overhead cost centers and the appropriate allocation factors used to determine the pharmacy use of the indirect (overhead) cost centers. The following questions have been used to calculate the pharmacy use of each of the overhead cost centers: The pharmacy use of the indirect (overhead) cost centers = (Number of pharmacy staff/total hospital staff) × (annual total cost) or the pharmacy use of the indirect (overhead) cost centers = (pharmacy floor area/total hospital floor area) × (annual total cost). Summing up all the allocations gave the total pharmacy use of the indirect (overhead) cost centers. Then the total pharmacy use of the indirect (overhead) cost centers multiplied by the inpatient proportion to get the inpatient pharmacy use of the indirect (overhead) cost centers. The results of this question divided by total annual number of (inpatient days) to get the inpatient pharmacy use cost per day. This unit cost in the question was then multiplied by (the length of stays) of investigated patient to get the inpatient pharmacy use cost per patient per day, Figure 1.

The pharmacy equipment cost (capital costs)
In this costing study the pharmacy capital costs comprised of all the purchased or donated equipments, furniture and vehicles in the last 5 years (RM 642,375.16). The information was obtained from the financial department in the hospital. The total capital cost has been divided by Annualization factor (4.32) at 5% discount rate [24]. The result (RM148, 697.95) has been multiplied by inpatient proportion (16%) which already determined by The UKMMC pharmacy office. Then the inpatient pharmacy capital asset costs (RM 23, 791.67) divided by the total number of inpatient days (193824) to get the capital assets cost per day. This unit cost (0.12) in the question was multiplied by length of stays of the investigated

Table 1 Overhead cost centers and the allocation key factors

No.	Allocation factor	
	Number of staff	Floor area
1	The administrative,	The maintenance
2	General store and consumable	Utility
3	IT centre	Cleaning Services
4	Library	Security
5	Tax and insurance	CSSD centers
6	Rent	
7	Telephone and fax centers	

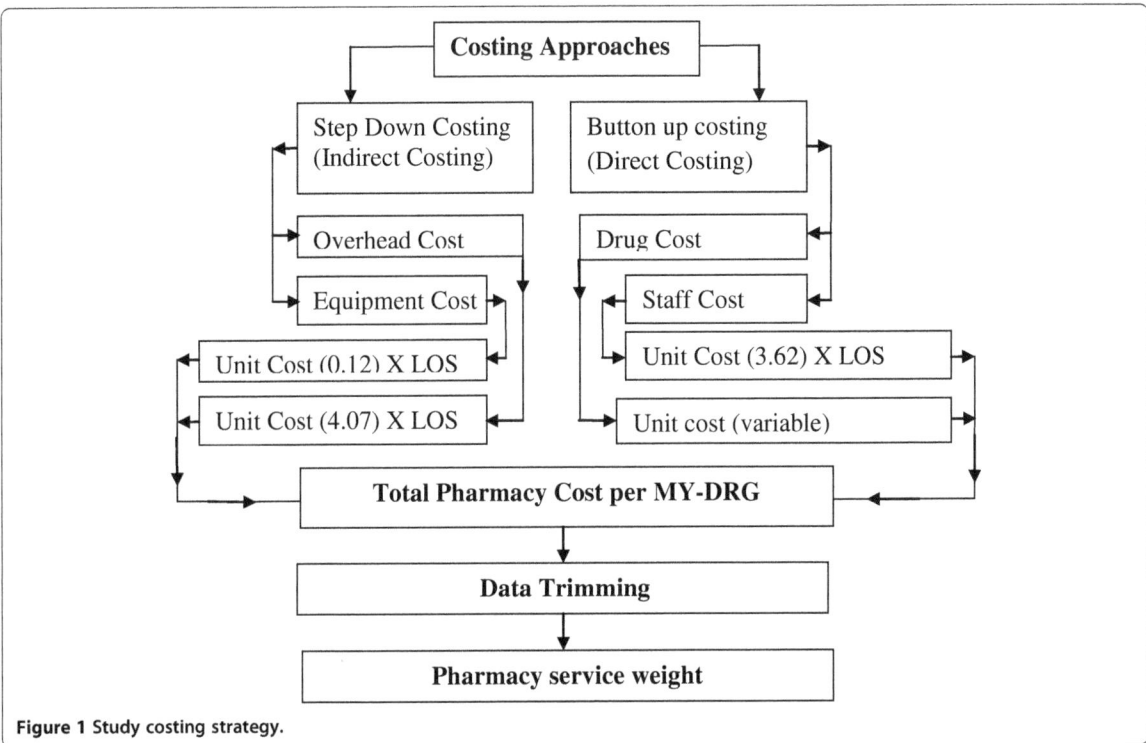

Figure 1 Study costing strategy.

patient to get the inpatient pharmacy capital assets cost per patient per day.

b. Bottom-up or Activity based costing and data collection:

The Bottom-up costing requires recording of every item of service that a patient receives, and changing them into costs. Bottom-up costing gives more accurate results, but it requires a large investment in time and resources [24,25]. In this study the bottom-up approach was used 1) to estimate drug and supply cost per episode and 2) to cost inpatient staff of the pharmacy per patient.

Costs of pharmacy staff serviced inpatients

Direct cost for staff cost covered all in-patient pharmacy staff responsible for supplying medications to all wards and units in UKMMC. Basic salaries and additional allowances, bonuses, contributions, payments were obtained from the staff directly and confirmed by hospital personnel services administrative records. Summing up all in-patient pharmacy staff costs gave the total staff cost (RM 702,030.48). Then the total staff cost was divided by total annual number of inpatient days (193824) to get staff cost per day. This unit cost (3.62) was then multiplied by (length of stay) of investigated patient to estimate staff cost per patient per day.

Cost of inpatient drugs/medicines and medical supplies

Information on the drugs/medicines, fluids and medical supplies prescribed to the patient was obtained from electronic-prescription system on Excel based file. Electronic prescribing refers to the ordering, administration and supply of drugs is completely supported by electronic systems. Each e-prescription defined as one episode (a period of inpatient care) [26] having data on registration number (MRN) which is a unique number given for each local and international client; name of the patient; e-prescription number; date of prescription; number of items, quantity, duration and name of the prescribed medicines, fluids and supplies. Drugs prescribed and purchased by patients for take home were excluded. List of acquisition unit costs (price) of each drug and supplies were obtained from the UKMMC pharmacy office. This unit cost was then multiplied by the quantity of the corresponding item to estimate cost per item. Then we summed up the cost of all items in one e-prescription to estimate drug cost per patient (per episode).

Calculation of patient level total pharmacy costs

The total pharmacy cost of each individual patient/episode would be the summing of total drugs and supplies cost plus the results of multiplying the unit cost of each of pharmacy use of overhead cost centers; the pharmacy equipment cost; pharmacy staff cost by the LOS of investigated patient/episode.

Step three: data trimming
The L3H3 method (Lower three Higher three), is data trimming method commonly used to ensure that the means reported more accurately represent the central tendency amongst cases analyzed [27]. For each DRG we calculated the total and the average pharmacy cost depending on the number of patients/episodes in that DRG. Trimming method mainly consists of using the average pharmacy cost for every MY-DRG having more than 20 patients/episodes divided by three as the low trim point and the average pharmacy cost multiplied by three as the high trim point. So, in term of distribution the normal cases in each MY-DRG lie inside the trim points and known as inliers. In contrast, the cases which lie outside the trim points considered skewed or outlier cases and have been excluded from analysis.

Step four: calculation the pharmacy service weight per each MY-DRG
Pharmacy service weight was defined as the burden of work or services performed by pharmacy component and the resources used for a patient compared to the burden of other services for others DRGs. The actual service weights are unit less numbers that express the expected cost for one visit in relation to average visit. The best way to calculate service weights is to use actual cost per inpatient case by assigning each DRG a relative value that reflects the cost of any one, or all, of the resources consumed (e.g. bed-days, theatre time, drugs, diagnostic procedures, physiotherapy and nursing treatment) in that respective DRG when compared with all DRGs [28,29]. In order to estimate the pharmacy service weight we need first to calculate the average pharmacy cost for all MY-DRGs. The closest average cost among all the MY-DRGs would be the base used to calculate the pharmacy service weight using the following question:

Pharmacy service weight of a MY-DRG = Average pharmacy cost of the investigated MY-DRG/Average of a specified MY-DRG (which usually the average pharmacy cost of all MY-DRGs).

Ethics
This study was approved by ethics committee of National University of Malaysia- Medical Center (UKMMC), code number (UNU-002- 2013) in 20 May 2013.

Results
The pharmacy component unit costs
Table 2 shows the estimated unit costs of the pharmacy components with exception of the drugs and supplies unit cost which is variable depending on the number of

Table 2 Unit costs of the four pharmacy components

No.	Pharmacy components	Unit cost (RM)
1	Total drugs and supplies cost	Episode/variable
2	Pharmacy staff cost	3.62
3	Pharmacy use of overhead cost centers	4.07
4	Pharmacy equipment cost	0.12

items and the quantity of drugs and supplies consumed by each patient (episode).

The pharmacy component
The total and the average pharmacy cost have been calculated for each MY-DRG using the estimated unit costs. Table 3 reports the frequency distribution of the average pharmacy components cost: Drugs and supplies were the main component (86.0%) of pharmacy cost compared to overhead cost centers (7.31%), staff cost (6.50%) and pharmacy equipments (0.22%) respectively.

After data trimming
After data trimming and excluding DRGs with less than 5 cases, 13,663 cases with ALOS of 7 days were available for analysis. There were 450 DRGs identified in the study, 5.6% of which had only 5 cases. DRG O-6-13-I, Vaginal Delivery with severity level one (5.0%) was the highest volume DRG identified in this study. Almost 61.3% of total separations were classified as medical and 39.7% of them were classified into the surgical partition.

Pharmacy service weight
Average pharmacy cost of all MY-DRGs was 484.48. MY-DRG F-4-16-III, Dementia and Other Organic Brain Disturbances Including Mental Retardation with severity level three was the closest average (486.08) among all other MY-DRGs. Thus this average was the base (denominator) used in the question to estimate the pharmacy service weight for all MY-DRGs. Table 4 shows the pharmacy service weight of the highest 20 MY-DRGs. MY-DRG case-mix group of Lymphoma & Chronic Leukemia group with severity level three (C-4-11-III) has the highest pharmacy service weight of 11.8 equivalents to average pharmacy cost of RM 5383.90. While the MY-DRG case-mix group for Circumcision with

Table 3 Frequency distribution of the average pharmacy components cost

No.	Pharmacy components	Average (RM)	%
1	Total drugs and supplies cost	315.15	85.98
2	Pharmacy staff cost	23.81	6.50
3	Pharmacy use of overhead cost centers	26.78	7.31
4	Pharmacy equipment cost	0.79	0.22
	Average total pharmacy cost (n = 20,192)	366.53	100

Table 4 Pharmacy service weights of the highest 20 MY-DRGs

No.	MY-DRG	No. of episodes per DRG	Total pharmacy cost per DRG	Average pharmacy cost per DRG	Pharmacy service weight
1	C-4-11-III	38	204588.16	5383.90	11.8
2	B-1-10-III	11	49817.84	4528.89	9.32
3	J-1-20-III	5	22178.34	4435.67	9.13
4	U-1-20-III	17	61664.92	3627.35	7.46
5	M-1-20-III	5	16848.74	3369.75	6.93
6	C-4-10-III	31	104232.86	3362.35	6.92
7	G-1-11-III	14	46170.40	3297.89	6.78
8	M-1-60-III	8	22978.67	2872.33	5.91
9	S-4-13-III	6	17148.36	2858.06	5.88
10	D-4-10-III	13	34282.24	2637.10	5.43
11	B-1-11-III	7	18080.84	2582.98	5.31
12	M-1-03-III	11	26994.90	2454.08	5.05
13	J-4-12-III	9	20444.37	2271.60	4.67
14	G-4-21-III	5	10925.50	2185.10	4.50
15	D-1-10-I	9	18569.22	2063.25	4.24
16	I-4-13-III	6	11693.31	1948.89	4.01
17	I-1-04-III	5	9550.77	1910.15	3.93
18	D-1-20-III	5	9455.59	1891.12	3.89
19	K-1-20-III	16	30134.09	1883.38	3.87
20	I-4-14-III	10	18375.21	1837.52	3.78

severity level one (V-1-15-I) has the lowest pharmacy service weight of 0.04 equivalents to average pharmacy Cost RM 17.83.

Limitation of study

This study has few areas of limitations. First of all, this study was not designed to cover a representative size of hospitals in Malaysia due to time and resource constraints in addition to the limited number of hospitals that implemented DRG system in Malaysia. Other limitation is related to (date) of e-prescription issue which was not always be the same date of patient admission. This limitation made the joining of e-prescription data to MY-DRG data base to be done manually.

Discussion

The main objective of this study was to develop the MY-DRG inpatient pharmacy service weight in UKMMC using E-prescription data and DRG data base in UKMMC. For this purpose a mixed approach of top-down and bottom-up costing methodology has been recruited jointly [24].

Although international literature indicated that there are several approaches to estimate the cost of providing services by health related institution including hospitals.

However, there is no unique, appropriate and acceptable methodology for costing hospital services [30]. Type of the service and reason for costing in addition to economical feasibility of cost calculation are the main determinants for selection of appropriate costing approach. Thus, the cost of a particular service can vary substantially according to the purpose of cost data for which it was generated [31].

This study indicated that the drugs and supplies made the highest component of the pharmacy cost. These findings come in line with other international and local studies considering the pharmacy services as ancillary services [27] and among the highest components of cost in the hospital [28,29,32]. To our knowledge, the pharmacy services and its related weights are commonly studied within the general hospital level costing and are rarely to be evaluated as an independent subject [27,33].

Costing study done in Philippine for selected hospitals used both the activity based and top down costing approaches found that medicines and supplies cost more than 25% of the total hospital cost [33]. In 2004, two studies done in UKMMC, and the costing analysis were conducted based on the case-mix concept of the top-down costing approach. The first one was to study the cost analysis for cardiology. This study found that the three biggest components of medical cardiology cases are ICU cost (38.0%), Pharmacy component (14.2%) and Ward Services (12.7%). In the Surgical Cardiology, the biggest component of cost was the Operation Theatre (27.9%), followed by ward Services (25.4%) and Pharmacy Component (8.5%) [15]. The other study was the cost analysis and cost weight for the treatment of orthopedic cases in HUKM. This study showed that the top three components of cost for the treatment of medical orthopedic was Pharmacy Services (22.3%), followed by Ward Services which was (20.7%) and Laboratory Services which was (12.1%), while the top three components of cost for treatment of surgical orthopedic was Operating Theatre Services which was (21.2%), followed by Pharmacy Services which was (17.6%) and Ward Services which was (16.3). It is noted that for both the medical and surgical partitions of cardiology and orthopedic cases, the pharmacy component services were among the top three contributors of the large portion of cost or resources [34].

Indeed, the actual drug costs and the pharmacy cost are being among the main objectives of much research in the health care economy [29,35]. Although there is considerable variation between countries, the developing countries (the upper middle-income, the lower middle-income and the low-income countries) contribute only to 21.5% of the total global pharmaceutical expenditures in 2006; however they spend proportionally more of their health budget on medicines than the developed countries [4,36].

This study shows that using of e-prescription data would greatly facilitate the activity based costing methodology to estimate the pharmacy service weight by identifying pharmacy services and the actual cost of care. In fact, the availability of pharmacy service weights or cost weights will enable a comparison is made between the treatments cost of various DRG cases within and between hospitals [17]. For the purpose of using DRG as a base of hospital payment, a price needs to be assigned to each DRG. This is usually done by assigning a cost relativity (or service weight) with a base price multiplier [13].

Conclusion

A mixed approach which is based partly on top-down and partly on bottom up costing methodology has been recruited to develop MY-DRG case-mix inpatient pharmacy service weight for 450 groups utilized by the UKMMC in 2011. This methodology can be used for calculating pharmacy service weight among Government Hospital such as General, District and private hospital in future. It is a hope that the results of this study will participate in the development of MY-DRG in UKMMC specifically in pharmacy services by identifying which DRG consumes the bulk of the resources. So, this can greatly support decision maker regarding budget planning of pharmacy services and patients' outcomes, and eventually will contribute in the quality of care and services improvement as well as an effective use of resources.

Abbreviations
MY-DRG: Malaysian Diagnosis Related Group; DRG: Diagnosis Related Group; UKMMC: University Kebangsaan Malaysia Medical center; HUKM: Hospital OF University Kebangsaan Malaysia; UMBI: Institute of Medical Molecular Research; ALOS: The average length of stay; L3H3: L three H three; IT: Information technology; CSSD: The Central Sterile Services Department.

Competing interests
The authors declare that they have no competing interests.

Authors' contributions
SAAJ: conceived study, collected, coded and analyzed the data, and wrote the first and final draft of the article. SA: advised and contributed to the study design and data analysis. AMN: advised and contributed to the data analysis. ZA: advised in the study design data collection. DV: advised and contributed to data collection. All authors have read and approved the final manuscript.

Acknowledgments
We are grateful to the heads of UKKMC Pharmacy and department of health information and all the pharmacy and department of health information staff for their unlimited cooperation and support in data collection process. Special thanks to all our colleagues in international center of casemix and clinical coding (ITCC).

Author details
[1]United Nations University-International Institute for Global Health (UNU-IIGH), Kuala Lumpur, Malaysia. [2]International Centre for Case-Mix and Clinical Coding (ITCC), University Kebangsaan Malaysia Medical Centre, Jalan Yaacob Latiff, 56000 Cheras, Kuala Lumpur, Malaysia. [3]Pharmacy of Hospital University Kebangsaan Malaysia Medical Centre, Jalan Yaacob Latiff, 56000 Cheras, Kuala Lumpur, Malaysia.

References
1. Hoffman JM, Shah ND, Vermeulen LC, Schumock GT, Grim P, Hunkler RJ, et al. Projecting future drug expenditures-2006. Am J Health-Syst Pharm. 2006;63:123–38.
2. The World Health Organization. The World Medicines Situation. 2004. Chapter 5 & Annex 2. http://apps.who.int/medicinedocs/pdf/s6160e/s6160e.pdf.
3. OECD. Pharmaceutical expenditure. In: Health at a Glance2011: OECD Indicators. OECD Publishing; 2011. http://dx.doi.org/10.1787/health_glance-2011-63-en.
4. Kaplan W, Mathers C. The world medicine situation 2011: medicine expenditure. In: 2011. http://www.who.int/medicines/areas/policy/world_medicines_situation/en/.
5. Falkenberg T, Tomson G. The World Bank and Pharmaceuticals. Health Policy Plan. 2000;15(1):52–8. http://heapol.oxfordjournals.org/content/15/1/52.long.
6. Abdollahiasl A, Kebriaeezadeh A, Dinarvand R, Abdollahi M, Cheraghali AM, Jaberidoost M, et al. A system dynamics model for national drug polic. DARU. 2014;22(4):34.
7. Heerey A, McGowan B, Ryan M, Barry M. Microcosting *versus* DRGs in the provision of cost estimates for use in pharmacoeconomic evaluation. Expert Rev Pharmacoeconomics Outcomes Res. 2002;2(1):29–33.
8. Aguado A, Guinó E, Mukherjee B, Sicras A, Serrat J, Acedo M, et al. Variability in prescription drug expenditures explained by adjusted clinical groups (ACG) case-mix: A cross-sectional study of patient electronic records in primary care. BMC Health Serv Res. 2008;8:53. http://www.biomedcentral.com/1472-6963/8/53.
9. Saperi BS, Amrizal MN, Rohaizat BY, Zafar A, Syed A. Implementation of case-mix in hospital UKM: the progress. MJPHM. 2005;5(Supplement 2):45–53.
10. Ali Jadoo SA, Sulku SN, Aljunid SM, Dastan I. Validity and reliability analysis of knowledge of, attitude toward and practice of a case-mix questionnaire among Turkish healthcare providers. JHEOR. 2014;2(1):96–107.
11. Jackson T. Using Computerized Patient-Level Costing Data for Setting DRG Weights: The Victorian (Australia) Cost Weight Studies. Health Policy. 2011;56(2):149–63. http://www.sciencedirect.com/science/article/pii/S0168851000001482#.
12. Palmer G, Aisbett C, Milis N, Xu C. The integration of the clinical and cost modeling approaches to case-mix costing. Case-mix Quarterly. 1998;0(1):1–10.
13. Luce BR, Manning WG, Siegel JE, Lipscomb J. Estimating costs in cost effectiveness analysis. In: Gold MR, Siege JE, Russe LB, Weinstein MC, editors. Cost Effectiveness in Health and Medicine. New York: Oxford University Press; 1996. p. 176–213.
14. Langenbrunner J, Cashin C, O'Dougherty S, editors. Designing and Implementing Health Care Provider Payment Systems: How to Manuals. Washington DC: The World Bank; 2009. http://siteresources.worldbank.org/HEALTHNUTRITIONANDPOPULATION/Resources/Peer-Reviewed-Publications/ProviderPaymentHowTo.pdf.
15. Amrizal MN, Rohaizat Y, Zafar A, Saperi, Syed A. Case-mix costing in Universiti Kebangsaan Malaysia hospital a top-down approach: cost analysis for cardiology cases. MJPHM. 2005;5(Supplement 2):33–44.
16. James CV. The top down approach to allocate hospital costs and to computing relative weights. MJPHM. 2005;5(Supplement 2):75–90.
17. Rohaizat Y. Proposed national health care financing mechanism for Malaysia: the role of case-mix. MJPHM. 2005;5(Supplement 2):91–8.
18. Kamaruddin MA. Universiti Kebangsaan Malaysia: Historical Background. Bangi: UKM Publisher; 2006.
19. University Kebangsaan Malaysia - Medical Centre (UKMMC), Department Of Health Information, Statistics; 2013. http://www.ppukm.ukm.my/wbppukmen/index.php/component/content/article/69-jabatan-jabatan/sokongan-klinikal/jabatan-maklumat-kesihatan/253-statistik
20. Drummond M, Manca A, Sculpher M. Increasing the generalizability of economic evaluations: recommendations for the design, analysis, and reporting of studies. Int J Technol Assess Health Care. 2005;21(2):165–71.
21. Hendriks ME, Kundu P, Boers AC, Bolarinwa OA, Te Pas MJ, Akande TM, et al. Step-by-step guideline for disease-specific costing studies in low- and

middle-income countries: a mixed methodology. Glob Health Action. 2014;7:23573. http://dx.doi.org/10.3402/gha.v7.23573.

22. Conteh L, Walker D. Cost and unit cost calculations using step-down accounting. Health Policy Plan. 2004;19(2):127–35.

23. Taghreed A, Evans DB, Murray CJL. Econometric estimation of country-specific hospital costs. Cost Effectiveness and Resource Allocation. 2003;1:3. http://www.resource-allocation.com/content/1/1/3.

24. Shepard DS, Hodgkin D, Anthony YE. Analysis of Hospital Costs: A Manual for Managers. Geneva: World Health Organization; 2000.

25. Negrini D, Kettle A, Sheppard L, Mills GH, Edbrooke DL. The cost of a hospital ward in Europe: is there a methodology available to accurately measure the costs? J Health Organ Manag. 2004;18(2–3):195–206.

26. Damberg CL, Sorbero ME, Hussey PS, Lovejoy S, Liu H, Mehrotra A. Exploring Episode-Based Approaches for Medicare Performance Measurement, Accountability and Payment- Final Report, WR-633-ASPE. Assistant Secretary for Planning and Evaluation, US Department of Health and Human Services; 2009. http://aspe.hhs.gov/health/reports/09/mcperform/report.pdf.

27. Duckett SJ. Casemix funding for acute hospital inpatient services in Australia. eMJA. 1998;19:s17–21. https://www.mja.com.au/journal/1998/169/8/casemix-funding-acute-hospital-inpatient-services-australia accessed 8/May/2014.

28. Heslop L. Status of costing hospital nursing work within Australian casemix activity-based funding policy. Int J Nurs Pract. 2012;18(1):2–6.

29. Mills AJ, Kapalamula J, Chisimbi S. The cost of the district hospital: a case study in Malawi. Bull World Health Organ. 1993;71:329–39.

30. Mogyorosy Z, Smith P. *The main methodological issues in costing health care services:* a literature review. University of York: Centre for Health Economics; 2005. http://www.york.ac.uk/media/che/documents/papers/researchpapers/rp7_Methodological_issues_in_costing_health_care_services.pdf.

31. Zimmerman JL. Accounting for Decision-Making and Control. 4th ed. Boston: McGraw-Hill Irwin; 2003. p. 29–75.

32. Centers for Medicare and Medicaid Services, National Health Expenditures Projections2011-2021. www.cms.gov/Research-Statistics-data-and-Systems/Statistics-Trends-and-Reports/NationalHealthExpendData/Downloads/Proj2011PDF.pdf

33. Tsilaajav T. Costing Study for Selected Hospitals in the Philippines, Final Report, technical assistance to the health sector policy support program in the Philippines. 2009. http://www.doh.gov.ph/sites/default/files/Costing%20Study%20for%20Selected%20Hospitals%20in%20the%20Philippines.pdf.

34. Rohaizat Y, Amrizl MN, Saperi S, Syed A. Cost analysis and cost weight for the treatment of orthopedic cases in a teaching hospital in Malaysia using the case-mix approach: the experience of Universiti Kebangsaan Malaysia hospital. MJPHM. 2005;5(Supplement 2):63–73.

35. Rivers PA, Hall NG, Frimpong J. Prescription drug spending: contribution to health care spending and cost containment strategies. J Health Care Finance. 2006;32(3):8–19.

36. Kebriaeezadeh A, Koopaei NN, Abdollahiasl A, Nikfar S, Mohamadi N. Trend analysis of the pharmaceutical market in Iran; 1997–2010; policy implications for developing countries. DARU J Pharm Sci. 2013;21:52.

10

Antinociceptive properties of new coumarin derivatives bearing substituted 3,4-dihydro-2*H*-benzothiazines

Masoumeh Alipour[1], Mehdi Khoobi[2], Saeed Emami[3], Saeed Fallah-Benakohal[2], Seyedeh Farnaz Ghasemi-Niri[2], Mohammad Abdollahi[4], Alireza Foroumadi[2] and Abbas Shafiee[2*]

Abstract

Background: Coumarins are an important class of widely distributed heterocyclic natural products exhibiting a broad pharmacological profile. In this work, a new series of coumarins bearing substituted 3,4-dihydro-2*H*-benzothiazines were described as potential analgesic agents. The clinical use of NSAIDs as traditional analgesics is associated with side effects such as gastrointestinal lesions and nephrotoxicity. Therefore, the discovery of new safer drugs represents a challenging goal for such a research area.

Results: The target compounds 3-(3-methyl-3,4-dihydro-2*H*-benzo[*b*][1,4]thiazin-3-yl)-2*H*-chromen-2-ones **2a-u** were synthesized and characterized by spectral data. The antinociceptive properties of target compounds were determined by formalin-induced test and acetic acid-induced writhing test in mice. Among the tested compounds, compound **2u** bearing 2-(4-(methylsulfonyl)benzoyl)- moiety on benzothiazine ring and 4-(methylsulfonyl)phenacyloxy- group on the 7 position of coumarin nucleus showed better profile of antinoceciept in both models. It was more effective than mefenamic acid during the late phase of formalin-induced test as well as in the acetic acid-induced writhing test.

Conclusion: Considering the significant antinoceceptive action of phenacyloxycoumarin derivatives, compound **2u** prototype might be further used as model to obtain new more potent analgesic drugs.

Keywords: Analgesic activity, Antinociception, Coumarin, Benzothiazine, Formalin test, Writhing test

Introduction

Pain is an uncomfortable sensation that alerts the human organs about a current or potential damage to tissues [1]. It has been accepted that pain can widely affect human life quality, and its management is considered as a main challenge in pharmacotherapy [2]. NSAIDs are one of major classes of traditional analgesics for treatment of pain. The clinical use of NSAIDs is associated with side effects such as gastrointestinal lesions and nephrotoxicity [3]. Therefore, the discovery of new safer drugs represents a challenging goal for such a research area.

Coumarins are an important class of widely distributed heterocyclic natural products exhibiting a broad pharmacological profile [4]. Several coumarin derivatives have been synthesized with diverse biological activities [5-9] especially analgesic/anti-inflammatory activity [10-13]. Recently, the synthesis and anti-inflammatory/analgesic activities of several coumarin derivatives with various substitutions on 3-position of coumarin nucleus have been reported [14-16]. On the other hand, benzothiazine derivatives are also important heterocyclic compounds with wide spectrum of biological activities [17,18]. In view of the above facts and in continuation of our research program on the synthesis of biologically active heterocyclic compounds [19,20], we introduced herein the new coumarin derivatives bearing substituted 3,4-dihydro-2*H*-benzothiazines as analgesic agents. The antinociceptive properties of target compounds were determined by formalin-induced paw licking test and

* Correspondence: ashafiee@ams.ac.ir
[2]Department of Medicinal Chemistry, Faculty of Pharmacy and Pharmaceutical Sciences Research Center, Tehran University of Medical Sciences, Tehran 14176, Iran
Full list of author information is available at the end of the article

acetic acid-induced writhing test in mice. Indeed, the formalin-induced paw licking method is used to investigate both peripheral and central mechanisms whereas the acetic acid test is believed to demonstrate the involvement of peripheral mechanisms in the control of pain [21,22].

Materials and methods
Chemistry
The target compounds 3-(3-methyl-3,4-dihydro-2*H*-benzo[*b*][1,4]thiazin-3-yl)-2*H*-chromen-2-ones **2a-r** (Additional file 1: Table S1) were synthesized according to the pathway outlined in Scheme 1 [23]. All reagents and chemicals were commercially available and used as received. Alumina-supported potassium fluoride (KF/Al$_2$O$_3$) was prepared by literature method [24]. The dihydrobenzothiazole derivatives **1** were prepared as reported method by us [19,20]. The synthesis of compounds **2a-d**, **2f-i** and **2p-r** was described in our previous paper [23]. Column chromatography was carried out on silica gel (70–230 mesh). TLC was conducted on silica gel 250 micron, F254 plates. Melting points were measured on a Kofler hot stage apparatus and are uncorrected. The IR spectra were taken using Nicolet FT-IR Magna 550 spectrographs (KBr disks). ^{1}H NMR spectra were recorded on a Bruker 400 or 500 MHz NMR instruments. The chemical shifts (δ) and coupling constants (*J*) are expressed in parts per million and Hertz, respectively. Mass spectra of the products were obtained with an HP (Agilent technologies) 5937 Mass Selective Detector. Elemental analyses were carried out by a CHN-Rapid Heraeus elemental analyzer. The results of elemental analyses (C, H, N) were within ± 0.4% of the calculated values.

General procedure for the synthesis of compounds 2
A suspension of dihydrobenzothiazole derivatives **1** (1.0 mmol), KF/Al$_2$O$_3$ (0.7 g), and quinine hydrochloride (10 mol%) in ethanol (3.0 mL) was stirred at room temperature for 5 min. Then, appropriate phenacyl halide (1.2 mmol) was added to the mixture and stirring was continued. After completion of the reaction (3–5 h), the solvent was removed under reduced pressure. The residue was mixed with ethyl acetate (5 mL) and the catalyst was filtered and washed with ethyl acetate (3 × 5 mL). After evaporation of the solvent at reduced pressure, the crude product was purified by column chromatography (*n*-hexane/ethyl acetate, 9:1) and crystallized from ethanol for further purification.

3-(2-(3,4-Dichlorobenzoyl)-3-methyl-3,4-dihydro-2H-benzo[b][1,4]thiazin-3-yl)-2H-chromen-2-one (2e)
Yellow solid (361 mg, 75%); *syn*-isomer; mp 91–93°C; IR (KBr, cm^{-1}) 3382 (NH), 1708 (C=O); ^{1}H NMR (500 MHz, CDCl$_3$) δ ^{1}H NMR (500 MHz, CDCl$_3$) δ 1.94 (s, 3H, CH$_3$ benzothiazine), 4.49 (s, 1H, NH), 5.77 (s, 1H, C-H benzothiazine), 6.75 (dt, *J* = 7.2 and 1.2 Hz, 1H, H$_7$ benzothiazine), 6.95 (m, 2H, H$_{5,8}$ benzothiazine), 7.14 (dt, *J* = 7.2 and 1.2 Hz, 1H, H$_6$ benzothiazine), 7.22 (t, *J* = 8.0 Hz, 1H, H$_6$ chromene), 7.28 (dd, *J* = 8.0 and 1.9 Hz, 1H, H$_5$ benzoyl), 7.33 (d, *J* = 8.0 Hz, 1H, H$_6$ benzoyl), 7.40 (m, 2H, H$_{5,8}$ chromene), 7.43 (d, *J* = 1.9, 1H, H$_3$ benzoyl), 7.49 (dt, *J* = 8.0 and 1.2 Hz, 1H, H$_7$ chromene), 7.77 (s, 1H, H$_4$ chromene); ^{13}C NMR (125 MHz, CDCl$_3$) δ 24.3, 42.9, 58.0, 110.9, 116.1, 117.1, 119.1, 119.3, 124.3, 127.0, 127.1, 128.4, 128.7, 130.1, 130.8, 131.2, 131.4, 132.0, 136.9, 137.1, 139.8, 141.0, 153.2, 160.9, 192.6; Anal. calcd for

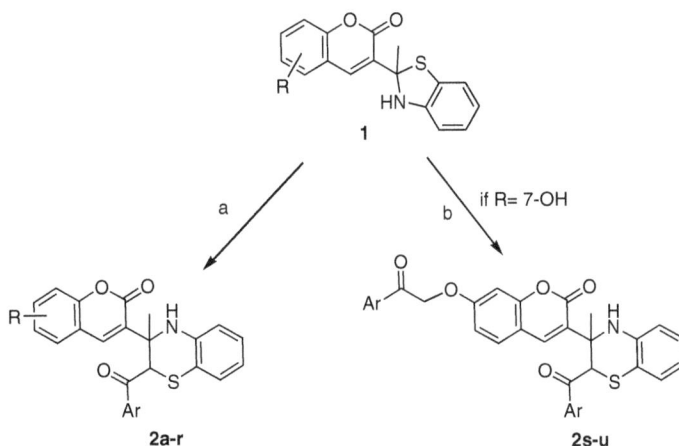

Scheme 1 Synthesis of coumarin based dihydrobenzothiazines 2a-u. Reagents and conditions: (a) phenacyl halide (1.2 mmol), KF/Al$_2$O$_3$ (0.7 g), quinine hydrochloride (10 mol%), EtOH (3 mL), r.t. (b) phenacyl halide (2.5 mmol), KF/Al$_2$O$_3$ (1.5 g), quinine hydrochloride (10 mol%), EtOH (3 mL), r.t.

$C_{25}H_{17}Cl_2NO_3S$: C, 62.25; H, 3.55; N, 2.90. Found: C, 62.41; H, 3.67; N, 3.15.

3-(2-(4-Fluorobenzoyl)-3-methyl-3,4-dihydro-2H-benzo[b] [1,4]thiazin-3-yl)-2H-chromen-2-one (2j)

Yellow solid (336 mg, 78%); syn-isomer; mp 161–163°C; IR (KBr, cm^{-1}) 3413 (NH), 1708 (C=O); ^{1}H NMR (500 MHz, CDCl$_3$) δ 1.76 (s, 3H, CH$_3$ benzothiazine), 4.50 (s, 1H, NH), 5.97 (s, 1H, C-H benzothiazine), 6.73 (t, J = 7.4 Hz, 1H, H$_7$ benzothiazine), 6.93 (m, 2H, H$_{5,6}$ benzothiazine), 7.14 (m, 3H, H$_8$ benzothiazine and H$_{3,5}$ benzoyl), 7.28 (t, J = 7.4 Hz, 1H, H$_6$ chromene), 7.35 (d, J = 7.4 Hz, 1H, H$_8$ chromene), 7.40 (d, J = 7.4 Hz, 1H, H$_5$ chromene), 7.50 (t, J = 7.4 Hz, 1H, H$_7$ chromene), 7.79 (s, 1H, H$_4$ chromene), 8.05 (m, 2H, H$_{2,6}$ benzoyl); ^{13}C NMR (125 MHz, CDCl$_3$) δ 24.6, 37.5, 57.6, 111.9, 115.7, 115.9, 116.1, 119.1, 119.4, 124.4, 126.7, 128.4, 128.5, 131.2, 131.3, 131.5, 133.2, 139.5, 141.1, 153.3, 161.3, 164.7, 166.7, 191.3; Anal. calcd for $C_{25}H_{18}FNO_3S$: C, 69.59; H, 4.20; N, 3.25. Found: C, 69.42; H, 4.03; N, 3.47.

3-(3-Methyl-2-(thiophene-2-carbonyl)-3,4-dihydro-2H-benzo [b][1,4]thiazin-3-yl)-2H-chromen-2-one (2k)

Yellow solid (356 mg, 85%); as mixture of diastereomers (anti/syn: 15/85); IR (KBr, cm^{-1}) 3389 (NH), 1707 (C=O); ^{1}H NMR (500 MHz, CDCl$_3$) δ 1.77$_{syn}$ (s, CH$_3$ benzo-thiazine), 1.87$_{anti}$ (s, CH$_3$ benzothiazine), 4.48$_{syn}$ (s, NH), 4.53$_{anti}$ (s, NH), 5.50$_{anti}$ (s, C-H benzothiazine), 5.87$_{syn}$ (s, C-H benzothiazine), 6.77$_{syn}$ (t, J = 8.0, H$_7$ benzothiazine), 6.81$_{anti}$ (t, J = 8.0, H$_7$ benzothiazine), 6.92$_{anti}$ (d, J = 8.0 Hz, H$_5$ benzothiazine), 6.95$_{syn}$ (d, J = 8.0 Hz, H$_5$ benzothiazine), 7.07-7.10$_{anti}$ (m, H$_{6,8}$ benzothiazine), 7.10-7.13$_{syn}$ (m, H$_{6,8}$ benzothiazine), 7.20$_{syn}$ (t, J = 7.6 Hz, H$_7$ chromene), 7.25$_{syn}$ (t, J = 7.6 Hz, H$_6$ chromene), 7.25-7.29$_{anti}$ (m, H$_4$ thiophene and H$_7$ chromene), 7.38$_{syn}$ (d, J = 7.6 Hz, H$_5$ chromene), 7.42$_{syn}$ (d, J = 7.6 Hz, H$_8$ chromene), 7.48-7.54 (m, H$_{5,7,8}$ chromene (anti) and H$_4$ thiophene (syn)), 7.56$_{anti}$ (d, J = 4.0, H$_3$ thiophene), 7.74$_{syn}$ (d, J = 4.0, H$_3$ thiophene), 7.79$_{anti}$ (d, J = 4.0, H$_5$ thiophene), 7.80$_{syn}$ (s, H$_4$ chromene), 7.97$_{syn}$ (d, J = 4.0, H$_5$ thiophene), 8.15$_{anti}$ (s, H$_4$ chromene); ^{13}C NMR (syn-isomer, 125 MHz, CDCl$_3$) δ 27.5, 45.3, 54.2, 116.1, 117.0, 118.6, 119.0, 120.1, 124.5, 126.2, 127.1, 128.2, 128.4, 131.4, 131.7, 132.2, 134.4, 140.2, 140.9, 143.5, 153.1, 160.1, 186.8; Anal. calcd for $C_{23}H_{17}NO_3S_2$: C, 65.85; H, 4.08; N, 3.34. Found: C, 65.92; H, 3.91; N, 3.29.

3-(2-(5-Bromothiophene-2-carbonyl)-3-methyl-3,4-dihydro-2H-benzo[b][1,4]thiazin-3-yl)-2H-chromen-2-one (2l)

Yellow solid (378 mg, 77%); as mixture of diastereomers (anti/syn: 26/74); IR (KBr, cm^{-1}) 3390 (NH), 1712 (C=O); ^{1}H NMR (500 MHz, CDCl$_3$) δ 1.75$_{syn}$ (s, CH$_3$ benzo-thiazine), 1.87$_{anti}$ (s, CH$_3$ benzothiazine), 4.45$_{syn}$ (s, NH), 4.55$_{anti}$ (s, NH), 5.48$_{anti}$ (s, C-H benzothiazine), 5.78$_{syn}$ (s, C-H benzothiazine), 6.76$_{syn}$ (t, J = 8.0, H$_7$ benzothiazine),

6.81$_{anti}$ (t, J = 8.0, H$_7$ benzothiazine), 6.92$_{syn}$ (d, J = 8.0 Hz, H$_5$ benzothiazine), 6.94$_{anti}$ (d, J = 8.0 Hz, H$_5$ benzothiazine), 6.92$_{anti}$ (d, J = 8.0 Hz, H$_8$ benzothiazine), 6.96$_{syn}$ (d, J = 8.0 Hz, H$_8$ benzothiazine), 7.09$_{anti}$ (t, J = 8.0 Hz, H$_6$ ben-zothiazine), 7.12$_{syn}$ (t, J = 8.0 Hz, H$_6$ benzothiazine), 7.16$_{syn}$ (d, J = 4.0 Hz, H$_4$ thiophene), 7.23$_{anti}$ (d, J = 4.0 Hz, H$_4$ thio-phene), 7.24$_{syn}$ (t, J = 7.5, H$_6$ chromene), 7.27-7.29$_{anti}$ (m, H$_{6,8}$ chromene), 7.36$_{syn}$ (d, J = 7.5 Hz, H$_8$ chromene), 7.40$_{syn}$ (d, J = 7.5 Hz, H$_5$ chromene), 7.50 $_{syn}$ (t, J = 7.5 Hz, H$_7$ chromene), 7.51-7.53$_{anti}$ (m, H$_{5,7}$ chromene), 7.56$_{anti}$ (d, J = 4.0, H$_3$ thiophene), 7.69$_{syn}$ (d, J = 4.0, H$_3$ thio-phene), 7.77$_{syn}$ (s, H$_4$ chromene), 8.15$_{anti}$ (s, H$_4$ chromene); ^{13}C NMR (syn-isomer, 125 MHz, CDCl$_3$) δ 24.8, 38.7, 57.4, 112.3, 116.1, 116.9, 119.1, 119.5, 123.6, 124.4, 126.6, 128.1, 128.4, 130.8, 131.5, 131.6, 132.4, 139.2, 141.0, 145.9, 153.3, 161.2, 185.6; MS, m/z (%) 499 ([M + 2]$^+$, 40%), 497 (M$^+$, 37), 375 (47), 373 (44), 308 (100), 294 (51), 280 (84); Anal. calcd for $C_{23}H_{16}BrNO_3S_2$: C, 55.43; H, 3.24; N, 2.81 Found: C, 55.22; H, 3.47; N, 2.73.

3-(3-Methyl-2-(thiophene-3-carbonyl)-3,4-dihydro-2H-benzo [b][1,4]thiazin-3-yl)-2H-chromen-2-one (2m)

Yellow solid (335 mg, 80%); as mixture of diastereomers (anti/syn: 32/68); IR (KBr, cm^{-1}) 3374 (NH), 1708 (C=O); ^{1}H NMR (500 MHz, CDCl$_3$) δ 1.77$_{syn}$ (s, CH$_3$ benzo-thiazine), 1.87$_{anti}$ (s, CH$_3$ benzothiazine), 4.50$_{anti}$ (s, NH), 4.55$_{syn}$ (s, NH), 5.48$_{anti}$ (s, C-H benzothiazine), 5.81$_{syn}$ (s, C-H benzothiazine), 6.74$_{syn}$ (t, J = 7.5, H$_7$ benzothiazine), 6.80$_{anti}$ (t, J = 7.5, H$_7$ benzothiazine), 6.93$_{anti}$ (d, J = 7.5 Hz, H$_5$ benzothiazine), 6.97$_{syn}$ (d, J = 7.5 Hz, H$_5$ benzothiazine), 7.08$_{anti}$ (d, J = 7.5 Hz, H$_8$ benzothiazine), 7.12$_{syn}$ (t, J = 7.5 Hz, H$_6$ benzothiazine), 7.13$_{syn}$ (t, J = 7.2 Hz, H$_6$ chromene), 7.24-7.25$_{syn}$ (m, H$_8$ benzothiazine and H$_8$ chromene), 7.26-7.29$_{anti}$ (m, H$_6$ benzothiazine and H$_{6,8}$ chromene), 7.35-7.37$_{syn}$ (m, H$_4$ thiophene and H$_{5,7}$ chro-mene), 7.37-7.40$_{anti}$ (m, H$_6$ chromene and H$_4$ thiophene), 7.50-7.53$_{anti}$ (m, H$_7$ chromene and H$_5$ thiophene), 7.58$_{syn}$ (d, J = 5.0 Hz, H$_5$ thiophene), 7.79$_{anti}$ (s, H$_2$ thiophene), 8.04$_{syn}$ (s, H$_2$ thiophene), 8.14$_{anti}$ (s, H$_4$ chromene), 8.25$_{syn}$ (s, H$_4$ chromene); ^{13}C NMR (syn-isomer, 125 MHz, CDCl$_3$) δ 27.8, 45.7, 54.4, 116.1, 116.8, 119.1, 119.9, 124.6, 126.3, 126.5, 127.3, 128.2, 128.4, 130.6, 131.5, 131.7, 132.6, 140.0, 140.2, 141.2, 153.1, 160.2, 187.7; MS, m/z (%) 419 (M$^+$, 68%), 404 (12), 386 (12), 308 (97), 295 (100), 280 (64), 111 (63); Anal. calcd for $C_{23}H_{17}NO_3S_2$: C, 65.85; H, 4.08; N, 3.34. Found: C, 65.98; H, 3.82; N, 3.60.

8-Methoxy-3-(3-methyl-2-(4-methylbenzoyl)-3,4-dihydro-2H-benzo[b][1,4]thiazin-3-yl)-2H-chromen-2-one (2n)

Yellow solid (343 mg, 75%); syn-isomer; mp 145–147°C; IR (KBr, cm^{-1}) 3360 (NH), 1700 (C=O); ^{1}H NMR (500 MHz, CDCl$_3$) δ 1.77 (s, 3H, CH$_3$ benzothiazine), 2.43 (s, 3H, CH$_3$ benzoyl), 3.90 (s, 3H, O-CH$_3$ chromene), 4.52 (s, 1H, NH), 6.00 (s, 1H, C-H benzothiazine), 6.78 (dt, J = 7.5 and

1.3 Hz, 1H, H_7 benzothiazine), 6.93 (dd, $J = 8.0$ and 1.3 Hz, 1H, H_7 chromene), 7.02-7.11 (m, 4H, $H_{5,6,8}$ benzothiazine and H_6 chromene), 7.18 (m, 3H, H_5 chromene and $H_{3,5}$ benzoyl), 7.74 (d, $J = 8.3$ Hz, 2H, $H_{2,6}$ benzoyl), 8.13 (s, 1H, H_4 chromene); ^{13}C NMR (125 MHz, CDCl$_3$) δ 21.6, 27.9, 43.6, 54.6, 56.1, 113.3, 114.8, 118.9, 119.4, 119.7, 119.9, 124.3, 126.3, 127.4, 128.5, 129.3, 131.1, 133.7, 140.0, 140.2, 142.8, 143.8, 146.7, 159.5, 192.9 cm^{-1}; Anal. calcd for $C_{27}H_{23}NO_4S$: C, 70.88; H, 5.07; N, 3.06. Found: C, 70.64; H, 5.23; N, 3.22.

3-(2-(4-Fluorobenzoyl)-3-methyl-3,4-dihydro-2H-benzo[b] [1,4]thiazin-3-yl)-8-methoxy-2H-chromen-2-one (2o)

Yellow solid (323 mg, 70%); syn-isomer; mp 236–238°C; IR (KBr, cm^{-1}) 3398 (NH), 1690 (C=O); ^1H NMR (500 MHz, CDCl$_3$) δ 1.78 (s, 3H, CH$_3$ benzothiazine), 3.98 (s, 3H, O-CH$_3$ chromene), 4.51 (s, 1H, NH), 5.98 (s, 1H, C-H benzothiazine), 6.74 (t, $J = 7.4$ Hz, 1H, H_7 benzothiazine), 6.93 (m, 2H, $H_{5,6}$ benzothiazine), 6.98 (d, $J = 8.0$ Hz, 1H, H_7 chromene), 7.05 (m, 2H, $H_{5,6}$ chromene), 7.16 (m, 3H, H_8 benzothiazine and $H_{3,5}$ benzoyl), 7.77 (s, 1H, H_4 chromene), 8.05 (m, 2H, $H_{2,6}$ benzoyl); ^{13}C NMR (125 MHz, CDCl$_3$) δ 24.5, 37.4, 56.3, 57.6, 111.9, 113.3, 115.7, 115.9, 116.9, 119.3, 119.8, 124.2, 126.7, 128.4, 131.2, 131.3, 131.4, 133.1, 139.5, 141.2, 146.8, 160.7, 164.7, 166.7, 191.2; Anal. calcd for $C_{26}H_{20}FNO_4S$: C, 67.67; H, 4.37; N, 3.04. Found: C, 67.43; H, 4.18; N, 3.25.

3-(2-(4-Bromobenzoyl)-3-methyl-3,4-dihydro-2H-benzo[b] [1,4]thiazin-3-yl)-7-(2-(4-bromophenyl)-2-oxoethoxy)-2H-chromen-2-one (2s)

Yellow solid (507 mg, 72%); as mixture of diasteromers (anti/syn: 18/82); IR (KBr, cm^{-1}) 3382 (NH), 1697 (C=O); ^1H NMR (500 MHz, CDCl$_3$) δ 1.74$_{syn}$ (s, CH$_3$ benzothiazine), 1.85$_{anti}$ (s, CH$_3$ benzothiazine), 4.48$_{anti}$ (s, NH), 4.51$_{syn}$ (s, NH), 5.29$_{anti}$ (s, O-CH$_2$), 5.31$_{syn}$ (s, O-CH$_2$), 5.60$_{anti}$ (s, C-H benzothiazine), 5.91$_{syn}$ (s, C-H benzothiazine), 6.71$_{anti}$ (t, $J = 7.5$, H_7 benzothiazine), 6.73$_{syn}$ (t, $J = 7.5$, H_7 benzothiazine), 6.80$_{anti}$ (s, H_8 chromene), 6.82$_{syn}$ (s, H_8 chromene), 6.87$_{syn}$ (d, $J = 8.5$, H_6 chromene), 6.90$_{anti}$ (d, $J = 8.5$, H_6 chromene), 6.93$_{syn}$ (d, $J = 8.0$ Hz, $H_{3,5}$ phenyl-2-oxoethoxy), 7.05$_{anti}$ (d, $J = 8.0$, $H_{3,5}$ phenyl-2-oxoethoxy), 7.07$_{anti}$ (t, $J = 7.5$, H_6 benzothiazine), 7.12$_{syn}$ (t, $J = 7.5$, H_6 benzothiazine), 7.33$_{syn}$ (d, $J = 8.5$, H_5 chromene), 7.44$_{anti}$ (d, $J = 8.5$, H_5 chromene), 7.52$_{anti}$ (d, $J = 8.5$, $H_{3,5}$ benzoyl), 7.63$_{syn}$ (d, $J = 8.0$ Hz, $H_{3,5}$ benzoyl), 7.64-7.67$_{anti}$ (m, $H_{5,8}$ benzothiazine), 7.68$_{syn}$ (m, $H_{5,8}$ benzothiazine), 7.72$_{syn}$ (s, H_4 chromene), 7.82-7.85$_{anti}$ (m, $H_{2,6}$ benzoyl and $H_{2,6}$ phenyl-2-oxoethoxy), 7.85-7.89$_{syn}$ (m, $H_{2,6}$ benzoyl and $H_{2,6}$ phenyl-2-oxoethoxy), 8.06$_{anti}$ (s, H_4 chromene); ^{13}C NMR (syn-isomer, 125 MHz, CDCl$_3$) δ 24.5, 37.6, 57.4, 70.6, 101.1, 111.8, 112.9, 116.9, 118.7, 119.3, 126.7, 128.3, 128.4, 129.5, 129.6, 129.9, 130.0, 131.9, 132.0, 132.3, 132.8, 135.5, 139.6, 140.9, 154.7, 160.6, 161.3,

191.6, 192.4; Anal. calcd for $C_{33}H_{23}Br_2NO_5S$: C, 56.19; H, 3.29; N, 1.99. Found: C, 56.21; H, 4.31; N, 2.09.

3-(3-Methyl-2-(4-methylbenzoyl)-3,4-dihydro-2H-benzo[b] [1,4]thiazin-3-yl)-7-(2-oxo-2-p-tolylethoxy)-2H-chromen-2-one (2t)

Yellow solid (397 mg, 70%); as mixture of diastereomers (anti/syn: 30/70); IR (KBr, cm^{-1}) 3397 (NH), 1702 (C=O); ^1H NMR (500 MHz, CDCl$_3$) δ 1.74$_{syn}$ (s, CH$_3$ benzothiazine), 1.85$_{anti}$ (s, CH$_3$ benzothiazine), 2.36$_{anti}$ (s, CH$_3$ phenyl-2-oxoethoxy), 2.42$_{syn}$ (s, CH$_3$ phenyl-2-oxoethoxy), 2.44$_{anti}$ (s, CH$_3$ benzoyl), 2.45$_{syn}$ (s, CH$_3$ benzoyl), 4.50$_{syn}$ (s, NH), 4.61$_{anti}$ (s, NH), 5.31$_{anti}$ (s, O-CH$_2$), 5.35$_{syn}$ (s, O-CH$_2$), 5.61$_{anti}$ (s, C-H benzothiazine), 5.96$_{syn}$ (s, C-H benzothiazine), 6.69$_{anti}$ (d, $J = 2.1$ Hz, H_8 chromene), 6.72$_{syn}$ (t, $J = 7.3$ Hz, H_7 benzothiazine), 6.75$_{anti}$ (t, $J = 7.3$ Hz, H_7 benzothiazine), 6.81$_{syn}$ (d, $J = 2.1$ Hz, H_8 chromene), 6.87$_{syn}$ (dd, $J = 8.0$ and 2.1 Hz, H_6 chromene), 6.90-6.93$_{syn/anti}$ (m, $H_{5,8}$ benzothiazine), 7.05$_{anti}$ (t, $J = 7.3$ Hz, H_6 benzothiazine), 7.11$_{syn}$ (t, $J = 7.3$ Hz, H_6 benzothiazine), 7.17$_{anti}$ (d, $J = 8.0$ Hz, $H_{3,5}$ phenyl-2-oxoethoxy), 7.28-7.33 (m, H_5 chromene (syn/anti), $H_{3,5}$ benzoyl (syn/anti) and $H_{3,5}$ phenyl-2-oxoethoxy (syn)), 7.34$_{anti}$ (d, $J = 8.0$ Hz, $H_{2,6}$ phenyl-2-oxoethoxy), 7.73$_{syn}$ (s, H_4 chromene), 7.79$_{anti}$ (d, $J = 8.0$ Hz, $H_{2,6}$ benzoyl), 7.87$_{syn}$ (d, $J = 8.0$ Hz, $H_{2,6}$ phenyl-2-oxoethoxy), 7.94$_{syn}$ (d, $J = 8.0$ Hz, $H_{2,6}$ benzoyl), 8.06$_{anti}$ (s, H_4 chromene); ^{13}C NMR (syn-isomer, 125 MHz, CDCl$_3$) δ 24.0, 27.7, 32.6, 43.3, 56.0, 80.2, 110.4, 110.6, 113.6, 116.1, 118.7, 118.9, 119.9, 122.4, 124.5, 126.2, 127.2, 128.4, 129.2, 131.6, 140.1, 154.2, 161.2, 161.4, 192.1, 192.6; MS, m/z (%) 575 (M$^+$, 8%), 557 (64), 542 (43), 410 (35), 264 (44), 239 (29), 119 (100); Anal. calcd for $C_{35}H_{29}NO_5S$: C, 73.02 ; H, 5.08; N, 2.43. Found: C, 73.21; H, 5.12; N, 2.54.

3-(3-Methyl-2-(4-(methylsulfonyl)benzoyl)-3,4-dihydro-2H-benzo[b][1,4]thiazin-3-yl)-7-(2-(4-(methylsulfonyl)phenyl)-2-oxoethoxy)-2H-chromen-2-one (2u)

Yellow solid (576 mg, 82%); as mixture of diastereomers (anti/syn: 28/72); IR (KBr, cm^{-1}) 3394 (NH), 1688 (C=O), 1320 (SO$_2$), 1153 (SO$_2$); ^1H NMR (500 MHz, CDCl$_3$) δ 1.78$_{syn}$ (s, CH$_3$ benzothiazine), 1.89$_{anti}$ (s, CH$_3$ benzothiazine), 3.02$_{anti}$ (s, SO$_2$-CH$_3$ phenyl-2-oxoethoxy), 3.04$_{anti}$ (s, SO$_2$-CH$_3$ benzoyl), 3.09$_{syn}$ (s, SO$_2$-CH$_3$ phenyl-2-oxoethoxy), 3.12$_{syn}$ (s, SO$_2$-CH$_3$ benzoyl), 4.50$_{anti}$ (s, NH), 4.69$_{syn}$ (s, NH), 5.37$_{syn}$ (s, O-CH$_2$), 5.41$_{anti}$(s, O-CH$_2$), 5.61$_{anti}$ (s, C-H benzothiazine), 5.95$_{syn}$ (s, C-H benzothiazine), 6.69$_{anti}$ (s, H_8 chromene), 6.74$_{syn}$ (t, $J = 7.5$, H_7 benzothiazine), 6.80$_{anti}$ (t, $J = 7.5$, H_7 benzothiazine), 6.83$_{syn}$ (s, H_8 chromene), 6.88-6.95$_{syn}$ (m, H_6 chromene and $H_{5,8}$ benzothiazine), 7.08$_{anti}$ (d, $J = 8.0$, H_6 chromene), 7.11$_{anti}$ (t, $J = 7.5$, H_6 benzothiazine), 7.13$_{syn}$ (t, $J = 7.5$ Hz, H_6 benzothiazine), 7.36$_{syn}$ (d, $J = 8.0$, H_5 chromene), 7.50$_{anti}$ (d, $J = 8.0$, H_5 chromene), 7.59$_{anti}$ (d, $J = 7.5$ Hz, H_8

benzothiazine), 7.74_{syn} (s, H_4 chromene), 7.82_{anti} (d, $J =$ 7.5 Hz, H_5 benzothiazine), 7.94_{anti} (s, H_4 chromene), 8.04-$8.19_{syn/anti}$ (m, $H_{2,3,5,6}$ phenyl-2-oxoethoxy and $H_{2,3,5,6}$ benzoyl); ^{13}C NMR (syn-isomer, 125 MHz, $CDCl_3$) δ 24.5, 44.2, 44.3, 57.5, 65.5, 70.9, 101.0, 110.9, 113.0, 116.9, 119.4, 126.9, 127.4, 127.9, 128.1, 128.5, 129.1, 129.3, 129.8, 138.0, 139.6, 140.8, 141.0, 143.9, 145.1, 154.7, 160.4, 161.2, 190.6, 192.6; Anal. calcd for $C_{35}H_{29}NO_9S_3$: C, 59.73 ; H, 4.15; N, 1.99. Found: C, 59.59; H, 4.31; N, 2.30.

Pharmacology

Animals

Male NMRI mice weighing 20–30 g were used for studying in vivo antinociceptive activities of target compounds. Animals were maintained under standard conditions (24 ± 2°C, 60-70% humidity) and allowed food and water *ad libitum*. They were housed in appropriate cages with 12 h light/dark cycle. Before each experiment animals randomly

selected and allocated into groups. The whole protocol was approved by the Ethics Committee of the Faculty of Pharmacy at Tehran University of Medical Sciences.

Formalin-induced pain test

All target compounds **2a-u** were subjected for testing their analgesic activity using formalin paw test [25]. The compounds or standard drug mefenamic acid were administered i.p. (30 mg/kg, 0.2 mL/20 g body weight) as a suspension in saline and tween 80 (4% w/v). Each group of mice (n = 6 animals per group) were pretreated by test compounds, mefenamic acid or vehicle, 30 minutes before injection of formalin (20 μL, 0.5%, s.c.) into the planar surface of the right hind paw. The amount of time that the animal spent licking injected paw was measured during the first 10 minutes (phase 1, neurogenic) and 10–30 minutes (phase 2, inflammatory) after formalin injection.

Table 1 Antinociception activity of target compounds 2a-u and mefenamic acid (30 mg/kg, i.p.) assessed by formalin test in mice

Compounds	Phase 1			Phase 2		
	Licking time[a]	Inhibition[b] (%)	Relative activity[c]	Licking time	Inhibition (%)	Relative activity
2a	58 ± 3.46	48.10**	0.54	37.33 ± 3.93	44.28**	0.52
2b	51.33 ± 2.96	54.06***	0.61	50.33 ± 4.91	24.88	0.29
2c	68.33 ± 4.05	38.85**	0.44	38 ± 1.73	43.28**	0.51
2d	55 ± 2.74	50.78***	0.57	57.33 ± 6.35	14.43	0.17
2e	44 ± 2.89	60.63***	0.68	54 ± 4.93	19.40	0.23
2f	60.33 ± 3.76	46.01**	0.52	38.33 ± 4.63	42.79**	0.50
2g	56.66 ± 8.74	49.29**	0.55	55.66 ± 3.92	16.92	0.20
2h	70.25 ± 2.95	37.14**	0.42	38 ± 1	43.28**	0.51
2i	51.33 ± 2.40	54.06***	0.61	37 ± 1.15	44.78**	0.53
2j	46.25 ± 2.56	58.61***	0.66	50.33 ± 0.33	24.88	0.29
2k	51.66 ± 2.18	53.77***	0.60	51.66 ± 5.54	22.89	0.27
2l	70 ± 11.13	37.36**	0.42	37 ± 4.35	44.78**	0.53
2m	63.33 ± 8.21	43.33**	0.49	18.33 ± 0.33	72.64***	0.85
2n	69 ± 9.16	38.26**	0.43	40.66 ± 1.20	39.30**	0.46
2o	53.8 ± 3.21	51.85**	0.58	65 ± 6.41	2.98	0.03
2p	53.9 ± 3.18	51.76**	0.58	64.8 ± 4.19	3.28	0.04
2q	61.33 ± 5.78	45.12**	0.51	49.5 ± 2.02	26.12	0.31
2r	94.4 ± 4.89	25.86**	0.29	11 ± 1.7	93.64***	1.1
2s	50 ± 3.22	33.33**	0.37	5.2 ± 2.78	96.99***	1.14
2t	46 ± 2.4	38.86**	0.43	3 ± 1.04	98.26***	1.15
2u	34.8 ± 2.65	53.6***	0.61	14.8 ± 1.92	91.44***	1.07
Control	111.75 ± 6.94	-	-	67 ± 3.14	-	-
Mefenamic acid	12.33 ± 3.93	88.96***	1	10 ± 2.52	85.07***	1

[a]Data are expressed as mean ± S.E.M (number of animals in each group, n = 6).
[b]The percentage inhibition was determined by using the following formula: Inhibition % = 100 × (control − experiment)/control. The asterisks denote the levels of significance in comparison with control groups (*P <0.05, **P <0.01 and ***P <0.001).
[c]Activity relative to mefenamic acid was determined by using the following formula: Relative Activity = Inhibition % of compound/Inhibition % of mefenamic acid.

Acetic acid-induced writhing test

The analgesic activity was also determined *in vivo* by the abdominal constriction test induced by acetic acid (0.6%; 0.1 mL/10 g) in mice [21]. An acetic acid solution was administered i.p. 30 minutes after administration of compounds or mefenamic acid. After the treatment, pairs of mice were placed in separate boxes and the numbers of constrictions of the abdominal muscles, together with stretching, were counted cumulatively over a period of 60 minutes. Antinociceptive activity was expressed as the percentage of inhibition of constrictions when compared with the vehicle control group.

Statistical analysis

The nociception data are expressed as means ± SEM. Variance analysis (ANOVA) followed by Bonferroni's test was used to compare means. *P*-values less than 0.05 were considered to be statistically significant.

Results and discussion

Chemistry

The dihydrobenzothiazole derivatives **1** were quantitatively obtained by reaction of 3-acetylcoumarins with 2-aminothiophenol derivatives in the presence of acetic acid under reflux condition or microwave irradiation [19,20]. The intramolecular Mannich-type reaction of compounds **1** with different phenacyl halides in the present of KF/Al_2O_3 and catalyzing by quinine hydrochloride in ethanol afforded 3,4-dihydro-2H-benzothiazine derivatives **2a-r** via a ring expansion. When 7-hydroxy-3-(benzothiazol-2-

yl) coumarin derivative **1e** was treated with 2.5 equivalents of phenacyl halides, without protection of hydroxyl group, O-phenacyl derivatives **2s-u** was obtained in excellent yields (Scheme 1). The physicochemical and spectral data of new compounds **2e**, **2j-o**, and **2s-u** are described in experimental section.

Biological activity

Formalin-induced nociception test

All target compounds **2a-u** were tested using formalin-induced pain test in mice [25]. The obtained results were reported as mean ± SEM of licking time and as percent of inhibition in Table 1. In general, the results showed that most of compounds were significantly able to reduce the licking time with percent of inhibition in the range of 25% to 60% at the first phase. The standard drug mefenamic acid showed 89% reduction of the licking time during the first phase. Amongst the tested compounds, **2a**, **2c**, **2f**, **2h**, **2i**, **2l-n** and **2r-u** significantly reduced the formalin induced licking time in the range of 39-98% as compared to mefenamic acid with 85% of inhibition during the second phase. Compounds **2m** and **2r-u** showed more effective antinociceptive activity in the second phase rather than first phase, indicating their ability to inhibit nociception associated with inflammatory response. Indeed, 7-hydroxy- and 7-phenacyloxy-coumarin derivatives (**2r** and **2s-u**, respectively) were more effective than mefenamic acid. Compounds **2s** and **2t** were the most effective compounds at the dose of 30 mg/kg.

Table 2 Antinociception activity of selected compounds in comparison with mefenamic acid (30 mg/kg, i.p.) assessed by acetic acid-induced writhing test in mice

Compound	Nociception (Mean ± SEM)	Inhibition (%)[a]	Relative activity[b]
2b	0.6 ± 0.24***	99	1.4
2c	38 ± 4.04***	49	0.7
2d	9.6 ± 2.54***	87	1.3
2g	3.5 ± 1.09***	96	1.37
2h	3 ± 1.84***	97	1.38
2i	4.6 ± 2***	94	1.34
2k	20 ± 2.48***	73	1.04
2o	6 ± 3.2***	92	1.31
2r	29 ± 2.12***	63	0.9
2s	14 ± 2.28***	80	1.14
2t	30 ± 7.6***	60	0.85
2u	2 ± 1.3***	98	1.4
Control[c]	75 ± 3.2		
Mefnamic acid	23 ± 1.3***	70	

[a]The percentage inhibition was determined by using the following formula: Inhibition% = 100 × (control – experiment)/control.
[b]Activity relative to mefenamic acid was determined by using the following formula: Relative Activity = Inhibition % of compound/Inhibition % of mefenamic acid.
[c]Tween 80 in saline (4% w/v).
***P <0.001 vs. control.

Acetic acid-induced writhing test

The analgesic activity of compounds **2b-d**, **2g-i**, **2k**, **2o** and **2r-s** was also evaluated in vivo by using abdominal constriction test induced by acetic acid in mice [21]. The abdominal constriction response induced by acetic acid is sensitive procedure to establish efficacy of peripherally acting analgesics. The analgesic activity was expressed as the percentage of inhibition of constrictions when compared with the control group. The results are summarized in Table 2.

Significant protection against writhing was observed in animals treated with all test compounds where the mean numbers of writhes after 1 h were less than 38 compared to 75 in the control group. The percent of inhibition was in the range of 49-99%. All tested compounds were more effective than standard drug mefenamic acid with the exception of **2c**, **2r** and **2t**. Compounds **2b** and **2u** with percent of inhibition ≥98% were the most effective compounds in acetic acid-induced writhing test. Moreover, compounds **2g-i** and **2o** exhibited high protection against writhing (percent of inhibition > 90%).

Structure–activity relationships

From the structure–activity relationships of unsubstituted coumarin series (compound **2a-m**) based on the late stage of formalin-induced test, it was inferred that 3-thienylcarbonyl group is more favorable for activity. By comparing the activity of 7-substituted coumarin compounds **2r-u** with those of other compounds it is appeared that the 7-hydroxy or 7-phenacyloxy groups dramatically increase the effectiveness of compounds and their ability to inhibit nociception associated with inflammatory response. On contrary, compounds **2r-u** showed low level of inhibition at early phase of formalin test.

By comparing the percent of inhibition of 4-(methylsulfonyl)benzoyl derivatives **2d**, **2r** and **2u**, it is revealed that the introduction of hydroxyl group on 7-position of coumarin ring diminished the antinociception activity, while the introduction of 4-(methylsulfonyl)phenacyloxy- group increased the activity as resulted from writhing test. In the 7-phenacyloxy-coumarin derivatives **2s-u**, methylsulfonyl substituent was more favorable than bromo and methyl groups. The observed results of unsubstituted coumarin derivatives in Table 2 demonstrate that electron donating or bulky groups (for example, methoxy or phenyl, respectively) can increase antinociceptive activity in writhing test.

Conclusion

In summary, a series of 3-(3-methyl-3,4-dihydro-2*H*-benzo[*b*][1,4]thiazin-3-yl)-2*H*-chromen-2-one derivatives **2a-u** bearing different aroyl group on the 2-position of benzothiazine ring were described as potential analgesic agents. The antinociceptive properties of target compounds were determined by formalin-induced test and

acetic acid-induced writhing test in mice. The effect of substituent on aroyl moiety was explored by introduction of various electron withdrawing, electron donating or bulky groups. Surprisingly, compound **2u** bearing 2-[4-(methylsulfonyl)benzoyl]- moiety on benzothiazine ring and 4-(methylsulfonyl)phenacyloxy- group on the 7 position of coumarin nucleus showed better profile of antinociception in both models. It was more effective than mefenamic acid during the late phase of formalin-induced test as well as in the acetic acid-induced writhing test. However, unsubstituted coumarin derivative **2b** containing 4-methylbenzoyl moiety on benzothiazine ring, fully protected animals against writhing and was moderately able to inhibit the both phases of the formalin test. Considering the significant antinociceptive action of phenacyloxy-coumarin derivatives, compound **2u** prototype might be further used as model to obtain new more potent analgesic drugs.

Additional file

Additional file 1: Table S1. Chemical structure of coumarin compounds **2a-u**.

Competing interests

The authors declare that they have no competing interests.

Authors' contributions

MA: Synthesis of target compounds. MK: Synthesis of target compounds. SE: Collaboration in identifying of the structures of target compounds, manuscript preparation. SF: Collaboration in determination of antinociceptive properties. SFG: Collaboration in determination of antinociceptive properties. MA: Supervision of the pharmacological part, AF: Collaboration in identifying of the structures of target compounds. AS: Design of target compounds and supervision of the synthetic and pharmacological parts. All authors read and approved the final manuscript.

Acknowledgments

This work was financially supported by grants from Research Council of Tehran University of Medical Sciences and INSF (Iran National Science Foundation).

Author details

[1]School of Chemistry, University College of Science, University of Tehran, P.O. Box 14155-6455, Tehran, Iran. [2]Department of Medicinal Chemistry, Faculty of Pharmacy and Pharmaceutical Sciences Research Center, Tehran University of Medical Sciences, Tehran 14176, Iran. [3]Department of Medicinal Chemistry and Pharmaceutical Sciences Research Center, Faculty of Pharmacy, Mazandaran University of Medical Sciences, Sari, Iran. [4]Department of Toxicology and Pharmacology, Pharmaceutical Sciences Research Center, Faculty of Pharmacy, Tehran University of Medical Sciences, Tehran 14176, Iran.

References

1.   Ruoff G, Lema M: **Strategies in pain management: new and potential indications for COX-2 specific inhibitors.** *J Pain Symptom Manage* 2003, 25:S21–S31.
2.   Giovannoni MP, Cesari N, Graziano A, Vergelli C, Biancalani C, Biagini P, Dal Piaz V: **Synthesis of pyrrolo[2,3-d]pyridazinones as potent, subtype selective PDE4 inhibitors.** *J Enzyme Inhib Med Chem* 2007, 22:309–318.

3. Cesari N, Biancalani C, Vergelli C, Dal Piaz V, Graziano A, Biagini P, Ghelardini C, Galeotti N, Giovannoni MP: **Arylpiperazinylalkylpyridazinones and analogues as potent and orally active antinociceptive agents: synthesis and studies on mechanism of action.** *J Med Chem* 2006, **49**:7826–7835.

4. Magiatis P, Melliou E, Skaltsounis AL, Mitaku S, Léonce S, Renard P, Pierré A, Atassi G: **Synthesis and cytotoxic activity of pyranocoumarins of the seselin and xanthyletin series.** *J Nat Prod* 1998, **61**:982–986.

5. Beillerot A, Domínguez JCR, Kirsch G, Bagrel D: **Synthesis and protective effects of coumarin derivatives against oxidative stress induced by doxorubicin.** *Bioorg Med Chem Lett* 2008, **18**:1102–1105.

6. Zhou X, Wang XB, Wang T, Kong LY: **Design, synthesis, and acetylcholinesterase inhibitory activity of novel coumarin analogues.** *Bioorg Med Chem* 2008, **16**:8011–8021.

7. Sashidhara KV, Kumar A, Kumar M, Sarkar J, Sinha S: **Synthesis and in vitro evaluation of novel coumarin–chalcone hybrids as potential anticancer agents.** *Bioorg Med Chem Lett* 2010, **20**:7205–7211.

8. Sashidhara KV, Kumar A, Kumar M, Srivastava A, Puri A: **Synthesis and antihyperlipidemic activity of novel coumarin bisindole derivatives.** *Bioorg Med Chem Lett* 2010, **20**:6504–6507.

9. Lee S, Sivakumar K, Shin WS, Xie F, Wang Q: **Synthesis and anti-angiogenesis activity of coumarin derivatives.** *Bioorg Med Chem Lett* 2006, **16**:4596–4599.

10. Leal LKAM, Ferreira AAG, Bezerra GA, Matos FJA, Viana GSB: **Antinociceptive, anti-inflammatory and bronchodilator activities of Brazilian medicinal plants containing coumarin: a comparative study.** *J Ethnopharmacol* 2000, **70**:151–159.

11. Keri RS, Hosamani KM, Shingalapur RV, Hugar MH: **Analgesic, anti-pyretic and DNA cleavage studies of novel pyrimidine derivatives of coumarin moiety.** *Eur J Med Chem* 2010, **45**:2597–2605.

12. Kalkhambkar RG, Kulkarni GM, Kamanavalli CM, Premkumar N, Asdaq SMB, Sun CM: **Synthesis and biological activities of some new fluorinated coumarins and 1-aza coumarins.** *Eur J Med Chem* 2008, **43**:2178–2188.

13. Ghate M, Kusanur RA, Kulkarni MV: **Synthesis and in vivo analgesic and anti-inflammatory activity of some bi heterocyclic coumarin derivatives.** *Eur J Med Chem* 2005, **40**:882–887.

14. Bolakatti GS, Maddi VS, Mamledesai SN, Ronad PM, Palkar MB, Swamy S: **Synthesis and evaluation of anti-inflammatory and analgesic activities of a novel series of coumarin mannich bases.** *Arzneim-Forsch/Drug Res* 2008, **58**:515–520.

15. Khode S, Maddi V, Aragade P, Palkar M, Ronad PK, Mamledesai S, Thippeswamy AHM, Satyanarayana D: **Synthesis and pharmacological evaluation of a novel series of 5-(substituted)aryl-3-(3-coumarinyl)-1-phenyl-2-pyrazolines as novel anti-inflammatory and analgesic agents.** *Eur J Med Chem* 2009, **44**:1682–1688.

16. Melagraki G, Afantitis A, Igglessi-Markopoulou O, Detsi A, Koufaki M, Kontogiorgis C, Hadjipavlou-Litina DJ: **Synthesis and evaluation of the antioxidant and anti-inflammatory activity of novel coumarin-3-aminoamides and their alpha-lipoic acid adducts.** *Eur J Med Chem* 2009, **44**:3020–3026.

17. Rathore BS, Kumar M: **Synthesis of 7-chloro-5-trifluoromethyl/7-fluoro/7-trifluoromethyl-4H-1,4-benzothiazines as antimicrobial agents.** *Bioorg Med Chem* 2006, **14**:5678–5682.

18. Trapani G, Reho A, Morlacchi F, Latrofa A, Marchini P, Venturi F, Cantalamessa F: **Synthesis and antiinflammatory activity of various 1,4-benzothiazine derivatives.** *Farmaco Sci* 1985, **40**:369–376.

19. Khoobi M, Emami S, Dehghan G, Foroumadi A, Ramazani A, Shafiee A: **Synthesis and free radical scavenging activity of coumarin derivatives containing a 2-methylbenzothiazoline motif.** *Arch Pharm* 2011, **344**:588–594.

20. Khoobi M, Ramazani A, Foroumadi A, Hamadi H, Hojjati Z, Shafiee A: **Efficient microwave-assisted synthesis of 3-benzothiazolo and 3-benzothiazolino coumarin derivatives catalyzed by heteropoly acids.** *J Iran Chem Soc* 2011, **8**:1036–1042.

21. Collier HDJ, Dinnin LC, Johnson CA, Schneider C: **The abdominal constriction response and its suppression by analgesic drugs in the mouse.** *Br J Pharmacol Chemother* 1968, **32**:295–310.

22. Tjolsen A, Berge OG, Hunskaar S, Rosland JH, Hole K: **The formalin test: an evaluation of the method.** *Pain* 1992, **51**:5–17.

23. Khoobi M, Ramazani A, Foroumadi A, Emami S, Jafarpour F, Mahyari A, Ślepokura K, Lis T, Shafiee A: **Highly *cis*-diastereoselective synthesis of coumarin-based 2,3-disubstituted dihydrobenzothiazines by organocatalysis.** *Helv Chim Acta* 2012, **95**:660–671.

24. Victoria FN, Radatz CS, Sachini M, Jacob RG, Perin G, da Silva WP, Lenard EJ: **KF/Al$_2$O$_3$ and PEG-400 as a recyclable medium for the selective α-selenation of aldehydes and ketones. Preparation of potential antimicrobial agents.** *Tetrahedron Lett* 2009, **50**:6761–6763.

25. Hunskaar S, Hole K: **The formalin test in mice: dissociation between inflammatory and non-inflammatory pain.** *Pain* 1987, **30**:103–114.

11

The release behavior and kinetic evaluation of tramadol HCl from chemically cross linked Ter polymeric hydrogels

Muhammad A Malana* and Rubab Zohra

Abstract

Background and the purpose of the study: Hydrogels, being stimuli responsive are considered to be effective for targeted and sustained drug delivery. The main purpose for this work was to study the release behavior and kinetic evaluation of Tramadol HCl from chemically cross linked ter polymeric hydrogels.

Methods: Ter-polymers of methacrylate, vinyl acetate and acrylic acid cross linked with ethylene glycol dimethacrylate (EGDMA) were prepared by free radical polymerization. The drug release rates, dynamic swelling behavior and pH sensitivity of hydrogels ranging in composition from 1-10 mol% EGDMA were studied. Tramadol HCl was used as model drug substance. The release behavior was investigated at pH 8 where all formulations exhibited non-Fickian diffusion mechanism.

Results and major conclusion: Absorbency was found to be more than 99% indicating good drug loading capability of these hydrogels towards the selected drug substance. Formulations designed with increasing amounts of EGDMA had a decreased equilibrium media content as well as media penetrating velocity and thus exhibited a slower drug release rate. Fitting of release data to different kinetic models indicate that the kinetic order shifts from the first to zero order as the concentration of drug was increased in the medium, showing gradual independency of drug release towards its concentration. Formulations with low drug content showed best fitness with Higuchi model whereas those with higher concentration of drug followed Hixson-Crowell model with better correlation values indicating that the drug release from these formulations depends more on change in surface area and diameter of tablets than that on concentration of the drug. Release exponent (n) derived from Korse-Meyer Peppas equation implied that the release of Tramadol HCl from these formulations was generally non-Fickian (n > 0.5 > 1) showing swelling controlled mechanism. The mechanical strength and controlled release capability of the systems indicate that these co-polymeric hydrogels have a great potential to be used as colon drug delivery device through oral administration.

Keywords: Tramadol HCl, Acrylic acid, Ter-polymer, Cross-linked, Release behavior

Introduction

Tramadol, a synthetic opioid of the amino-cyclohexanol group, exhibiting weak opioid agonist properties, is a centrally acting analgesic and has been observed to be effective in both experimental and clinical pain and additionally causes no serious cardiovascular or respiratory side effects [1]. The usual oral dosage requirement of the drug is 50 to 100 mg every 4 to 6 hours with a maximum dosage of 400 mg per day [2]. A sustained-release formulation of tramadol is required to improve patient compliance and to reduce the administration frequency. To modulate the drug release, the most commonly used method is to include it in a matrix system [3]. As hydrophilic polymer matrix systems are proved to be flexible to obtain a desirable drug release profile, these are widely used in oral controlled drug delivery [4]. Using a hydrophilic matrix system to release the drug for extended duration, especially, for highly water-soluble drugs, is restricted to rapid diffusion of the dissolved drug through the hydrophilic gel structures. For such highly soluble drug substances, chemically cross linked hydrogels are considered suitable as matrixing agents

* Correspondence: aslam.malana2@gmail.com
Chemistry Department, Bahauddin Zakarya University, Multan, Pakistan

for developing sustained-release dosage forms. This extensive use corresponds to the non-toxicity, high drug loading capacity and pH-sensitivity of the network structure. Moreover, a problem, frequently, encountered with the oral administration of these formulations, is inability to increase the resistance time in stomach and proximal portion of small intestine [5]. To overcome this problem, it becomes necessary to prolong the dosage form either in the stomach or somewhere in the upper small intestine until all the drug is released over the desired period of time [6,7].

These polymer matrices can be either chemically cross linked having covalent bonding or physically cross linked through hydrogen bonds depending on the monomers, polymerization methods and the mode of application [8]. Advance research has flashed over synthesizing and characterizing hydrogels having particular mechanical properties such as strength and modulus, environmental sensitivity to temperature, electric field, pH or ionic strength and mass transport control that can be "tuned" to get special pharmacological application including reduced toxic "burst" effects of a drug, protections of fragile drugs in their dosage environment and location specific dosage etc. [9].

In the present work, the main objective was to study the release behavior and kinetic evaluation of a model drug tramadol HCl from chemically cross linked (Vinylacetate-co-methacrylate-co-acrylic acid) (VA-co-MA-co-AA) co-polymeric ternary systems. The preliminary swelling studies [10] are indicative of the fact that these hydrogels may be able to face the problems related to sustained drug delivery. For this purpose chemically cross linked co-polymeric hydrogels were prepared with a range of cross linker concentration. Effect of the concentration of the cross linker on various swelling parameters and the drug release profiles was estimated. Influence of amount of drug loaded on drug release rate was also studied in detail. Different release models were applied to evaluate the release kinetics of the drug from the optimized formulation.

Experimental

Materials and polymer preparation

Two hydrophobic monomers, methacrylate (MA) (MERCK, 99%) and vinylacetate (VA) 9Fluka, 99%) were mixed with a hydrophilic monomer, acrylic acid (AA) (fluka, 99%) to prepare the polymer for this study. Copolymers of MA, VA and AA were prepared according to the previously reported method by free radical polymerization [10] using Benzoylperoxide (BPO) (MERCK, 100%) as the initiator and ethanol as solvent. Different grades (E_1, E_2, E_3, E_4 having 1, 3.5, 6.5, 10 mol% respectively) of the cross linker Ethylene glycoldimethacrylate (EGDMA) (Fluka, 100%) were added to prepare chemically cross linked co-polymeric networks.

Swelling studies

The dried hydrogel disks were immersed in excess of the swelling medium (50ml) having a pH range from 1-8 at 37°C. At regular intervals of time, the disks were removed from the solution and weighed after excess solution on the surface was blotted. The experiment was performed in triplicate and the swelling parameters like media penetration velocity (v), equilibrium media content (Q_e) and diffusion exponent were calculated using following equations [10]:

$$\%S \ = \ m_t-m_o/m_o \ \times 100 \tag{1}$$

Where m_t is the mass of the swollen hydrogel and m_o is the mass of xerogel.

$$1n \ W_t/W_e \ = \ 1nk \ + \ n \ 1nt \tag{2}$$

Where W_t is the dynamic media content at time t and W_e is the equilibrium media content, n stands for diffusion exponent and k is the rate constant.

Drug loading

The dried polymer disks were loaded with Tramadol HCl by soaking them in various drug solutions (T_1, T_2, T_3, T_4, T_5, T_6 having 0.8, 1.6, 2.4, 3.2, 4.0, 4.8 mg/ml respectively) in phosphate buffer solutions of pH 8.0 at 37°C till the equilibrium swelling was attained. This method was preferred to in situ drug loading to avoid any probable degradation of the drug substance or undesirable drug-polymer reaction when high temperature was applied during the synthesis process. The wet drug loaded polymers were dried at room temperature through simple evaporation. The drug loaded dried polymer disks were cloudy when compared to similar disks without the drug. The absorbency of tramadol by the hydrogels was calculated using the following equation [11]:

$$Absorbency \ (Q) \ = \ (C_1V_1-C_2V_2)/m_o \tag{3}$$

Where Q (mg/g) is the absorbency of tramadol by the xerogel; C_1 (mg/ml) is the initial concentration of tramadol solution; V_1 (ml) represents the initial volume of tramadol solution; C_2 (mg/ml) is the concentration of tramdol after absorption by the xerogel; V_2 (ml) is the volume of tramadol solution after absorption by the polymer; and m_o is the mass of the polymer in dry state.

In vitro drug release studies

In vitro drug release of Tramadol HCl from co-polymeric hydrogels was evaluated in triplicate using UV-Visible spectrophotometry. The dried drug loaded disks were transferred into the fixed volume of buffer solution of pH 8 at 37°C. At specified time intervals, 3 ml of aliquots were removed from every buffer solution and the absorbance was noted using UV-visible spectrophotometer at the maximum absorption wave length (240nm) already measured using a stock solution of Tramadol HCl in phosphate buffer of pH 8. Three aliquots of various solutions were studied for any single point of release curve. After absorbance measurements, aliquots were returned to the original solution, so that the volume may be kept constant. To transform absorbance determinations into concentrations, calibration curve was used [12].

Release kinetics

To study the release kinetics of Tramadol HCl from the matrix tablets, the release data were fitted to the following equations:

Zero order equation [13]:

$$Q_t = k_o t \qquad (4)$$

Where Q_t stands for the percentage of drug released at time t and k_o is the release rate constant;

First order equation [14]:

$$1n\ (100 - Q_t) = 1n100 - k_1 t \qquad (5)$$

Where k_1 stands for release rate constant for the first order kinetics;

Higuchi's equation [15]:

$$Q_t = k_H t^{1/2} \qquad (6)$$

Where k_H represents the Higuchi release rate constant;

Hixson-Crowell model [16]:

$$(100 - Q_t)^{1/2} = 100^{1/3} - k_{HC} t \qquad (7)$$

Where, k_{HC} stands for Hixson-Crowell rate constant.

Moreover, for better characterization of the drug release mechanisms, the Korsmeyer-Peppas [17] semi-empirical model was applied:

$$Q_t/Q_e = k_{KP} t^n \qquad (8)$$

Where Q_t/Q_e is the fraction of the drug released at time t, k_{KP} is a constant corresponding to the structural and geometric characteristics of the device and n is the release exponent which is indicative of the mechanism of the drug release. In case of cylindrical geometries such as tablets, for fitting the data to the equations, only the points within the interval 10-70% were used. In case of Hixson-Crowell and korsmeyer-Peppas models, the data taken was within 10-60% drug release.

Mechanical strength

Mechanical strength of dried as well as hydrogels swollen at different pH values up to equilibrium point was determined applying the weight on them until the hydrogels were fractured [18,19].

DSC/TGA analysis

Thermal degradation of the hydrogel systems was studied using a thermo-gravimetric analyzer [TA Instruments SDT Q. 600 V20 .9 Build 20 simultaneous TGA-DSC], by heating them from room temperature to 600°C at a heating rate of 10°C/min under a nitrogen flow.

Discussion

Media penetration velocity and equilibrium media content

Figures 1 and 2 show the influence of the copolymer composition and the media pH on the dynamic swelling behavior of the copolymers. As the concentration of EGDMA in the polymer network increased, the rate of sorption and equilibrium water content was decreased. This is not surprising since AA is hydrophilic and EGDMA binds AA to increase the cross link density in the hydrogels which lowers the average molecular weight between the cross links and this curtails the free volumes accessible to the penetrant water molecules [18]. As far as pH of the medium is concerned, the highest swelling rate and equilibrium media content were observed at pH 8. It has already been reported that acidic hydrogels show greater media sorption rate in basic medium where most of the free carboxylic groups get ionized to produce negatively charged carboxylate ions which cause repulsions ultimately resulting in higher swelling rate as well as equilibrium media content [20].

The rate of advancement of glassy to rubbery front from the surface to the center of the polymer disk was determined by calculating the media penetration velocity (v),

$$v = 1/2\rho A\ \delta w/\delta t \qquad (9)$$

Where "ρ" is the density of the medium, "A" represents the area of the one disk face, "w" is the mass

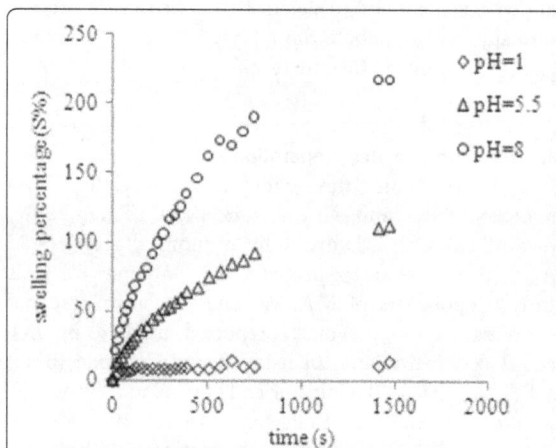

Figure 1 Media sorption profile for optimized concentration of the cross linker (3.5 mol%) exhibting effect of pH.

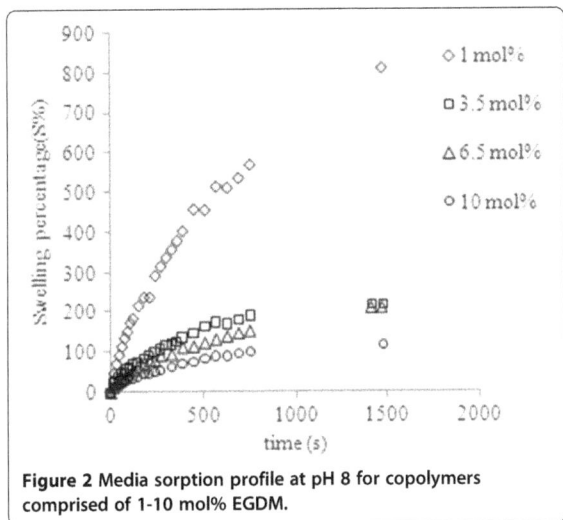

Figure 2 Media sorption profile at pH 8 for copolymers comprised of 1-10 mol% EGDM.

gained by the polymer and "t" is the time. The early time data (t<15 min) were used to calculate the media penetration velocity. It has been reported, as the media penetrates the glassy polymer, the solvent swells the polymer and produces a rubbery region [21]. Figure 3 shows that the media penetration velocity decreased by 75% at pH 5.5 and 73% at pH8 and on the other hand the equilibrium media content also decreased by an order of magnitude as the concentration of EGDMA was increased from 1-10 mol % at all the pH values. A similar degree of decrease in media penetration velocity was observed in other hydrophobic-hydrophilic copolymers like poly (HEMA-co-MMA) as the proportion of hydrophobic monomer MMA was increased from 0-40% [21,22].

The change in media penetration velocity with increasing EGDMA content may be due to two possible mechanisms: first if the media travelled primarily through the hydrophilic AA regions of these copolymers, the increasing number of cross link domains might keep AA content busy in building the cross links that could obstruct the media diffusive path way for diffusion; secondly, the increased cross linker's concentration may also inhibit polymer chain relaxation, thus reducing the free volume through which the media can travel [23].

However, the media penetration velocity increased (46.6%) when the concentration of EGDMA was increased at pH=1. It is assumed that pK_a value of AA (4.75) appeared to have a great impact on penetration velocity. It was concluded that the equilibrium media content was directly proportional to the media penetration velocity at the pH higher than pK_a value of AA (Figure 4). This trend has also been observed in poly (NIPA-co-FOSA) copolymers [24]. This relationship is also important because it suggests that from the media penetration velocity, the equilibrium media content can be predicted in very short experimental time (i.e on the order of minutes vs hours or days) at a specific pH. But below pK_a value the inverse relationship was observed between the media penetration velocity and equilibrium media content. The most probable reason for this unexpected behavior for these polymeric systems may be that the carbonyl oxygen atom of the EGDMA present on the surface of disks should facilitate the intermolecular hydrogen bonds with surrounding water molecules during early times of exposure of hydrogels. However, as a continuous column of water is developed from outside to inside of the disk, the increased crosslink density predominates to cause a usual decrease in equilibrium media content. The formation of hydrogen bonds by carbonyl oxygen with water molecules contributing an

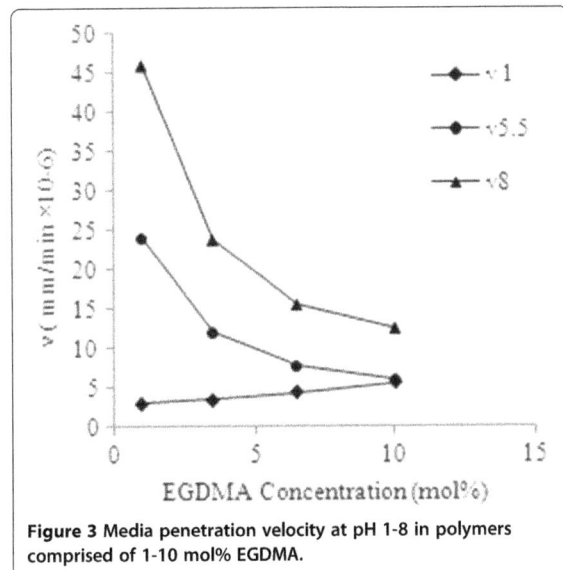

Figure 3 Media penetration velocity at pH 1-8 in polymers comprised of 1-10 mol% EGDMA.

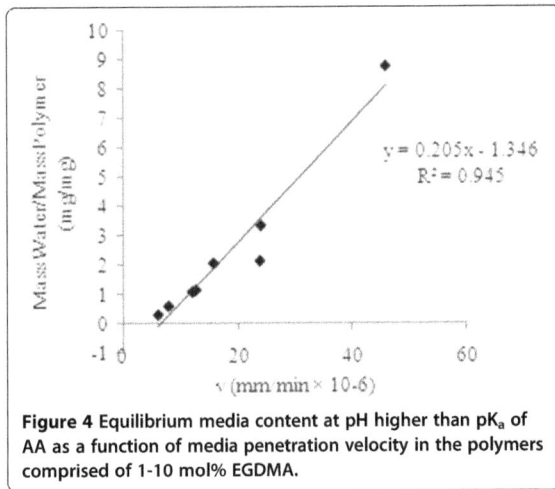

Figure 4 Equilibrium media content at pH higher than pK_a of AA as a function of media penetration velocity in the polymers comprised of 1-10 mol% EGDMA.

increase in media penetration velocity has also been suggested by Hajimi et al. [25].

Media diffusion mechanism

The mechanism of the media sorption was estimated by calculating the diffusion exponent (n) using Korsmeyer-Peppas model [10]. The values are tabulated in Table 1. It was found that all formulations followed Fickian mode of media sorption (values of "n" are ranging from 0.100 to 0.407) at pH below pK_a value of AA content, whereas the values of "n" were greater than 0.5 above pK_a. It was observed that increased pH values shifts the mechanism from diffusion-controlled to an anomalous transport in which both the concentration gradient and erosion are governing the diffusion mechanism. It is suggested that the polymer matrix maintains its structure in acidic conditions and the media sorption is mainly controlled by diffusion, whereas the polymer chains get relaxed in the basic media. It has been reported that in the anionic hydrogels like having carboxylic groups attached with the polymeric chains, the H^+ ions can combine with OH^- ions present in the basic solution to produce water. The cations joined with other hydroxyl groups, may compensate the charge, going into the polymeric network, thus leading to an osmotic pressure increase which is responsible for the swelling of the hydrogels [11]. At swelling equilibrium, the recovery elastic force is equal to the osmotic pressure [26,27].

Table 1 Summary of media penetration velocities, equilibrium media contents, mechanical strength and power law parameters for the polymers

Sample	Media penetration velocity	Equilibrium media sorbed	Mechanical strength	Fick's model	
	(mm/min×10^{-6})	(mg media/ mg polymer)	(gm)	n	R^2
pH =1					
E$_1$	3.027	0.1923		0.407	0.965
E$_2$	3.47	0.1336		0.290	0.925
E$_3$	4.46	0.0782		0.189	0.911
E$_4$	5.67	0.06923		0.206	0.721
pH =5.5					
E$_1$	24	3.713		0.671	0.996
E$_2$	12	1.114		0.557	0.976
E$_3$	7.8	0.630		0.558	0.976
E$_4$	6	0.3342		0.507	0.991
pH =8					
E$_1$	45.99	8.79	452	0.662	0.999
E$_2$	23.85	8.79	490	0.572	0.996
E$_3$	15.6	2.085	560	0.603	0.996
E$_4$	12.6	1.173	634	0.571	0.992

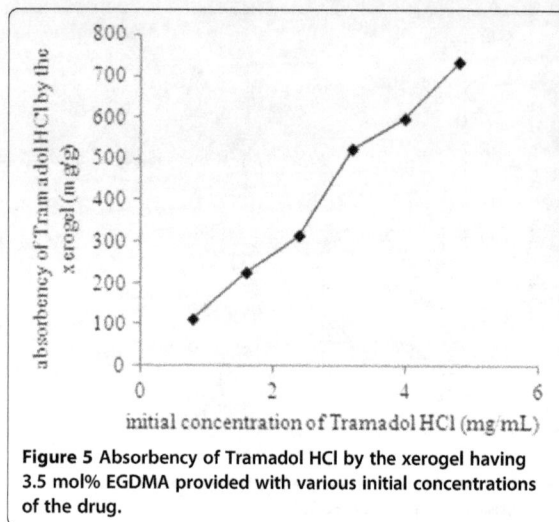

Figure 5 Absorbency of Tramadol HCl by the xerogel having 3.5 mol% EGDMA provided with various initial concentrations of the drug.

In vitro release of tramadol HCl from the copolymer

Owing to preliminary swelling studies, the drug loading and release studies were carried out at pH 8 and 37°C where all the formulations attained the highest rate of sorption and equilibrium media content. Figure 5 exhibits the absorbency of Tramadol HCl by the xerogel with different EGDMA content as well as drug concentration. As the mol% of the cross linker in the copolymer hydrogels increases, less tramadol was absorbed because of low water up take. The amount of the drug loaded in the hydrogel has a close relation with the cross link density of the hydrogels. As the increased concentration of the cross linker increases the cross link density, so the amount of tramadol loaded decreases as also reported by other authors [28].

Drug release studies were performed with respect to the concentration of the cross linker (Figure 6) and the drug

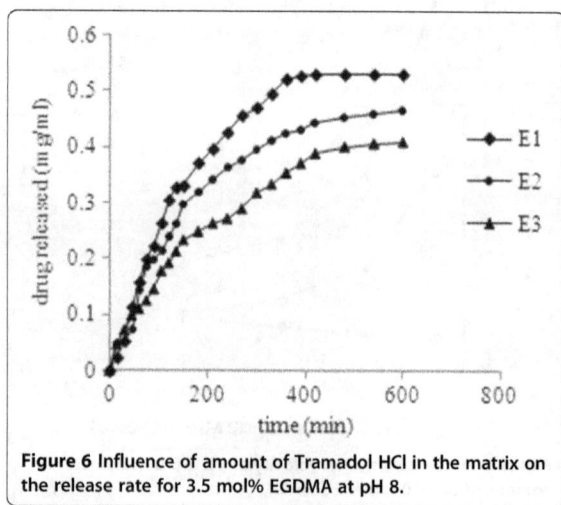

Figure 6 Influence of amount of Tramadol HCl in the matrix on the release rate for 3.5 mol% EGDMA at pH 8.

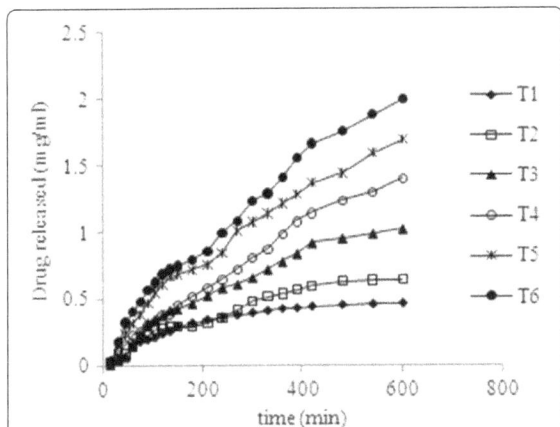

Figure 7 Influence of the concentration of the cross linking agent on the release rate of Tramadol HCl.

reported by other authors [20]. On the other hand, the release rate was enhanced by the amount of the drug loaded in the polymer networks. The optimized formulation (E_2) was used to study the effect of amount of the drug loaded in the system as shown in the Figure 7.

In initial stages the effect was not pronounced. The difference was negligible up to 1.6 mg/ml initially prepared drug concentration solution. However, for higher drug loading concentrations, the amount of the drug release as well as the drug release rate were increased significantly. The root cause for the observed effect might be the higher concentration gradient which is responsible for a more efficient diffusion of the drug substance through the polymer network, keeping all other conditions the same. Hence, variation in drug loading concentration offers a real probability of controlling the drug release [30].

Various mathematical equations have been proposed to describe the kinetics of the drug release from the controlled release formulations. The zero order model equation (Eq. 4) describes the systems, where the drug release does not depend on its concentration [13]. The first order release kinetics describes the dependency on the drug concentration in the polymeric networks [14]. Higuchi model proposes a direct relation of the drug release from the matrix to a square root of time and is based on the Fickian diffusion [15]. The Hixson-Crowell cube root law describes the release rate from the systems depending on the change in surface area and diameter of the particles or tablets and specifically is applied for the systems which erode over time [16].

To describe drug release mechanism more precisely, there is a more comprehensive but still very simple semi-empirical formula, called the Korsmeyer-Peppas power law (Eq. 10). So the drug release data were fitted to these kinetic models (Figures 8, 9, 10 and 11) to analyze the release kinetics and the mechanism from the hydrogels. Based on the best correlation coefficient values, the most appropriate model was selected to explain the release behavior of the drug. The values of the release exponent (n),

content available to be released by the system (Figure 7), because it has been reported that the chemical structure and dissolution in water do not show a significant influence on the drug release rate from the hydrogel networks; on the other hand the cross link density and the amount of the drug loaded determine the drug release from the system [29]. The drug release data are shown in the Table 2.

To analyze the effect of the concentration of the cross linker on the release behavior of the drug, only three samples E_1, E_2 and E_3 were used for experiment as the sample E_4 was collapsed during the loading process (Figure 6). The most probable explanation for the behavior of E_4 may be that there is some type of repulsive interaction between the material of the drug loaded and the highly cross linked dense polymeric matrix. Figure 6 is showing the release profile for influence of the cross linking agent concentration. As predicted from swelling studies, the drug release rate decreased with increase in the cross link density. Same effect of the cross linker's concentration on the drug release rate has also been

Table 2 Kinetic parameters of tramadol HCl release from the matrix tablets

Formulation	Zero-order		First-order		Higuchi		Hixson-Crowell		Korsmeyer-Peppas		
	k_o (%min^{-1})	R^2	k_1 (min^{-1})	R^2	k_H (%min$^{-1/2}$)	R^2	k_{HC} (%min^{-1})	R^2	n	R^2	k_{KP} (%min^{-n})
E_1	0.339	0.957	0.007	0.990	7.715	0.989	0.009	0.965	0.907	0.987	7.15
E_2	0.332	0.941	0.006	0.987	6.68	0.980	0.008	0.974	0.982	0.893	4.52
E_3	0.23	0.942	0.004	0.981	4.921	0.983	0.005	0.974	0.691	0.990	16.0
T1	0.332	0.941	0.006	0.987	6.83	0.980	0.008	0.974	0.982	0.893	4.52
T2	0.131	0.963	0.002	0.973	3.803	0.967	0.003	0.949	0.713	0.914	9.18
T3	0.123	0.978	0.002	0.986	3.827	0.989	0.002	0.984	0.748	0.969	7.019
T4	0.146	0.996	0.002	0.973	4.309	0.978	0.003	0.990	0.832	0.994	4.13
T5	0.096	0.991	0.001	0.989	3.155	0.983	0.002	0.990	0.688	0.988	7.99
T6	0.0127	0.985	0.002	0.989	3.701	0.989	0.002	0.991	0.733	0.979	7.73

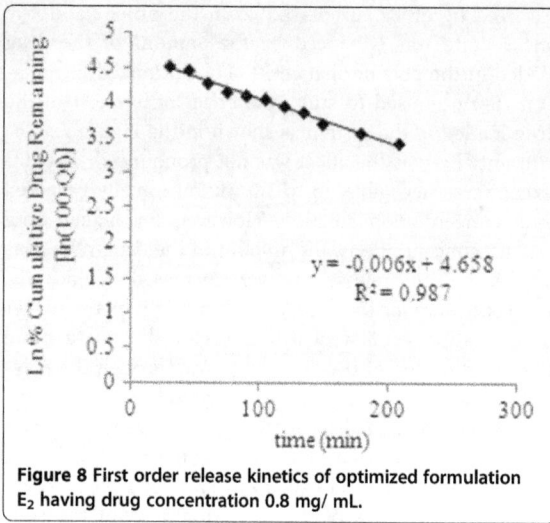

Figure 8 First order release kinetics of optimized formulation E_2 having drug concentration 0.8 mg/ mL.

kinetic rate constant (k) and the correlation coefficient (R^2) are tabulated in the Table 2. Generally speaking, the formulations with varying concentration of the cross linker (E_1, E_2 and E_3) did not seem to obey a zero order kinetics based on the low R^2 values obtained compared to those of the first order profiles of the drug release. On the other hand the values obtained from other models were found to be very close to each other throughout the whole series of formulations investigated. Nevertheless, with higher concentration of drug loaded, the hydrogels (T_4, T_5 and T_6) were either following the zero order profile or exhibiting very close R^2 values to those of first order kinetics. It was concluded that these formulations show drug concentration dependency up to a certain limit of drug loaded

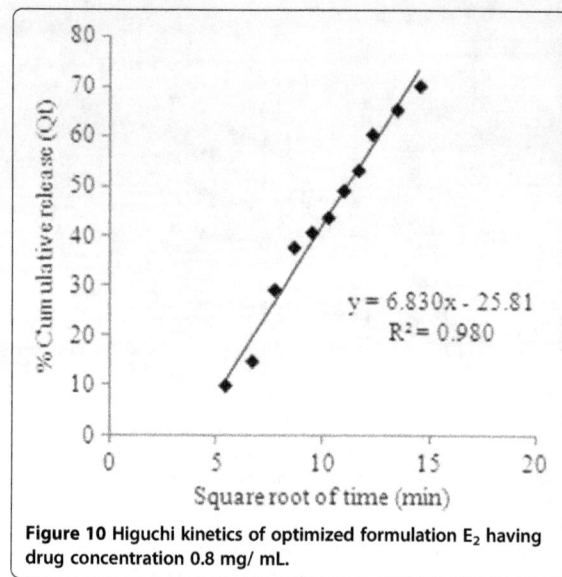

Figure 9 Zero order release kinetics of optimized formulaion having 3.5 mol% EGDMA at pH 8, having drug concentration of 3.2 mg/mL.

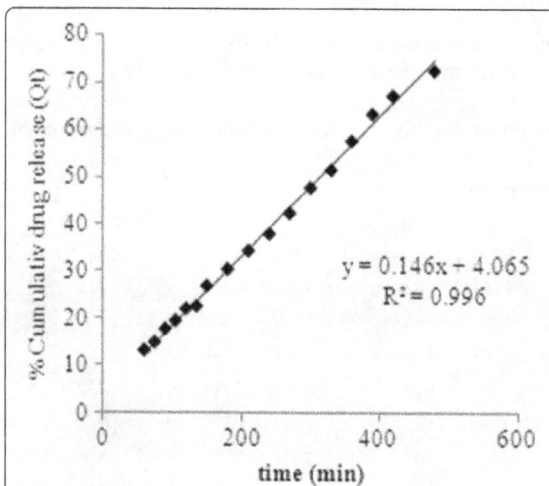

Figure 10 Higuchi kinetics of optimized formulation E_2 having drug concentration 0.8 mg/ mL.

(T_1, T_2 and T_3). After that threshold concentration of the drug loaded, the release kinetics is observed by other factors like cross link density, chain relaxation and osmotic pressure. Applicability of Hixson-Crowell model to the formulations (T_4, T_5 and T_6) indicated a change in surface area and diameter of the tablets with a progressive dissolution of matrix as a function of time [31]. This result was similar to that obtained when the release behavior of diltiazem HCl from matrix tablets was analyzed by Crohel et al. [32].

The values of "n" determined for chemically cross linked hydrogels studied, ranged from 0.688 to 0.982 as tabulated in the Table 2. The results indicated that all the formulations exhibited anomalous transport (i.e non-Fickian diffusion mechanism), so the drug release was governed by

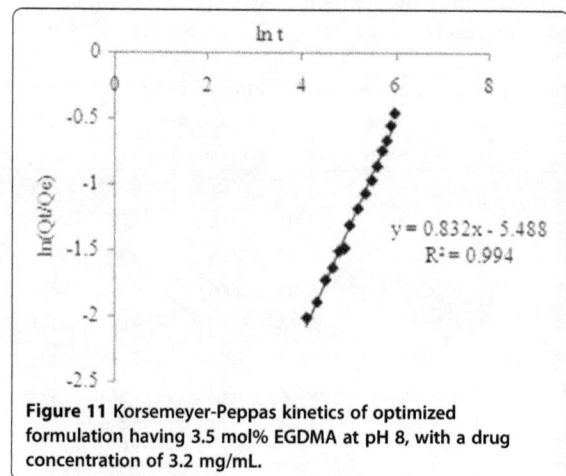

Figure 11 Korsemeyer-Peppas kinetics of optimized formulation having 3.5 mol% EGDMA at pH 8, with a drug concentration of 3.2 mg/mL.

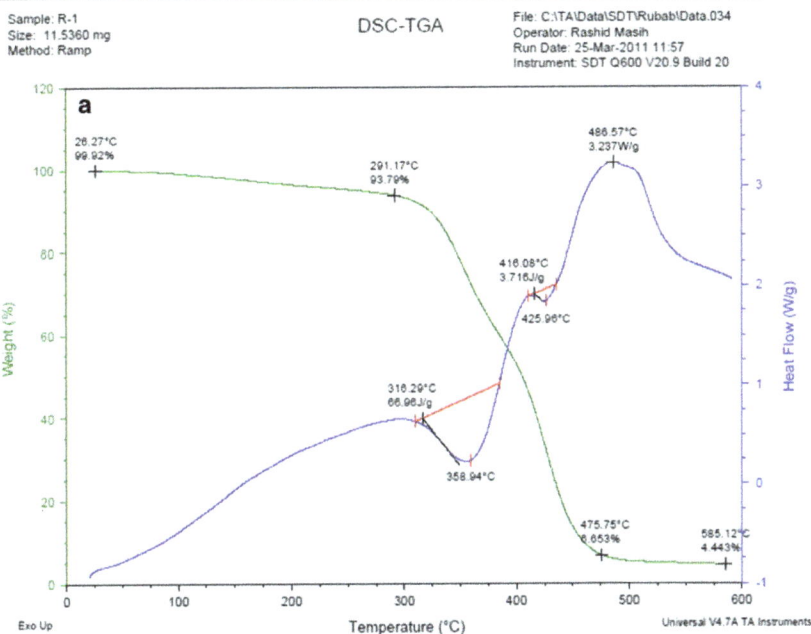

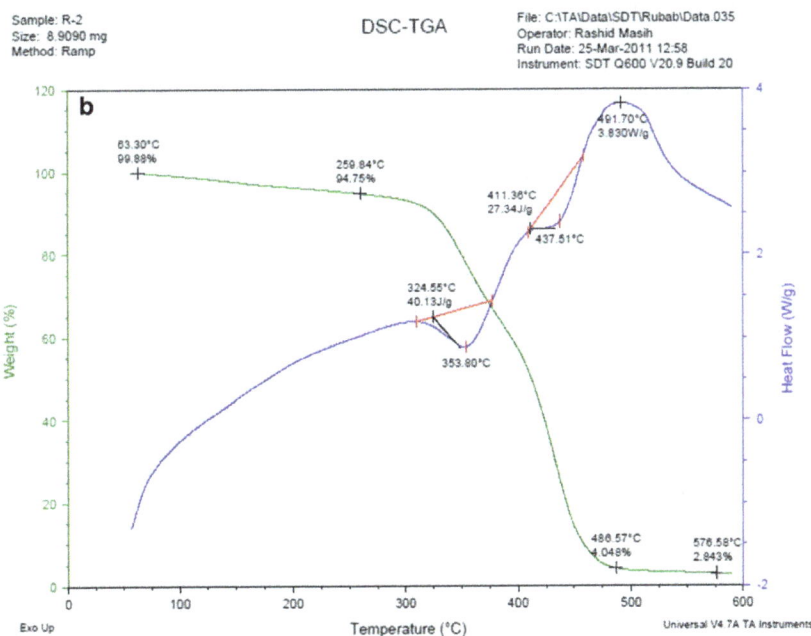

Figure 12 a. DSC/TGA for E1. b. DSC/TGA for E2.

both diffusion of the drug and dissolution of the polymeric network. In fact all the tablets started to erode during the first two hours of their introduction into a fixed volume of phosphate buffer solutions. Even the samples with higher drug concentrations were collapsed during the first hour of exposure of the formulations to the dissolution medium.

Mechanical strength

The mechanical strength of the xerogels was determined, applying a maximum weight on them. Surprisingly, not a single disk was broken down even the maximum force was applied on them. However, the polymers with low concentration of the cross linker showed a little strain in them by equal increase in their diameter, thus decreasing their thickness; but the observed strain was vanished away within a few minutes after the applied stress was released. The fully swollen hydrogels up to their equilibrium point, exhibited a regular increase in the mechanical strength with the concentration of the cross linker (Table 1). Similar effect of the cross linker on the mechanical strength was also observed by other authors [20].

DSC and TGA

In Figure 12, the DSC/TGA curves of the two samples E_1 and E_2 before swelling are observed. It is observed that T_g of both the samples are not appeared in the thermo gram. If we compare both the samples, it is clear that a rapid increase occurs in heat flow in E_1 having low mol percent of the cross linker. In TGA curve three steps with difference in weight loss at respective temperatures are observable. The first step in both samples is almost similar showing the presence of almost equal amount of un-reacted volatile monomers as well solvent trapped inside the polymer network. Moreover, a reasonable quantity of moisture may also be present which is removed in the first step. After the removal of moisture and other volatile materials from the samples, side chain decomposition takes place in the range of 300-3.75°C and after that up to 475°C, the back bone degradation is observed. It is clear that most of the weight loss occurred in the second step in a narrow range of temperature (from 300-475°C). After 475°C, up to 600°C, round about, horizontal curve is exhibited by both samples. At the end higher percentage of residue was left behind in E_1 as compared to E_2. Exothermic peak after 485°C, in both the samples, indicates phase change taking place in the residual material. The overall analysis indicates that the concentration of the cross linker has no significant effect on thermo gravimetric behavior of these specific systems.

Conclusions

The chemically cross linked hydrogel copolymer comprised of VA-co-MA-co-AA and EGDMA has proven to be effective controlling the desorption rate of the drug substance from its matrix. The introduction of the higher cross link density decreased (1) the media penetration velocity through the hydrogels in basic media (2) the equilibrium media content in the hydrogels (3) the absorbency of the drug into the polymeric material and (4) the drug release rate from the hydrogels. The shift of the mechanism from diffusion controlled to an anomalous transport changing the pH of the medium from acidic to basic conditions and the mechanical strength indicate that the polymer matrix not only can maintain its structure in the acidic medium of the stomach but also can resist peristaltic movements of the digestive tract, thus preventing the drug release until the target has been achieved. The ability of these ter-polymeric hydrogels systems to load

and deliver a drug substance at a controlled rate suggests that these hydrogels show a great promise as a drug delivery system.

Competing interests
The authors declare that they have no competing interests.

Authors' contribution
The main purpose of this paper is to study the drug release behavior of ternary copolymer poly (AAm-co-MA-co-AA). Novelty of the work is Interpretation of media penetration velocity at different pH the media. The relationship of media penetration velocity with equilibrium media sorbed. The effect of crosslinker concentration on above parameters and mechanism of the diffusion. The effect of cross linker concentration on the drug release rate of a model drug. The effect of drug concentration on release behavior. Mechanical strength. DSC/TGA analysis. Application various models to drug release rates. All authors have read and approved this version of the article, and no part of this paper has been published nor is it submitted for publication elsewhere and will not be submitted elsewhere. All authors read and approved the final manuscript.

References
1. Lehmann KA: **Tramadol in acute pain.** Drug 1997, **53**(suppl 2):25–33.
2. Scott LJ, Perry CM: **Tramadol: a review of its use in perioperative pain.** Drug 2002, **60**(1):139–176.
3. Salsa T, Veiga F: Pina ME. **Oral controlled release dosage form. I. Cellulose ether polymers in hydrophilic matrices.** Drug Dev Ind Pharm 1997, **23**:929–938.
4. Alderman DA: **A reviw of cellulose ethers in hydrophilic matrices for oral controlled release dosage forms.** Int J Pharm Tech Prod Mfr 1984, **5**:1–9.
5. El-Gibaly I: **Development and in vitro evaluation of novel floating chitosan microcapsules for oral use: comparison with non-floating chitosan microspheres.** Int J Pharm 2002, **249**:7–21.
6. Qiu Y, Park K: **Environment sensitive hydrogels for drug delivery.** Adv Drug Delivery Rev 2001, **53**:321–339.
7. Karadag E, Uzam OB, Saraydin D: **Swelling equilibrium and the absorption studies of chemically cross linked super sorbent acrylamide/maleic acid hydrogels.** Eur Polym J 2002, **38**:2133–2141.
8. Hoffman AS: **Hydrogels for biomedical applications.** Adv Drug Delivery Rev 2002, **43**:3–12.
9. Blanco MD, Gomez C, Gracia O, Teijon JM: **Polymer gels network.** 1998, **6**:57–69.
10. Zafar ZI, Malana MA, Pervez HM, Shad A, Momina K: **Synthesis and swelling kinetics of a cross-linked pH-sensitive ternary co-polymer gel system.** Polym. (Korea) 2008, **32**:1–11.
11. Xinming L, Yingde CUI: **Study on synthesis and chloramphenicol release of poly (2-hydroxymethylmethacrylate-co-acrylamide) hydrogels.** Chin J Chem Eng 2008, **16**(4):640–645.
12. Gomez ML, Williams RJJ, Montejano HA, Previtali CM: **Influence of the ionic character of the drug on its release rate from hydrogels based on 2-hydroxymethylmethacrylate and acrylamide synthesized by photo polymerization.** eXPRESS Polym Lett 2012, **6**(3):189–197.
13. Najib N, Suleiman M: **The kinetics of drug release from ethyl cellulose solid dispersions.** Drug Dev Ind Pharm 1985, **11**:2169–2181.
14. Desai SJ, Singh P, Simonelli AP, Higuchi WI: **Investigation of factors influencing release of solid drug dispersed in wax matrices III. Quantitative studies involving polyethylene plastic matrices.** J Pharm Sci 1966, :1230–1234.
15. Higuchi T: **Mechanism of sustained action medication. Theoretical analysis of rate of solid drugs dispersed in solid matrices.** J Pharm Sci 1963, **52**:1145–1149.
16. Hixson AW, Crowell JH: **Dependence of reaction velocity upon surface and agitation.** Ind Eng Chem 1931, **23**:923–931.
17. Korsmeyer RW, Gurny R, Doelker E, Buri P, Peppas NA: **Mechanism of solute release from porous hydrophilic polymers.** Ind J Pharm 1983, **15**:25–35.
18. Chen J, Belvins WE, Park H, Park K: **Gastric retention properties of superporous hydrogel components.** J Contrl Release 2000, **64**(1–4):39–51.

19. Chen J, Park K: **Synthesis and characterization of superporous hydrogel composites.** *J Control Release* 2000, **65**(1–2):73–82.

20. Kumar A, Pandey M, Koshi MK, Saraf SA: **Synthesis of fast swelling superporous hydrogel: effect of concentration of cross linker and acdisol on swelling ratio and mechanical strength.** *Int. J Drug Deliv* 2010, **2**:135–140.

21. Davidson R, Peppas NA: **Solute and penetrant diffusion in swelling polymers V. Relaxation control transport in P (HEMA-co-MMA) copolymers.** *J Control Release* 1986, **3**:243–258.

22. Brazel CS, Peppas NA: **Dimensionless analysis of swelling of hydrophilic glassy polymers with subsequent release of drug from relaxing structures.** *Biomaterials* 1999, **20**:721–732.

23. Chen LLH: **Kinetic modeling for macromolecular loading into cross linked polyacrylamide hydrogel matrix by swelling.** *Pharm Dev Technol* 1998, **3**:241–249.

24. Tia Q, Zhao Z, Tang X, Zhang Y: **Hydrophobic association and temperature and pH sensitivity of hydrophobically modified poly (n-isopropylacrylamide-co-acrylamide) gels.** *J Applied Polym Sci* 2003, **87**:2406–2413.

25. Hajimi M, Ishida K, Tamaki E, Satoh M: *Polymer* 2002, **43**:103–110.

26. Hiratani H, Mizutani Y, Alvarez-Lorenzo C: **Controlling drug release from imprinted hydrogels by modifying the characteristics of the imprinted cavities.** *Macromol Biosci* 2005, **5**:728–733.

27. Li CC, Chauhan A: **Modeling ophthalmic drug delivery by soaked contact lenses.** *Ind Eng Chem Res* 2006, **45**:3718–3734.

28. Sung-Eun P, Young-Chang N, Hyung K: **Preparaion of poly (ethylene gl ycolmethacrylate-co-acrylic acid) hydrogels by radiations and their physical properties.** *Rad Phy Chem* 2002, :221–227.

29. Landner WD, Mockel JE, Lippold BC: **Controlled release of drugs from hydrocolloid embedding.** *Pharmazei* 1996, **51**:263–272.

30. Dimitrov M, Lambov N, Shencov S, Dossevav-Baranovski V: **Hydrogels based on chemically cross linked polyacrylic acid: biopharmaceutical chacterization.** *Acta Pharm* 2003, **53**:25–31.

31. Mehrgan H, Mortazavi SA: **The release behavior and kinetic evaluation of diltiazem HCl from various hydrophilic and plastic based matrices.** *Iran J Pharm Sci* 2005, **3**:137–146.

32. Crohel MC, Amin AF, Patel KV, Pamchal MK: **Studies of release behavior of diltiazem HCl from matrix tablets containing hydroxyl propyl methyl cellulose and xanthan gum.** *Boll Chin Farm* 2002, **141**:21–28.

12

Novel heteroaryl phosphonicdiamides PTPs inhibitors as anti-hyperglycemic agents

Kuruva Chandra Sekhar[1], Rasheed Syed[1], Madhava Golla[1], Jyothi Kumar MV[2], Nanda Kumar Yellapu[3], Appa Rao Chippada[4] and Naga Raju Chamarthi[1*]

Abstract

Background: Chronic and oral administration of benzylamine improves glucose tolerance. Picolylamine is a selective functional antagonist of the human adenosine A_{2B} receptor. Phosphonic diamide derivatives enhance the cellular permeability and in turn their biological activities.

Methods: A series of heteroaryl phosphonicdiamide derivatives were designed as therapeutics to control and manage type2 diabetes. Initially defined Lipinski parameters encouraged them as safer drugs. Molecular docking of these compounds against Protein tyrosine phosphatase (PTP), the potential therapeutic target of type 2 diabetes, revealed their potential binding ability explaining their anti-diabetic activity in terms of PTP inhibition. Human intestinal absorption, Caco-2 cell permeability, MDCK cell permeability, BBB penetration, skin permeability and plasma protein binding abilities of the title compounds were calculated by PreADMET server. A convenient method has been developed for the synthesis of title compounds through the formation of 1-ethoxy-N,N'-bis (4-fluorobenzyl/pyridin-3-ylmethyl)phosphinediamine by the reaction of 4-fluorobenzylamine/ 3-picolylamine with ethyldichlorophosphite, subsequently reacted with heteroaryl halides using lanthanum(III) chloride as a catalyst.

Results: All the compounds exhibited significant *in vitro* anti-oxidant activity and *in vivo* evaluation in streptozotocin induced diabetic rat models revealed that the normal glycemic levels were observed on 12th day by **9a** and 20th day by **5b**, **5c**, **9e** and **9f**. The remaining compounds also exhibited normal glycemic levels by 25th day.

Conclusion: The results from molecular modeling, *in vitro* and *in vivo* studies are suggesting them as safer and effective therapeutic agents against type2 diabetes.

Background

The stipulation of anti-diabetic drugs is snowballing hastily, due to millions of people is distressing about diabetes. Several budding essential mechanisms for diabetes are characterized by elevation of blood glucose levels caused by decreased production of the hormone insulin and/or increased resistance to the action of insulin by certain cells. Tyrosine phosphorylation is associated with a group of enzymes which are mainly involved in the negative regulation of insulin signaling and intertwined in the insulin resistance, complementary to type 2 diabetes [1,2]. Protein tyrosine phosphatase-1B (PTP-1B) is one of the PTP enzymes a major negative regulator in both insulin

and leptin signaling. It has been observed to serve as an outstanding target for the treatment of cancer, diabetes and obesity [3]. Mice lacking the PTP-1B have enhanced insulin sensitivity which certifies that the inhibition activity of PTP-1B could be a novel way of treating type 2 diabetes and obesity [1,2]. Thus insulin action will be enhanced by persuading the activity of cellular PTPases and glucose production can be reduced [4,5]. This study created an interest in designing the new drugs by structural modification of existing drugs (Figures 1 and 2).

The study of the reported drugs **i-vii** reveals that they are ideal for anti-diabetic activity due to the thiazolidine-2, 4-dione (**i, ii, iii**), pyridinyl (**i,ii**), quinolone (**iv**), urea and amide (**v, vii**), Flouro substituted, heteroaryl pyrazine (**vi**) and benzyl amine (**vii**). Compound **xiii** is a α-aminophosphonate with established anti-diabetic property which gave an idea to focus on phosphorus containing drugs.

* Correspondence: rajuchamarthi10@gmail.com
[1]Department of Chemistry, Sri Venkateswara University, Tirupati 517 502, India
Full list of author information is available at the end of the article

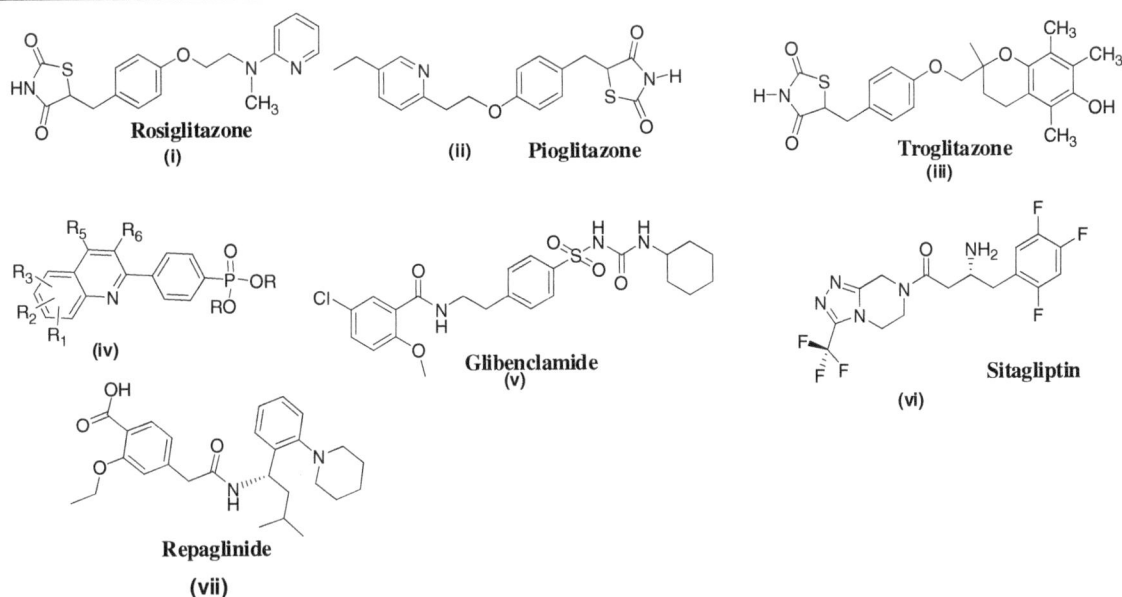

Figure 1 A few anti-diabetic drugs.

Benzylamine is used to treat diabetes in traditional medicine. Chronic and oral administration of benzylamine improves glucose tolerance and the circulating lipid profile without increasing oxidative stress in overweight and pre-diabetic mice [12]. The stipulation of picolylamine was attested in the synthesis of various pharmacological compounds such as ^{99m}Tc(I)-complexes [13] and selective functional antagonists of the human adenosine A_{2B} receptor [14]. When compared to normal benzyl amine analogues, picolylamine analogues are exhibiting the potential pharmacological activity [15]. Among the 2-picolyl, 3-picolyl and 4-picolyl amines, the performance of 3-picolyl amines are virtuous [16].

Phosphonic diamide derivatives enhance the cellular permeability and in turn their activities akin to the analogous phosphoric diamide prodrugs of 3′-azido-3′-

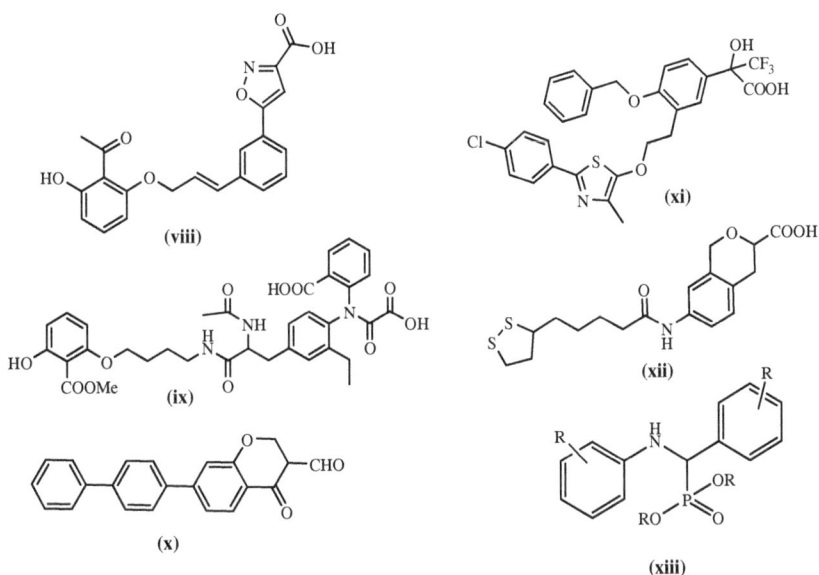

Figure 2 Some of the PTP1B inhibitors Ref [6-11].

deoxythymidine (AZT) monophosphate with AZT [17], glycine methyl ester phosphonic diamide of a 9-[2-(phosphonomethoxy)ethyl]-adenine (PMEA) analogue [18], and diamides of 9-[2-(phosphonomethoxy)ethyl]-N6-(cyclopropyl)-2-aminoadenine [19]. If phosphonic diamides hydrolyze *in vivo* to produce phosphonic acids benzyl amine itself act as antidiabetic agent [12]. Phosphonic diamide derivatives are used as prodrugs to improve the membrane permeability of drugs. P-C bond is playing an important role in preserving so many syndromes and in the synthesis of numerous anticancer [20], antiviral [21], antimicrobial [22], anti-diabetic [23], and antioxidant agents [24]. If the carbon in the P-C bond is aromatic, it acts better than the aliphatic carbon. Quinolines are expressed as LXR mediate disease inhibitors [25]. Quinoline phosphonicdiesters are known for preventing hypercholesterolemia and diabetes [26]. There are number of patents which are dependent on this type of drugs.

Lipinski parameters help in preclinical trials to avoid the tedious and costly procedures that can define them as drugs and to avoid the failure rates. Lipinski parameters suggest the potency of the compounds with a variety of molecular descriptors [27]. The *in silico* studies involving construction, optimization and molecular dynamics will generate the stable conformations of the molecules. It is also an important task to find out the structure based intermolecular interactions of the compounds with the biologically meaningful and effective targets at specified conditions [28]. This helps to predict the inhibitory activity and the strength of the molecule to form a stable complex with the target. The identification of binding orientations of the compounds in the binding site of target will provide fruitful information on their reactivity. Hence, in the present study we applied Lipinski parameters and molecular docking studies to predict the drug likeliness and binding ability of the compounds to the protein tyrosine phosphatase.

Although several synthetic methods are described for the preparation of such P-C bond containing compounds, one of them is the Michaelis–Arbuzov reaction. Unfortunately, it has some drawbacks when use classical conditions such as length of reaction time, high temperature and removal of the trialkyl phosphite used in a large excess. These drastic conditions may be responsible for side reactions, low yields and limits the application of such reactions to sensitive substrates. Recently, researchers focused on rare earth elemental catalysts due to their high catalytic properties and also act as Lewis acids. In this connection, we selected Lanthanum (III) chloride as an efficient catalyst for nucleophilic substitution on hetero aromatic ring for the synthesis of heteroaryl phosphonicdiamide derivatives *via* Michaelis-Arbuzov reaction.

The improved production and ineffective scavenging of reactive oxygen species (ROS) cause chemical changes in virtually all cellular components, leading to lipid peroxidation. The enhanced production of free radicals and oxidative stress is central event to the development of diabetic complications. This was supported by demonstration of increased levels of indicators of oxidative stress in diabetic individuals suffering from complications [29]. Oxidative stress is involved in the pathogenesis of diabetes and its complications. Use of antioxidants reduces oxidative stress and alleviates diabetic complications [30]. There are many reports on effects of antioxidants in the management of diabetes [31,32]. So the *in vitro* antioxidant activity was carried out as preliminary test for all the title compounds. The results of antioxidant activity supported for the reduction of oxidative stress. Finally, title compounds were screened for their *in vivo* anti-diabetic activity on mice. Most of the title compounds are effective and satisfactory in reducing glucose levels in both the tests.

Materials and methods
Chemistry
Chemicals were procured from Sigma–Aldrich and Merck were used as such without further purification. All solvents used for spectroscopic and other physical studies were reagent grade and were further purified by literature methods [33]. Melting points (m p) were determined by Guna Digital Melting Point apparatus using a calibrated thermometer. They expressed in degrees centigrade (°C) and are uncorrected. Infrared spectra (IR) were obtained on a Perkin-Elmer Model 281-B spectrophotometer. Samples were analyzed as potassium bromide (KBr) disks. Absorptions were reported in wave numbers (cm^{-1}). ^{1}H and ^{13}C NMR spectra were recorded as solutions in DMSO-d_6 on a Bruker AMX 400 MHz spectrometer operating at 400 MHz for ^{1}H, 100 MHz for ^{13}C and 161.9 MHz for ^{31}P NMR. The ^{1}H and ^{13}C chemical shifts were expressed in parts per million (ppm) with reference to tetramethylsilane (TMS) and ^{31}P chemical shifts to 85% H_3PO_4. LCMS mass spectra were recorded on a Jeol SX 102 DA/600 Mass spectrometer.

Synthesis of N,N'-di(4-fluorobenzyl)(2-pyrazinyl)phosphonic diamide (5a)
To a stirred solution of 4-fluorobenzylamine (0.002 mol) in dry tetrahydrofuran (THF) (10 mL), ethyldichlorophosphite (0.001 mol) was added at 0°C in the presence of triethylamine (TEA) (0.002 mol) under N$_2$ atmosphere. After completion of the addition, the reaction mixture was heated to 30°C and stirred for 2 h to form the intermediate 1-ethoxy-N,N'-bis(4-fluorobenzyl)phosphinediamine (3). The reaction progress was monitored by thin layer chromatography (TLC) using ethyl acetate: hexane (1:1) as mobile phase. After completion of the reaction,

it was filtered to remove triethylamine hydrochloride. 2-Chloropyrazine (**4a**) (0.001 mol) in dry THF (10 mL) was added to the filtrate under N_2 atmosphere in the presence of La(III)Cl$_3$.7H$_2$O (20 mol%) and the reaction mixture was refluxed for 3 h. The progress of the reaction was monitored by TLC using ethyl acetate: hexane (1:1) as mobile phase. After completion of the reaction, catalyst was removed by filtration and the filtrate was concentrated in vacuum to afford the crude product. It was purified by silica gel column chromatography eluting with ethyl acetate: hexane (1:2) mixture to afford the title compound, *N,N'*-di(4-fluorobenzyl)(2-pyrazinyl) phosphonic diamide (**5a**). The same experimental procedure was adopted for the preparation of the remaining title compounds **5b-f** (Scheme 1).

Spectral data

N,N'-Di(4-fluorobenzyl)(2-pyrazinyl)phosphonic diamide (5a)

Yield: 72%; mp: 162-164°C; IR (KBr): ῡ 3378 (N-H), 1252 (P = O), 1018 (P-C$_{Ar}$) cm^{-1}; ^{1}H NMR (400 MHz, DMSO-d_6): δ 8.52-6.84 (11H, m, Ar), 5.12 (2H, brs, H-8), 4.08-3.83 (4H, m, H-7); ^{13}C NMR (100 MHz, DMSO-d_6): δ 161.3 (C-4), 154.3 (C-1), 152.2 (C-1'), 148.9 (C-6'), 145.6 (C-3'), 147.9 (C-4'), 122.4-121.5 (C-2 & C-6), 117.4-116.2 (C-3 & C-5), 31.2 (C-7); ^{31}P NMR (161.9 MHz, DMSO-d_6): δ 28.9; LC MS (%): m/z 375.7 (100%) [MH$^{+•}$]; Anal.

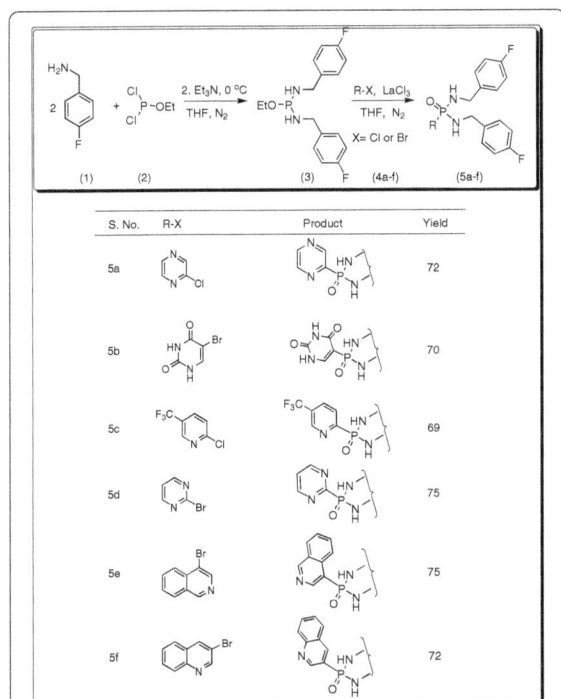

Scheme 1 Synthesis of substituted heteroaryl-N,N'-di(4-fluorobenzyl) phosphonicdiamides (5a-f).

Calcd. for C$_{18}$H$_{17}$N$_4$F$_2$OP: C 57.76; H 4.58; N 14.97; Found: C 57.63; H 4.39; N 14.77.

2,4-Dioxo-1,2,3,4-tetrahydro-5-pyrimidinyl-N,N'-di(4-fluorobenzyl) phosphonic diamide (5b)

Yield: 70%; mp: 189-191°C; IR (KBr): ῡ 3386 (N-H), 1238 (P = O), 992 (P-C$_{Ar}$) cm^{-1}; ^{1}H NMR (400 MHz, DMSO-d_6): δ 9.06 (1H, brs, H-3'), 8.32-6.74 (9H, m, Ar), 5.73-5.68 (1H, s, H-5'), 5.15 (2H, brs, H-8), 3.83-4.08 (4H, m, H-7); ^{13}C NMR (100 MHz, DMSO-d_6): δ 169.6 (C-2'), 161.6 (C-4), 161.3 (C-4'), 158.2 (C-1'), 155.4 (C-1), 141.9 (C-6'), 122.6-121.8 (C-2 & C-6), 117.8-116.8 (C-3 &C-5), 30.9 (C-7); ^{31}P NMR (161.9 MHz, DMSO-d_6): δ 27.6; LC MS (%): m/z 407.8 (100%) [MH$^{+•}$]; Anal. Calcd. for C$_{18}$H$_{17}$N$_4$F$_2$O$_3$P: C 53.21; H 4.22; N 13.79; Found: C 53.08; H 4.12; N 13.55.

N,N'-Di(4-fluorobenzyl)[5-(trifluoromethyl)-2-pyridyl] phosphonic diamide (5c)

Yield: 69%; mp: 202-204°C; IR (KBr): ῡ 3354 (N-H), 1261 (P = O), 1010 (P-C$_{Ar}$) cm^{-1}; ^{1}H NMR (400 MHz, DMSO-d_6): δ 7.65-6.50 (11H, m, Ar), 5.12 (2H, brs, H-8), 4.06-3.83 (4H, m, H-7); ^{13}C NMR (100 MHz, DMSO-d_6): δ 159.1 (C-4), 155.9 (C-1'), 154.8 (C-3'), 154.0 (C-1), 133.6 (C-5'), 133.5 (C-4'), 122.2-121.1 (C-2 & C-6), 119.6 (C-6'), 118.9 (C-7'), 117.7-116.6 (C-3 & C-5), 30.9 (C-7); ^{31}P NMR (161.9 MHz, DMSO-d_6): δ 28.7; LC MS (%): m/z 442.8 (100%) [MH$^{+•}$]; Anal. Calcd. for C$_{20}$H$_{17}$F$_5$N$_3$OP: C 54.43; H 3.88; N 9.52; Found: 54.15; H 3.51; N 9.22.

N,N'-Di(4-fluorobenzyl)(2-pyrimidinyl)phosphonic diamide (5d)

Yield: 75%; mp: 167-169°C; IR (KBr): ῡ 3346 (N-H), 1268 (P = O), 996 (P-C$_{Ar}$) cm^{-1}; ^{1}H NMR (400 MHz, DMSO-d_6): δ 8.55-6.79 (11H, m, Ar), 5.14 (2H, brs, H-8), 4.08-3.83 (4H, m, H-7); ^{13}C NMR (100 MHz, DMSO-d_6): δ 162.5 (C-1'), 161.9 (C-4), 155.1 (C-1), 154.3 (C-3' & C-5'), 124.4 (C-4'), 121.8-121.1 (C-2 & C-6), 117.6-116.4 (C-3 & C-5), 31.4 (C-7); ^{31}P NMR (161.9 MHz, DMSO-d_6): δ 28.2; LC MS (%): m/z 375.4 (100%) [MH$^{+•}$]; Anal. Calcd. for C$_{18}$H$_{17}$F$_2$N$_4$OP: C 57.76; H 4.58; N 14.97; Found: 57.62; H 4.41; N 14.82.

N,N'-Di(4-fluorobenzyl)(4-isoquinolyl)phosphonic diamide (5e)

Yield: 75%; mp: 221-224°C; IR (KBr): 3364 (N-H), 1274 (P = O), 986 (P-C$_{Ar}$) cm^{-1}; ^{1}H NMR (400 MHz, DMSO-d_6): δ 8.65-6.76 (14H, m, Ar), 5.16 (2H, brs, H-8), 4.06-3.84 (4H, m, H-7); ^{13}C NMR (100 MHz, DMSO-d_6): δ 161.6 (C-4), 156.2 (C-4'), 155.2 (C-1), 142.6 (C-2'), 135.9 (C-9'), 129.5 (C-7'), 129.2 (C-10'), 127.5 (C-5'), 127.1 (C-8'), 126.9 (C-6'), 126.2 (C-1'), 122.3-121.5 (C-2 & C-6), 117.7-116.6 (C-3 & C-5), 30.7 (C-7); ^{31}P NMR (161.9 MHz, DMSO-d_6): δ 27.8; LC MS (%): m/z 424.5

(100%) [MH$^{+\bullet}$]; Anal. Calcd. for $C_{23}H_{20}F_2N_3OP$: C 65.25; H 4.76; N 9.92; Found: C 65.09; H 4.57; N 9.71.

N,N'-Di(4-fluorobenzyl)(3-quinolyl)phosphonic diamide (5f)

Yield: 72%; mp: 179-181°C; IR (KBr): 3372 (N-H), 1259 (P = O), 1012 (P-C$_{Ar}$) cm^{-1}; ^{1}H NMR (400 MHz, DMSO-d_6): δ 8.63-6.92 (14H, m, Ar), 5.13 (2H, brs, H-8), 4.08-3.83 (4H, m, H-7); ^{13}C NMR (100 MHz, DMSO-d_6): δ 161.5 (C-4), 157.2 (C-9'), 154.5 (C-1), 148.4 (C-2'), 136.8 (C-3'), 131.7 (C-6'), 128.5 (C-4'), 127.3 (C-7'), 126.8 (C-10'), 126.7 (C-5'), 123.6 (C-8'), 122.1-121.3 (C-2 & C-6), 117.8-116.2 (C-3 & C-5), 30.5 (C-7); ^{31}P NMR (161.9 MHz, DMSO-d$_6$): δ 28.9; LC MS (%): m/z 424.6 (100%) [MH$^{+\bullet}$]; Anal. Calcd. for $C_{23}H_{20}F_2N_3OP$: C 65.25; H 4.76; N 9.92; Found: C 65.08; H 4.51; N 9.84.

Synthesis of 4,6-dimethoxy-1,3,5-triazin-2-yl-N,N'-di (3-pyridylmethyl)phosphonicdiamide (9a)

To a stirred solution of 3-picolylamine (6) (0. 002 mol) in dry tetrahydrofuran (THF) (10 mL), ethyldichlorophosphite (2) (0.001 mol) was added at 0°C in the presence of triethylamine (TEA) (0.002 mol) under N$_2$ atmosphere. After completion of the addition, the reaction mixture was raised to 30°C and stirred for 2 h to form the intermediate 1-ethoxy-N,N'-bis(pyridin-3-ylmethyl) phosphinediamine (7). The reaction progress was monitored by thin layer chromatography (TLC) using ethyl acetate: hexane (1:1) as mobile phase. After completion of the reaction, it was filtered to remove triethylamine hydrochloride. 2-Chloro-4,6-dimethoxy-1,3,5-triazine (8a) (0.001 mol) in dry THF (10 mL) was added to the filtrate under N$_2$ atmosphere at 20°C in the presence of La(III) Cl$_3$.7H$_2$O (20 mol%) and the reaction mixture was refluxed for 3 h. The progress of the reaction was monitored by TLC using ethyl acetate: hexane (1:1). After completion of the reaction, catalyst was removed by filtration and the filtrate was concentrated in rota-evaporator to afford the crude product. It was purified by silica gel column chromatography eluting with ethyl acetate: hexane (1:2) mixture to afford the title compound, 4,6-dimethoxy-1,3,5-triazin-2-yl-N,N'-di(3-pyridylmethyl)phosphonic diamide (9a). The same experimental procedure was adopted for the preparation of the remaining title compounds 9b-f (Scheme 2).

Spectral data

4,6-Dimethoxy-1,3,5-triazin-2-yl-N,N'-di(3-pyridylmethyl) phosphonic diamide (9a)

Yield: 70%; mp: 198-200°C; IR (KBr): ῡ 3371 (N-H), 1242 (P = O), 989 (P-C$_{Ar}$) cm^{-1}; ^{1}H NMR (400 MHz, DMSO-d_6): δ 8.92-7.26 (8H, m, Ar), 5.63 (2H, brs, H-8), 4.39-4.35 (4H, d, H-7), 3.72 (6H, s, -OMe); ^{13}C NMR (100 MHz, DMSO-d_6): δ 178.3 (C-3' & C-5'), 169.2 (C-1'), 149.5 (C-2), 148.1 (C-4), 145.8 (C-1), 135.3 (C-6),

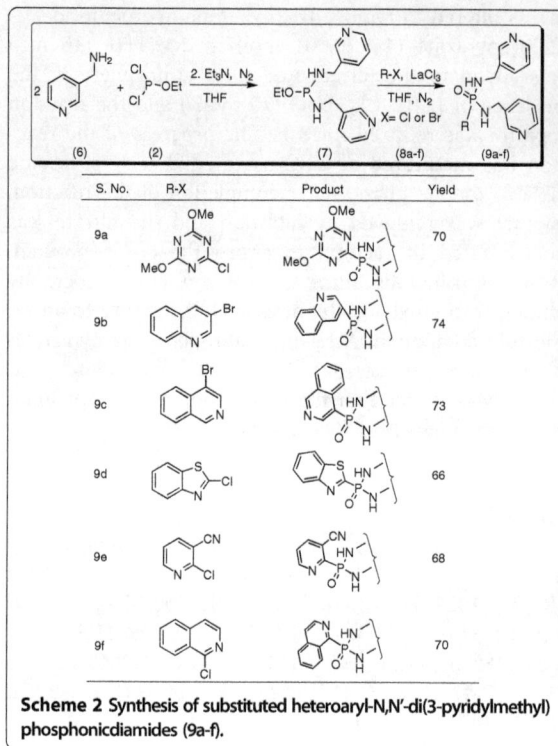

Scheme 2 Synthesis of substituted heteroaryl-N,N'-di(3-pyridylmethyl) phosphonicdiamides (9a-f).

121.5 (C-5), 51.9 (C-OMe), 38.6 (C-7); ^{31}P NMR (161.9 MHz, DMSO-d$_6$): δ 21.6; LC MS (%): m/z 402.5 (100%) [MH$^{+\bullet}$]; Anal. Calcd. for $C_{17}H_{20}N_7O_3P$: C 50.87; H 5.02; N 24.43; Found: C 50.66; H 4.81; N 24.23.

N,N'-Di(3-pyridylmethyl)(3-quinolyl)phosphonic diamide (9b)

Yield: 74%; mp: 206-208°C; IR (KBr): 3376 (N-H), 1247 (P = O), 1005 (P-C$_{Ar}$) cm^{-1}; ^{1}H NMR (400 MHz, DMSO-d_6): δ 8.61-7.46 (14H, m, Ar), 5.64 (2H, brs, H-8), 4.35-4.31 (4H, d, H-7); ^{13}C NMR (100 MHz, DMSO-d_6): δ 149.4 (C-2), 148.9 (C-4), 147.5 (C-2'), 145.2 (C-9'), 135.3 (C-6), 134.6 (C-1), 132.3 (C-3'), 131.7 (C-6'), 128.9 (C-4'), 127.5 (C-5'), 127.3 (C-10'), 126.1 (C-7'), 122.5 (C-8'), 121.7 (C-5), 38.8 (C-7); ^{31}P NMR (161.9 MHz, DMSO-d$_6$): δ 20.2; LC MS (%): m/z 390.3 (100%) [MH$^{+\bullet}$]; Anal. Calcd. for $C_{21}H_{20}N_5OP$: C 64.77; H 5.18; N 17.99; Found: C 64.51; H 5.03; N 17.81.

4-Isoquinolyl-N,N'-di(3-pyridylmethyl)phosphonic diamide (9c)

Yield: 73%; mp: 166-169°C; IR (KBr): ῡ 3379 (N-H), 1253 (P = O), 995 (P-C$_{Ar}$) cm^{-1}; ^{1}H NMR (400 MHz, DMSO-d_6): δ 8.63-7.45 (14H, m, Ar), 5.62 (2H, brs, H-8), 4.37-4.34 (4H, d, H-7); ^{13}C NMR (100 MHz, DMSO-d_6): δ 152.5 (C-4'), 149.1 (C-2), 148.5 (C-4), 145.2 (C-1), 143.9 (C-2'), 135.1 (C-6), 134.5 (C-9'), 130.2 (C-10'), 129.5 (C-7'), 128.2 (C-6'), 127.4 (C-5'), 127.1 (C-8'), 125.9

(C-1'), 121.3 (C-5), 38.4 (C-7); ^{31}P NMR (161.9 MHz, DMSO-d_6): δ 19.1; LC MS (%): m/z 390.5 (100%) [MH$^{+\bullet}$]; Anal. Calcd. for $C_{21}H_{20}N_5OP$: C 64.77; H 5.18; N 17.99; Found: C 64.68; H 5.12; N 17.85.

1,3-Benzothiazol-2-yl-N,N'-di(3-pyridylmethyl)phosphonic diamide (9d)

Yield: 66%; mp: 175-177°C; IR (KBr): ṽ 3383 (N-H), 1245 (P = O), 1013 (P-C$_{Ar}$) cm^{-1}; ^{1}H NMR (400 MHz, DMSO-d_6): δ 8.48-7.44 (12H, m, Ar), 5.62 (2H, brs, H-8), 4.35-4.31 (4H, d, H-7); ^{13}C NMR (100 MHz, DMSO-d_6): δ 162.2 (C-1'), 155.3 (C-8'), 149.2 (C-2), 148.9 (C-4), 145.5 (C-1), 135.8 (C-6), 134.3 (C-9'), 129.5 (C-4'), 127.1 (C-5'), 125.9 (C-6'), 125.7 (C-3'), 121.2 (C-5), 38.3 (C-7); ^{31}P NMR (161.9 MHz, DMSO-d$_6$): δ 21.6; LC MS (%): m/z 396.5 (100%) [MH$^{+\bullet}$]; Anal. Calcd. for $C_{19}H_{18}N_5OPS$: C 57.71; H 4.59; N 17.71; Found: C 57.62; H 4.41; N 17.58.

3-Cyano-2-pyridyl-N,N'-di(3-pyridylmethyl)phosphonic diamide (9e)

Yield: 68%; mp: 172-174°C; IR (KBr): ṽ 3388 (N-H), 1258 (P = O), 1018 (P-C$_{Ar}$) cm^{-1}; ^{1}H NMR (400 MHz, DMSO-d_6): δ 8.66-7.41 (11H, m, Ar), 5.63 (2H, brs, H-8), 4.32-4.30 (4H, d, H-7); ^{13}C NMR (100 MHz, DMSO-d_6): δ 157.3 (C-1'), 156.3 (C-3'), 149.3 (C-2), 148.8 (C-4), 145.5 (C-1), 138.4 (C-5'), 135.9 (C-4'), 135.8 (C-6), 121.4 (C-5), 118.3 (C-7'), 113.6 (C-6'), 38.2 (C-7); ^{31}P NMR (161.9 MHz, DMSO-d$_6$): δ 22.7; LC MS (%): m/z 365.7 (100%) [MH$^{+\bullet}$]; Anal. Calcd. for $C_{18}H_{17}N_6OP$: C 59.34; H 4.70; N 23.07; Found: C 59.19; H 4.48; N 22.91.

1-Isoquinolyl-N,N'-di(3-pyridylmethyl)phosphonic diamide (9f)

Yield: 73%; mp: 185-187°C; IR (KBr): ṽ 3387 (N-H), 1261 (P = O), 1010 (P-C$_{Ar}$) cm^{-1}; ^{1}H NMR (400 MHz, DMSO-d_6): δ 8.61-7.48 (14H, m, Ar), 5.64 (2H, brs, H-8), 4.34-4.31 (4H, d, H-7); ^{13}C NMR (100 MHz, DMSO-d_6): δ 159.3 (C-1'), 149.1 (C-2), 148.5 (C-4), 145.9 (C-1), 144.8 (C-3'), 135.9 (C-10'), 135.3 (C-6), 129.7 (C-6'), 129.5 (C-9'), 129.1 (C-8'), 128.5 (C-7'), 127.3 (C-5'), 122.6 (C-4'), 121.7 (C-5), 38.4 (C-7); ^{31}P NMR (161.9 MHz, DMSO-d$_6$): δ 18.9; LC MS (%): m/z 390.2 (100%) [MH$^{+\bullet}$]; Anal. Calcd. for $C_{21}H_{20}N_5OP$: C 64.77; H 5.18; N 17.99; Found: C 64.55; H 5.02; N 17.75.

Molecular modeling

All the *in silico* studies were carried out in the Molecular Operating Environment (MOE) software tool [34].

Protein preparation and processing

The three dimensional X-Ray Crystallographic structure of Protein tyrosine phosphatase (PTP) was retrieved from Protein Data Bank (PDB ID: 2F71). The structure was loaded into the MOE working environment ignoring the water molecules and hetero atoms. Polar hydrogens were added to the protein and subjected protonation followed by energy minimization in the implicit solvated environment in MMFF94x force field at a gradient cut off value of 0.05. A stabilized conformation of the protein was obtained after energy minimization and it was used for docking study.

Molecular docking

The above obtained stable conformation of the protein was preceded with molecular docking process. The binding site was defined with Arg 24, Asp 181, Ser 216, Ala 217, Gly 220, Arg 221 and Arg 254 residues. These are all the residues that were found to be interacting with the previously reported sulfamic acid inhibitor and hence considered for the docking of library of the present novel compounds. All the ligands were docked into the specified binding site using alpha triangle placement methodology where the Poses are generated by superposition of ligand atom triplets and triplets of receptor site points. A random triplet of ligand atoms and a random triplet of alpha sphere centers are used to determine the binding pose at each interaction. The free energy of binding of each compound from each pose generated after docking process is determined by London dG scoring function. A total of 30 conformations were generated for each compound and they were refined and rescored again using the same scoring function. The pose with lowest binding score was selected for further analysis and to analyze the binding mode orientations of the ligands in the binding site.

ADMET study

Pharmacokinetic parameters like absorption, distribution, metabolism and excretion of compounds designates their disposition. Such parameters influence the pharmacokinetics of the drug in the body and in turn influence their performance and pharmacological activity [35]. In that sequence we have predicted some ADMET properties for the designed compounds to define them as drug candidates at their significant conditions. The parameters such as Caco-2 (colon adeno carcinoma) cell permeability, MDCK (Madin-Darby canine kidney) cell permeability, BBB (blood-brain barrier) penetration, HIA (human intestinal absorption), skin permeability and plasma protein binding ability were predicted by submitting the structures to PreADMET online software tool (http://preadmet.bmdrc.org/index.php?option=com_content&view=frontpage&Itemid=1) a web-based application server for predicting ADMET.

Pharmacology

Compounds **5a-f** and **9a-f** were screened for *in vitro* antioxidant activity by DPPH (2,2-diphenyl-1-picrylhydrazyl), NO and H_2O_2 methods where Ascorbic acid and

BHT (Butylated hydroxytoluene) as standards. Subsequently all the title compounds were screened for their *in vivo* antihyperglycemic activity in twenty five days period and examined for every four days. The experimental procedures are described below.

Antioxidant activity
DPPH radical scavenging activity
The DPPH radical scavenging activity was measured from the bleaching of the purple colored methanol solution of 2,2-diphenyl-1-picrylhydrazyl (DPPH). Initially 1 mL of various concentrations of test compounds (50, 75, 100 and 150 µg/ mL) in methanol were added to 4 mL of 0.004% (w/v) methanol solution of DPPH. The resultant test solutions were incubated for 30 min period at room temperature and absorbance was read against blank at 517 nm. All the tests were carried out in triplicate. The % of inhibition (I%) of free radical production from DPPH was calculated by following equation.

$$I\% = \left[(A_{control} - A_{sample}) / A_{control} \right] X100$$

Nitric oxide (NO) scavenging activity
NO scavenging activity action was measured by slightly modified method of Green et al. and Marcocci et al. [36]. The mixture of 1 mL of sodium nitro prusside (10 mM) and 1.5 mL of phosphate buffer saline (0.2 M, pH 7.4) were tested to different concentrations (50, 75, 100 and 150 µg/mL) of the test compounds and incubated for 150 min at 25°C and treated with 1 mL of Griess reagent and absorbance of the chromophore was measured at 546 nm. Butylated hydroxyl toluene was used as the standard in the present method. Tests were carried out in triplicate. Nitric oxide scavenging activity was calculated by the following equation.

$$\% \text{ of scavenging} = \left[(A_{control} - A_{sample}) / A_{control} \right] X100$$

Hydrogen peroxide (H₂O₂) scavenging activity
Radical scavenging activity of the title compounds was screened against H_2O_2 through the method of Ruch et al. [37]. A solution of H_2O_2 (40 mM) in phosphate buffer (P^H 7.4) was prepared, 0.6 mL of prepared H_2O_2 solution was added to the test compounds at different concentrations (50, 75, 100 and 150 µg/mL) and the absorbance value for the reaction mixture was recorded at 230 nm for every test sample in average of triplicate. Tests were carried out in triplicate. The per cent of scavenging of H_2O_2 was calculated by the following equation.

$$\% \text{ of scavenging} = \left[(A_{control} - A_{sample}) / A_{control} \right] X100$$

Where $A_{control}$ is the absorbance of the control reaction (containing all reagents except the test compound)

and A_{sample} is the absorbance of the test compound and Acetate buffer as A_{blank}.

In vivo antihyperglycemic activity
Induction of diabetes
Male wistar albino rats (body weight 180-200 grams) were subjected to intra-peritoneal administration of Streptozotocin dissolved in freshly prepared 0.01M ice-cold citrate buffer (P^H 4.3) at a dose of 50 mg/Kg body weight. After 72 hours, the animals with fasting blood glucose levels ≥350 mg/dL were used to evaluate the anti-diabetic activity of title compounds. Blood glucose levels were measured with the help of Accuchec Glucometer (Glucose oxidase method). All the animals were maintained in ventilated cages provided with standard pellet diet and water in light/dark cycle of (12h/12h) [38]. All of animal experiments were carried out according to the guidelines of the Sri Venkateswara University's Institutional Animal Care and Use Committee (No./02 (i)/a/CPCSCA/IAEC/SVU/TV).

Experimental design
The animals were divided into fifteen groups and each group maintained six rats. Group 1 as normal rats Untreated, Group 2 as diabetic rats Untreated, Group 3 as Diabetic rats treated with standard Glibenclamide (25 mg/kg b.w.) and Group 4-15 as Diabetic rats treated with title compounds (25 mg/kg b.w.) from **5a-f** and **9a-f** respectively for each group. After an overnight fast, the drug dissolved in DMSO (25 mg/kg b.w.) was fed to 4-15 group rats by gastric intubation using force feeding needle. Normal untreated and diabetic untreated rats were fed with normal diet and distilled water alone. Group 3 diabetic rats were treated with Glibenclamide 25 mg/kg b.w. Blood samples were collected to measure blood glucose levels from the tail vein on 1st, 4th, 8th, 12th, 16th, 20th and 25th days after the administration of drug and blood glucose levels were determined by glucose oxidase–peroxidase method [39].

Results
Chemistry
The IR spectra of **5a-f** showed the expected absorption bands at 998-1008, 3350–3330 and 1255–1233 cm^{-1} for the P-C$_{(Ar)}$, NH and P = O stretching vibrations respectively [40]. The signals in δ 5.12-5.16 of **5a-f** and δ 5.63-5.64 of **9a-f** are representing the NH protons attached to the phosphorus atom. All ^{13}C signal of aromatic carbon attached to the phosphorus is observed in between the range of δ 128-139 and δ 152-169. ^{31}P NMR signals appeared in the range of 27.3 to 28.6 ppm as expected for the P = O group of the title compounds.

Prediction of Lipinski parameters

The three dimensional structures were constructed for all the compounds and their stable conformations were obtained after optimization. These conformations were used to study their Lipinski parameters and the results showed that all of them are showing best properties with good agreement to Lipinski rule suggesting them as safer drugs. All the compounds have the molecular weight less than 500 Da, the lowest molecular weight of 364 Da was found with **9e** and the highest molecular weight of 441 Da was found with **5c**. The number of hydrogen bond donors is found to be less than 5 and the hydrogen bond acceptors is less than 10 for all the compounds. The logP values observed below 5 are themselves indicating that they are all non-toxic to the host system. The molar refractivity is also found to be in the optimal range of 40-150. The remaining descriptors like surface area, volume, hydration energy, polarizability and energy levels are also encouraging them with suitable features to bind and inhibit the target, there by better results can be expected and promotes them as safer and effective drugs (Table 1).

Molecular docking

A total of 30 binding pose conformations were generated for each compound from docking simulations using MOE dock system. The free energy of binding of each ligand was ranked and assessed by London dG scoring function. The binding energies and hydrogen bond interactions of each Receptor-Ligand complexes were studied and the information is tabulated in Table 2. The best lowest docking score -11.810 Kcal/mol was observed for the compound **9e** and second the highest docking score of -9.813 Kcal/mol was observed for **9a**. The remaining compounds are also showing better docking scores

indicating the good affinity levels between the receptor and compounds. The binding mode orientations of **9e** ligand-receptor complex are showing that the ligand is interacting with the binding site with the help of a single arene cat ionic interaction with Arg24 residue. Hydrogen bond interactions were not seen for **9e** in the complex. It was observed from all docking complexes that Arg24 residue is playing a major role in interacting with almost all of the compounds. In addition with **9e**, the arene cat ionic interaction was also observed with the compounds **5d**, **9b**, **9c**, **9d** and **9f**. More over in all of these complexes the arene cat ionic interaction was contributed by Arg24 residue only. This indicates that the aromatic rings of the compounds are highly influencing them to interact with the Arginine residue. The hydrogen bond interactions were not observed for **9d** and **9e** where as such bonds were observed in the remaining docking complexes (Figure 3 and Additional file 1: Figure S1-S12). However, **9d** and **9e** are also showing satisfactory docking scores along with remaining compounds. So, finally it can be predicted from these studies that all these compounds have the ability to bind with PTP-1B and inhibits its activity.

ADMET results

Human intestinal absorption, Caco-2 cell permeability, MDCK cell permeability, BBB penetration, skin permeability and plasma protein binding abilities of the title compounds were calculated by PreADMET server and the results presented in Figure 4.

The HIA results demonstrate the best absorption of the title compounds **5a-f** and **9a-f** into Human Intestine. Weak plasma protein binding results represent their virtuous properties such as diffusion or transport across cell membranes, interaction with a pharmacological

Table 1 Lipinski parameters of the title compounds 5a-f and 9a-f

Ligand	Molecular Weight (Daltans)	Hydrogen Bond Donors	Hydrogen Bond Acceptors	LogP	Molar Refractivity (A^{o3})	Surface area (A^{o2})	Volume (A^{o3})	Hydration energy (K.cal/mol)	Polarizability (A^{o3})	Gradient energy (K.cal/molA°)	Total energy (K.cal/mol)
5a	374	2	5	4.5	103.11	672.40	1175.38	−4.06	37.40	0.086231	157.989
5b	406	4	5	2.6	106.25	691.18	1199.19	−14.33	39.78	0.092319	142.533
5c	441	2	7	3.32	110.60	653.20	1247.31	−2.86	40.55	0.087467	168.395
5d	374	2	5	2.31	103.41	685.33	1177.04	−4.18	38.50	0.082136	158.398
5e	423	2	4	3.50	123.12	732.44	1318.93	−2.41	45.55	0.094976	196.071
5f	423	2	4	3.58	124.45	748.81	1328.20	−3.87	45.55	0.097266	190.509
9a	401	2	8	1.8	102.18	715.05	1257.28	−17.30	42.18	0.099135	166.626
9b	389	2	4	4.3	112.33	697.94	1253.43	−10.04	44.77	0.091709	166.626
9c	389	2	4	4.2	111.00	696.31	1259.79	−9.42	44.77	0.095766	188.333
9d	395	2	4	4.3	109.77	704.82	1243.68	−8.45	44.10	0.091985	170.187
9e	364	2	4	2.9	98.20	685.29	1201.59	−11.42	41.39	0.096933	245.03
9f	389	2	4	4.2	111.00	702.04	1267.84	−8.75	44.77	0.090542	186.537

Table 2 Molecular docking of the title compounds (5a-f and 9a-f) into the PTP biding domain

Ligand	Docking score (Kcal/mol)	No.H-bonds	Interacting residues	H-bond length (Å)
5a	−10.5251	2	Arg 24	2.4
			Ala 27	2.8
		Arene cat ionic interaction	Arg 24	
5b	−11.3541	1	Gln262	3.2
5c	−10.2642	2	Arg24	3.2
			Arg254	3.0
5d	−10.1672	1	Arg24	2.6
		Arene cat ionic interaction	Arg24	
5e	−10.3299	2	Arg24	2.8
			Arg24	2.9
5f	−11.4417	1	Arg24	2.5
			His25	2.3
9a	−9.8136	1	Arg24	2.3
9b	−11.4253	1	Arg24	2.8
		Arene cat ionic interaction	Arg24	
9c	−10.1006	1	Arg24	2.7
		Arene cat ionic interaction	Arg24	
9d	−11.2717	Arene cat ionic interaction	Arg24	
9e	−11.8104	Arene cat ionic interaction	Arg24	
9f	−10.5172	1	Arg24	2.0
		Arene cat ionic interaction	Arg254	

Major strength of interaction is contributed by arene cat ionic interactions.

target and excretion. This is due to, generally the drugs less bound to plasma protein exist freely for diffusion or transport across cell membranes and also for interaction with a pharmacological target. The title compounds 9a-j, altogether showed moderate cellular permeability against Caco-2 cells. The compound 5b exhibited medium MDCK cellular permeability. In turn all the above parameters represent their good excretion, disposition and efficacy values in the human body.

The Blood-Brain Barrier (BBB) penetration is represented as BB = [Brain]/[Blood], where [Brain] and [Blood] are the steady-state concentration of radio labeled compound in brain and peripheral blood. Predicting BBB penetration helps to know whether the compounds able to pass across the blood-brain barrier or not. This parameter expresses the BBB penetration capacity and absorption rate of compound to CNS. All the compounds were observed to be having moderate absorption to CNS.

The skin permeability is a crucial parameter that can define the transdermal delivery of the compound as the risk assessment during accidental contact with the skin. The skin permeability values are defined as logKp, cm/hr for all the compounds, where Kp = Km*D/h. **Km** is distribution coefficient between stratum corneum and vehicle, **D** is average diffusion coefficient (cm^2/h) and **h** is thickness of skin (cm) [41].

Pharmacology
The title compounds were assessed for anti-oxidant and anti-hyperglycemic activity. The detailed discussion regarding the assessment method is demonstrated as follows.

Antioxidant activity
Free radical 2,2-diphenyl-1-picrylhydrazyl (DPPH) scavenging activity
DPPH is usually used as a reagent to evaluate free radical scavenging activity of antioxidants [42]. DPPH is a stable free radical and accepts an electron or hydrogen radical to become a stable diamagnetic molecule [43]. The reduction capability of DPPH radical is determined by the decrease in absorbance at 517 nm induced by antioxidants. In the present study, Ascorbic acid was used as a standard, the title compounds 5a-f and 9a-f were able to reduce the stable radical DPPH to the yellow-colored diphenylpicrylhydrazine. The compounds were evaluated at four different concentrations of 50 μg/mL, 75 μg/mL, 100 μg/mL and 150 μg/mL and the IC_{50} values were determined from these evaluations. The scavenging effect of title compounds as compared to standard with the DPPH radical is in the following order 5f >5e >9f > Ascorbic acid >5c >9c and the remaining compounds showed less effect than these compounds. The compounds showed almost all same order at all concentrations and the complete results are given in Additional file 1. The IC_{50} value of each compound was considered as the concentration (μg/mL) of the compound at which 50% of DPPH reduction was observed. These results are presented in Figure 5 and in Additional file 1: Table S5.

Assay of Nitric oxide radicals scavenging activity
In the current investigation, newly synthesized compounds exhibited an excellent NO radicals scavenging activity. The compounds were evaluated at four different concentrations of 50 μg/mL, 75 μg/mL, 100 μg/mL and 150 μg/mL and the IC_{50} values were determined from these evaluations. Amongst the title compounds 5e > BHT >5f >5a >5c >9f have exerted significant inhibitory activity and the remaining compounds exhibited less effect than these compounds on radicals that are generated *in vitro* and the complete results are given in Additional file 1.

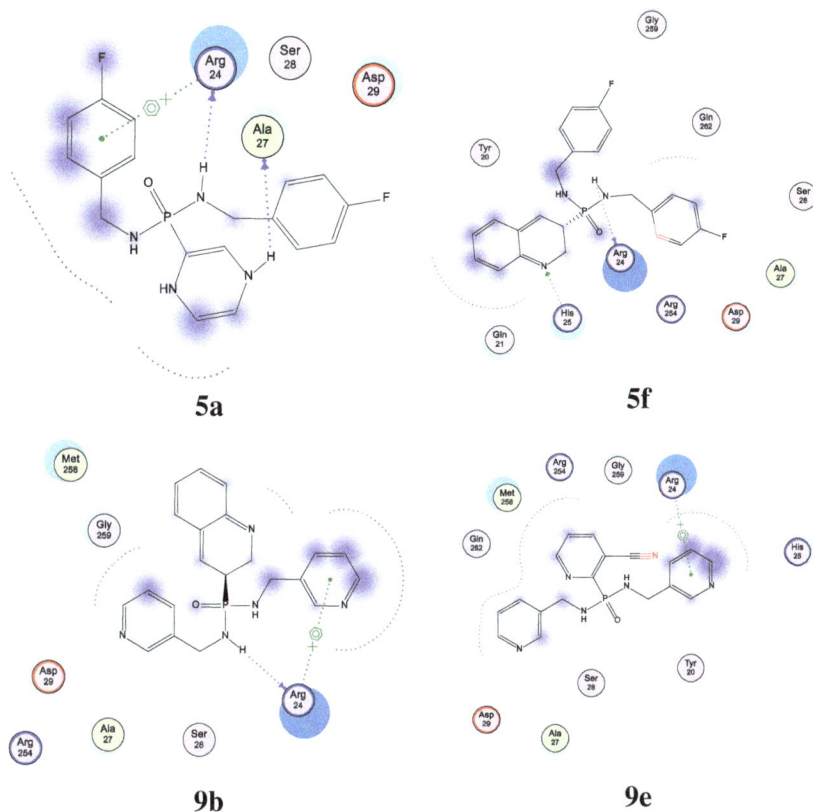

Figure 3 Molecular docking complexes of 5a, 5f and 9b and 9e with PTP (PDB ID: 2F71)

The IC$_{50}$ value of each compound was considered as the concentration (µg/mL) of the compound at which 50% of NO reduction was observed. These results are presented in Figure 5 and in Additional file 1: Table S6.

Assay of superoxide radical (O$_2^-$) scavenging activity

Superoxide radical is known to be a very harmful species to cellular components as a precursor of more reactive oxygen species [44]. The superoxide radical is known to be produced *in vivo* and can result in the formation of H$_2$O$_2$ *via* dismutation reaction. Moreover, the conversion of superoxide and H$_2$O$_2$ into more reactive species, for instance, the hydroxyl radical, has been thought to be one of the unfavorable effects caused by superoxide radicals [45]. The newly synthesized compounds are efficient scavengers for the superoxide radical generated in riboflavin−NBT−light system *in vitro* and their activity is in comparable to that of Ascorbic acid. The compounds were evaluated for their scavenging effects at four different concentrations of 50 µg/mL, 75 µg/mL, 100 µg/mL and 150 µg/mL and the IC$_{50}$ values were determined from these evaluations. The scavenging effects of the compounds are in the following order

5e >5f >9f >9c > Ascorbic acid and the remaining compounds exhibited less scavenging effect than these compounds on radicals that are generated *in vitro*. The compounds exhibited almost all same order at all concentrations and the complete results are presented in Additional file 1. This result clearly indicates that the tested compounds have a noticeable effect on scavenging superoxide radical. The IC$_{50}$ value of each compound was considered as the concentration (µg/mL) of the compound at which 50% of NO reduction was observed. These results are presented in Figure 5 and in Additional file 1: Table S7.

In over view of observation, the compounds **5e, 5f, 9c, 9f** are showing the better antioxidant activity, it may be due to the presence of quinolone group in the structures of the title compounds. These results are supported by the previous reports of Shridhar et al. of the antioxidant activity of eight substituted quinolines [46].

The proposed mechanism for the DPPH radical scavenging activity with the title compounds

All the title compounds are containing atleast two N-H functional groups in their structure. These N-H groups

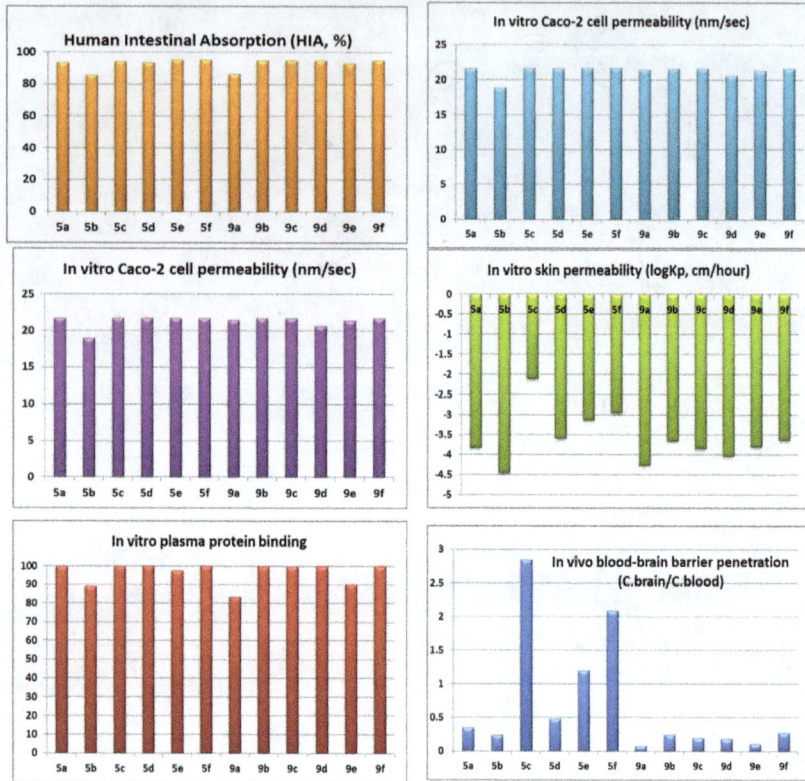

Figure 4 ADMET results of title compounds 5a-f and 9a-f.

are playng the main role in the abridging of free radicals, there by oxidative stress decreases. This mechanisim was supported by previous reports. This reduction of oxidative stress is the basis for mechanism for the antihyperglycemic actitivity (Figure 6).

Anti-hyperglycemic activity

All the title compounds showed significant anti-diabetic activity in the diabetes-induced rats when compared with the standard Glibenclamide. All the rats were kept in the observation for 25 days and seasoned the glycemic

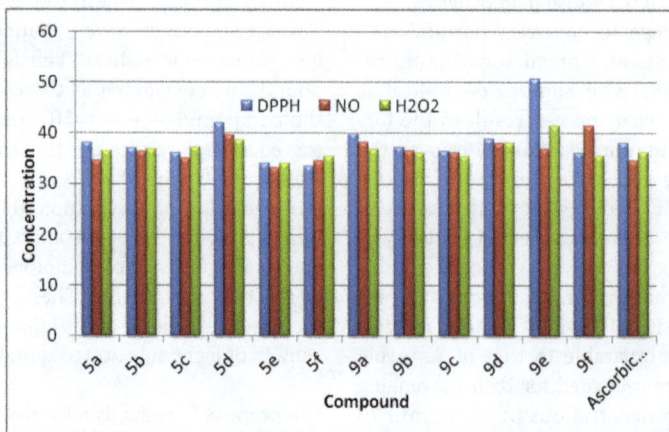

Figure 5 IC$_{50}$ values in µg/mL of the title compounds on DPPH scavenging activity, Nitric oxide radical scavenging activity and superoxide radical (O$_2{}^-$) scavenging activity.

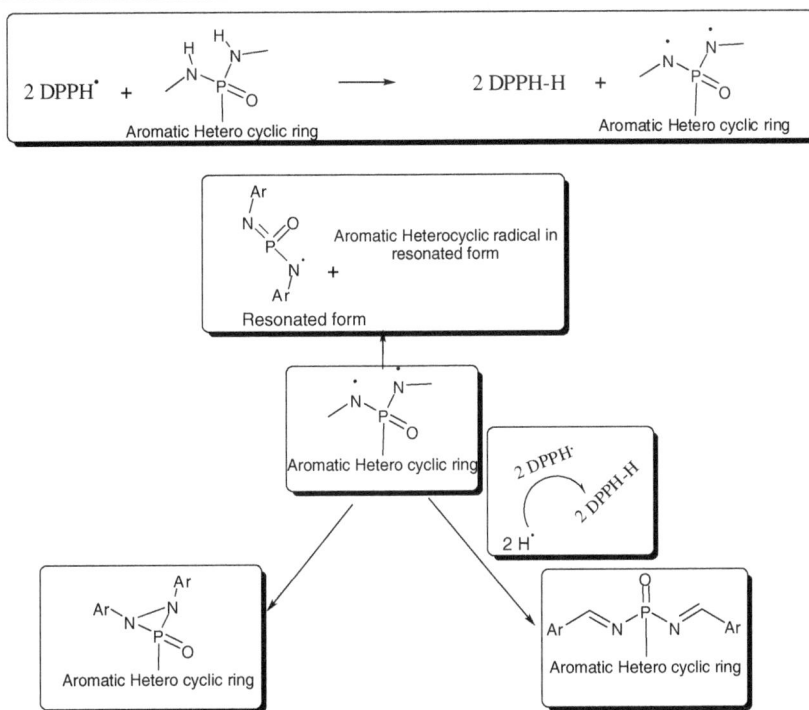

Figure 6 The proposed mechanism for the DPPH radical scavenging activity with the title compounds [47].

levels (mg/dL) for every four days after administration of drug. The diabetic rats showing glucose levels ≥350 mg/dL were taken for the experiment on the first day. On the fourth day, the glucose levels were almost all decreased i.e 221 ± 3.25 (**9a**) <242 ± 3.42 (**9f**) <244 ± 2.35 (**5f**) <245 ± 2.56 (Standard) <245 ± 4.86 (**9b**) <250 ± 3.24 (**5c**). On the eighth day the compounds **9a** (152 ± 3.46) and **9f** (195 ± 3.48) showed the least glycemic levels than the other compounds. On the 12th day, the compound **9a** induced rats showed the normal glycemic levels (120 ± 3.15) and compound **9b** (146 ± 1.95), **9f** (153 ± 2.32), **5c** (165 ± 2.76), Glibenclamide (166 ± 2.46) and **9e** (168 ± 2.68) induced rats gave moderate glycemic levels. On the 16th day only the compound **9a** (103 ± 1.47) gave the good result. The remaining compounds gave the moderate glycemic levels except **5a, 5d, 5e** and **9c**. On the 20th day all the compounds showed normal glycemic levels but **9d** gave moderate and **5a, 5d, 5e** and **9c** gave the high glycemic levels. Finally on the last day, all the title compounds gave excellent results with glycemic levels in between 82 ± 1.58 (**9a**) to 109 ± 1.23 (**9d**) apart from **5a, 5d, 5e** and **9c**. The detailed observation of results of all title compounds are reproduced in Table 3 (Figure 7).

The molecules which were bound at Arg24 of Protein tyrosine phosphatase (PTP) gave the potential anti-hyperglycemic properties against Diabetic rats. From

these results, compound **9a** can be stated as an effective anti-hyperglycemic compound among all as it exerted its effect in the earlier days among all. This may be due to the presence of two methoxy groups on the triazine moiety which are binding at Arg24 of PTP that can make it more reactive and effective. On the 20th day **5b, 5c, 9a, 9e** and **9f** compounds gave normal glycemic levels, it may be due to the presence of structural moieties like uracil, trifluoromethyl, dimethoxytriazine, nicotinonitrile and quinoline moieties respectively. On the othe other hand the same ligand groups are binding with PTP at Arg24. But a few compounds exhibited moderate results though they contain the quinoline and isoquinoline structures. On an overall, all the compounds have shown good anti-diabetic activities by 25th day except **5a, 5d, 5e** and **9c**. Over again, these results from molecular docking studies and in vivo assays of the title compounds supporting for previous reports that development of PTPs inhibitors is very ease for diabetes prevention [48].

Conclusion

Lanthanum (III) chloride is stated as an efficient catalyst for the Michaelis-Arbuzov reaction and for the synthesis of the title compounds **5a-f** and **9a-f** by two-step reaction. The molecular descriptors of all the compounds from

Table 3 Anti-diabetic activity of compounds 5a-f and 9a-f in STZ induced diabetic rats

Compound	Glycemic levels(mg/dL) at different time intervals after drug administration to mice						
	1st day	4day	8th day	12th day	16th day	20th day	25th day
N	98 ± 1.42^{g}	97 ± 1.42^{g}	98 ± 1.42^{g}	98 ± 1.42^{g}	99 ± 1.42^{g}	99 ± 1.42^{g}	98 ± 1.42^{g}
D	365 ± 3.22^{ng}	364 ± 2.85^{ng}	366 ± 4.54^{ng}	360 ± 3.72^{ng}	364 ± 2.18^{ng}	362 ± 4.36^{ng}	361 ± 1.68^{ng}
5a	355 ± 2.55^{n}	280 ± 4.85^{ng}	225 ± 4.58^{ng}	198 ± 4.25^{ng}	172 ± 3.25^{ng}	165 ± 3.85^{ng}	145 ± 2.76^{ng}
5b	360 ± 3.44^{n}	270 ± 3.95^{ng}	210 ± 4.34^{n}	179 ± 3.25^{ng}	135 ± 1.22^{n}	110 ± 1.85^{n}	105 ± 2.32^{n}
5c	372 ± 4.22^{ng}	250 ± 3.24^{n}	208 ± 2.85^{n}	165 ± 2.76^{n}	138 ± 2.44^{n}	116 ± 3.08^{n}	95 ± 2.25
5d	356 ± 4.44^{n}	312 ± 4.21^{ng}	250 ± 3.59^{ng}	221 ± 2.65^{ng}	200 ± 3.26^{ng}	193 ± 2.44^{ng}	178 ± 1.42^{ng}
5e	364 ± 3.88^{n}	272 ± 2.66^{ng}	236 ± 2.88^{ng}	202 ± 3.11^{ng}	182 ± 1.35^{ng}	169 ± 2.52^{ng}	152 ± 1.43^{ng}
5f	355 ± 3.14^{n}	244 ± 2.35^{n}	212 ± 3.16^{n}	173 ± 2.42^{ng}	142 ± 2.35^{ng}	125 ± 1.56^{n}	108 ± 1.34^{n}
9a	359 ± 2.37^{n}	221 ± 3.25^{ng}	152 ± 3.46^{ng}	120 ± 3.15^{ng}	103 ± 1.47^{g}	95 ± 1.25^{g}	82 ± 1.58^{ng}
9b	362 ± 4.92^{n}	245 ± 4.86^{n}	205 ± 2.83^{n}	146 ± 1.95^{ng}	132 ± 2.2^{ng}	123 ± 2.63^{n}	105 ± 1.73
9c	365 ± 5.22^{ng}	306 ± 3.58^{ng}	295 ± 3.64^{ng}	222 ± 2.95^{ng}	193 ± 1.45^{ng}	162 ± 1.73^{ng}	135 ± 1.34^{ng}
9d	362 ± 1.85^{n}	274 ± 4.23^{ng}	224 ± 2.62^{ng}	183 ± 3.18^{ng}	152 ± 1.36^{ng}	132 ± 1.8^{ng}	109 ± 1.23^{ng}
9e	357 ± 2.33^{n}	255 ± 3.82^{ng}	205 ± 2.47^{n}	168 ± 2.68^{n}	132 ± 1.45^{ng}	114 ± 1.37^{n}	98 ± 1.3
9f	363 ± 3.09^{n}	242 ± 3.42^{n}	195 ± 3.48^{ng}	153 ± 2.32^{ng}	131 ± 1.76^{ng}	108 ± 1.92^{ng}	92 ± 1.54^{ng}
G	357 ± 2.95^{n}	245 ± 2.56^{n}	210 ± 2.45^{n}	166 ± 2.46^{n}	137 ± 1.95^{n}	118 ± 1.83^{n}	95 ± 2.15^{n}

with N = Normal rats untreated, D = Diabetic rats untreated G = Glibenclamide.
[n]Represents significant difference on the respective day with normal rat group at $p < 0.05$.
[g]Represents significant difference on the respective day with glibenclimade rat group at $p < 0.05$.
The data values were analyzed using one way ANOVA.

Lipinski parameters explained their drug likeliness and suggesting them as safer drugs. The descriptors also indicate that they are all not harmful to the host system because of their optimal logP values. The molecular docking study revealed their strong ability to interact with the target and inhibits its activity, there by predicting their antidiabetic activity. PreADMET results demonstrated that the title compounds exhibit good absorption, permeability, penetration abilities in the human body. This prediction is confirmed by *in vivo* screening of these compounds in the diabetic induced rat models where the test compounds exhibited significant antihyperglycemic activity comparative to the standard Glibenclamide. Almost all the compounds brought the glycemic levels to normal on the 25th day. Especially, **9a** was shown normal glycemic levels on 12th day. On the 20th day **5c, 5b, 9a, 9e** and **9f** were shown normal glycemic levels. All the compounds exhibited good diabetic levels on 25th day except **5a, 5d, 5e** and **9c**.

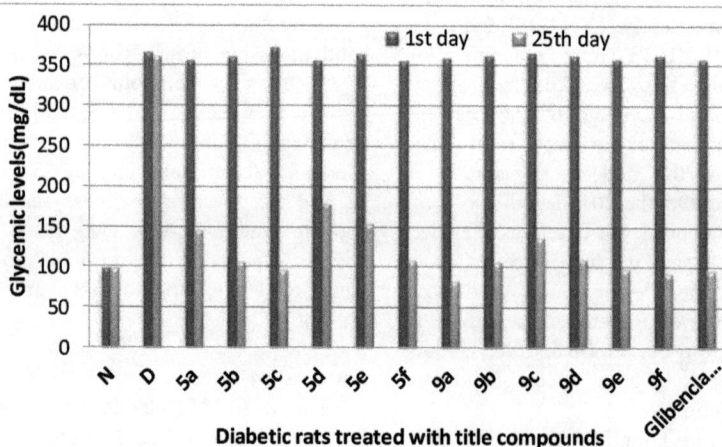

Figure 7 Anti-diabetic activity of compounds 5a-f and 9a-f in STZ induced diabetic rats.

Additional file

Additional file 1: Construction of 3D-models and ligand database of the compounds. Lipinski Descriptors. **Table S5.** DPPH radical scavenging activity of the compounds **5a-f** and **9a-f. Table S6.** Nitric oxide (NO)scavenging activity of the compounds **5a-f** and **9a-f. Table S7.** Hydrogen peroxide (H$_2$O$_2$) scavenging activity of the compounds **5a-f** and **9a-f. Figure S1:** molecuar docking complex of **5a. Figure S2:** molecuar docking complex of **5b. Figure S3:** molecuar docking complex of **5c. Figure S4:** molecuar docking complex of **5d. Figure S5:** molecuar docking complex of **5e. Figure S6:** molecuar docking complex of **5f. Figure S7:** molecuar docking complex of **9a. Figure S8:** molecuar docking complex of **9b. Figure S9:** molecuar docking complex of **9c. Figure S10:** molecuar docking complex of **9d. Figure S11:** molecuar docking complex of **9e. Figure S12:** molecuar docking complex of **9f.**

Competing interests
The authors declare that they have no competing interests.

Authors' contributions
CSK carried out synthesis and structural elucidation of title compounds, involved in screening of molecular modeling studies of designed compounds and drafted the manuscript. NKY had screen molecular modeling and ADMET studies of title compounds. JKMV was carried out Pharmacological studies of title compounds. ARC and NRC were provided the lab facilities and guidance in all aspects of this work. RS and MG were cooperated by their partial involvement in this work. All authors read and approved the final manuscript.

Acknowledgements
The authors express their grateful thanks to BRNS (DAE) for sanctioning research project (2012/37C/21/BRNS/785), Mumbai, India for providing financial assistance through the project.

Author details
[1]Department of Chemistry, Sri Venkateswara University, Tirupati 517 502, India. [2]Department of Biotechnology, Sri Venkateswara University, Tirupati 517 502, India. [3]Biomedical informatics Center, Vector Control Research Centre, Indian Council of Medical Research, Puducherry 605006, India. [4]Department of Biochemistry, Sri Venkateswara University, Tirupati 517 502, India.

References
1. Kennedy BP, Ramachandran C: Protein tyrosine phosphatase-1B in diabetes. *Biochem Pharmacol* 2000, **60:**877–883.
2. Johnson TO, Ermolieff J, Jirousek MR: Protein tyrosine phosphatase 1B inhibitors for diabetes. *Nat Rev Drug Disc* 2002, **1:**696–709.
3. Wang Q, Gao J, Liu Y, Liu C: Molecular dynamics simulation of the interaction between protein tyrosine phosphatase 1B and aryl diketoacid derivatives. *J Mol Graph Model* 2012, **38:**186–193.
4. Evans JL, Jallal B: Protein tyrosine phosphatases: their role in insulin action and potential as drug targets. *Exp Opin Invest Drugs* 1999, **8:**139–160.
5. Cheng A, Dube N, Gu F, Tremblay ML: Coordinated action of protein tyrosine phosphatases in insulin signal transduction. *Eur J Biochem* 2002, **269:**1050–1059.
6. Liu G, Xin Z, Liang H, Zapatero CA, Hajduk PJ, Janowick DA, Szczepankiewicz BG, Pei Z, Hutchins CW, Ballaron SJ, Stashko MA, Lubben TH, Berg CE, Rondinone CM, Trevillyan JM, Jirousek MR: Selective protein tyrosine phosphatase-1B inhibitors: targeting the second

phosphotyrosine binding site with non-carboxylic acid-containing ligands. *J Med Chem* 2003, **46:**3437–3440.
7. Wan ZK, Lee J, Xu W, Erbe DV, McCarthy DJ, Follows BC, Zhang Y: Monocyclic thiophenes as protein tyrosine phosphatase-1B inhibitors: capturing interactions with Asp48. *Bioorg Med Chem Lett* 2006, **16:**4941–4945.
8. Liu G, Xin Z, Pei Z, Hajduk PJ, Zapatero CA, Hutchins CW, Hongyu ZH, Lubben TH, Ballaron SJ, Haasch DL, Kaszubska W, Rondinone CM, Trevillyan JM, Jirousek MR: Selective protein tyrosine phosphatase-1B inhibitors: targeting the second phosphotyrosine binding site with non-carboxylic acid-containing ligands. *J Med Chem* 2003, **46:**4232–4235.
9. Shim YS, Kim KC, Chi DY, Lee KH, Cho H: Formylchromone derivatives as a novel class of protein tyrosine phosphatase-1B inhibitors. *Bioorg Med Chem Lett* 2003, **13:**2561–2563.
10. Adams DR, Abraham A, Asano J, Breslin C, Dick CAJ, Lxkes U, Johnston BF, Johnston D, Kewnay J, Mackay SP, Mackenzie SJ, Mcfarlane M, Mitchell L, Takano Y: 2-Aryl-3,3,3-trifluoro-2-hydroxypropionic acids: a new class of protein tyrosine phosphatase-1B inhibitors. *Bioorg Med Chem Lett* 2007, **17:**6579–6583.
11. Qingming W, Miaoli Z, Ruiting Z, Liping L, Caixia Y, Shu X, Xueqi F, Yuhua M, Qingwei H: Exploration of α-aminophosphonate N-derivatives as novel, potent and selective inhibitors of protein tyrosine phosphatases. *Eur J Med Chem* 2012, **49:**354–364.
12. Zsuzsa I, Estelle W, Almudena L, Maria PP, Federica P, Eva S, Sandy B, John W, Fermin IM, Alfredo Martinez J, Philippe V, Christian C: Chronic benzylamine administration in the drinking water improves glucose tolerance, reduces body weight gain and circulating cholesterol in high-fat diet-fed mice. *Pharmacol Res Off J Italian Pharmacol Soc* 2010, **61:**355–363.
13. Stefan M, Robert W, Bernhard S, Susanne K, Roger A: Picolylamine-methylphosphonic acid esters as tridentate ligands for the labeling of alcohols with the fac-[M(CO)3]+ core (M = 99mTc, Re): synthesis and biodistribution of model compounds and of a 99mTc-labeled cobinamide. *Nuclear Med Biol* 2005, **32:**473–484.
14. Simon TB, Karen RB, Teresa B, Ijen C, Mike C, Sarah D, Tim H, Allan MJ, Guy AK, Anthony RK, Burkhard K, Loic L, Angela M, Anil M, Sean L, Anthony P, Karine P, Mark R, Heather S, Melanie W, Ian AY: Discovery and optimization of potent and selective functional antagonists of the human adenosine A2B receptor. *Bioorg Med Chem Lett* 2009, **19:**5945–5949.
15. Phillip JK, Thomas MB, Patrick RG, John TB, Alexander SK, Carrie KJ, Ashley EB, Jana KS, Jeffrey CP, Craig WL: Synthesis and structure–activity relationships of allosteric potentiators of the M4 muscarinic acetylcholine receptor. *Chem Med Chem* 2009, **4:**1600–1607.
16. Y Patrick YSL, Yu R, Prabhakar KJ, Paul EA, George VD, Charles JE, Chong HC, George E, Edward RH, Wayne FD, Liangzhù L, Pat NC, Robert JM, Qi H, Renhua L, Jay AM, Steven PS, Thomas RS, Lee TB, Marlene MR, Ronald MK, Linyee S, Dean LW, David MK, David AJ, Erickson-Viitanen S, Nicholas Hodge C: Cyclic HIV protease inhibitors: synthesis, conformational analysis, P2/P2¢ structure-activity relationship and molecular recognition of cyclic ureas. *J Med Chem* 1996, **39:**3514–3525.
17. Jones BCNM, McGuigan C, O'Connor TJ, Jeffries DJ, Kinchington D: Synthesis and anti-HIV activity of some novel phosphoradiamidate derivatives of 3'-azido-3'-deoxythymidine (AZT). *AntiVir Chem Chemother* 1991, **2:**35–39.
18. Serafinowska HT, Ashton RJ, Bailey S, Harnden MR, Jackson SM, Sutton D: Synthesis and in vivo evaluation of prodrugs of 9-[2-(phosphono-methoxy)ethoxy] adenine. *J Med Chem* 1995, **38:**1372–1379.
19. Keith KA, Hitchcock MJ, Lee WA, Holy A, Kern ER: Evaluation of nucleoside phosphonates and their analogs and prodrugs for inhibition of orthopoxvirus replication. *Antimicrob Agents Chemother* 2003, **47:**2193–2198.
20. Petr J, Ondrej B, Martin D, Ivan V, Zdenek Z, Gina B, George S, Tomas C, Richard M, Antonin H, Zlatko J: A novel and efficient one-pot synthesis of symmetrical diamide (bis-amidate) prodrugs of acyclic nucleoside phosphonates and evaluation of their biological activities. *Eur J Med Chem* 2008, **46:**3748–3754.
21. Qun D, Rao KS, Tao J, Kevin F, Yan L, Frank T, William S, Daniel KC, Reddy KR, Paul DP, James MF, Scott CP, Mark DE: Discovery of phosphonicdiamideprodrugs and their use for the oral delivery of a series of fructose 1,6-bisphosphatase inhibitors. *J Med Chem* 2008, **51:**4331–4339.
22. Claude G, Nicolas B, Chantal F, Raphael ED: Synthesis and antibacterial activity of novel enolphosphate derivatives. *Bioorg Med Chem* 2010, **38:**218–223.
23. Asish KB, Florian S, Schmidt R: Design and synthesis of aryl/hetarylmethylphosphonate-UMP derivatives as potential glucosyltransferase inhibitors. *Tetrahedron Lett* 2001, **42:**5393–5395.

24. Salkeeva LK, Nurmaganbetova MT, Minaeva EV, Kokzhalova BZ: **Reactions of tert-Butyl N, N-Diethyl-N -(4-phenylthiazol-2-yl)-phosphorodiamidite with electrophilic reagents.** *Russ J Gen Chem* 2006, **76**:1397–1400.

25. Michael DC, Robert RS, Baihua H, James WJ, Robrt LM, David HK, Miller CP, Ullrich JW, Unwalla RJ, Wrobel JE, Quinet E, Nambai P, Bernotas RC, Elloso M: *Anticholesterol Agents; Antidiabetic Agents; Cardiovascular Disorders; Antiarthritic Agents,* US7576215 B2; 2009.

26. Miyata K, Shoji Y, Tsuda Y, Tsutsumi K, Kamisaka E, Inoue Y: **Inoue, JP-A-5043589.** In 1993. http://www.wikipatents.com/JP-Patent-5043589/quinoline-derivative.

27. Nallusamy S, Samuel S: **QSAR studies on HIV-1 protease inhibitors using Non-linearly transformed descriptors.** *Curr Comput Aided Drug Des* 2012, **8**:10–49.

28. Valasani KR, Hu G, Chaney MO, Yan SS: **Structure-based design and synthesis of benzothiazole phosphonate analogues with inhibitors of human ABAD-Aβ for treatment of Alzheimer's disease.** *Chem Biol Drug Des* 2013, **81**(2):238–249.

29. Ehsaneh T, Mahmoud D, Ahmad S, Ali MM, Djazayeri A, Qorbani M: **The relationship between the activates of antioxidant enzymes in red blood cells and body mass index in Iranian type 2 diabetes and healthy subjects.** *J Diab Metabol Disord* 2012, **11**:1–5.

30. Roja R, Shekoufeh N, Bagher L, Mohammad A: **A review on the role of antioxidants in the management of diabetes and its complications.** *Biomed Pharmacother* 2005, **59**:365–373.

31. Suresh K, Sunil S, Vasudeva N, Varun R: *In vivo* **anti-hyperglycemic and antioxidant potentials of ethanolic extract from Tecomella undulate.** *Diabetol Metabol Syndrome* 2012, **4**:1–7.

32. V Jan V, Marek J, Travnicek Z, Racanska E, Muselik J, Svajlenova O: **Synthesis, structural characterization, antiradical and antidiabetic activities of copper(II) and Zinc(II) Schiff's base complexes derived from salicylaldehyde and β-alanine.** *J Inorg Biochem* 2008, **102**:595–605.

33. Armarego WLF, Perrin DD: *Purification of Laboratory Chemicals.* 4th edition. Heinemann, Oxford: Butterworth; 1997.

34. Molecular Operating Environment (MOE): 1010 Sherbooke St. West, Suite #910, Montreal, QC, Canada, H3A 2R7: 2011.10; Chemical Computing Group Inc; 2011.

35. Beresford AP, Selick HE, Tarbit MH: **The emerging importance of predictive ADME simulation in drug discovery.** *Drug Discov Today* 2002, **7**(2):109–116.

36. Marcocci L, Maguire JJ, Droy Lefaix MT, Packer L: **The nitric oxide-scavenging properties of ginkgo biloba extract EGb 761.** *Biochem Biophys Res Commun* 1994, **201**:748–755.

37. Ruch RJ, Cheng SJ: **Klaunig: prevention of cytotoxicity and inhibition of intercellular communication by antioxidant catechins isolated from Chinese green tea.** *Carcinogenesis* 1989, **10**:1003–1008.

38. Magid AFA, Carson KG, Harris BD, Maryanoff CA, Shah RD: **Reductive amination of aldehydes and ketones with sodium triacetoxyborohydride. studies on direct and indirect reductive amination procedures.** *J Org Chem* 1996, **61**:3849–3862.

39. Kesari AN, Gupta RK, Singh SK, Diwakar S, Watal G: **Hypoglycemic and anti-hyperglycemic activity of Aeglemarmelos seed extract in normal and diabetic rats.** *J Ethnopharmacol* 2006, **107**:374–379.

40. Thomas LCP: *Interpretation of the Infrared Spectra of Organophosphorus Compounds.* London: Hyden and Son Ltd; 1974.

41. Rao VK, Michael OC, Victor WD, Yan SS: **Acetylcholinesterase inhibitors: structure based design, synthesis, pharmacophore modeling, and virtual screening.** *J Chem Inf Model* 2013, **53**(8):2033–2046.

42. Gulcin I, Bursal E, Hilal M, Ehitoglu S, Bilsel M, Goren AC: **Polyphenol contents and antioxidant activity of lyophilized aqueous extract of propolis from Erzurum, Turkey.** *Food Chem Toxic* 2010, **48**:2227–2230.

43. Soares JR, Dins TCP, Cunha AP, Ameida LM: **Antioxidant activity of some extracts of Thymus zygis.** *Free Rad Res* 1986, **26**:469–478.

44. B Halliwell B, Gutteridge JMC: *In Free Radicals, Ageing, and Disease, Free Radicals in Biology and Medicine.* 4th edition. Oxford: Clarendron Press; 2007.

45. Halliwell B: **Reactive oxygen species in living systems source, biochemistry, and role in human disease.** *Am J Med* 1991, **91**:14–22.

46. Shridhar AH, Keshavayya J, Peethambar SK, Hoskeri JH: **Synthesis and Biological activity of Bis alkyl 1,3,4-oxadiazole incorporated azo dye derivatives.** Arab J Chem 2012. http://dx.doi.org/10.1016/j.arabjc.2012.04.018.

47. Osman H, Arshad A, Lam CK, Bagley MC: **Microwave assisted synthesis and antioxidant properties of hydrazinylthiazolylcoumarin derivatives.** *Chem Centr J* 2012, **6**:32–41.

48. Safavi M, Foroumadi A, Abdollahi M: **The importance of synthetic drugs for type 2 diabetes drug discovery.** *Expert Opin Drug Discov* 2013, **8**(11):1339–1363.

13

Effects of atorvastatin on plasma matrix metalloproteinase-9 concentration after glial tumor resection

Niayesh Mohebbi[1], Alireza Khoshnevisan[2], Soheil Naderi[2], Sina Abdollahzade[2], Jamshid Salamzadeh[3], Mohammadreza Javadi[1], Mojtaba Mojtahedzadeh[1] and Kheirollah Gholami[1*]

Abstract

Background: Neurosurgical procedures such as craniotomy and brain tumor resection could potentially lead to unavoidable cerebral injuries. Matrix metalloproteinase-9 (MMP-9) is up-regulated in neurological injuries. Statins have been suggested to reduce MMP- 9 level and lead to neuroprotection. Atorvastatin preoperatively administered to evaluate its neuroprotective effects and outcome assessment in neurosurgical-induced brain injuries after glial tumor resection. In this prospective, randomized, double-blind, placebo-controlled trial, 42 patients undergoing glial tumor surgery randomly received 40 mg atorvastatin or placebo twice daily from seven days prior to operation and continued for a 3 weeks period. Plasma MMP-9 concentration measured 4 times, immediately before starting atorvastatin or placebo, immediately before surgery, 24 hours and two weeks after the surgery. Karnofsky performance score was assessed before first dose of atorvastatin as a baseline and 2 months after the surgery.

Results: Karnofsky performance scale after surgery raised significantly more in Atorvastatin group (11.43 +/− 10.62 vs. 4.00 +/− 8.21) (p = 0.03). Atorvastatin did not significantly reduce MMP-9 plasma concentration 24 hours after surgery in comparison to placebo. No statistical significance detected regarding length of hospital stay among the groups. Significant reduction in MMP-9 plasma concentration was recorded in atorvastatin group two weeks after surgery (p = 0.048).

Conclusions: Significant statistical differences detected with atorvastatin group regarding MMP-9 plasma concentration, clinical outcome and Karnofsky performance score. Consequently, atorvastatin use may lead to better outcome after neurosurgical procedures.

Keywords: Atorvastatin, Matrix metalloproteinase-9, Neuroprotective effects, Brain injuries, Glial tumor resection

Introduction

Neurosurgical procedures could be complicated by a diverse spectrum of factors, such as direct trauma, hemorrhage, brain retraction, and electrocautery with subsequent morbidity and mortality. Blood–brain barrier (BBB) disruption and brain edema is one of the proposed causalities [1,2]. Discovering novel neuro-protective agents and suggesting pre-operative regimen can result in better outcome after

brain surgeries. The matrix metalloproteinases (MMPs) are enzymes that play important roles in physiologic and pathophysiologic processes. These enzymes' levels mostly are not detectable, and increase in response to transcriptional regulators [3,4]. MMP-9 (Gelatinase B) is up-regulated in neurological injuries such as cerebral ischemia, BBB disruption, edema formation, and hemorrhagic transformation [5-8]. Different explanations provided to clarify relation of this enzyme and neurotoxicity [9-11]. In particular MMP-9 level rises in acute neurological injuries, so this enzyme proposed to be closely related to neurological impairments [3,12,13]. On the other hand,

* Correspondence: khgholami@tums.ac.ir
[1]Department of Clinical Pharmacy, Faculty of Pharmacy, Tehran University of Medical Sciences, Tehran, Iran
Full list of author information is available at the end of the article

blockade of MMP-9 activity have shown to be neuroprotective, and appropriate for the treatment of acute brain injuries [14-16]. Experimental studies suggest that preoperative inhibition of MMP-9 reduce brain injuries following neurosurgical procedures [1,2].

Statins not only lower cholesterol effectively [17] but also have other properties called "pleiotropic effects." Several clinical trials have indicated that statins suppress inflammatory reactions, recover neurological injuries, decrease the incidence of ischemic stroke, improve endothelial function, inhibit platelet activation, control vasospasm following subarachnoid hemorrhage, have neuroprotective activity in spinal cord injury, and prevent progression of Alzheimer's disease [18-30]. There are published documents claiming that statins decrease MMP-9 levels [30-32]. Many of these evidences are related to atorvastatin, a potent member of this family. This study was designed to evaluate atorvastatin effects on plasma MMP-9 concentration in neurosurgical- induced brain injuries after glial tumor resection. To minimize confounding factors Patients with gliomas grade 1, 2 and 3 which pathologically do not increase MMP-9 plasma levels substantially were entered the study and patients with Glioblastomamultiforme (GBM) were excluded.

Methods

This is a randomized, double blind, placebo-controlled prospective clinical trial performed in neurosurgery ward of a tertiary care Hospital from March 2011 to December 2012. The protocol was approved by the ethics committee of Tehran University of Medical Sciences (TUMS). This clinical trial was registered at Iranian Registry of Clinical Trial (IRCT) with the registration ID of "IRCT201203039196N1". For detecting any significant changes of MMP-9 concentration as main endpoint a sample size was calculated to be 21 patients at each group. Standard deviation for plasma MMP9 in human was supposed 23 ng/ml and 20 ng/ml was accepted as significant rise in MMP9 level, with $\alpha = 0.05$ and $\beta = 0.20$. [$n = 2(Z1- \alpha/2+ Z1-\beta)2$ $S2/d2$, i.e. $n = 2(1.96 + 0.84)2 \times 232/202$, $n = 21$] Patients undergoing elective surgery as therapeutic approach for tumor resection with diagnosis of glial tumor based on radiographic findings were included in this study. Patients excluded from the study with any atorvastatin contraindications such as, atorvastatin sensitivity, active hepatic disease, pregnancy and lactation; elevated liver enzymes; history of serious adverse reaction induced by atorvastatin; severe renal or hepatic failure; concurrent infectious disease; use of atorvastatin or other statins before the study; pathology report of other type of tumors instead of glioma grade 1,2 and 3; serious interaction between patients medications and atorvastatin; MAP < 70 mmHg; Na < 130 mEq/L; Hematocrit < 28%.

After obtaining informed consent, using permuted-block randomization patients were randomly assigned to atorvastatin or placebo group. Patients received atorvastatin or placebo 40 mg oral tablets, twice daily (totally 80 mg) for 3 weeks, from one week before to 2 weeks after surgery. Standard therapeutic regimen and supportive care, such as antibiotic prophylaxis, seizure prophylaxis, fluid therapy, and gastro intestinal ulcer prophylaxis have been used for both groups. This standard therapeutic regimen was including cefazolin as antibiotic prophylaxis, phenytoin for seizure prophylaxis, appropriate fluid therapy with normal saline, ranitidine as gastrointestinal ulcer prophylaxis, and dexamethasone for controlling brain edema after surgery.

At the beginning of the study, patients' demographic data such as age, sex, weight, comorbidity (having any concurrent disease other than glial tumor), history of hypertension, drug history, and neurological exam were collected on pre-designed questionnaires. Laboratory data recorded at baseline, were as follow: Fasting blood sugar (FBS), creatinin (Cr), blood urea nitrogen (BUN), white blood cell count (WBC count), hemoglobin, erythrocyte sedimentation rate (ESR), C-reactive protein (CRP), liver function tests (LFTs), lipid profile (including total cholesterol, LDL Cholesterol, HDL Cholesterol, and triglycerides). For detection of plasma MMP-9 concentration blood samples collected 4 times from each patient: immediately before starting atorvastatin or placebo, immediately before surgery, 24 hours and two weeks after the surgery. The plasma MMP-9 measured by enzyme-linked immunosorbent assay (ELISA) kits, Quantikine®, manufactured by R&D Systems, United States of America. Based on the kit catalog recommendations blood samples carried with heparinized tubes on ice. To separate plasma, blood centrifuged for 15 minutes at $1000 \times g$ within 30 minutes of collection. Following the above an additional centrifugation step of the plasma at $10,000 \times g$ for 10 minutes at 2 - 8°C performed for complete platelet removal, then all samples stored at −80°C till the assay day. This kit uses the quantitative sandwich enzyme immunoassay technique to assay MMP-9 levels. A monoclonal antibody specific for MMP-9 has been pre-coated on a microplate. All Standard samples and study samples are pipetted into the wells, and MMP-9 is bound by the immobilized antibody. Following washing away unbound substances, an enzyme-linked polyclonal antibody specific for MMP-9 is added to the wells. After a wash to eliminate unbound antibody-enzyme reagent, a substrate solution is added to the wells and color develops in proportion to the quantity of MMP-9 bound in the primary step. The color expansion is stopped and the intensity of the color is measured.

Clinical outcome were assessed with Karnofsky performance score at the baseline (one week before surgery) and 2 months after the surgery by the same examiner. Type and grade of tumors recorded after pathology report. Hospital stay defined as number of nights patient spent at the hospital. Our patients were closely observed for atorvastatin adverse effects, by interviewing patients during hospitalization and also after discharge in the clinic. Baseline and LFTs was measured in all patients and recheck CPK in any patient with symptoms suggestive of myopathy and also repeat transaminase levels when clinically indicated thereafter was about to be done. High rate reported adverse reactions such as diarrhea, arthralgia, limb pain, myalgia, muscle spasms, musculoskeletal pain, insomnia, nausea, and dyspepsia was asked from each patient specifically.

Statistical analyses were executed with the Statistical Package for Social Sciences (SPSS version 17; SPSS Inc., Chicago, IL, USA) and significance level was defined as p-value less than 0.05. The normal distribution of quantitative data was assessed with one sample Kolmogorov-Smirnov test. Data with a normal distribution were expressed as means ± standard deviations (SDs) and student t-test as well as paired t-test was used to compare quantitative variables between or within groups, respectively. The Mann–Whitney U test and Wilcoxon test were applied to compare non-normally distributed data (expressed as median (inter quartile range) to assess differences between and within groups, respectively. Regarding qualitative variables (categorical data), the chi-square or Fisher's exact test were performed.

Results

Forty- two patients, (25 males and 17 females) randomly assigned to 21 in atorvastatin group and 21 in placebo group. Patients' demographic data is presented in Table 1.

Patients mean ± SD age were 53.62 ± 15 years for atorvastatin group, and 40.43 ± 13.09 years in placebo group (p = 0.006, 95% CI: - 22.31- -4.08).

There were no statistically significant difference in regard to baseline parameters such as sex, weight, comorbidity (11 patients with hypertension [26%], 5 patients with ischemic heart disease [12%], 2 patients with gastrointestinal diseases [4.7%], one with lumbar herniated disc [2.4%], a patient with inherited neurofibromyalgia[2.4%], a patient with cataract [2.4%], and one patient with glaucoma [2.4%]), hypertension, concurrent drug therapy, and laboratory data such as FBS, Cr, BUN, WBC count, ESR, CRP (Table 1). The drug history of each patient obtained carefully, and there was no significant difference among the groups regarding medications. Considering drugs that may affect level of MMP-9 just 6 (3 patients in atorvastatin and 3 in placebo group) patients took low doses of aspirin (81 mg) to suppress platelet function. Dexamethasone as a part of standard post-operative protocol administered to all of the patients, 8 mg three times daily.

There were significant differences between baseline lipid profile (total cholesterol (p = 0.006), LDL Cholesterol (p = 0.009), and triglycerides (p = 0.04)) of the study groups. Lipid levels were higher in atorvastatin group; however, in both groups patients were not categorized as hyperlipidemic (Table 1).

Baseline plasma MMP-9 concentration, Karnofsky performance score, type of tumor, and grade of tumor among the groups were not significantly different (Table 1). Pathologic reports indicated grade 1, 2, 3 of glial tumor including, ependymoma grade 1 and 2, pilomyxoid astrocytoma, grade 2 astrocytoma, oligodendroglioma, ganglioglioma, anaplastic astrocytoma, and anaplastic oligodendroglioma.

Comparison of Karnofsky performance scale before and 2 months after surgery showed no significant difference among the groups (p = 0.07), however by further exploration of patients leading to exclusion of just one patient as outlier, significant difference showed up (p = 0.03). Atorvastatin group showed significantly better improvement of Karnofsky performance scale after surgery (11.43 ± 10.62 vs. 4.00 ± 8.21).

MMP-9 plasma level changes, immediately before surgery and 24 hours after surgery was not significantly different among the groups (p = 0.38).

In within group statistical analysis Karnofsky performance score showed significant increase in both atorvastatin (P = 0.001) and placebo (P = 0.03) groups. However, as it is depicted in Table 2 more progression was seen in atorvastatin group. MMP-9 plasma concentration levels increased significantly 24 hours after surgery in placebo group (P = 0.02). Nevertheless, there was no significant rise in MMP-9 levels in the atorvastatin group (P = 0.42). Comparison of MMP-9 plasma levels before surgery and 2 weeks after surgery revealed no significant changes in any of the groups, however there were an increasing trend in the placebo group and a decreasing trend in the atorvastatin group (Table 2).

Comparison of MMP –9 plasma level changes just before surgery with 2 weeks after surgery demonstrated significant difference among the groups (p = 0.048). Increase in MMP-9 levels 2 weeks after surgery was less in atorvastatin group. Atorvastatin and placebo groups MMP-9 plasma level changes between the first week of drug therapy and before surgery (1st and 2nd measurements), and changes between 3rd and 4th measurements indicated no significant difference. Likewise, comparison of ESR and CRP measurements before and after surgery did not indicate any significance in response to atorvastatin treatment.

Length of hospital stay was slightly in favor of atorvastatin group, but not to a significant degree (8.52 ± 6.77 days for drug group, and 11.29 ± 11.50 days for placebo group). There was no significant relation between

Table 1 Distribution of the baseline demographic and medical characteristics of patients in atorvastatin and placebo groups

Parameter	Atorvastatin group	Placebo group	P value
Sex			0.12
Male	15	10	
Female	6	11	
Age	53.62 ± 15	40.43 ± 13.09	0.006(95% CI: - 22.31- -4.08)
Weight	75.95 ± 12.35	72.43 ± 16.63	0.44(95% CI: - 12.66- 5.61)
Comorbidity	14	8	0.06
Hypertension	8	3	0.08
Concurrent drug therapy	14	8	0.06
FBS	94.57 ± 17.72	94.43 ± 24.16	0.98(95% CI: -13.36 – 13.07)
Cr	0.93 ± 0.19	0.81 ± 0.15	0.03 (95% CI: -0.23 – -0.01)
BUN	19.90 ± 6.36	15.48 ± 5.44	0.02(95% CI: -8.12 – -074)
WBC count	7400.48 ± 2857.89	7968.57 ± 379.129	0.98
ESR	20.24 ± 8.54	23.00 ± 10.29	0.35(95% CI: -3.13 – 8.66)
CRP	10.52 ± 10.96	11.62 ± 10.28	0.50
Total cholesterol	198.86 ± 33.45	173.52 ± 31.88	0.006
LDL cholesterol	129.62 ± 30.69	107.76 ± 31.73	0.009
Triglycerides	153.14 ± 50.58	173.52 ± 31.88	0.04
Plasma MMP-9 concentration	256.24 ± 279.81	130.95 ± 78.50	0.33
Karnofsky performance scale	82.38 ± 17.29	76.67 ± 19.32	0.25
Grade of tumor			0.80
Grade 1	4	3	
Grade 2	15	15	
Grade 3	2	3	
Type of tumor			0.73
Ependymoma grade 1	0	1	
Ependymoma grade 2	4	2	
Pilomyxoid astrocytoma	0	2	
Astrocytoma grade 2	5	7	
Oligodendroglioma	3	4	
Ganglioglioma	3	0	
Anaplastic astrocytoma	2	1	
Anaplastic oligodendroglioma	0	2	

age and Karnofsky performance score, MMP9 level changes, or hospital stay in any of the groups. BUN and Cr level changes were not significantly different between two groups. No adverse drug reaction reported by atorvastatin group.

Discussion

Neurosurgical procedures can induce serious neurological injuries [1,2]. Different medications such as diuretics, osmotic agents, and corticosteroids are suggested to decrease ameliorating brain edema induced by operation,

Table 2 Mean ± SD of outcome indicators in atorvastatin (drug) and placebo group

Variable	Plasma MMP-9 concentration before surgery	Plasma MMP-9 concentration 24 hours after surgery	Plasma MMP-9 concentration 2 weeks after surgery	Karnofsky performance scale before surgery	Karnofsky performance scale 2 months after surgery
Drug group	190.14 ± 197.74	236.38 ±225.08	164.95 ± 126.68	82.38 ± 17.29	93.81 ± 9.73
Placebo group	130.19 ± 83.04	184.81 ± 107.04	180.81 ± 115.93	76.67 ± 19.32	82.86 ± 14.88

but there is no clinical study in this regard [33]. Immuno-histochemical evidences specified that MMP-9 increases surrounding surgical induced brain injury areas [2]. Two experimental studies have demonstrated that MMP inhibitors preserve the BBB, attenuate brain edema, and act as a neuroprotectant after brain surgery [1,2].

There is some evidence that suggesting statins decrease MMP-9 levels [30-32]. Various retrospective and prospective clinical trials, meta-analysis, and researches evaluated pleiotropic effects of statins on surgical outcome. In cardiac, vascular, or non cardiovascular operations, irrespective to the type of surgery, positive effects and reduction of undesirable postoperative outcomes, such as mortality, morbidity, length of hospital and ICU stay have been reported following statin therapy [34-38]. Neuro-protective effects of statins were established in many studies [19-30].

In this prospective, randomized, double blind, controlled trial, 42 patients underwent glial tumor surgery, atorvastatin 40 mg or placebo used two times daily. Since most of the studies use full dose of statins to evaluate surgical induced injuries, 80 mg atorvastatin as a full dose is used in this study. Results demonstrated significant reduction in MMP-9 plasma level in atorvastatin patients after two weeks. Regarding clinical endpoint (Karnofsky performance scale at 2 months after surgery), better outcome observed in atorvastatin group. Length of hospital stay was less in patients who had received atorvastatin, but not to a statistical significant degree.

Plasma MMP9 changes followed the anticipated pattern. No significant change observed in the baseline measurement and second measurement (immediately before surgery), since there was no neuronal injury happened before surgery. Plasma MMP9 increased 24 hours after surgery as expected confirming the hypothesis of MMP9 surge after surgery. There was decrease in the MMP9 plasma concentration 2 weeks after surgery indicating improvement in patients. Between groups, statistical analyses demonstrated that atorvastatin group had significantly more reduction in MMP9 level after two weeks in comparison with placebo.

Within group statistical analyses revealed that atorvastatin diminished MMP-9 peak 24 hours after surgery. This outcome improvement was also confirmed by better neurological outcome as assessed with Karnofsky performance score in atorvastatin group. Despite no significant change in MMP-9 plasma concentration 2 weeks after surgery in within group statistical analyses, mean level increased in placebo group and decreased in atorvastatin group. All these findings indicate beneficial effects of atorvastatin in these patients.

Anti-inflammatory effects and MMP9 suppression appear to be irrelevant to concomitant medications. Although age of two patient groups was significantly different, there was no significant relation between age and outcome variables (i.e. karnofsky performance score, MMP9 level changes, or hospital stay).

Atorvastatin administration was well tolerated during the study period. No adverse drug reaction detected same as other studies on statins [37,38]. Acute kidney injuries were recently reported with high doses of statins [39-42]; therefore renal laboratory values were carefully monitored in this study. There were no significant changes in renal laboratory values between two groups. There is even a retrospective cohort of 98,939 patients who underwent various operations including; major open abdominal, cardiac, thoracic, or vascular procedure between 2000 and 2010 claims that statin use before surgery reduce risk of postoperative acute kidney injury [42]. Preoperative statin therapy decreased the need for postoperative renal replacement therapy [34].

Study had some limitations due to complexity of neurologic, physiologic and pathologic of human brain. Due to diversity of functioning regions of brain each glioma can cause different symptoms and debilities in different functioning parts of human brain within and or between different groups of patients pre and postoperatively. Due to complexity of circuits of brain (mostly unknown) different people suffer from different disabilities even when the glioma is operated on, in same area of brain; different surgical approaches caused different complications that could have been misinterpreted as effect of drug while being merely surgical.

Conclusion

Pre-operative atorvastatin administration resulted in reduction of MMP-9 level 2 weeks postoperatively and improvement of Karnofsky performance scale 2 month after surgery. Larger trials, longer duration of statin therapy, retrospective analysis of neurosurgical procedures in patients with long term statins use, could be helpful for decisive evidence.

Competing interests
All authors declare that they have no competing interests.

Authors' contributions
All authors participated in study design. KG and AK wrote the study protocol, and supervised all the stages of the research. KG managed supplying drug and placebo. AK performed surgeries. NM as a clinical pharmacist was involved in every steps of the project including literature review, writing the proposal, performing randomization and keeping it secret, collecting demographic data, design and filling the questionnaire, analyzing blood samples and providing article draft. SN and SA did neurological physical examination of patients, involved in blood sample collection, and assessed Karnofsky performance score. JS did all statistical analyses. MM and MJ consulted us in different stages of the project. KG, AK, JS, SA, and SN edited the draft. All authors read and approved the final manuscript.

Acknowledgements
We would like to thank Tehran University of Medical Sciences for providing the research fund. We also gratefully appreciate all attendants, residents,

nurses and staffs of the neurosurgery ward at Shariati hospital for their supports in this project.

Author details

[1]Department of Clinical Pharmacy, Faculty of Pharmacy, Tehran University of Medical Sciences, Tehran, Iran. [2]Department of Neurosurgery, Tehran University of Medical Sciences, Tehran, Iran. [3]Department of Clinical Pharmacy, Shahid Beheshti University of Medical Sciences, Tehran, Iran.

References

1. Jadhav V, Yamaguchi M, Obenaus A, Zhang JH: Matrix metalloproteinase inhibition attenuates brain edema after surgical brain injury. *Acta Neurochir Suppl* 2005, **105:**357–361.
2. Jadhav V, Yamaguchi M, Obenaus A, Zhang JH: Matrix metalloproteinase inhibition attenuates brain edema in an *in vivo* model of surgically-induced brain injury. *Neurosurg* 2007, **61:**1067–1076.
3. Yong VW, Agrawal SM, Stirling DP: Targeting MMPs in acute and chronic neurological conditions. *Neurother* 2007, **4:**580–589.
4. Liu W, Hendren J, Qin XJ, Shen J, Liu KJ: Normobarichyperoxia attenuates early blood–brain barrier disruption by inhibiting MMP-9-mediated occludin degradation in focal cerebral ischemia. *J Neurochem* 2009, **108:**811–820.
5. Rosenberg GA, Estrada EY, Dencoff JE: Matrix metalloproteinases and TIMPs are associated with blood–brain barrier opening after reperfusion in rat brain. *Stroke* 1998, **29:**2189–2195.
6. Noble LJ, Donovan F, Igarashi T, Goussev S, Werb Z: Matrix metalloproteinases limit functional recovery after spinal cord injury by modulation of early vascular events. *J Neurosci* 2002, **22:**7526–7535.
7. Pfefferkorn T, Rosenberg GA: Closure of the blood–brain barrier by matrix metalloproteinase inhibition reduces rtPA-mediated mortality in cerebral ischemia with delayed reperfusion. *Stroke* 2003, **34:**2025–2030.
8. Sumii T, Lo EH: Involvement of matrix metalloproteinase in thrombolysis-associated hemorrhagic transformation after embolic focal ischemia in rats. *Stroke* 2002, **33:**831–836.
9. Gu Z, Kaul M, Yan B, Kridel SJ, Cui J, Strongin A, Smith JW, Liddington RC, Lipton SA: Snitrosylation of matrix metalloproteinases: signaling pathway to neuronal cell death. *Science* 2002, **297:**1186–1190.
10. Xue M, Hollenberg M, Yong VW: Combination of thrombin and matrix metalloproteinase-9 exacerbates neurotoxicity in cell culture and intracerebral hemorrhage in mice. *J Neurosci* 2006, **26:**10281–10291.
11. Van den Steen PE, Proost P, Wuyts A, Van Damme J, Opdenakker G: Neutrophil gelatinase B potentiates interleukin-8 tenfold by aminoterminal processing, whereas it degrades CTAP-III, PF-4, and GRO-alpha and leaves RANTES and MCP-2 intact. *Blood* 2000, **96:**2673–2681.
12. Alvarez-Sabin J, Delgado P, Abilleira S, Molina CA, Arenillas J, Ribó M, Santamarina E, Quintana M, Monasterio J, Montaner J: Temporal profile of matrix metalloproteinases and their inhibitors after spontaneous intracerebral hemorrhage relationship to clinical and radiological outcome. *Stroke* 2004, **35:**1316–1322.
13. Abilleira S, Montaner J, Molina CA, Monasterio J, Castillo J, Alvarez-Sabı'n J: Matrix metalloproteinase concentration after spontaneous intracerebral hemorrhage. *J Neurosurg* 2003, **99:**65–70.
14. Wang J, Tsirka SE: Neuroprotection by inhibition of matrix metalloproteinases in a mouse model of intracerebralhaemorrhage. *Brain* 2005, **128:**1622–1633.
15. Rosenberg GA, Navratil M: Metalloproteinase inhibition blocks edema in intracerebral hemorrhage in the rat. *Neurol* 1997, **48:**921–926.
16. Rosenberg GA, Kornfeld M, Estrada E, Kelley RO, Liotta LA, Stetler-Stevenson WG: TIMP-2 reduces proteolytic opening of blood–brain barrier by type IV collagenase. *Brain Res* 1992, **576:**203–207.
17. Gotto AM: Management of dyslipidemia. *Am J Med* 2002, **112**(Suppl 1):10–18.
18. Chopp M, Zhang ZG, Jiang Q: Neurogenesis, angiogenesis, and MRI indices of functional recovery from stroke. *Stroke* 2007, **38:**827–831.
19. Khoshnevisan A, Mardani A, Kamali S: An overview of pharmacological approaches for management and repair of spinal cord injuries. *Iran J Psychiatry* 2010, **5:**119–127.
20. Chen J, Chopp M: Neurorestorative Treatment of Stroke: Cell and Pharmacological Approaches. *NeuroRx* 2006, **3:**466–473.
21. Chen J, Zhang ZG, Li Y, Wang Y, Wang L, Jiang H, Zhang C, Lu M, Katakowski M, Feldkamp CS, Chopp M: Statins induce angiogenesis, neurogenesis, and synaptogenesis after stroke. *Ann Neurol* 2003, **53:**743–751.
22. Endres M, Laufs U, Huang Z, Nakamura T, Huang P, Moskowitz MA, Liao JK: Stroke protection by 3-hydroxy- 3-methylglutaryl (HMG)-CoA reductase inhibitors mediated by endothelial nitric oxide synthase. *ProcNatl AcadSci U S A* 1998, **95:**8880–8885.
23. Laufs U, Gertz K, Dirnagl U, Bohm M, Nickenig G, Endres M: Rosuvastatin, a new HMG-CoA reductase inhibitor, upregulates endothelial nitric oxide synthase and protects from ischemic stroke in mice. *Brain Res* 2002, **942:**23–30.
24. Aslanyan S, Weir CJ, McInnes GT, Reid JL, Walters MR, Lees KR: Statin administration prior to ischaemic stroke onset and survival: exploratory evidence from matched treatment-control study. *Eur J Neurol* 2005, **12:**493–498.
25. Elkind MS, Flint AC, Sciacca RR, Sacco RL: Lipid-lowering agent use at ischemic stroke onset is associated with decreased mortality. *Neurol* 2005, **65:**253–258.
26. McGirt MJ, Garces Ambrossi GL, Huang J, Tamargo RJ: Simvastatin for the prevention of symptomatic cerebral vasospasm following aneurysmal subarachnoid hemorrhage: a single-institution prospective cohort study. *J Neurosurg* 2009, **110:**968–674.
27. Miida T, Takahashi A, Ikeuchi T: Prevention of stroke and dementia by statin therapy: experimental and clinical evidence of their pleiotropic effects. *PharmacolTher* 2007, **113:**378–393.
28. Amarenco P, Bogousslavsky J, Callahan AS, Goldstein L, Hennerici M, Sillsen H, Welch MA, Zivin J: Design and baseline characteristics of the stroke prevention by aggressive reduction in cholesterol levels (SPARCL) study. *Cerebrovasc Dis* 2003, **16:**389–395.
29. Chen J, Zacharek A, Li A, Zhang C, Ding J, Roberts C, Lu M, Kapke A, Chopp M: Vascular endothelial growth factor mediates atorvastatin-induced mammalian achaete-scute homologue-1 gene expression and neuronal differentiation after stroke in retired breeder rats. *Neurosci* 2006, **141:**737–744.
30. Kwak BR, Mulhaupt F, Mach F: Atherosclerosis: anti-inflammatory and immunomodulatory activities of statins. *Autoimmun Rev* 2003, **2:**332–338.
31. Corsini A, Bellosta S, Baetta R, Fumagalli R, Paoletti R, Bernini F: New insights into the pharmacodynamic and pharmacokinetic properties of statins. *PharmacolTher* 1999, **84:**413–428.
32. Bellosta S, Via D, Canavesi M, Pfister P, Fumagalli R, Paoletti R, Bernini F: HMG-CoA reductase inhibitors reduce MMP-9 secretion by macrophages. *Arterioscler Thromb Vasc Biol* 1998, **18:**1671–1678.
33. Menon D: Critical care medicine: management of raised intracranial pressure. In *Oxford textbook of medicine*. Volume 24th edition. Edited by Warrell DA, Cox TM, Firth JD. New York: Oxford University Press; 2003:1256.
34. Singh Singh I, Rajagopalan S, Srinivasan A, Achuthan S, Dhamija P, Hota D, Chakrabarti A: Preoperative statin therapy is associated with lower requirement of renal replacement therapy in patients undergoing cardiac surgery: a meta-analysis of observational studies. *Int Cardiov Thorac Surg* 2013, **17:**345–352.
35. Hindler K, Shaw AD, Samuels J, Fulton S, Collard CD, Riedel B: Improved postoperative outcomes associated with preoperative statin therapy. *Anesthesiol* 2006, **105:**1260–1272.
36. Chopra V, Wesorick DH, Sussman JB, Greene T, Rogers M, Froehlich JB, Eagle KA, Saint S: Effect of perioperative statins on death, myocardial infarction, atrial fibrillation, and length of stay: a systematic review and meta-analysis. *Arch Surg* 2012, **147:**181–189.
37. Liakopoulos OJ, Kuhn EW, Slottosch I, Wassmer G, Wahlers T: Preoperative statin therapy for patients undergoing cardiac surgery. *Cochrane Database Syst Rev* 2012, **4:**CD008493.
38. Sanders RD, Nicholson A, Lewis SR, Smith AF, Alderson P: Perioperative statin therapy for improving outcomes during and after noncardiac vascular surgery. *Cochrane Database Syst Rev* 2013, **3**(7):CD009971.
39. Sarma A, Cannon CP, Wiviott SD, Sabatine MS, Pfeffer MA, Hoffman EB, Guo J: The incidence of kidney injury for patients treated with intensive versus less potent statin therapy after an acute coronary syndrome [abstract]. *Circulation* 2013, **128:**00–00. 10.1161/CIR.0b013e31829ecc16.
40. Carney EF: Acute kidney injury: high-potency statin therapy and risk of acute kidney injury. *Nat Rev Nephrol* 2013, **9:**309. 10.1038/nrneph.2013.68.

41. Dormuth CR, Hemmelgarn BR, Paterson JM, James MT, Teare GF, Raymond CB, Lafrance J-P, Levy A, Garg AX, Ernst P: **Use of high potency statins and rates of admission for acute kidney injury: multicenter, retrospective observational analysis of administrative databases.** *BMJ* 2013, **346**. http://dx.doi.org/10.1136/bmj.f880.

42. Brunelli SM, Waikar SS, Bateman BT, Chang TI, Lii J, Garg AX, Winkelmayer WC, Choudhry NK: **Preoperative statin use and postoperative acute kidney injury.** *Am J Med* 2012, **125**:1195–1204.

14

Effect of IMOD™ on the inflammatory process after acute ischemic stroke

Mehdi Farhoudi[1], Mahdi Najafi-Nesheli[1*], Mazyar Hashemilar[1], Ata Mahmoodpoor[2], Ehsan Sharifipour[3], Behzad Baradaran[1], Aliakbar Taheraghdam[1], Daryoush Savadi-Oskouei[1], Homayoun Sadeghi-Bazargani[1], Elyar Sadeghi-hokmabadi[3], Hosein Akbari[3] and Reza Rikhtegar[3]

Abstract

Background and purpose of the study: Considering the role of inflammation in acute cerebrovascular accidents, anti-inflammatory treatment has been considered as an option in cerebrovascular diseases. Regarding the properties of Setarud (IMOD™) in immune regulation, the aim of the present study was to evaluate the role of this medication in treating patients with acute ischemic stroke.

Methods: In this randomized clinical trial, 99 patients with their first ever acute ischemic stroke were divided into two groups of IMOD™ (n = 49) and control (n = 50). The control group underwent routine treatment and the intervention group underwent routine treatment plus daily intermittent infusion of IMOD™ (250mg on the first day and then 375mg into DW5% serum during a 30-minute period for 7 days). The serum levels of inflammatory markers were evaluated on the first day (baseline) and on 4th and 7th days. Data were analyzed and the results were compared.

Results and major conclusion: 58 males (58.6%) and 41 females (41.4%) with a mean age of 67.00 ± 8.82 years, who had their first ever stroke attack, were enrolled in this trial. Treatment with IMOD™ showed a decreasing trend in IL-6 levels compared to the control group (p = 0.04). In addition, the treatment resulted in the control of increasing serum levels of hsCRP after 7 days compared to the control group (p = 0.02). There was an insignificant decrease in TNF-α and IL-1 levels in the IMOD™ group. Considering the prominent role of inflammation after an ischemic cerebral damage, it appears that treatment with IMOD™ improves the inflammatory profile. Therefore, IMOD™ (Setarud) might be considered as a therapeutic option in the acute ischemic stroke. However, future studies are necessary on its long-term results and clinical efficacy.

Keywords: Ischemic cerebro-vascular accident, IMOD™, Inflammatory markers

Background

Cerebrovascular accident is the main etiologic factor for disability in adults and the second most important cause of death worldwide [1]. Based on available evidence, a strong inflammatory reaction is induced subsequent to acute CVA, which has a great role in cerebral injury, demonstrating a significant interaction between the immune and nervous systems [2,3].

This inflammatory reaction is mediated by various cells, molecules and cytokines [3]; cytokines are upregulated in the brain after the stroke and are expressed not only in the immunologic cells but also in the glial cells and neurons [4].

The most extensively studied cytokines associated with stroke are IL-1β, IL-10, IL-6 and TNF-α. IL-1β and TNF-α, proinflammatory cytokines secreted by the activated immune cells in the ischemic area, induce the inflammatory process and facilitate the inflammatory cascade by inducing the expression of inflammatory molecules. These molecules recruit more leukocytes to the affected ischemic area, give rise to the loss of more nerve cells, cause cerebral tissue and expand cerebral infarction [5,6].

Considering the role of cytokines in neurologic inflammation, these inflammatory mediators can be the target of

* Correspondence: mnajafi_md@yahoo.com
[1]Neuroscience Research Center (NSRC), Imam Reza Hospital, Tabriz University of Medical Sciences, Tabriz, Iran
Full list of author information is available at the end of the article

neuroimmunomodulatory treatment [7]. Immunomodulatory medication is a substance that alters the ability of the immune system to produce antibodies or sensitized cells that recognize and react with the antigens that have initiated their production.

Setarud (IMOD™) is a combination of the extracts of Tanacetum vulgare, Rosa canina and Urtica dioica plant species, which has been enriched with selenium. The plant content of this medication has anti-inflammatory and immunoregulatory properties and selenium has a protective effect against oxidative stress. Extracts from Urtica dioica may prevent maturation of myeloid dendritic cells and reduce T cell responses. Multiple in vitro and in vivo studies in animal models and also in human has shown that it decreases TNF-α, IFN-γ and IL-2 levels and its effect in some clinical situations, such as experimental inflammatory bowel diseases, immunogenic type-1 diabetes in mouse and also in patients with sepsis and in HIV patients, has been evaluated due to its immunoregulatory properties [8-15]. Shirazi and colleagues in an in vitro study concluded that the dose-dependent inhibitory effect of Setarud on TLR stimulated B lymphocytes implies its potential therapeutic implication in B lymphocyte mediated autoimmune diseases and B-cell malignancies [16]. In addition, the herbal content of this medication can exhibit anti-inflammatory, anti-viral and immonomodulatory effects [17-20].

Considering the inflammatory changes during the acute phase of ischemic stroke and its central role on disease outcome, anti-inflammatory treatment might be an appropriate option in such patients; in addition, considering the role of IMOD™ in immunoregulation, the aim of the present study was to evaluate the effect of this medication on chief inflammatory biomarkers in patients with acute ischemic cerebrovascular accidents.

Methods

After approval of the ethics committee of Tabriz University of Medical Sciences, 99 patients with first attack of acute ischemic stroke (AIS), hospitalized in Tabriz Imam Reza and Razi Hospitals from September 2011 to March 2012, were enrolled in the study (using convenient sampling), and were randomly divided into two groups, with an allocation sequence based on a block size of fifty, generated with computer random-number generator. Allocation was concealed by use of sequentially numbered black envelopes. (IRCT No: IRCT 201108202195N2)

The AIS was initially diagnosed using Cincinnati Prehospital Stroke Scale (Facial droop, Arm drift and Speech) and confirmed based on clinical criteria and imaging techniques as used in TOAST Subtype Classification System [21]. The exclusion criteria were: age over 80 or under 18; previous history of stroke; a previous neurological deficit of any cause; cancer or any other severe disease; a rapid improvement in signs and symptoms before the institution of treatment; a baseline NIHSS (National Institutes of Health Stroke Scale) below5; elapse of less than 3 hours and more than 24 hours after the appearance of signs and symptoms; refusal to sign an informed consent form and a history of taking immunomodulatory medications such as immunoglobulin's or steroids.

All the patients who were available during the specified time interval and had the inclusion criteria were enrolled in the study. Since it was not possible to use placebo because of technical and ethical limitations, blinding was carried out through masked evaluation and any unmasked condition was taken into account during statistical analysis.

In the present study the subjects were divided into two randomized groups of case and control using stratified block randomization technique. The subjects in the control groups underwent a routine treatment protocol (according to the protocol of the University Department of Neurology); the subjects in the case group underwent routine treatment protocol plus daily intermittent infusion of IMOD™ (250mg on the first day and 375mg on the subsequent days into DW5% serum) during 30 minutes for 7 days. Previous studies showed that IMOD didn't have any side effect and only one case of phlebitis was reported [9]. So we used DW5% for its dilution and a duration of 30 minutes time for IMOD injection to reduce the probability of phlebitis. Both groups equally received routine therapeutic, supportive and rehabilitative measures. All study participants had blood samples taken at the first, fourth and seventh day of admission. Non-fasting blood was collected and within 30 minutes, the blood was centrifuged for 15 minutes at 3000 rotations per minute at room temperature. Subsequently, U-CyTech kit was used for determination of serum inflammatory markers by ELISA method. The levels of TNF-α, IL-6 and IL-1, and also platelets, WBC and High-sensitive CRP were determined on the first day of disease presentation (before treatment) and on the 4th and 7th days, by laboratory procedures in the hospital immunology department.

Informed consent was obtained from all the subjects. All the subjects were thoroughly under supervision in relation to the occurrence of any complication and all the equipment necessary for the control of acute conditions were available in the department.

Statistical analysis

STATA 11® statistical software was used to provide a randomization list in two equal 50-member blocks. Data were analyzed using SPSS 16® statistical software. Independent t-test, or as required Mann–Whitney U test, was used for quantitative variables. Repeated measures ANOVA were used to evaluate changes in quantitative variables throughout the study. Statistical significance was defined at $P < 0.05$.

Results

In the present study, 99 patients with their first ever stroke consisting of 58 males (58.6%) and 41 females (41.4%) with a mean age of 67.00 ± 8.82 years, were enrolled. Forty-nine patients (49.5%) were randomly placed in the IMOD™ group and 50 patients (50.5%) were placed in the control group. Tables 1 and 2 presents the baseline data of the two groups. As it is shown the two groups were matched in relation to all the baseline findings.

The mean duration of time between the appearance of signs and symptoms and the institution of treatment was 12.92 ± 3.80 hours in the IMOD™ group, with a median of 13 hours. The shortest and longest times were 5 and 21 hours, respectively. The patients in the IMOD™ group were aware, lethargic, obtunded and stuporous in 85.7%, 8.20%, 2% and 4.10% of cases, respectively at the time of referral; the percentages above were 70%, 16%, 4% and 6%, respectively, in the control group, with 4% of comatose patients in this group. In relation to stroke types in the TOAST classification [21], in the IMOD™ group the vessel involvements were as follows: 26 cases (53.1%) of large vessels, 5 cases (10.2%) of cardioembolic and 18 cases (36.7%) of lacunar; in the control group the percentages above were as follows, respectively: 26 cases (52%), 6 cases (12%) and 18 cases (36%). No significant differences were observed between the two groups (p = 0.93).No major adverse effect of IMOD injection was seen except for three cases of superficial phlebitis that resolved by conservative measures.

Table 1 Baseline findings in the two groups under study

	IMOD™ group	Control group	P value
Age	67.00 ± 8.16	67.00 ± 9.50	0.90
Gender (male)	30 (61.2%)	28 (56.0%)	0.68
IHD	15(30.6%)	13 (26.0%)	0.66
HTN	38(77.6%)	35 (70.0%)	0.49
DM	6(12.2%)	10(20.0%)	0.41
CHF	1(2.0%)	2(4.0%)	0.90
Smoking	9(18.4%)	15(30.0%)	0.24
Atrial Fibrillation	3(6.1%)	4(8.0%)	0.9
Hyperlipidemia	7(14.3%)	13(26.0%)	0.21
ASA use	18(36.7%)	20(40.0%)	0.77
ACEI/ARB use	28(57.1%)	26(52.0%)	0.72
Statin use	7(14.3%)	13(26.0%)	0.21

DM: Diabetes Mellitus, CHF: Congestive Heart Failure, IHD: Ischemic Heart Failure, HTN: Hypertension.
ACEI/ARB: Angiotensin Converting Enzyme Inhibitors/Angiotensin Receptor Blockers.
Data are mean ± SE.

Table 2 Baseline clinical characteristics based on NIHSS in the two groups under study

	IMOD™ group	Control group	P value
NIHSS	10.59 ± 5.56	11.04 ± 6.56	0.71
Facial weakness	1.57 ± 0.54	1.50 ± 0.54	0.51
Arm weakness	2.33 ± 1.12	2.30 ± 1.24	0.91
Leg weakness	2.02 ± 1.14	1.96 ± 1.27	0.80
Speech difficulty	1.33 ± 0.47	1.36 ± 0.56	0.75

NIHSS: National Institute of Health Stroke Scale.
Data are mean ± SE.

Considering the differences in the laboratory findings between the two groups (insignificant at baseline), the effects of the medications were evaluated by assessing the changes observed.

Figure 1 shows changes in IL-1 levels in the two groups during the study. As the figure shows IL-1 exhibited a decreasing trend in the IMOD™ group; however, it exhibited almost constant variations in the control group. No significant differences were observed between the two groups (p = 0.20).

As shown in Figure 1, IL-6 levels increased significantly in the control group until the 7th day. However, treatment successfully decreased the levels of this marker (p = 0.04).

Figure 1 also shows changes in TNF-α level in the two groups; TNF-α levels exhibited a mild increase in the control group by the 7th day but decreased in the IMOD™ group; however, treatment did not significantly decrease TNF-α levels (p = 0.10).

Figure 2 shows variations in hsCRP levels in the two groups of study; hsCRP levels exhibited an almost constant level after Setarud was administered and then decreased. However, in the control group an increasing trend was observed before the 7th day. Treatment successfully controlled increasing hsCRP levels (p = 0.02).

As shown in Figure 2, WBC and platelet counts increased in both groups throughout the 7 days period, indicating that treatment did not influence these two markers (p = 0.71 and p = 0.13, respectively).

Patients in each group were divided into two groups of NIHSS ≥ 15 and NIHSS < 15 based on NIHSS scores. Laboratory findings in the IMOD™ group showed that only hsCRP levels were significantly higher in patients with NIHSS ≥ 15 at the time of referral (9.07 ± 1.75 vs. 21.92 ± 5.38) and 4 days after the treatment was instituted (10.95 ± 1.73 vs. 22.00 ± 4.69) (p = 0.01 and p = 0.02, respectively). Evaluation of laboratory findings in the control group also revealed that only hsCRP levels were significantly higher at the time of referral (9.84 ± 2.03 vs. 18.54 ± 96) and 4 days after the institution of treatment (27.57 ± 3.98 vs. 16.05 ± 2.38) in patients with NIHSS ≥ 15 (p = 0.04 and p = 0.04, respectively).

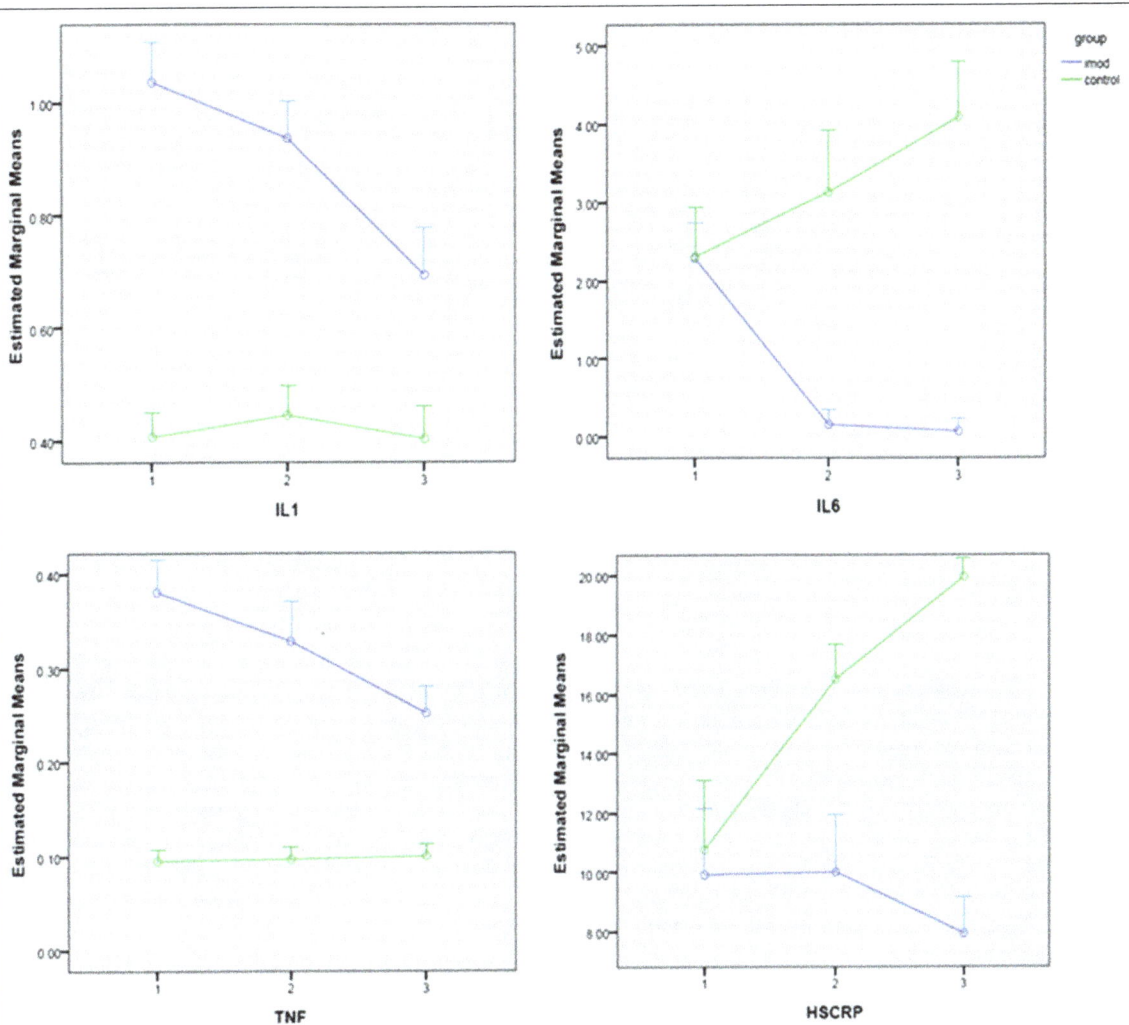

Figure 1 Changes in serum levels of TNF-α, IL-1, IL-6 and hsCRP in different days of study. Data are mean ± SE. Difference between two groups is not significant for TNF-α (P = 0.10) and IL-1 (P = 0.20) but is significant for IL-6 (P = 0.04) and hsCRP (P = 0.02).

Considering the difference in biomarker levels during treatment in each group, just the decrease of first day's serum IL6 level in comparison to 4th and 7th days' serum IL6 level in treatment group was significant (p = 0.023 and p = 0.049, respectively) and also treatment successfully controlled increasing hsCRP level.

Discussion

Inflammation is a pathological hallmark of ischemic stroke and impairs outcome in patients via mechanisms which are poorly understood [22]. Central nervous system and the immune system interact in complex ways. Neuron destruction due to cerebral ischemia induces an immune response which is necessary to remove cell debris and initiate the regenerative process; however, this inflammatory response can exacerbate cerebral damage, resulting in secondary cerebral injuries [23,24]. Circulating inflammatory mediators can activate cerebrovascular endothelium or glial cells in the brain and impact on ischemic brain injury [22-25]. Cytokines are important inflammatory mediators and it is well established that both in vivo and in vitro ischemic challenges increase the release of a large number of cytokines which are involved in the necrosis of neuronal cells [26-29].

Among the large number of cytokines, TNF-α, IL-1 and IL-6, modulate tissue injury in experimental stroke and are therefore potential targets in stroke therapy. The effect of these cytokines on infarct evolution depends on their availability in the ischemic penumbra in the early phase after stroke onset [29]. Many neuroprotective

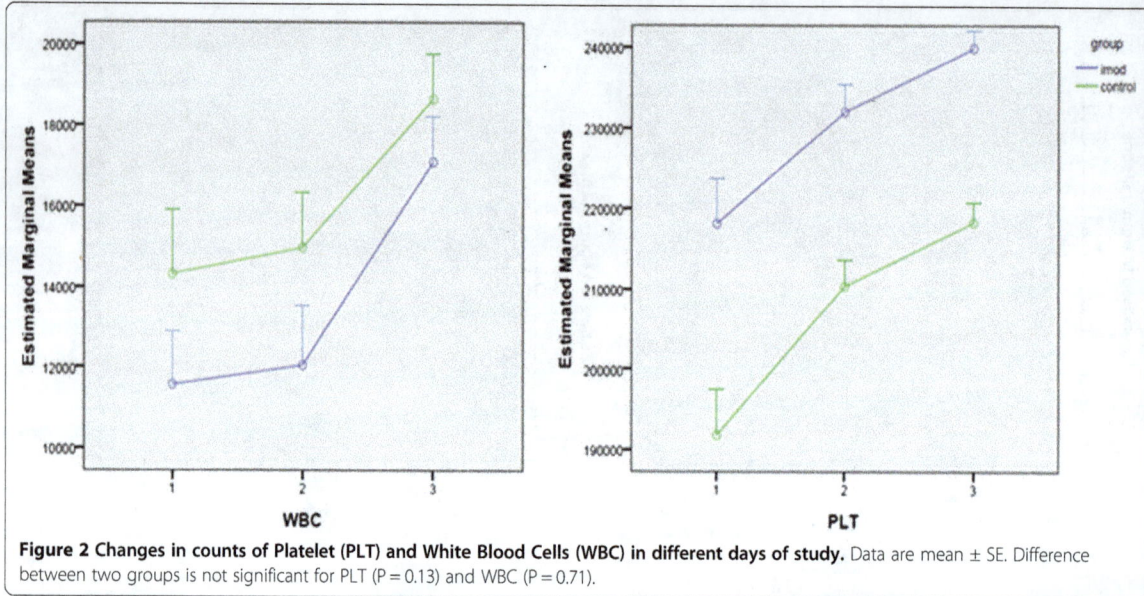

Figure 2 Changes in counts of Platelet (PLT) and White Blood Cells (WBC) in different days of study. Data are mean ± SE. Difference between two groups is not significant for PLT (P = 0.13) and WBC (P = 0.71).

agents have been effective in experimental stroke, yet few have translated into clinical application. One reason for this may be failure to consider clinical co-morbidities/risk factors in experimental models [30].

Therefore, attempts are aimed at controlling the principle inflammatory markers in acute ischemic stroke patients. Several efforts are performed to design and undertake trials of strategies that can modulate inflammation to improve outcomes of ischemic stroke patients. Multiple studies has been conducted to evaluate the effect of different medications on inflammation in AIS.

IL-1 is an established mediator of inflammation and damage in central nervous system (CNS) diseases in experimental studies. The IL-1 family consists of three main ligands: the agonists IL-1α and IL-1β, and the endogenous antagonist, IL-1Ra [31]. Denes et al. demonstrated that inhibition of IL-1 has beneficial effects on a variety of experimental paradigms of acute brain injury and is a promising clinical target in stroke. They proposed that blockade of IL-1 could be therapeutically useful in several diseases which are risk factors for stroke, and there is already considerable pre-clinical and clinical evidence that inhibition of IL-1 by IL-1 receptor antagonist may be valuable in the management of acute stroke [32]. Pradillo et al., have shown that a naturally occurring interleukin-1 receptor antagonist (IL-1Ra) is protective against ischemic brain damage in healthy animals. However, protective effects of IL-1Ra have not been determined in comorbid animals [30]. Shin et al. reported that the extent of complications and disease severity decrease with suppression of TNF-α and IL-1β [33].

Vinychuk et al., tested IL-6 in serum of 109 patients with ischemic stroke on the 1st day and 7 days after developing the disease. The decrease in concentration of IL-6 on the 7th day was found after a complex therapy with Flogensim in the study group in comparison with the control group where a traditional therapy was used. They found considerable difference in consequences of the ischemic stroke in 21 days among patients pertaining to different groups: the number of patients of the study group, with better results, increased and number of the patients of this group with no dynamic or even worsening in neurological status decreased [34].

De Aguilar-Nascimento et al. demonstrated enteral formula containing whey protein may decrease inflammation and increase antioxidant defenses in elderly patients with ischemic stroke, compared to casein-containing formula [35]. Montaner et al. in a pilot, double-blind, randomized, multicenter clinical trial to study the efficacy of Simvastatin in the acute phase of ischemic stroke, evaluated the evolution of several inflammation markers [IL-6, IL-8, IL-10, monocyte chemoattractant protein-1, intercellular adhesion molecule-1, vascular cell adhesion molecule-1, C-reactive protein, sApo/Fas, tumor necrosis factor-alpha, E-selectin, L-selectin and nitrites + nitrates] and neurological outcome at baseline, day 1, 3, 5, 7 and 90. They found no differences among the biomarkers studied regarding treatment allocation. But the outcome of their patients was improved [36]. Raju et al. performed a pilot randomized controlled trial comparing the effect of colchicines (1 mg per day) with placebo on high sensitivity C-reactive protein (hsCRP) levels and platelet function in 80 patients with acute coronary syndrome or acute ischemic stroke who were followed for 30 days. Their study provided no evidence that colchicine suppresses inflammation in patients with acute coronary syndrome or acute ischemic stroke [37].

IMOD^{TM}, which is a combination of plant extracts enriched with selenium and has exhibited anti-inflammatory and immunoregulatory properties, has been studied in several trials evaluating its effects on different clinical situations. In a study by Mahmoodpoor et al., the effect of IMOD^{TM} on controlling signs and symptoms and treatment of patients with sepsis was evaluated and it was reported that TNF-α levels, as a chief inflammatory mediator involved in sepsis, significantly decreased after treatment with IMOD^{TM} compared to the control group [11]. Another study by Eslami et al. showed that Septimeb (IMOD^{TM}) had positive effects on survival of patients with severe sepsis. Considering withdrawal of Activated Protein C from market, IMOD^{TM} might be considered as an adjuvant therapy for standard treatment of sepsis [38]. In addition, Baghaei et al. evaluated the effect of IMOD^{TM} on inflammatory bowel disease in rats and reported that the medication significantly decreased TNF-α and IL-1β levels, resulting in a decrease in macroscopic tissue damage [12]. Also, the potential effects of IMOD^{TM} have been shown in initial evaluations in HIV patients on decreasing TNF-α levels and decreasing TNF-α and IL-2 levels during patenting processes [39]. These studies showed that IMOD has anti-inflammatory effects.

In this context, IMOD^{TM} as an immunomodulatory medication may be a therapeutic option in AIS. Vafaee et al. studied the neuroprotective effect of Setarud (IMOD^{TM}) on cerebral ischemia in male rats. In this randomized controlled animal study, rats intraperitoneally administered with Setarud after Middle Cerebral Artery occlusion. The study showed that Setarud could reduce infarct volume of subjected rats. The medication could alleviate degenerative changes in cortical neurons and also improved motor function of rats with cerebral ischemia [40].

In the present randomized clinical trial designed to assess the effect of IMOD^{TM} on main inflammatory biomarkers, as reflexives of neuroinflammation in AIS, 99 patients with their first ischemic stroke attack were divided into two groups of control and IMOD^{TM} and evaluated in relation to the levels of inflammatory markers in the first days of symptom initiation. The results showed that IMOD^{TM} had a significant effect on some inflammatory markers, such as IL-6 and hsCRP, which was consistent with the clinical situation of patients in the case of hsCRP. In addition, the medication decreased TNF-α and IL-1 levels, although with no statistical significance. Previous studies have shown that IMOD^{TM} can significantly reduce TNF-α and IL-1 levels [11,12,39],but insignificant effect of IMOD^{TM} on these biomarkers in present study may be due to different amount or source of secretion of various

biomarkers in AIS; although, further studies measuring biomarkers in serum and CSF may be needed to test this hypothesis. This study shows that IMOD^{TM} has immunomodulatory effects as shown in previous studies.

Several studies have shown that C-reactive protein (CRP), an inflammatory marker, is associated with stroke severity and outcome [41]. Dewan et al., demonstrated that high CRP level is associated with stroke severity at admission and is an independent predictor of early seven-day mortality after ischemic stroke [42]. Hasan et al. showed three biomarkers (C-reactive protein, P-selectin and homocysteine) significantly differentiated between ischemic stroke and healthy control subjects [43]. Similarly, in a study by Idicula et al., a significant relationship was reported between a high CRP Level, a high NIHSS score and high mortality rate [44]. Rajeshwar et al. showed that hsCRP and NO levels predict the incidence of ischemic stroke and hsCRP is an independent prognostic factor of poor outcome at 3 months [45]. In the present study, there was a significant relationship between disease severity (NIHSS)at referral and an increase in hsCRP level on the first and the 4th days in both groups.

As in previous studies, we observed no major side effect of IMOD injection except for few cases of superficial phlebitis that resolved by conservative measures. In a study by Mahmoodpoor et al., it was shown that IMOD^{TM} had no side effects on coagulatory factors such as platelets, prothrombin time, partial thromboplastin time, fibrinogen and D-dimer [10]. In our study changes in WBC and platelet counts subsequent to receiving IMOD^{TM} were not significant, so, present study supports the safety of the drug.

Limitation of the study

First, the number of included patients was small (limitation of eligible patients in that period of time). Second, a potential random error can't be eliminated completely and our results remained to be confirmed. Third, placebo was not used in present study because of technical and ethical limitations.

Conclusion

Considering the role of inflammation in the induction of ischemic cerebral damage, it appears that treatment with IMOD^{TM} improves the profiles of main inflammatory markers; therefore, it might be considered as a therapeutic option in ischemic strokes. However, it is necessary to match laboratory findings with clinical findings and follow them in the long term to further elucidate such an effect. We recommend future multicenter studies with larger sample size and long duration period. Evaluation of the effect of the drug on the inflammatory profile in the cerebrospinal fluid (CSF) of experimental models may provide more localizing data about the effect of IMOD^{TM}.

Competing interests

The authors reported no competing interest.

Authors' contributions

MF: Manuscript preparing, approved the final manuscript. MN-N: Study conduct, Manuscript preparation, approved the final manuscript. AM: Literature Review, Manuscript preparation, approved the final manuscript. MH: study conduct, approved the final manuscript. ES: study conduct, approved the final manuscript. BB: Analysis of biomarkers, approved the final manuscript. AT: Data analysis, approved the final manuscript. DS-O: Data analysis, approved the final manuscript. HS-B: Study conduct, approved the final manuscript. ES-h: Study conduct, approved the final manuscript. HA: Study conduct, approved the final manuscript. RR: Study conduct, approved the final manuscript. All authors read and approved the final manuscript.

Acknowledgment

Thanks for Pars Roos company for their cooperation in providing IMOD.

Author details

[1]Neuroscience Research Center (NSRC), Imam Reza Hospital, Tabriz University of Medical Sciences, Tabriz, Iran. [2]Department of Anesthesiology and critical care medicine, Imam Reza Hospital, Tabriz University of Medical Sciences, Tabriz, Iran. [3]Student Research Committee, Tabriz University of Medical Sciences, Tabriz, Iran.

References

1. Lopez AD, Mathers CD, Ezzati M, Jamison DT, Murray CJ: Global and regional burden of disease and risk factors, 2001: systematic analysis of population health data. *Lancet* 2006, 367:1747–1757.
2. McColl BW, Allan SM, Rothwell NJ: Systemic infection, inflammation and acute ischemic stroke. *Neuroscience* 2009, 158:1049–1061.
3. Wang Q, Tang XN, Yenari MA: The inflammatory response in stroke. *J Neuroimmunol* 2007, 184:53–68.
4. Sairanen T, Carpen O, Karjalainen-Lindsberg ML, Paetau A, Turpeinen U, Kaste M, Lindsberg PJ: Evolution of cerebral tumor necrosis factor-alpha production during human ischemic stroke. *Stroke* 2001, 32:1750–1758.
5. Feuerstein GZ, Wang X, Barone FC: The role of cytokines in the neuropathology of stroke and neurotrauma. *Neuroimmunomodulation* 1998, 5:143–159.
6. Stoll G, Jander S, Schroeter M: Inflammation and glial responses in ischemic brain lesions. *ProgNeurobiol* 1998, 56:149–171.
7. Jordán J, Segura T, Brea D, Galindo MF, Castillo J: Inflammation as Therapeutic Objective in Stroke. *Current Pharm Design* 2008, 14:3549–3564.
8. Khorram Khorshid HR, Novitsky YA, Abdollahi M, Shahhosseiny MH, Sadeghi B, Madani H, Rahimi R, Farzamfar B: Studies on potential mutagenic and genotoxic activity of Setarud. *DARU* 2008, 16:223–228.
9. Khairandish P, Mohraz M, Farzamfar B, Abdollahi M, Shahhosseiny MH, Madani H, Sadeghi B, Heshmat R, Gharibdust F, Khorram-Khorshid HR: Preclinical and phase 1 clinical safety of Setarud (IMOD™), a novel immunomodulator. *DARU* 2009, 17:148–156.
10. Paydary K, Emamzadeh-Fard S, Khorram Khorshid HR, Kamali K, SeyedAlinaghi S, Mohraz M: Safety and efficacy of Setarud (IMOD TM) among people living with HIV/AIDS: a review. *Recent Pat Antiinfect Drug Discov* 2012, 7(1):66–72.
11. Mahmoodpoor A, Eslami K, Mojtahedzadeh M, Najafi A, Ahmadi A, Dehnadi-Moghadam A, Mohammadirad A, Baeeri M, Abdollahi M: Examination of Setarud (IMOD™) in the management of patients with severe sepsis. *DARU* 2010, 18:23–28.
12. Baghaei A, Esmaily H, Abdolghaffari AH, Baeeri M, Gharibdoost F, Abdollahi M: Efficacy of Setarud (IMod), a novel drug with potent anti-toxic stress potential in rat inflammatory bowel disease and comparison with dexamethasone and infliximab. *Indian J Biochem Biophys* 2010, 47(4):219–226.
13. Look MP, Rockstroh JK, Rao GS, Barton S, Lemoch H, Kaiser R, Kupfer B, Sudhop T, Spengler U, Sauerbruch T: Sodium selenite and N-acetylcysteine in antiretroviral-naive HIV-1-infected patients: a randomized, controlled pilot study. *Eur J Clin Invest* 1998, 28:389–397.

14. Ogunro PS, Ogungbamigbe TO, Elemie PO: EgbewaleBE, Adewole TA. Plasma selenium concentration and glutathione peroxidase activity in HIV-1/AIDS infected patients: a correlation with the disease progression. *Niger Postgrad Med J* 2006, 13:1–5.
15. Mohseni-Salehi-Monfared SS, Habibollahzadeh E, Sadeghi H, Baeeri M, Abdollahi M: Efficacy of Setarud (IMOD™), a novel electromagnetically-treated multi-herbal compound, in mouse immunogenic type-1 diabetes. *Arch Med Sci.* 2010, 6(5):663–669. doi: 10.5114/aoms.2010.17078. Epub 2010 Oct 26.
16. Shirazi FG, Raoufi A, Yousefi M, Asgarian-Omran H, Memarian A, Khoshnoodi J, Younesi V, Shokri F: In vitro immunoinhibitory effects of Setarud on human B lymphocyte. *J Medicinal Plants Research* 2011, 5(11):2223–2231.
17. Schinella GR, Giner RM, Mordujovich BP, Rhos JL: Anti-inflammatory effects of South American Tanacetumvulgare. *J Pharm Pharmacol* 1998, 50:1069–1074.
18. Karata SD, Arda N, Candan A: Some medicinal plants as immunostimulant for fish. *J Ethnopharmacol* 2003, 88(1):99–106.
19. Abdollahi M, Rahmat-Jirdeh N, Soltaninejad K: Protection by selenium of lead-acetate-induced alterations on rat submandibular gland function. *Hum ExpToxicol* 2001, 20:28–33.
20. Rayman MP: The importance of selenium to human health. *Lancet* 2000, 356:233–241.
21. Adams HP, Bendixen BH, Kappelle J, Biller J, Love B, Gordon MD, Marsh EE: TheTOAST Investigators. Classification of subtypes of acute ischemic stroke. *Stroke* 1993, 24:35–41.
22. Dénes A, Ferenczi S, Kovács KJ: Systemic inflammatory challenges compromise survival after experimental stroke via augmenting brain inflammation, blood- brain barrier damage and brain oedema independently of infarct size. *J Neuroinflammation* 2011, 8:164.
23. Kamel H, Iadecola C: Brain-immune interactions and ischemic stroke: clinical implications. *Arch Neurol* 2012, 69:576–581.
24. Brea D, Sobrino T, Ramos-Cabrer P, Castillo J: Inflammatory and neuroimmunomodulatory Changes in Acute Cerebral Ischemia. *Cerebrovasc Dis* 2009, 27:48–64.
25. Benakis C, Vaslin A, Pasquali C, Hirt L: Neuroprotection by inhibiting the c-Jun N-terminal kinase pathway after cerebral ischemia occurs independently of interleukin-6 and keratinocyte-derived chemokine (KC/CXCL1) secretion. *J Neuroinflammation* 2012, 9:76.
26. O'Neill MJ, Astles PC, Allan SM, Anthony DC: Anti-inflammatory modulators in stroke. *Drug disc today* 2004, 1:59–67.
27. Hamishehkar H, Beigmohammadi MT, Abdollahi M, Ahmadi A, Mahmoodpour A, Mirjalili MR, Abrishami R, Khoshayand MR, Eslami K, Kanani H, et al: Identification of enhanced cytokine generation following sepsis. Dream of magic bullet for mortality prediction and therapeutic evaluation. *DARU* 2010, 18:155–162.
28. Najafi A, Mojtahedzadeh M, Mahmoodpoor A, Aghamohammadi M, Ahmadi A, Nahreini S, Pazuki M, Khajavi MR, Abdollahi M: Effect of N-Acetyl cysteine on microalbuminuria in patients with acute respiratory distress syndrome. *Arc Med Sci* 2009, 3:1–7.
29. Lambertsen KL, Biber K, Finsen B: Inflammatory cytokines in experimental and human stroke. *J Cereb Blood Flow Metab* 2012, 32:1677–1698.
30. Pradillo JM, Denes A, Greenhalgh AD, Boutin H, Drake C, McColl BW, Barton E, Proctor SD, Russell JC, Rothwell NJ, Allan SM: Delayed administration of interleukin-1 receptor antagonist reduces ischemic brain damage and inflammation in comorbid rats. *J Cereb Blood Flow* 2012, 39:1810–1819.
31. Chen CJ, Kono H, Golenbock D, Reed G, Akira S, Rock KL: Identification of a key pathway required for the sterile inflammatoryresponse triggered by dying cells. *Naturemedicine* 2007, 13:851–856.
32. Denes A, Pinteaux E, Rothwell NJ, Allan SM: Interleukin-1 and stroke: biomarker, harbinger of damage, and therapeutic target. *Cerebrovasc Dis* 2011, 32:517–527.
33. Shin JA, Lee H, Lim YK, Koh Y, Choi JH, Park EM: Therapeutic effects of resveratrol during acute periods following experimental ischemic stroke. *J Neuroimmunol* 2010, 227:93–100.
34. Vinychuk SM, Cheren'ko TM: Effect of flogensim in the treatment of postischemic inflammation (according to results of using interleukin-6 in patients with acute brain infarction). *LikSprava* 2007, 3:80–84.
35. De Aguilar-Nascimento JE, Prado Silveira BR, Dock-Nascimento DB: Early enteral nutrition with whey protein or casein in elderly patients with acute ischemic stroke: a double-blind randomized trial. *Nutrition* 2011, 27:440–444.

36. Montaner J, Chacón P, Krupinski J, Rubio F, Millán M, Molina CA, Hereu P, Quintana M, Alvarez SJ: **Simvastatin in the acute phase of ischemic stroke: a safety and efficacy pilot trial.** *Eur J Neurol* 2008, **15**:82–90.

37. Raju NC, Yi Q, Nidorf M, Fagel ND, Hiralal R, Eikelboom JW: **Effect of colchicine compared with placebo on high sensitivity C-reactive protein in patients with acute coronary syndrome or acute stroke: a pilot randomized controlled trial.** *J ThrombThrombolysis* 2012, **33**:88–94.

38. Eslami K, Mahmoodpoor A, Ahmadi A, Abdollahi M, Kamali K, Mousavi S, Najafi A, Baeeri M, Hamishehkar H, Kouti L, *et al*: **Positive effect of septimeb on mortality rate in severe sepsis: a novel non antibiotic strategy.** *DARU* 2012, **20**:40.

39. Novitsky YA, Madani H, Gharibdoust F, Farhadi M, Farzamfar B, Mohraz M: *Use of a combination of ethanolic Rosa sp., Urtica Dioica and Tanacetum Vulgare extracts, further comprising selenium and urea and having been exposed to a pulsed electromagnetic field, for the preparation of a medicament for immunostimulation and/or treatment of HIV infections. USPTO Patent Application 20090208598; EU Patent Application 087825.* International Application PCT/EP2006/000820; 2007. http://www.google.com/patents/US20090208598.

40. Vafaee F, Zangiabadi N, Pour FM, Dehghanian F, Asadi-Shekaari M, Afshar HK: **Neuroprotective effects of the immunomodulatory drug Setarud on cerebral ischemia in male rats.** *Neural Regen Res* 2012, **7**(27):2085–2091.

41. Tuttolomondo A, Di Raimondo D, Pecoraro R, Arnao V, Pinto A, Licata G: **Inflammation in Ischemic Stroke Subtypes.** *Curr Pharm Des* 2012, **29** [Epub ahead of print].

42. Dewan KR, Rana PV: **C-reactive Protein and Early Mortality in Acute Ischemic Stroke.** *Kathmandu Univ Med J* 2011, **9**:252–5.

43. Hasan N, McColgan P, Bentley P, Edwards RJ, Sharma P: **Towards the identification of blood biomarkers for acute stroke in humans: a comprehensive systematic review.** *Br J ClinPharmacol.* 2012, **74**:230–40.

44. Idicula TT, Brogger J, Naess H, Waje-Andreassen U, Thomassen L: **Admission C – reactive protein after acute ischemic stroke is associated with stroke severity and mortality: the 'Bergen stroke study.** *BMC Neurol* 2009, **9**:18.

45. Rajeshwar K, Kaul S, Al-Hazzani A, Babu MS, Balakrishna N, Sharma V, Jyothy A, Munshi A: **C-reactive protein and nitric oxide levels in ischemic stroke and its subtypes: correlation with clinical outcome.** *Inflammation* 2012, **35**(3):978–84.

15

A preliminary investigation of anticholinesterase activity of some Iranian medicinal plants commonly used in traditional medicine

Seyed Behzad Jazayeri[1,2], Arash Amanlou[2], Naghmeh Ghanadian[3], Parvin Pasalar[3] and Massoud Amanlou[2*]

Abstract

Background: The aim of this study was to evaluate acetylcholinesterase inhibitory activity of some commonly used herbal medicine in Iran to introduce a new source for management of Alzheimer's disease. A total of 18 aqueous-methanolic extract (1:1; v/v) from the following plants: *Brassica alba, Brassica nigra, Camellia sinensis, Cinchona officinalis, Citrus aurantifolia, Citrus x aurantium, Ferula assafoetida, Humulus lupulus, Juglans regia, Juniperus sabina, Myristica fragrans, Pelargonium graveolens, Pistacia vera, Punica granatum, Rheum officinale, Rosa damascena, Salix alba, and Zizyphus vulgaris* were prepared and screened for their acetylcholinesterase inhibitory activity using *in vitro* Ellman spectrophotometric method.

Results: According to the obtained results, the order of inhibitory activity (IC$_{50}$ values, µg /ml) of extracts from highest to the lowest was: *C. sinensis* (5.96), *C. aurantifolia* (19.57), *Z. vulgaris* (24.37), *B. nigra* (84.30) and *R. damascena* (93.1).

Conclusions: The results indicated and confirmed the traditional use of these herbs for management of central nervous system disorders. *C. sinensis* showed the highest activity in inhibition of acetylcholinesterase. However, further investigations on identification of active components in the extracts are needed.

Keywords: Plant extracts, Acetylcholinesterase inhibitor, Alzheimer's disease, Camellia sinensis, Citrus aurantifolia

Finding

Alzheimer's disease (AD) is a an age related neurodegenerative disorder with clinical characteristic and pathological features associated with loss of neurons in certain brain areas leading to impairment of memory, cognitive dysfunction, behavioral disturbances, deficits in activities of daily living, which eventually leads to death [1-3]. In 2010, approximately 35 million people worldwide were suffering from AD and this number is believed to reach 65.7 million by 2030 [4].

Although the underlying pathophysiological mechanisms are not clear, AD is firmly associated with impairment in cholinergic pathway, which results in decreased level of acetylcholine in certain areas of brain [1,2,5,6].

The management of AD focuses on slowing disease progression, symptomatic treatment, maintaining functional status and improving quality of life, and decreasing caregiver stress [5]. Acetylcholine, a neurotransmitter, which is hydrolyzed by acetylcholinesterase (AChE) and butyrylcholinesterase (BuChE) is considered to play an important role in the pathology of AD [1,2,7].

The treatment of AD has progressed and shifted since the late 1970s to a transmitter replacement strategy. Elevation of acetylcholine levels in brain through the use of AChE inhibitors has been accepted as the most effective treatment strategy against AD [3,8]. Therefore, AChE and/or BuChE inhibitors have become the drug of choice in management of AD [9]. Several AChE inhibitors named as "cognitive enhancers "are being investigated for the symptomatic treatment of Alzheimer's disease but few have been approved by the Food and Drug Administration in the United States [2,8,10,11]. The few drugs that have received regulatory approval

* Correspondence: amanlou@tums.ac.ir
[2]Department of Medicinal Chemistry, Faculty of Pharmacy and Medicinal Plants Research Center, Tehran University of Medical Sciences, Tehran, Iran
Full list of author information is available at the end of the article

to this date include: donepezil, rivastigmine and gal-antamine, all three working through increasing the concentration of acetylcholine at the neurotransmitter sites or acts by regulating activity at nicotinic receptors [2,5].

However, studies investigating the use of medications for AD have not been consistently supportive [12-17]. Various side effects of medications reported in clinical trials include: nausea, vomiting, diarrhea, syncope and bradycardia. Consequently, a need for development and utilization of alternative anticholinesterase compounds with fewer side effects leads to investigation on plants as a possible source of treatment [18-26]. Plants have been used since antiquity in the treatment of various diseases including cognitive disorders, such as AD.

Considering the importance of plant-driven compounds in drug discovery, the present study was undertaken to evaluate the anticholinesterase activity of a number of se-lected medicinal plants with various ethnobotanical uses, aiming to discover new candidates for anticholinesterase activity to be used in management of AD.

Material and methods

Plant materials

Eighteen medicinal plants, which are listed in Table 1 were chosen randomly from local herbal market in September 2010, Tehran and identified by Dr. Faraz Mojab. Voucher specimens were kept in the Herbarium of Faculty of Pharmacy, Shahid Beheshti University of Medical Sciences, Tehran, Iran.

Table 1 List of medicinal plants, traditional use and anticholinesterase activity against electric eel acetylcholinesterase

Botanical name	Plant family	Parts tested	Common name	Traditional uses[*]	Percent of inhibition (IC$_{50}$); μg/ml
Brassica alba	Brassicaceae	Seed	White mustard	Chest congestion, bronchitis, swollen joints, rheumatism	84.3 ± 1.36
Brassica nigra	Brassicaceae	Seed	Mustard	Common cold, painful joints and muscles, arthritis	135.0 ± 5.91
Camellia sinensis	Theaceae	Leaf	Tea	Relieve mental and physical fatigue, antioxidant	5.96 + 0.73
Cinchona officinalis	Rubiaceae	Bark	Quina-quina	Muscle relaxant, anti-malaria, palpitations, anemia, diarrhea	187.6 ± 4.25
Citrus aurantifolia	Rutaceae	Fruit	Key lime	Alertness, anti-flatulent, uplifting and cheering the spirit, common cold, anti- inflammatory	19.57 ± 2.66
Citrus x aurantium	Rutaceae	Flower	Bitter orange	Digestive aid and sedative, regulating fertility	226.1 ± 7.41
Ferula assafoetida	Apiaceae	Gum	Asafoetida	Anti-inflammatory, antispasmodic, cancer, colitis	281.3 ± 5.23
Humulus lupulus	Cannabaceae	Flower	Hop	Sedative, stimulate digestion, insomnia, anti-anxiety	369.6 ± 9.82
Juglans regia	Juglandaceae	External shell	Walnut	Antimicrobial, antihelminthic, astringent, keratolytic	647.5 ± 8.61
Juniperus sabina	Cupressaceae	Fruit	Savin	Antifertility, antioxidant, anti-inflammatory	379.9 ± 9.38
Myristica fragrans	Myristicaceae	Seed	Nutmeg	Diarrhea, mouth sores, and insomnia	1024. ±11.02
Pelargonium graveolens	Geraniaceae	Areal parts	Rose geranium	Reducing stress and tension, easing pain,	196.9 ± 7.25
Pistacia vera	Anacardiaceae	Hull	Pistachio	Antiviral, antifungal, antiprotozoal, anti-inflammatory activity	204.1 ± 6.33
Punica granatum	Lythraceae	Fruit	Pomegranate	Gastrointestinal disorders, astringent, diarrhea, oral aphthous, hematopoiesis	408.2 ± 5.72
Rheum officinale	Polygonaceae	Root	Rhubarb	Astringent, antibacterial, laxative	341.7 ± 3.88
Rosa damascena	Rosaceae	Flower	Damask rose	Cardiovascular stimulant, mild laxative, anti-inflammatory, cough suppressant	93.1 ± 2.88
Salix alba	Salicaceae	Bark	White willow	Chronic diarrhea, reduction of fevers, menstrual irregularities	989.1 ± 4.29
Zizyphus vulgaris	Rhamnaceae	Fruit	Jujube	Aphrodisiac, hypnotic-sedative, anxiolytic, anti-inflammatory	24.37 ± 2.33

* Traditional uses mentioned in this table are obtained from Avicenna's cannon of medicine, herbal shops instructions, and general usages in traditional medicine of Iran.

Chemicals

Acetylthiocholine iodide (ATCI), 5,5'–dithio-bis-2-nitro-benzoic acid (DTNB), bovine serum albumin (BSA) and electric eel AChE (AChE; EC 3.1.17; lyophilized, 500 U/vial solid, 65U/mg) were purchased from Sigma (St. Louis, MO). Physostigmine was used as the standard drug. Buffers and other chemical were of extra pure analytical grade. The following buffers were used: Buffer A: 50 mM Tris–HCl, pH 8, containing 0.1% BSA; Buffer B: 50 mM Tris- HCl, pH 8 containing 0.1 M NaCl, 0.02 M MgCl2 × 6H2O.

Preparation of extracts

Each plant sample was individually powdered and 1 g of each sample was extracted by maceration method under shaking at room temperature with aqueous methanol (20 mL; 1:1 v/v) for 24 h. After filtration, organic layer was distilled under reduced pressure at 25°C and then freeze-dried to dryness. The crude extracts were stored at −20°C until analysis. Determination of fifty percent inhibitory concentrations (IC_{50}) at 100 µg/mL dissolved in aqueous methanol was accurately defined.

Anticholinesterase inhibitory activity

Ellman's method was employed for determination of AChE inhibitory activity [26-28]. Acetylthiocholine was used as a substrate and hydrolysis of acetylthiocholine was determined by monitoring the formation of the yellow 5-thio-2-nitrobenzoate anion as a result of the reaction with 5,5'–dithio-bis-2-nitrobenzoic acid with thiocholine, catalyzed by enzymes at a wavelength of 412 nm.

Briefly, 25 µl of 15 mM ATCI, (43 mg/10 mL in Millipore water), 125 µl of 3 mM DTNB, (11.9 mg/10 mL buffer B), 50 µl of buffer A and 20 µl of plant extract at concentration of 100 µ g/ml were added to 96 well plates and the absorbance was measured at 412 nm every 13 s for five times. After adding 25 µl of 0.22 U/ml enzyme, (0.34 mg AChE dissolved in 100 mL buffer A), the absorbance was read again every 13 seconds for five times. The absorbance was measured using a Synergy H4 Hybrid Multi-Mode Microplate Reader (BioTek Instruments Inc., United States). Percentage of inhibition was calculated by comparing rates of the sample with the blank (aqueous methanol), control samples contained all components except the tested extract. Physostigmine was used as positive control. Then, the mean ofthree measurements for each concentration was determined (n = 3). Inhibitory concentration (IC_{50} value) was calculated according to Michaelis–Menten model by using EZ-Fit. Enzyme Inhibition Kinetic Analysis program (EZ-Fit: Enzyme Kinetics Software, Perrella Scientific Inc., Amshert, USA).

Statistical method

The assays were conducted in triplicate (n = 3) and after calculating the mean ± SD, the results were compared using Student's t-test. A P value of less than 0.05 was considered significant.

Results and discussion

Eighteen plant species belonging to 16 plant families (*Anacardiaceae*, *Apiaceae*, *Brassicaceae*, *Cannabaceae*, *Cupressaceae*, *Geraniaceae*, *Juglandaceae*, *Lythraceae*, *Myristicaceae*, *Polygonaceae*, *Rhamnaceae*, *Rosaceae*, *Rubiaceae*, *Rutaceae*, *Salicaceae*, and *Theaceae*) were obtained from Tehran local herbal market and a total of 18 extracts were screened for AChE inhibitory activity using Ellman's spectrophotometric method in 96-well microplate. Table 1 gives the names of the plants investigated, their families, their traditional uses, and acetyl-cholinesterase inhibitory concentration (IC_{50}) respectively. IC_{50} of physostigmine (positive control) was estimated 0.093 µM against AChE. At the test extracts concentration (100 µg/ml), physostigmine showed complete inhibition of enzyme activity.

Camellia sinensis

Results showed that AChE inhibitory concentration (IC_{50}) of leaves of C. sinensis (5.96 µg/ml) was less than the inhibitory concentration (IC_{50}) of the other tested extracts (Table 1). An inhibitory activity has been reported for green leaves of C. sinensis previously [29]. The occurrence of flavonoid saponins, polyphenols, and catechins is well documented in different preparations of C. sinensis. Quantitative concentrations of these compounds in tea infusion might be different due to impact of preparation method, cultivar, and agricultural divergences, which might explain the observed difference in AChE inhibitory activity between different types of C. sinensis [30].

Citrus aurantifolia

In this study C. aurantifolia presented an IC_{50} inhibitory effect of AChE in concentration of 19.57 (µ g/ml). Report by Chaiyana and Okonogi [31] revealed inhibition of cholinesterase by essential oil of leaf and fruit peel of C. aurantifolia. Phytochemical investigations of C. aurantifolia revealed the occurrence of limonene, l-camphor, citronellol, o-cymene and 1,8-cineole as the major constituents [31]; A group of compounds reported to have AChE inhibitory activity [31]. Essential oils from same family have been reported to posses promising AChE inhibitory activity [32]. However, there is no AChE inhibitory activity in blooms of C. aurantifolia.

Zizyphus vulgaris

The extract from Z. vulgaris fruit showed moderate AChE inhibitory activity (IC_{50} = 24.37 µg/ml) in this study, which is similar to the results of previous studies [33,34]. The AChE inhibitory activity of Z. vulgaris can be explained by the presence of alkaloids, saponins, and flavonoids in the extract [33].

Rosa damascena

We found AChE inhibitor activity from *R. damascena* floret extract (IC_{50} = 93.10 μg/ml) that is not in supported in previous investigations [25]. The *R. damascena* floret jam is used traditionally as a sweetener to tea to increase memory and wellness.

Brassica nigra

There is limited data on seeds of *B. nigra*. This study shows that seeds of *B. nigra* present AChE inhibitory activity with an IC_{50} of 135.0 (IC_{50} = 93.10 μg/ml). This finding suggests a moderate inhibitory activity for *B. nigra* seeds. Though further investigation in active components of the extract is needed.

The promising finding of the study shows that most of the plant-extracts screened in this study had some degrees of inhibitory activity against AChE (Table 1), but five species showed the most active inhibitory property (*C. sinensis, C. aurantifolia, Z. vulgaris, B. nigra,* and *R. damascena*) and had lowest inhibitory concentration below 100 μg/ml ranging between 5.96 to 93.10 against electric eel AChE. The extract of the herbs alone or in combination of other herbal productions such as essential oil could be considered in herbal remedies of AD management. Since the most strong synthetic or natural product driven AChE inhibitors are known to contain nitrogen, the promising activity of reported medicinal plants could be due to their high alkaloidal contents [35-40]. Alkaloids are the major compounds isolated from plants and show inhibitory activity for AChE [35-40] but only one out of each five most potent species contains alkaloids.

The search performed using Chemical Abstracts, Biological Abstracts and Scopus database shows that AChE inhibitory activity is not only limited to alkaloids but also other compounds such as flavonoid, coumarins and essential oils are reported to have AChE inhibitory activity [35-41]. The finding of this study shows that the four most active herbal extracts contained not only nitorgenic compound such as alkaloid but also these extracts also contain rich components of saponin, flavonoid, and essential oils [29-34]. The new area of interest in research involves both AChE inhibitors and BuChE inhibitors after recognition of BuChE activity in hippocampus of patients with AD [33,42,43]. Recent studies have work on dual inhibitors of AChE and BuChE [42,43]. In these studies synthesized chemical compounds have shown promising inhibitory effect on both AChE and BuChE [42-44]. However, the present study was limited to the screening of AChE inhibitory properties of selected plants. Thus, further studies should focus on BuChE inhibitory activity of herbal products of the plants used in this study and other potent plants.

Conclusions

A primary screening process was run to investigate AChE inhibitory properties of medicinal plants of Iran. The primary findings of this study suggest that all herbs used in this study exhibited some degree of AChE inhibitory properties. Among the selected plants of this report *C. sinensis* had the most active components with inhibitory properties on AChE. Further researches should investigate more on the chemical composition and mechanism of actions of these herbal extract including *in vitro* and *in vivo* studies.

Abbreviations
AChE: Acetylcholinesterase; AD: Alzheimer's disease.; BuChE: Butyrylcholinesterase.

Competing interests
The authors declare that they have no competing interests.

Authors' contributions
All authors contributed to the concept and design, making and analysis of data, drafting, revising and final approval. MA and PP are responsible for the study registration. SBJ, AA and NG carried out plant extraction and enzymatic tests and drafted manuscript. SBJ, PP and MA participated in collection and/or assembly of data, data analysis, interpretation and manuscript writing. All authors read and approved the final manuscript.

Acknowledgements
This research was supported by a grant from the Research Council of Tehran University of Medical Sciences.

Author details
[1]Students' Scientific Research Center, Tehran University of Medical Sciences, Tehran, Iran. [2]Department of Medicinal Chemistry, Faculty of Pharmacy and Medicinal Plants Research Center, Tehran University of Medical Sciences, Tehran, Iran. [3]Department of Clinical Biochemistry, Faculty of Medicine, Tehran University of Medical Sciences, Tehran, Iran.

References
1. Thies W, Bleiler L: Alzheimer's disease facts and figures. *Alzheimer's and Dementia* 2012, 8:131–168.
2. Zarotsky V, Sramek JJ, Culter NR: Galanthamine hydrobromide: an agent for Alzheimer's disease. *Am J Health- System Pharmacist* 2003, 60:446–452.
3. Schneider JA, Arvanitakis Z, Bang W, Bennett DA: Mixed brain. Pathologies account for most dementia cases in community-dwelling older persons. *Neurology* 2007, 69:2197–2204.
4. World Alzheimer Report 2010: The Global Economic Impact of Dementia. Available at http://www.alz.co.uk/research/files/WorldAlzheimerReport2010.pdf Accessed January 2014
5. Tricco AC, Vandervaart S, Soobiah C, Lillie E, Perrier L, Chen MH, Hemmelgarn B, Majumdar SR, Straus SE: Efficacy of cognitive enhancers for Alzheimer's disease: protocol for a systematic review and network meta-analysis. *Syst Rev* 2012, 28:1–31.
6. Perry N, Court G, Bidet N, Court J, Perry E: European herbs with cholinergic activities: Potential in dementia therapy. *Int J Geriatr Psychiatry* 1996, 11:1063–1069.
7. Hebert LE, Scherr PA, Beckeff LA: Age-specific incidence of Alzheimer's disease in a community population. *JAMA* 1995, 273:1354–1359.
8. Arnold SE, Kumar A: Reversible dementias. *Med Clin Nort Am* 1993, 77:215–225.

9. Adams RL, Crai PL, Parsons OA: **Neuropsychology of dementia.** *Neurol Clin* 1984, **4**:387–405.

10. Adams M, Gmünder F, Hamburger M: **Plants traditionally used in age related brain disorders - A survey of ethnobotanical literature.** *J Ethnopharmacology* 2007, **113**:363–381.

11. Anon: **FDA-approved treatments for Alzheimer's.** 2012. Available at http://www.alz.org/national/documents/topicsheet_treatments.pdf.

12. Aisen PS, Davis KL: **The search for disease-modifying treatment for Alzheimer's Disease.** *Neurology* 1997, **48**:35–41.

13. Schneider LS: **Treatment of Alzheimer's disease with cholinesterase inhibitors.** *Clin Geriatric Med* 2001, **17**:337–358.

14. Aazza S, Lyoussi B, Miguel MG: **Antioxidant and antiacetylcholinesterase activities of some commercial essential oils and their major compounds.** *Molecules* 2011, **16**:7672–7690.

15. Houghton PJ, Ren Y, Howes MJ: **Acetylcholinesterase inhibitors from plants and fungi.** *NatProd Rep* 2006, **23**:181–199.

16. Lahiri DK, Farlow MR, Greig NH, Sambamurti K: **Current drug targets for Alzheimer's disease treatment.** *Drug Dev Res* 2002, **56**:267–281.

17. Darvesh S, Walsh R, Kumar R, Caines A, Roberts S, Magee D, *et al*: **Inhibition of human cholinesterases by drugs used to treat Alzheimer's disease.** *Alzheimer Dis Assoc Disord* 2003, **17**:117–126.

18. Adhami HR, Farsam H, Krenn L: **Screening of medicinal plants from Iranian traditional medicine for acetylcholinesterase inhibition.** *Phytother Res* 2011, **25**:1148–1152.

19. Adsersen A, Gauguin B, Gudiksen L, Jager AK: **Screening of plants used in Danish folk medicine to treat memory dysfunction for acetylcholinesterase inhibitory activity.** *J Ethnopharmacology* 2005, **104**:118–122.

20. Akhondzadeh S, Noroozian M, Mohammadi M, Ohadinia S, Jamshidi AH, Khani M: **Salvia officinalis extract in the treatment of patients with mild to moderate Alzheimer's disease: a double blind, randomized and placebo-controlled trial.** *J Clin Pharm Ther* 2003, **28**:53–59.

21. Akhondzadeh S, Abbasi SH: **Herbal medicine in the treatment of Alzheimer's disease.** *Am J Alzheimers Dis Other Demen* 2006, **21**:113–118.

22. Benamar H, Rached W, Derdour A, Marouf A: **Screening of Algerian medicinal plants for acetylcholinesterase inhibitory activity.** *J Bio Sci* 2010, **10**:1–9.

23. Howes MR, Perry NSL, Houghton PJ: **Plants with traditional uses and activities, relevant to the management of Alzheimer's disease and other cognitive disorders.** *Phytother Res* 2003, **17**:1–18.

24. Howes MR, Houghton PJ: **Plants used in Chinese and Indian traditional medicine for improvement of memory and cognitive function.** *Pharmacol Biochem Behav* 2003, **75**:513–527.

25. Ferreira A, Proença C, Serralheiro ML, Araújo ME: **The in vitro screening for acetylcholinesterase inhibition and antioxidant activity of medicinal plants from Portugal.** *J Ethnopharmacol* 2006, **108**:31–37.

26. Gholamhoseinian A, Moradi MN, Sharifi-Far F: **Screening the methanol extracts of some Iranian plants for acetylcholinesterase inhibitory activity.** *Res Pharm Sci* 2009, **4**:105–112.

27. Ellman GL, Courtney KD, Andres V Jr, Featherstone RM: **A new and rapid colorimetric determination of acetylcholinesterase activity.** *Biochem Pharmacol* 1961, **7**:88–95.

28. Nadri H, Pirali-Hamedani M, Shekarchi M, Abdollahi M, Sheibani V, Amanlou M, *et al*: **Design, synthesis and anticholinesterase activity of a novel series of 1-benzyl-4-((6-alkoxy-3-oxobenzofuran-2(3H)-ylidene) methyl) pyridinium derivatives.** *Bioorg Med Chem* 2010, **18**:6360–6366.

29. Bakthira H, Awadh Ali NA, Arnold N, Teichert A, Wessjohann L: **Anticholinesterase activity of endemic plant extracts from soqotra.** *Afr J Tradit Complement Altern Med* 2011, **8**:296–299.

30. Kwak JH, Jeong CH, Kim JH, Choi GN, Shin Y, Lee SC, *et al*: **Acetylcholinesterase inhibitory effect of green tea extracts according to storage condition.** *Korean J Food Sci Technol* 2009, **41**:435–440.

31. Lee EN, Song JH, Lee JS: **Screening of a potent antidementia acetylcholinesterase inhibitor-containing fruits and optimal extraction conditions.** *Korean J Food Nutr* 2010, **23**:318–323.

32. Chaiyana W, Okonogi S: **Inhibition of cholinesterase by essential oil from food plant.** *Phytomedicine* 2012, **19**:836–839.

33. Orhan I, Sener B, Choudhary MI, Khalid A: **Acetylcholinesterase and butyrylcholinesterase inhibitory activity of some Turkish medicinal plants.** *J Ethnopharmacol* 2004, **91**:57–60.

34. Mahajan RT, Chopda MZ: **Phyto-Pharmacology of *Ziziphus jujuba* Mill, A plant review.** *Phcog Rev* 2009, **3**:320–329.

35. Gomes NG, Campos MG, Orfão JM, Ribeiro CA: **Plants with neurobiological activity as potential targets for drug discovery.** *Prog Neuropsychopharmacol Biol Psychiatry* 2009, **33**:1372–1389.

36. Mantle D, Pickering AT, Perry EK: **Medicinal plant extracts for the treatment of dementia: A review of their pharmacology, efficacy and tolerability.** *CNS Drugs* 2000, **13**:201–213.

37. Martinez A, Castro A: **Novel cholinesterase inhibitors as future effective drugs for the treatment of Alzheimer's disease.** *Expert Opin Invest Drugs* 2006, **15**:1–12.

38. Mukherjee PK, Kumar V, Mal M, Houghton PJ: **Acetylcholinesterase inhibitors from plants.** *Phytomedicine* 2007, **14**:289–300.

39. Oh MH, Houghton PJ, Whang WK, Cho JH: **Screening of Korean herbal medicines used to improve cognitive function for anti-cholinesterase activity.** *Phytomedicine* 2004, **11**:544–548.

40. Sarris J: **Herbal medicines in the treatment of psychiatric disorders: a systematic review.** *Phytother Res* 2007, **21**:703–716.

41. Schultes RE: **Plants in treating senile dementia in the Northwest Amazon.** *J Ethnopharmacology* 1993, **38**:129–135.

42. Nadri H, Pirali-Hamedani M, Moradi A, Sakhteman A, Vahidi A, Sheibani V, *et al*: **5,6-Dimethoxybenzofuran-3-one derivatives: a novel series of dual Acetylcholinesterase/Butyrylcholinesterase inhibitors bearing benzyl pyridinium moiety.** *Daru* 2013, **21**:15.

43. Gholivand K, Abdollahi M, Mojahed F, Alizadehgan AM, Dehghan G: **Acetylcholinesterase/butyrylcholinesterase inhibition activity of some new carbacylamidophosphate derivatives.** *J Enzyme Inhib Med Chem* 2009, **24**:566–576.

44. Gholivand K, Alizadehgan AM, Mojahed F, Dehghan G, Mohammadirad A, Abdollahi M: **Some new carbacylamidophosphates as inhibitors of acetylcholinesterase and butyrylcholinesterase.** *Z Naturforsch C* 2008, **63**:241–250.

16

Synthesis and anti-proliferative activity evaluation of N3-acyl-N5-aryl-3,5-diaminoindazole analogues as anti-head and neck cancer agent

Jinho Lee[1*], Jina Kim[1], Victor Sukbong Hong[1] and Jong-Wook Park[2]

Abstract

Background: Head and neck squamous cell carcinoma (HNSCC) is the 11th leading cancer by incidence worldwide. Surgery and radiotherapy have been the major treatment for patients with HNSCC while chemotherapy has become an important treatment option for locally advanced HNSCC. Understanding of the molecular mechanisms underlying HNSCC impelled the development of targeted therapeutic agents. The development and combinations of targeted therapies in different cellular pathways may be needed to fulfill the unmet needs of current HNSCC chemotherapy.

Results: A series of N3-acyl-N5-aryl-3,5-diaminoindazoles were synthesized and their anti-proliferative activities were evaluated against human cancer cell lines, Caki, A549, AMC-HN1, AMC-HN3, AMC-HN4, AMC-HN6, and SNU449. The cellular selectivity of compound was obtained by the modification of substituent at N5-aryl group of 3,5-diaminoindazole. Compound 9a and 9b showed more than 7-fold selectivity for AMC-HN4 and AMC-HN3, respectively.

Conclusions: N3-acyl-N5-aryl-3,5-diaminoindazole analogues can be used as hits in the development of anticancer drug for HNSCC.

Keywords: Indazole, 3,5-diaminoindazole, Anticancer, HNSCC

Background

Head and neck squamous cell carcinoma (HNSCC) is the 11th leading cancer by incidence worldwide [1]. The 5-year survival for all stages combined on the basis of Surveillance Epidemiology and End Results (SEER) data is about 60% [2]. The primary risk factors are smoking, smokeless tobacco product, alcohol consumption, and the infection with human papillomavirus (HPV) [3].

Surgery and radiotherapy have been the major treatment for patients with HNSCC. Surgery is a standard treatment but is frequently limited by resectability of tumor and desire for organ preservation. Radiotherapy is used as a single treatment option in early-stage cancers and as an adjuvant treatment. A combination of radiotherapy and chemotherapy has increasingly been used for the treatment of HNSCC. Ten year follow up study of the Head and Neck trials showed that the concomitant non-platinum chemotherapy and radiotherapy reduce recurrences, new tumors, and deaths in patients who have not undergone previous surgery [4]. Chemotherapy has become an important treatment option for locally advanced HNSCC. Bleomycin, taxanes, cisplatin, carboplatin, methotrexate, and 5-fluorouracil (5-FU) are used as chemotherapy regimen in patients with recurrent or metastatic HNSCC and produce response rates from 10% to 40% [2].

Advances in molecular biology increased the knowledge about molecular mechanisms underlying HNSCC and led to the development of targeted therapeutics. Increased EGFR protein expression is observed over 90% of HNSCC. Overexpression of EGFR has been associated with disease recurrence and poor prognosis [5]. Along with the approval of cetuximab (BMS and Merck), monoclonal antibody that blocks the EGFR signaling, clinical trials using small molecular EGFR tyrosine kinase inhibitors have actively been performed. Gefitinib (AstraZeneca) showed a response rate of 10.6% in a phase II study for recurrent/metastatic HNSCC while erlotinib (Roche) demonstrated

* Correspondence: jinho@kmu.ac.kr
[1]Department of Chemistry, Keimyung University, Daegu 704-701, Korea
Full list of author information is available at the end of the article

a response rate of 4.3% in patients with recurrent/ metastatic HNSCC. Lapatinib (GSK) in combination with concurrent radiation and cisplatin showed increased complete response rate in phase II/III studies [6]. Lessons learned from clinical studies of EGFR inhibitors suggested the direction for the development of targeted agents for HNSCC. Inhibition of a single growth signaling pathway may not be enough to provide a clinically significant response for HNSCC. Therefore, development and combinations of targeted therapies in different cellular pathways may be needed to fulfill the unmet needs of current HNSCC chemotherapy.

In addition to EGFR overexpression, cyclin D1 overexpression and p53 mutation are frequently occurred in HNSCC. This abnormality may provide cancer cells with limitless replicative potential. Mutations in PI3K-PTEN-AKT signaling pathways are also found in about 10-20% of HNSCC. Activating mutations in PI3K and inactivating mutations of PTEN activate downstream signaling molecules such as Akt/protein kinase B (PKB), mammalian target of rapamycin (mTOR) and ribosomal protein S6 kinase (S6K). It was reported that AKT activation causes reduction of apoptosis as well as increased migration and invasion [7]. Therefore, new therapeutic agents targeting these pathways may provide synergistic effect with clinically advanced EGFR inhibitors when used in combination.

3-Aminoindazole-based small molecular inhibitors showed strong inhibitory activities against several kinases including CDK1 & 2 [8], KDR, cKIT, FLT3 [9], PDK1 [10] and exhibited potent anti-cancer activity [11]. The structures of representative compound are shown in Figure 1.

Previously, we reported that the treatment of HNSCC cell lines, AMC-HN4 and AMC-HN6, with compound B induced apoptosis in association with growth inhibition, cell cycle arrest, caspase-3 activation, and cytochrome C release [12]. While the compound B showed strong inhibitory effects on cancer cell growth, it had low selectivity, which may pose potential toxicity in *in vivo* studies. As

part of our ongoing effort to discover potent and selective kinase inhibitors as potential anticancer agents, a series of 3-aminoindazole derivatives were synthesized and tested for their cancer cell line selectivity.

Methods
Chemistry
^{1}H- NMR and ^{13}C-NMR spectra were recorded on a Bruker AVANEC 400 (400 MHz) spectrometer and chemical shifts (δ) are reported in ppm using tetramethyl-silane (TMS) as an internal standard. Mass spectra were obtained using Waters ACQUITY UPLC, Micromass Quattro microTM API. TLC was performed on E. Merck silica gel 60 F254 plates (0.25mm). Silica gel column chromatography was performed using Merck silica gel 60 (230-400 mesh). Unless otherwise noted, all starting materials were obtained from commercially available sources and they were used without further purification. Tetrahydrofuran (THF) was freshly distilled from sodium and benzophenone. All reactions were performed under a nitrogen atmosphere.

5-Bromo-1H-indazol-3-ylamine (2)
To a solution of 5-bromo-2-fluorobenzonitrile (3.0 g, 15 mmol) in *n*-butanol (20 mL) was added hydrazine (4.7 mL, 150 mmol). The reaction mixture was refluxed for 6 h. *n*-Butanol was then evaporated, and the residue was dissolved in ethyl acetate. The resulting solution was washed with saturated aqueous Na_2CO_3 solution and dried over $MgSO_4$. Removal of solvent gave the title compound (2.97 g, 93.4%). ^{1}H NMR (DMSO-d_6, 400 MHz) δ 11.58 (s, 1H, NH$_{indazole}$), 7.92 (s, 1H, H$_{phenyl}$), 7.30 (d, J = 8.8 Hz, 1H, H$_{phenyl}$), 7.20 (d, J = 8.8 Hz, 1H, H$_{phenyl}$), 5.44 (s, 2H, NH$_{2\ indazole}$).

N-(5-Bromo-1 H-indazol-3-yl)-2-(4-ethoxyphenyl)acetamide (3b)
To a solution of compound **2** (0.80 g, 3.8 mmol) in THF (10 mL) was added 4-ethoxyphenylacetyl chloride (1.9 g, 9.5 mmol). The reaction mixture was refluxed for 10 h under N_2 atmosphere. After cooled to room temperature, 1N NaOH (14 mL) was added and the reaction mixture was stirred for 2 h. The precipitate formed during evaporation of solvent was collected by filtration and washed with H_2O. The product was dried in vacuo and obtained 1.2 g in 84.4% yield: ^{1}H NMR (DMSO-d_6, 400 MHz) δ 12.88 (s, 1H, NH$_{indazole}$), 10.70 (s, 1H, NH$_{amide}$), 7.97 (s, 1H, H$_{phenyl}$), 7.42 (s, 1H, H$_{phenyl}$), 7.28 (d, J = 8.4 Hz, 2H, H$_{phenyl}$), 6.89 (d, J = 8.4 Hz, 2H, H$_{phenyl}$), 4.00 (q, J = 6.8 Hz, 2H, CH$_2$-O), 3.64 (s, 2H, CH$_2$), 1.32 (t, J =6.8 Hz, 3H, CH$_3$CH$_2$-O).

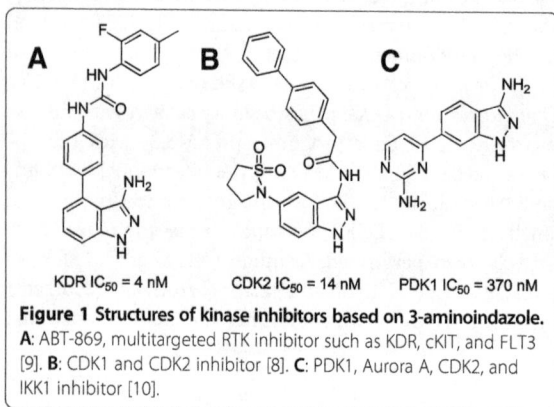

Figure 1 Structures of kinase inhibitors based on 3-aminoindazole. **A**: ABT-869, multitargeted RTK inhibitor such as KDR, cKIT, and FLT3 [9]. **B**: CDK1 and CDK2 inhibitor [8]. **C**: PDK1, Aurora A, CDK2, and IKK1 inhibitor [10].

KDR IC$_{50}$ = 4 nM   CDK2 IC$_{50}$ = 14 nM   PDK1 IC$_{50}$ = 370 nM

N-(5-Bromo-1-trityl-1H-indazol-3-yl)-2-(4-ethoxyphenyl) acetamide (4b)

To a solution of compound **3a** (0.070 g, 0.19 mmol) in CH$_3$CN (20 mL) were added K$_2$CO$_3$ (0.040 g, 0.28 mmol) and trityl chloride (0.080 g, 0.28 mmol) and the reaction mixture was refluxed for 12 h. Acetonitrile was then evaporated, and the residue was dissolved in ethyl acetate. The resulting solution was washed with brine and dried over MgSO$_4$. The crude product was purified by flash chromatography with a hexane:ethyl acetate (3:1) mixture to provide the title compound (0.060 g, 51%). ^{1}H NMR (CDCl$_3$, 400 MHz) δ 8.16 (s, 1H, NH$_{amide}$), 7.71 (s, 1H, H$_{phenyl}$), 7.26-7.15 (m, 17H, H$_{phenyl}$), 7.01 (d, J = 9.2 Hz, 1H), 6.89 (d, J = 8.4 Hz, 2H, H$_{phenyl}$), 6.21 (d, J = 9.2 Hz, 1H, H$_{phenyl}$), 4.07 (q, J = 6.8 Hz, 2H, CH$_2$-O), 3.67 (s, 2H, CH$_2$), 1.41 (t, J = 6.8 Hz, 3H, CH$_3$CH$_2$-O).

2-(4-Ethoxyphenyl)-N-[5-(2-fluorophenylamino)-1-trityl-1H-indazol-3-yl]acetamide (5b)

To a solution of compound **4a** (0.040 g, 0.065 mmol) in toluene (2 mL) were added 2-fluoroaniline (0.008 mL, 0.08 mmol), sodium *tert*-butoxide (0.013 g, 0.14 mmol), Pd$_2$(dba)$_3$ (0.001 g, 0.001 mmol), and (R)-BINAP (0.0015 g, 0.0023 mmol). The reaction mixture was refluxed for 4 h under N$_2$ atmosphere. Solvents were evaporated, and the residue was treated with ethyl acetate. The resulting mixture was washed with brine and dried over MgSO$_4$. The crude product was purified by flash chromatography with a hexane:ethyl acetate (3:1) mixture to provide the title compound (0.016 g, 38%). ^{1}H NMR (CDCl$_3$, 400 MHz) δ 7.93 (d, J = 7.6 Hz, 1H, H$_{phenyl}$), 7.82 (s, 1H, H$_{phenyl}$), 7.23-7.20 (m, 19H, H$_{phenyl}$), 7.00-6.94 (m, 2H, H$_{phenyl}$), 6.87 (d, J = 6.8 Hz, 2H, H$_{phenyl}$), 6.36 (d, J = 8.4 Hz, 1H, H$_{phenyl}$), 4.01 (q, J = 6.8 Hz, 2H, CH$_2$-O), 3.66 (s, 2H, CH$_2$), 1.42 (t, J = 6.8 Hz, 3H, CH$_3$CH$_2$-O).

2-(4-Ethoxyphenyl)-N-[5-(2-fluorophenylamino)-1H-indazol-3-yl] acetamide (6b)

To a solution of compound **5a** (0.040 g, 0.062 mmol) in CH$_2$Cl$_2$ (5 mL) were added trifluoroacetic acid (0.16 mL), phenol (0.013 mL), water (0.014 mL), and triisopropylsilane (0.007 mL) and the reaction mixture was stirred for 4 h at room temperature. Solvents were then evaporated, and the residue was dissolved in ethyl acetate. The resulting solution was washed with saturated aqueous Na$_2$CO$_3$ solution and dried over MgSO$_4$. The crude product was purified by flash chromatography with a dichloromethane: methanol (95:5) mixture to provide the title compound (0.01 g, 40 %). ^{1}H NMR (CDCl$_3$, 400 MHz) δ 7.77 (s, 1H, H$_{phenyl}$), 7.66 (s, 1H, H$_{phenyl}$), 7.28-7.23 (m, 2H, H$_{phenyl}$), 7.13-7.04 (m, 2H, H$_{phenyl}$), 6.97 (t, J = 7.2 Hz, 1H, H$_{phenyl}$), 6.90 (d, J = 7.6 Hz, 2H, H$_{phenyl}$), 6.77 (m, 1H, H$_{phenyl}$), 5.87 (s, 1H, H$_{phenyl}$), 4.02 (q, J = 6.8 Hz, 2H, CH$_2$-O), 3.75 (s, 2H, CH$_2$), 1.42 (t, J = 6.8 Hz, 3H,

CH$_3$CH$_2$-O); ^{13}C NMR (CDCl$_3$, 100 MHz) δ 169.9 (CO), 158.6 (C$_{phenyl}$), 151.0 (C$_{phenyl}$), 140.3 (C$_{phenyl}$), 138.8 (C$_{phenyl}$), 134.8 (C$_{phenyl}$), 130.7 (CH$_{phenyl}$), 127.6 (C$_{phenyl}$), 126.0 (C$_{phenyl}$), 124.4 (CH$_{phenyl}$), 124.2 (CH$_{phenyl}$), 119.2 (CH$_{phenyl}$), 119.1 (CH$_{phenyl}$), 116.9 (C$_{phenyl}$), 115.3 (CH$_{phenyl}$), 115.1 (CH$_{phenyl}$), 113.3 (CH$_{phenyl}$), 110.6 (CH$_{phenyl}$), 63.5 (CH$_2$-O), 43.2 (CH$_2$), 14.8 (CH$_3$).

2-(1,1'-Biphenyl-4-yl)-N-(5-(2-fluorophenylamino)-1H-indazol-3-yl)acetamide (6a)

The title compound was synthesized using the same procedure used for the synthesis of **6b**.

^{1}H NMR (DMSO-d$_6$, 400 MHz) δ 12.17(s, 1H, NH$_{indazole}$), 10.58 (s, 1H, NH$_{amide}$), 8.10 (s, 1H, H$_{phenyl}$), 7.66-7.59 (m, 4H, H$_{phenyl}$), 7.47-7.43 (m, 4H, H$_{phenyl}$), 7.36-7.32 (m, 2H, H$_{phenyl}$), 7.25-7.20 (m, 1H, H$_{phenyl}$), 7.11 (t, J = 7.6 Hz, 1H, H$_{phenyl}$), 6.99-6.94 (m, 1H, H$_{phenyl}$), 6.79-6.76 (m, 2H, H$_{phenyl}$), 3.74 (s, 1H, CH$_2$); ^{13}C NMR (DMSO-d$_6$, 100 MHz): δ 169.4 (CO), 169.3 (C$_{phenyl}$), 155.7 (C$_{phenyl}$), 153.3 (C$_{phenyl}$), 143.2 (C$_{phenyl}$), 143.1 (C$_{phenyl}$), 140.8 (C$_{phenyl}$), 140.6 (CH$_{phenyl}$), 138.9 (CH$_{phenyl}$), 136.0 (CH$_{phenyl}$), 131.2 (C$_{phenyl}$), 130.2 (CH$_{phenyl}$), 129.4 (CH$_{phenyl}$), 127.8 (CH$_{phenyl}$), 127.1 (CH$_{phenyl}$), 125.3 (CH$_{phenyl}$), 123.5 (CH$_{phenyl}$), 122.7 (C$_{phenyl}$), 121.3 (CH$_{phenyl}$), 116.6 (CH$_{phenyl}$), 113.3 (CH$_{phenyl}$), 111.0 (C$_{phenyl}$), 93.8 (C$_{phenyl}$), 42.4 (CH$_2$).

General procedure for the synthesis of compound **9a** to **9h**.

5-Nitro-1H-indazol-3-ylamine

To a solution of 2-fluoro-5-nitrobenzonitrile (5 g, 30.1 mmol) in *n*-butanol (20 mL) was added hydrazine (2.8 mL, 90 mmol). The reaction mixture was refluxed for 4 h, and *n*-butanol was evaporated. The precipitate formed during evaporation was collected by filtration and washed with H$_2$O. The product was dried in vacuo and obtained 5.0 g in 93.2 % yield. ^{1}H NMR (DMSO-d$_6$, 400 MHz) δ 12.18 (s, 1H, NH$_{indazole}$), 8.90 (s, 1H, H$_{phenyl}$), 8.05 (d, J = 9.0 Hz, 1H, H$_{phenyl}$), 7.34 (d, J = 9.0 Hz, 1H, H$_{phenyl}$), 6.01 (s, 2H, NH$_{2\ indazole}$).

2-(4-Ethoxyphenyl)-N-(5-nitro-1H-indazol-3-yl)acetamide

To a solution of 5-nitro-1H-indazol-3-ylamine (5.0 g, 28 mmol) in THF (20 mL) was added 4-ethoxyphenylacetyl chloride (11.1 g, 56 mmol). The reaction mixture was refluxed for 5 h under N$_2$ atmosphere. After cooled to room temperature, 2N NaOH (40 mL) was added and the reaction mixture was stirred for 2 h. The precipitate formed during evaporation was collected by filtration and washed with H$_2$O. The product was dried in vacuo and obtained 7.2 g in 75.6% yield. ^{1}H NMR (DMSO-d$_6$, 400 MHz) δ 11.05 (s, 1H, NH$_{indazole}$), 9.00 (d, J = 2.2 Hz, 1H, H$_{phenyl}$), 8.14 (dd, J = 2.2, 9.2 Hz, 1H, H$_{phenyl}$), 7.60 (d, J = 9.2 Hz, 1H, H$_{phenyl}$), 7.29 (d, J = 8.4 Hz, 2H,

H$_{phenyl}$), 6.89 (d, J = 8.4 Hz, 2H, H$_{phenyl}$), 3.99 (q, J = 6.8 Hz, 2H, CH$_2$-O), 3.70 (s, 2H, CH$_2$), 1.31 (t, J = 6.8 Hz, 3H, CH$_3$CH$_2$-O).

2-(4-Ethoxyphenyl)-N-(5-nitro-1-trityl-1H-indazol-3-yl) acetamide

To a solution of 2-(4-ethoxyphenyl)-N-(5-nitro-1H-indazol-3-yl)acetamide (7.2 g, 21 mmol) in CH$_3$CN (100 mL) were added triethylamine (8.8 mL, 63 mmol) and trityl chloride (8.8 g, 32 mmol). The resulting mixture was heated to reflux for 3 h. The precipitate formed during evaporation of solvent was collected. The crude product was purified by recrystallization using a mixture of dichloromethane and hexane to provide the title compound (9.18 g, 75%). ^{1}H NMR (CDCl$_3$, 400 MHz) δ 7.90 (s, 1H, H$_{phenyl}$), 7.80 (dd, J = 2, 9.5 Hz, 1H, H$_{phenyl}$), 7.31-7.13 (m, 17H, H$_{phenyl}$), 6.90 (d, J = 8 Hz, 2H, H$_{phenyl}$), 6.37 (d, J = 9.5 Hz, 1H, H$_{phenyl}$), 4.03 (q, J = 6.8 Hz, 2H, CH$_2$-O), 3.73 (s, 2H, CH$_2$), 1.26 (t, J = 6.8 Hz, 3H, CH$_3$CH$_2$-O).

N-(5-Amino-1-trityl-1H-indazol-3-yl)-2-(4-ethoxyphenyl) acetamide (7)

To a solution of 2-(4-Ethoxyphenyl)-N-(5-nitro-1-trityl-1H-indazol-3-yl)acetamide (3.45 g, 5.9 mmol) in methanol:dichloromethane (7:1) mixture was added catalytic amount of Pd/C. The resulting mixture was stirred for 12 h under H$_2$ atmosphere. The reaction mixture was filtered through a plug of celite and purified by flash chromatography with hexane:ethyl acetate (1:1) mixture to provide the title compound (2.2 g, 67.5%). ^{1}H NMR (CDCl$_3$, 400 MHz) δ 7.25-7.18 (m, 17H, H$_{phenyl}$), 7.09 (d, J = 1.8 Hz, 1H, H$_{phenyl}$), 6.87 (d, J = 8.8 Hz, 2H, H$_{phenyl}$), 6.42 (dd, J = 1.8, 9.1 Hz, 1H, H$_{phenyl}$), 6.15 (d, J = 9.1 Hz, 1H, H$_{phenyl}$), 4.02 (q, J = 7.0 Hz, 2H, CH$_2$-O), 3.65 (s, 2H, CH$_2$), 1.41 (t, J = 7.0 Hz, 3H, CH$_3$CH$_2$-O).

4-{3-[2-(4-Ethoxyphenyl)acetylamino]-1-trityl-1H-indazol-5-ylamino}-3-fluorobenzoic acid ethyl ester

To a solution of compound 7 (2.0 g, 3.6 mmol) in toluene (10 mL) were added ethyl 4-bromo-3-fluorobenzoate (1.34 g, 5.4 mmol), sodium *tert*-butoxide (0.70 g, 7.2 mmol), Pd$_2$(dba)$_3$ (0.10 g, 0.11 mmol), and (R)-BINAP (0.10 g, 0.16 mmol). The reaction mixture was refluxed for 6 h under N$_2$ atmosphere. Solvents were evaporated, and the crude product was purified by flash chromatography with a hexane:ethyl acetate (3:1) mixture to provide the title compound (1.57 g, 60.3%). ^{1}H NMR (CDCl$_3$, 400 MHz): δ 7.80 (s, 1H, H$_{phenyl}$), 7.68-7.63 (m, 2H, H$_{phenyl}$), 7.17-7.15 (m, 15H, H$_{phenyl}$), 7.02 (d, J = 8.2 Hz, 2H, H$_{phenyl}$), 6.83 (d, J = 9.0 Hz, 1H, H$_{phenyl}$), 6.70 (d, J = 8.2 Hz, 2H, H$_{phenyl}$), 6.36 (d, J = 9.0 Hz, 1H, H$_{phenyl}$), 6.31 (s, 1H, H$_{phenyl}$), 4.27 (q, J = 6.8 Hz, 2H, CH$_2$-OCO), 3.83 (q, J = 6.8 Hz, 2H, CH$_2$-O), 3.31 (s, 2H, CH$_2$), 1.31 (t, J = 6.8 Hz, 6H, CH$_3$CH$_2$-O).

4-{3-[2-(4-Ethoxyphenyl)acetylamido]-1-trityl-1H-indazol-5-ylamino}-3-fluorobenzoic acid (8)

To a solution of 4-{3-[2-(4-Ethoxyphenyl)acetylamido]-1-trityl-1H-indazol-5-ylamino}-3-fluorobenzoic acid ethyl ester (1.3 g, 1.8 mmol) in THF:methanol:H$_2$O (3:1:1) mixture was added LiOH · H$_2$O (0.4 g, 10 mmol). The resulting mixture was refluxed for 2 hr. Solvents were evaporated and the crude product was purified by flash chromatography with hexane:ethyl acetate(1:2) mixture to provide the title compound (0.89 g, 71.6%). ^{1}H NMR (CDCl$_3$, 400 MHz) δ 7.74 (s, 1H, H$_{phenyl}$), 7.68-7.65 (m, 2H, H$_{phenyl}$), 7.24-7.20 (m, 17H, H$_{phenyl}$), 7.04 (t, J = 8.4 Hz, 1H, H$_{phenyl}$), 6.89 (dd, J = 1.6, 9.2 Hz, 1H, H$_{phenyl}$), 6.83 (d, J = 8.4 Hz, 2H, H$_{phenyl}$), 6.38 (d, J = 9.2 Hz, 1H, H$_{phenyl}$), 3.97 (q, J = 6.8 Hz, 2H, CH$_2$-O), 3.59 (s, 2H, CH$_2$), 1.37 (t, J = 6.8 Hz, 3H, CH$_3$CH$_2$-O).

2-(4-Ethoxyphenyl)-N-{5-[2-fluoro-4-(morpholine-4-carbonyl)phenylamino]-1-trityl-1H-indazol-3-yl}acetamide

To a solution of compound 8 (0.1 g, 0.15 mmol) in DMF (10 mL) were added morpholine (0.015 mL, 0.17 mmol), EDC (0.058 g, 0.3 mmol), and HOBt (0.041 g, 0.3 mmol). The resulting solution was stirred for 9 h at room temperature. Solvents were then evaporated, and the residue was dissolved in ethyl acetate. The resulting solution was washed with saturated aqueous Na$_2$CO$_3$ solution and dried over MgSO$_4$. The crude product was purified by flash chromatography with a dichloromethane:methanol (95:5) mixture to provide the title compound (0.10 g, 88 %). ^{1}H NMR (CDCl$_3$, 400 MHz): δ 8.35 (s, 1H, H$_{phenyl}$), 7.73 (s, 1H, H$_{phenyl}$), 7.20-7.17 (m, 15H, H$_{phenyl}$), 7.12 (d, J = 8.8 Hz, 2H, H$_{phenyl}$), 7.05-7.01 (m, 1H, H$_{phenyl}$), 6.83 (dd, J = 2.4, 9.2 Hz, 1H, H$_{phenyl}$), 6.78 (d, J = 8.4 Hz, 2H, H$_{phenyl}$), 6.32 (d, J = 9.2 Hz, 1H, H$_{phenyl}$), 6.06 (d, J = 2.4 Hz, 1H, H$_{phenyl}$), 3.93 (q, J = 7.2 Hz, 2H, CH$_2$-O), 3.65-3.60 (m, 8H, CH$_2$ morpholine), 3.47 (s, 2H, CH$_2$), 1.36 (t, J = 6.8 Hz, 3H, CH$_3$CH$_2$-O).

2-(4-Ethoxyphenyl)-N-{5-[2-fluoro-4-(morpholine-4-carbonyl)phenylamino]-1H-indazol-3-yl}acetamide (9a)

Trityl protecting group was removed using the method which was used for the synthesis of compound 6b. The product was obtained in 73% yield (0.050 g). ^{1}H NMR (CDCl$_3$ + CD$_3$OD, 400 MHz) δ 7.49 (s, 1H, H$_{phenyl}$), 7.41 (d, J = 8.8 Hz, 1H, H$_{phenyl}$), 7.27 (d, J = 8.8 Hz, 2H, H$_{phenyl}$), 7.25-7.18 (m, 2H, H$_{phenyl}$), 7.11 (t, J = 8.4 Hz, 1H, H$_{phenyl}$), 7.04 (d, J = 8.4 Hz, 1H, H$_{phenyl}$), 6.82 (d, J = 8.4 Hz, aromatic, 2H, H$_{phenyl}$), 3.96 (q, J = 6.8 Hz, 2H, CH$_2$-O), 3.64 (m, 10H, CH$_2$, CH$_2$ morpholine), 1.34 (t, J = 6.8 Hz, 3H, CH$_3$CH$_2$-O); ^{13}C NMR (CDCl$_3$ + CD$_3$OD, 100 MHz) δ 172.1 (CONH), 170.4 (COmorpholine), 158.1 (C$_{phenyl}$), 152.3 (C$_{phenyl}$), 149.9 (C$_{phenyl}$), 139.3 (C$_{phenyl}$), 138.7 (C$_{phenyl}$), 136.5 (C$_{phenyl}$), 133.8 (C$_{phenyl}$), 129.8 (CH$_{phenyl}$), 127.1

CH_{phenyl}), 124.1 (CH_{phenyl}), 123.7 (C_{phenyl}), 116.9 (C_{phenyl}), 114.6 (CH_{phenyl}), 114.3 (CH_{phenyl}), 113.3 (CH_{phenyl}), 112.3 (CH_{phenyl}), 110.9 (CH_{phenyl}), 66.4 ($O\text{-}CH_2$ $_{morpholine}$), 63.1 (CH_2-O), 48.5 (CH_2), 41.6 ($N\text{-}CH_2$ $_{morpholine}$), 13.8 (CH_3); ESI MS: m/z = 518 [M + H]$^+$.

2-(4-Ethoxyphenyl)-N-{5-[2-fluoro-4-(4-methylpiperazine-1-carbonyl)phenylamino]-1H-indazol-3-yl}acetamide (9b)

^{1}H NMR ($CDCl_3$ + CD_3OD, 400 MHz) δ 7.49 (s, 1H, H_{phenyl}), 7.42 (d, J = 8.8 Hz, 1H, H_{phenyl}), 7.28 (d, J = 8.6 Hz, 2H, H_{phenyl}), 7.25 (dd, J = 1.6, 8.4 Hz, 1H, H_{phenyl}), 7.19 (dd, J = 1.2, 8.8 Hz, 1H, H_{phenyl}), 7.12 (t, J = 8.4 Hz, 1H, H_{phenyl}), 7.05 (dd, J = 1.6, 8.4 Hz, 1H, H_{phenyl}), 6.84 (d, J = 8.6 Hz, 2H, H_{phenyl}), 3.98 (q, J = 7.2 Hz, 2H, CH_2-O), 3.67-3.65 (m, 6H, CH_2), 2.45 (s, 4H, CH_2), 2.31 (s, 3H, CH_3-N), 1.35 (t, J = 7.2 Hz, 3H, CH_3CH_2-O); ^{13}C NMR ($CDCl_3$ + CD_3OD, 100 MHz) δ 172.1 (CONH), 170.3 (COmorpholine), 158.1 (C_{phenyl}), 152.3 (C_{phenyl}), 149.9 (C_{phenyl}), 139.3 (C_{phenyl}), 138.7 (C_{phenyl}), 136.5 (C_{phenyl}), 133.9 (C_{phenyl}), 130.3 (CH_{phenyl}), 129.3 (CH_{phenyl}), 127.2 (CH_{phenyl}), 124.6 (CH_{phenyl}), 123.8 (CH_{phenyl}), 116.9 (CH_{phenyl}), 114.4 (CH_{phenyl}), 112.8 (CH_{phenyl}), 111.6 (C_{phenyl}), 110.31 (C_{phenyl}), 63.1 (CH_2-O), 54.4 (CH_2-N), 48.8 (CH_2-N), 44.6 (CH_3-N), 41.6 (CH_2), 13.8 (CH_3); ESI MS: m/z = 531 [M + H]$^+$.

N-(2-Dimethylaminoethyl)-4-{3-[2-(4-ethoxyphenyl)acetylamido]-1H-indazol-5-ylamino}-3-fluorobenzamide (9c)

^{1}H NMR(CD_3OD, 400 MHz) δ 7.58 (d, J = 12.8 Hz, 1H, H_{phenyl}), 7.50 (s, 1H, H_{phenyl}), 7.47 (d, J = 10 Hz, 1H, H_{phenyl}), 7.43 (d, J = 8.8 Hz, 1H, H_{phenyl}), 7.29 (d, J = 8.6 Hz, 2H, H_{phenyl}), 7.26 (d, J = 10 Hz, 1H, H_{phenyl}), 7.08 (t, J = 8.4 Hz, 1H, H_{phenyl}), 6.83 (d, J = 8.6 Hz, 2H, H_{phenyl}), 3.95 (q, J = 6.8 Hz, 2H, CH_2-O), 3.68 (s, methylenic, 2H, CH_2), 3.50 (t, J = 6.8 Hz, 2H, CH_2-N), 2.59 (t, J = 6.8 Hz, 2H, CH_2-N), 2,33 (s, 6H, CH_3-N), 1.34 (t, J = 6.8 Hz, 3H, CH_3CH_2-O); ^{13}C NMR(CD_3OD, 100 MHz) δ 172.2 (CONH), 167.5 (CONH), 158.1 (C_{phenyl}), 152.3 (C_{phenyl}), 150.0 (C_{phenyl}), 139.3 (C_{phenyl}), 138.8 (C_{phenyl}), 137.6 (C_{phenyl}), 133.7 (C_{phenyl}), 130.3 (CH_{phenyl}), 129.3 (CH_{phenyl}), 127.1 (CH_{phenyl}), 124.2 (C_{phenyl}), 123.2 (CH_{phenyl}), 116.9 (CH_{phenyl}), 114.3 (CH_{phenyl}), 113.2 (CH_{phenyl}), 111.4 (CH_{phenyl}), 110.4 (C_{phenyl}), 63.0 (CH_2-O), 57.9 (CH_2-N), 44.0 (CH_2-N), 41.6 (CH_2), 37.0 (CH_3-N), 13.8 (CH_3); ESI MS: m/z = 519 [M + H]$^+$.

N-(2-Diethylaminoethyl)-4-{3-[2-(4-ethoxyphenyl)acetylamido]-1H-indazol-5-ylamino}-3-fluorobenzamide (9d)

^{1}H NMR (CD_3OD, 400 MHz) δ 7.57 (d, J = 12.8 Hz, 1H, H_{phenyl}), 7.50 (s, 1H, H_{phenyl}), 7.47 (d, J = 9.2 Hz, 1H, H_{phenyl}), 7.44 (d, J = 8.8 Hz, 1H, H_{phenyl}), 7.31-7.25 (m, 3H, H_{phenyl}), 7.10 (t, J = 8.8 Hz, 1H, H_{phenyl}), 6.84 (d, J = 8.4 Hz, 2H, H_{phenyl}), 3.97 (q, J = 6.8 Hz, 2H,

CH_2-O), 3.69 (s, 2H, CH_2), 3.49 (t, J = 7.2 Hz, 2H, CH_2-NCO), 2.75-2.66 (m, 6H, CH_2-N), 1.35 (t, J = 6.8 Hz, 3H, CH_3CH_2-O), 1.11 (t, J = 7.2 Hz, 6H, CH_3CH_2-N); ^{13}C NMR (CD_3OD, 100 MHz) δ 172.2 (CONH), 167.5 (CONH), 158.1 (C_{phenyl}), 152.3 (C_{phenyl}), 149.9 (C_{phenyl}), 139.3 (C_{phenyl}), 138.8 (C_{phenyl}), 137.6 (C_{phenyl}), 133.6 (C_{phenyl}), 130.3 (CH_{phenyl}), 129.3 (CH_{phenyl}), 127.1 (CH_{phenyl}), 124.2 (C_{phenyl}), 123.1 (CH_{phenyl}), 116.9 (CH_{phenyl}), 114.7 (CH_{phenyl}), 113.3 (CH_{phenyl}), 110.4 (CH_{phenyl}), 110.3 (C_{phenyl}), 63.0 (CH_2-O), 51.3 (CH_2-N), 46.2 (CH_2-N), 41.6 (CH_2), 36.7 (CH_2-N), 13.8 (CH_3), 10.0 (CH_3); ESI MS: m/z = 547 [M + H]$^+$.

4-{3-[2-(4-Ethoxyphenyl)acetylamido]-1H-indazol-5-ylamino}-3-fluoro-N-(2-morpholin-4-yl-ethyl)benzamide (9e)

^{1}H NMR (CD_3OD, 400 MHz) δ 7.56 (d, J = 12.4 Hz, 1H, H_{phenyl}), 7.51 (s, 1H, H_{phenyl}), 7.44 (d, J = 8.8 Hz, 1H, H_{phenyl}), 7.40 (d, J = 9.2 Hz, 1H, H_{phenyl}), 7.27-7.22 (m, 3H, H_{phenyl}), 7.07 (t, J = 8.4 Hz, 1H, H_{phenyl}), 6.79 (d, J = 8.4 Hz, 2H, H_{phenyl}), 3.91 (q, J = 6.8 Hz, 2H, CH_2-O), 3.68-3.66 (m, 6H, CH_2), 3.48 (t, J = 6.8 Hz, 2H, CH_2), 2.54 (t, J = 6.8 Hz, 2H, CH_2), 2.49 (s, 4H, CH_2), 1.31 (t, J = 6.8 Hz, 3H, CH_3CH_2-O); ^{13}C NMR (CD_3OD, 100 MHz) δ 172.2 (CONH), 167.5 (CONH), 158.1 (C_{phenyl}), 152.3 (C_{phenyl}), 149.9 (C_{phenyl}), 139.6 (C_{phenyl}), 137.6 (C_{phenyl}), 133.6 (CH_{phenyl}), 129.8 (CH_{phenyl}), 128.2 (C_{phenyl}), 127.1 (CH_{phenyl}), 124.2 (CH_{phenyl}), 123.7 (CH_{phenyl}), 123.2 (C_{phenyl}), 116.9 (CH_{phenyl}), 114.3 (CH_{phenyl}), 113.4 (C_{phenyl}), 112.7 (CH_{phenyl}), 110.9 (CH_{phenyl}), 67.3 (CH_2-$O_{morpholine}$), 63.0 (CH_2-O), 57.4 (CH_2-$N_{morpholine}$), 53.3 (CH_2-N), 41.6 (CH_2), 36.23 (CH_2-NCO), 13.8(CH_3); ESI MS: m/z = 561 [M + H]$^+$.

N-(3-Dimethylaminopropyl)-4-{3-[2-(4-ethoxyphenyl)acetylamido]-1H-indazol-5-ylamino}-3-fluorobenzamide (9f)

^{1}H NMR (CD_3OD, 400 MHz) δ 7.56 (dd, J = 2.0, 12.6 Hz, 1H, H_{phenyl}), 7.55 (d, J = 1.6 Hz, 1H, H_{phenyl}), 7.45 (dd, J = 1.6, 8.4 Hz, 1H, H_{phenyl}), 7.41 (d, J = 9.2 Hz, 1H, H_{phenyl}), 7.27 (d, J = 8.4 Hz, 2H, H_{phenyl}), 7.26-7.23 (m, 1H, H_{phenyl}), 7.08 (t, J = 8.8 Hz, 1H, H_{phenyl}), 6.81 (d, J = 8.8 Hz, 2H, H_{phenyl}), 3.93 (q, J = 7.2 Hz, 2H, CH_2-O), 3.67 (s, 2H, CH_2), 3.36 (t, J = 6.8 Hz, 2H, CH_2), 2.44 (t, J = 7.2 Hz, 2H, CH_2), 2.28 (s, 6H, CH_3-N), 1.78 (m, 2H, CH_2), 1.33 (t, J = 7.2 Hz, 3H, CH_3CH_2-O); ^{13}C NMR (CD_3OD, 100 MHz) δ 172.2 (CONH), 167.4 (CONH), 158.1 (C_{phenyl}), 152.3 (C_{phenyl}), 149.9 (C_{phenyl}), 139.3 (C_{phenyl}), 138.8 (C_{phenyl}), 137.6 (C_{phenyl}), 133.6 (C_{phenyl}), 130.3 (CH_{phenyl}), 129.3 (CH_{phenyl}), 127.1 (CH_{phenyl}), 124.2 (C_{phenyl}), 123.3 (CH_{phenyl}), 116.9 (CH_{phenyl}), 114.3 (CH_{phenyl}), 113.3 (CH_{phenyl}), 111.4 (CH_{phenyl}), 110.4 (C_{phenyl}), 63.0 (CH_2-O), 56.8 (CH_2), 43.9 (CH_2), 41.6 (CH_2), 37.7 (CH_2), 26.7 (CH_2), 13.8 (CH_3); ESI MS: m/z = 533 [M + H]$^+$.

N-(3-Diethylaminopropyl)-4-{3-[2-(4-ethoxyphenyl) acetylamido]-1H-indazol-5-ylamino}-3-fluorobenzamide (9g)

^{1}H NMR (CD$_3$OD, 400 MHz) δ 7.56 (dd, J = 2.0, 12.6 Hz, 1H, H$_{phenyl}$), 7.50 (s, 1H, H$_{phenyl}$), 7.45 (d, J = 8.4 Hz, 1H, H$_{phenyl}$), 7.42 (d, J = 9.2 Hz, 1H, H$_{phenyl}$), 7.28-7.23 (m, 3H, H$_{phenyl}$), 7.09 (t, J = 8.4 Hz, 1H, H$_{phenyl}$), 6.81 (d, J = 8.8 Hz, 2H, H$_{phenyl}$), 3.94 (q, J = 7.2 Hz, 2H, CH$_2$-O), 3.67 (s, 2H, CH$_2$), 3.37-3.35 (m, 2H, CH$_2$), 2.61-2.55 (m, 6H, CH$_2$), 1.77 (m, 2H, CH$_2$), 1.33 (t, J = 7.2 Hz, 3H, CH$_3$CH$_2$-O), 1.04 (t, J = 7.2 Hz, 6H, CH$_3$); ^{13}C NMR (CD$_3$OD, 100 MHz) δ 172.2 (CONH), 167.4 (CONH), 158.1 (C$_{phenyl}$), 152.3 (C$_{phenyl}$), 149.9 (C$_{phenyl}$), 139.3 (C$_{phenyl}$), 138.8 (C$_{phenyl}$), 137.6 (C$_{phenyl}$), 133.6 (C$_{phenyl}$), 130.3 (CH$_{phenyl}$), 129.3 (CH$_{phenyl}$), 127.1 (CH$_{phenyl}$), 124.2 (C$_{phenyl}$), 123.3 (CH$_{phenyl}$), 116.9 (CH$_{phenyl}$), 114.5 (CH$_{phenyl}$), 113.2 (CH$_{phenyl}$), 111.4 (CH$_{phenyl}$), 110.3 (C$_{phenyl}$), 63.0 (CH$_2$-O), 50.0 (CH$_2$), 46.3 (CH$_2$), 41.6 (CH$_2$), 38.1 (CH$_2$), 25.5 (CH$_2$), 13.3 (CH$_3$), 9.8(CH$_3$); ESI MS: m/z = 561 [M + H]$^+$.

N-(3-Dimethylaminopropyl)-4-{3-[2-(4-ethoxyphenyl) acetylamido]-1H-indazol-5-ylamino}-3-fluoro-N-methylbenzamide (9h)

^{1}H NMR (CD$_3$OD, 400 MHz) δ 7.49 (s, 1H, H$_{phenyl}$), 7.43 (d, J = 8.8 Hz, 1H, H$_{phenyl}$), 7.29 (d, J = 8.4 Hz, 2H, H$_{phenyl}$), 7.26 (d, J = 10.4 Hz, 1H, H$_{phenyl}$), 7.19 (d, J = 12.4 Hz, 1H, H$_{phenyl}$), 7.13 (t, J = 8.4 Hz, 1H, H$_{phenyl}$), 7.07 (m, 1H, H$_{phenyl}$), 6.85 (d, J = 8.4 Hz, 2H, H$_{phenyl}$), 3.99 (q, J = 7.0 Hz, 2H, CH$_2$-O), 3.68(s, 2H, CH$_2$), 3.06 (s, 3H, CH$_3$), 2.30-2.15 (m, 8H, CH$_2$, CH$_3$), 1.83 (m, 2H, CH$_2$), 1.35 (t, J = 7.0 Hz, 3H, CH$_3$CH$_2$-O), 1.28 (s, 2H, CH$_2$); ^{13}C NMR (CD$_3$OD, 100 MHz) δ 170.0 (CONH), 157.7 (CONH), 152.3 (C$_{phenyl}$), 149.9 (C$_{phenyl}$), 140.1 (C$_{phenyl}$), 138.6 (C$_{phenyl}$), 135.5 (C$_{phenyl}$), 133.8 (CH$_{phenyl}$), 131.0 (CH$_{phenyl}$), 130.0 (CH$_{phenyl}$), 128.3 (CH$_{phenyl}$), 126.5

(C$_{phenyl}$), 124.1 (C$_{phenyl}$), 117.1 (CH$_{phenyl}$), 115.1 (CH$_{phenyl}$), 114.2 (CH$_{phenyl}$), 113.4 (C$_{phenyl}$), 111.8 (CH$_{phenyl}$), 110.8 (C$_{phenyl}$), 63.4 (CH$_2$-O), 56.7 (CH$_2$-N), 46.3 (CH$_2$-NCO), 45.7 (CH$_3$-N), 45.2 (CH$_2$), 41.8 (CH$_3$-NCO), 15.5 (CH$_2$), 14.8 (CH$_3$); ESI MS: m/z = 547 [M + H]$^+$.

Biological assay

Cell growth inhibition assay (SRB assay)

The sulforhodamine B (SRB) assay was carried out as previously described [13]. Briefly, the cells were plated in 96-well culture plates at a density of 3,000 cells/well in phenol red free-medium and allowed to attach for 10 h. After 24 h or 48 h treatment of compounds, culture media were removed. 0.07 mL of 0.4% (w/v) SRB (Sigma) in 1% acetic acid solution were added to each well and left at room temperature for 20 min. SRB was removed and the plates washed 5 times with 1% acetic acid before air drying. Bound SRB was solubilized with 0.2 mL of 10 mM unbuffered Tris-base solution (Sigma) and plates were left on a plate shaker for at least 10 min. Absorbance was read in a 96-well plate reader at 492 nm subtracting the background measurement at 620 nm. The test optical density (OD) value was defined as the absorbance of each individual well, minus the blank value ('blank' is the mean OD of the background control wells).

Results and discussion

N3-Acyl-N5-aryl-3,5-diaminoindazole derivatives were synthesized using two different procedures (Figures 2 and 3). Figure 2 was used to synthesize compound 6a and 6b which had no additional substitution at 2-fluoroaniline ring. 3-Amino-5-bromoindazole was synthesized from 5-bromo-2-fluoronitrile and hydrazine. Mono-acylation

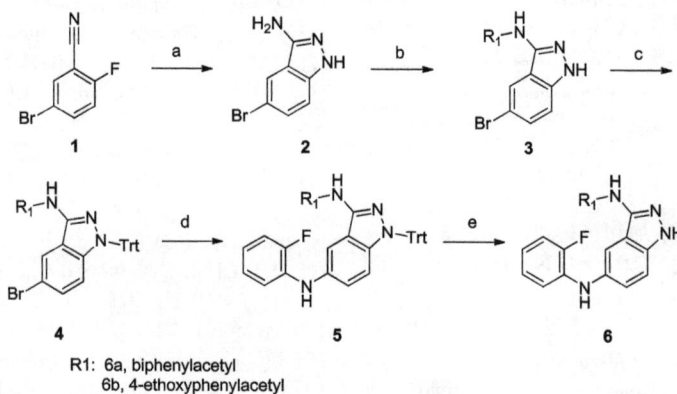

Figure 2 Synthetic scheme for compound 6a and 6b. Reagents and experimental conditions: **a)** H$_2$NNH$_2$, n-BuOH, reflux, **b)** i) 4-C$_2$H$_5$OC$_6$H$_4$ CH$_2$COCl (or 4-PhC$_6$H$_4$CH$_2$COCl), THF, reflux, ii) 2N NaOH, **c)** TrtCl, K$_2$CO$_3$, CH$_3$CN, reflux, **d)** 2-FC$_6$H$_4$NH$_2$, Pd$_2$(dba)$_3$, (R)-BINAP, NaOBu-t, toluene, reflux, **e)** TFA:Phenol:H$_2$O:TIPS (88:5:5:2), DCM.

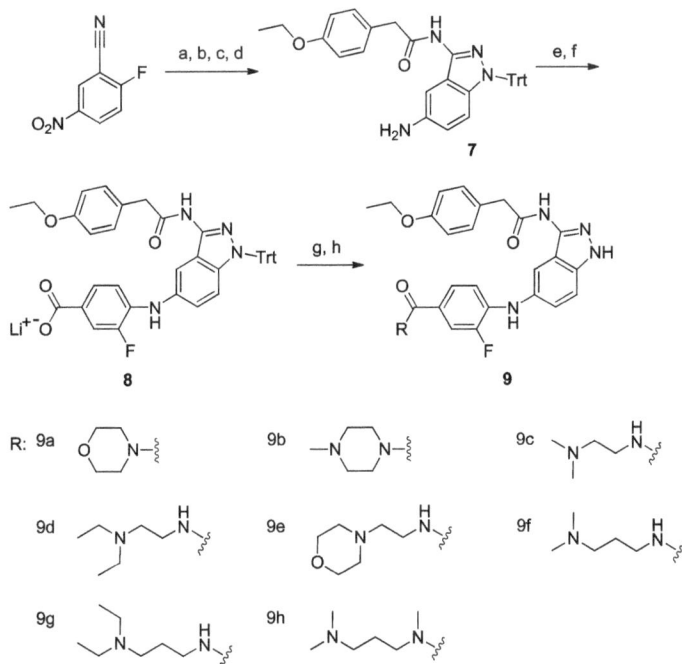

Figure 3 Synthetic scheme for compound 9a to 9h. Reagents and experimental conditions: **a)** H_2NNH_2, *n*-BuOH, reflux, **b)** i) *p*-$C_2H_5OC_6H_4CH_2$ COCl, THF, reflux, ii) 2N NaOH **c)** TrtCl, Et$_3$N, CH$_3$CN, reflux, **d)** Pd/C, H$_2$, MeOH/DCM, **e)** 2-F-4-EtO$_2$CC$_6$H$_3$Br, Pd$_2$(dba)$_3$, (R)-BINAP, NaOBu-*t*, toluene, reflux, **f)** LiOH, THF:H$_2$O:MeOH (3:1:1), reflux, **g)** RH, EDC, HOBT, DMF, **h)** TFA, DCM.

at 3-amino position of indazole was performed by consecutive diacylation and deacylation reaction. Buchwald-Hartwig palladium catalyzed amination and deprotection provided 3,5-diaminoindazole **6a, b**.

Syntheses of indazole substituted with 4-amino-3-fluorobenzamide derivatives were carried out with 2-fluoro-5-nitrobenzonitrile as shown in Figure 3. Various amines were introduced to 3-fluorobenzoic acid moiety which is at *N*5 position of 3,5-diaminoindazole while keeping 4-ethoxyphenylacetyl group at *N*3 position. After Buchwald-Hartwig palladium catalyzed amination with ethyl 4-bromo-3-fluorobenzoate, derivatized compound was obtained by ester hydrolysis followed by amide coupling. The structures of the synthesized compounds were characterized by ^{1}H NMR, ^{13}C NMR and ESI-MS [See Additional file 1].

The *in vitro* anti-proliferative activities of the synthesized compounds were evaluated by SRB assay [13] against human cancer cell lines and the results are shown in Table 1.

Modification of substituent at 5-position of indazole was performed based on the previous results that substituent structure at 3-position of indazole influenced on the potency but not the selectivity between cancer cell lines

Table 1 Anti-proliferative activity of the synthesized compounds against human cancer cell lines

	IC$_{50}$ (µM)^a			
	AMC-HN4	A549	Caki	SNU-449
Compd B^b	93%	91%	81%	-
Adriamycin^b	89%	52%	65%	-
5-FU	>10	4.9 ± 1.5	>10	>10
6a	0.37 ± 0.10	1.0 ± 0.1	7.2 ± 1.4	1.7 ± 0.5
6b	0.71 ± 0.17	1.3 ± 0.2	>10	3.8 ± 1.0
9a	0.21 ± 0.04	1.5 ± 0.2	11.0 ± 0.1	3.1 ± 1.3
9b	2.5 ± 0.3	>10	> > 10^c	>10
9c	2.9 ± 0.6	>10	> > 10^c	> > 10^c
9d	2.6 ± 0.4	>10	> > 10^c	> > 10^c
9e	>10	> > 10^c	> > 10^c	>10
9f	>10	> > 10^c	> > 10^c	> > 10^c
9g	5.5 ± 1.3	> > 10^c	> > 10^c	> > 10^c
9h	2.0 ± 0.5	> > 10^c	> > 10^c	>10

^{a}Data are mean of three independent experiments ± standard deviation.
^{b}% inhibition at 0.75 µM.
^{c}No inhibition up to 10 µM.

[8]. As a first step, 2-fluoroaniline was introduced instead of $1\lambda^6$-isothiazolidine-1,1-dione at 5-position of indazole. This approach improved the cell selectivity but resulted in reduction of inhibitory activity, (**B** vs. **6a**). When 1,1′-biphenyl group was replaced with 4-ethoxyphenyl group, the selectivity over Caki cell was enhanced, (**6a** vs. **6b**).

A good dependency between the structure and selectivity was obtained by changing the substituent on 2-fluoroaniline. Also, subtle structural differences in carboxamide at 2-fluoroaniline brought a significant change on the growth inhibitory activity. The compound with morpholine **9a** showed high potency on AMC-HN4 with more than 7-fold selectivity over other cancer cells. AMC-HN4 was known less sensitive to 5-FU which is widely used for the treatment of HNSCC, while a little prone to Adriamycin.

Though the activity was dropped by an order of magnitude by switching morpholine to 4-methylpiperazine, the selectivity for AMC-HN4 was not diminished, (**9a** vs. **9b**). Structurally similar substituents such as 2-(dimethylamino)ethylamine **9c** and 2-(diethylamino) ethylamine **9d** showed similar activity and selectivity while 2-molpholinoethylamine **9e** resulted in drastic loss of activity. The activity difference between 3-(dimethylamino) propylamine **9f**, 3-(diethylamino)propylamine **9g** and 3-(dimethylamino)propyl(methyl)amine **9h** may be understood as the target and its structural information are elucidated. Compounds **6b**, **9a**, and **9b** showed the growth inhibition of other HNSCCs (Table 2). Even though both **9a** and **9b** showed similar potency to AMC-HN3, only **9b** showed high selectivity to AMC-HN3 compared to other cancer cell lines.

The alterations in the function of Epidermal Growth Factor Receptor (EGFR) have been linked to tumor development and progression. Numerous EGFR inhibitors are currently in clinical trials based on the previous studies that EGFR overexpression is detected in 40% ~ 90% of HNSCCs [6]. Phase II trials of gefitinib, selective EGFR tyrosine kinase inhibitor, for recurrent/metastatic HNSCC have shown antineoplastic activity. However, in a phase III study, gefitinib did not improve the response rates or overall survival. The resistance of the EGFR-targeted therapy with gefitinib had been linked with the overexpression of cyclin D1 [14]. It was suggested that

the combination of CDK inhibitors with EGFR inhibitors might be a useful therapeutic strategy for HNSCC. Both AMC-HN3 and AMC-HN4 cell have mutations delivering inactivation of p16 and overexpression of cyclin D1 [15]. As a result, the compound showing selective potency to either AMC-HN3 or AMC-HN4 has high potential to show synergistic effect with EGFR inhibitors.

Small molecular drugs that have been used in HNSCC therapy or clinical trial have relatively low cellular potency. For example, 5-FU has $IC_{50} > 10$ μM (Table 1) while cis-platin has IC_{50} values between 2.7 to 36.7 μM [16]. The IC_{50} values of gefitinib are in the range of 0.4 and 14.4 μM [14]. A series of compounds tested in this research displayed comparable AMC-HN4 cellular activity to 5-FU, cis-platin and gefitinib. They also have a high level of AMC-HN3 selectivity over other cancer cell lines.

Conclusions

In summary, we have designed and synthesized a series of N3-acyl-N5-aryl-3,5-diaminoindazole derivatives, and evaluated their anti-proliferative activity against human cancer cell lines, Caki, A549, AMC-HN1, 3, 4, and 6, and SNU449. The study of structure and activity relationship showed that the selectivity against cell lines could be achieved by modification of substituents at N5-aryl group of 3,5-diaminoindazole. Compound **9a** was the most potent compound with about 7-fold selectivity against cancer cell lines tested. Other compounds such as **9b**, **c**, **d**, and **h** showed lower potency but increased selectivity. For example, **9b** was very selective for AMC-HN3. It is notable that N3-acyl-N5-aryl-3,5-diaminoindazole analogues can be used as hits in the development of anticancer drug for HNSCC.

Competing interests
The authors declare that they have no competing interests.

Authors' contributions
JL: Design of target compounds and supervision of the synthetic and pharmacological parts. JK: Design and synthesis of target compounds. VH: collaboration in manuscript preparation. JP: Supervision of biological tests. All authors read and approved the final manuscript.

Author details
[1]Department of Chemistry, Keimyung University, Daegu 704-701, Korea. [2]Department of Immunology, Keimyung University School of Medicine, Daegu 704-701, Korea.

Table 2 Anti-proliferative activity of the synthesized compounds against HNSCC

	IC_{50} (μM)[a]		
	AMC-HN1	AMC-HN3	AMC-HN6
6b	0.63 ± 0.04	0.58 ± 0.04	3.6 ± 1.1
9a	0.19 ± 0.03	0.23 ± 0.04	2.8 ± 0.9
9b	1.3 ± 1.0	0.34 ± 0.12	>> 10[b]

[a]Data are mean of three independent experiments ± standard deviation.
[b]No inhibition up to 10 μM.

References
1.   Jemal A, Bray F, Center MM, Ferlay J, Ward E, Forman D: Global cancer statistics. *CA Cancer J Clin* 2011, **61**:69–90.

2. Argiris A, Karamouzis MV, Raben D, Ferris RL: **Head and neck cancer.** *Lancet* 2008, **371:**1695–1709.

3. Molinolo AA, Amornphimoltham P, Squarize CH, Castilho RM, Patel V, Gutkind JS: **Dysregulated molecular networks in head and neck carcinogenesis.** *Oral Oncol* 2009, **45:**324–334.

4. Tobias JS, Monson K, Gupta N, MacDougall H, Glaholm J, Hutchison I, Kadalayil L, Hackshaw A: **Chemoradiotherapy for locally advanced head and neck cancer: 10-year follow-up of the UK Head and Neck (UKHAN1) trial.** *Lancet Oncol* 2010, **11:**66–74.

5. Le Tourneau C, Faivre S, Siu LL: **Molecular targeted therapy of head and neck cancer: review and clinical development challenges.** *Eur J Cancer* 2007, **43:**2457–2466.

6. Rao SD, Fury MG, Pfister DG: **Molecular-targeted therapies in head and neck cancer.** *Semin Radiat Oncol* 2012, **22:**207–213.

7. Leemans CR, Braakhuis BJM, Brakenhoff RH: **The molecular biology of head and neck cancer.** *Nat Rev Cancer* 2011, **11:**9–22.

8. Lee J, Choi H, Kim K-H, Jeong S, Park J-W, Baek C-S, Lee S-H: **Synthesis and biological evaluation of 3,5-diaminoindazoles as cyclin-dependent kinase inhibitors.** *Bioorg Med Chem Lett* 2008, **18:**2292–2295.

9. Dai Y, Hartandi K, Ji Z, Ahmed AA, Albert DH, Bauch JL, Bouska JJ, Bousquet PF, Cunha GA, Glaser KB, *et al:* **Discovery of N-(4-(3-amino-1H-indazol-4-yl) phenyl)-N′-(2-fluoro-5-methylphenyl)urea (ABT-869), a 3-aminoindazole-based orally active multitargeted receptor tyrosine kinase inhibitor.** *J Med Chem* 2007, **50:**1584–1597.

10. Medina JR, Blackledge CW, Heerding DA, Campobasso N, Ward P, Briand J, Wright L, Axten JM: **Aminoindazole PDK1 inhibitors: a case study in fragment-based drug discovery.** *ACS Med Chem Lett* 2010, **1:**439–442.

11. Raffa D, Maggio B, Cascioferro S, Raimondi MV, Schillaci D, Gallo G, Daidone G, Plescia S, Meneghetti F, Bombieri G, *et al:* **Synthesis and antiproliferative activity of 3-amino-N-phenyl-1H-indazole-1-carboxamides.** *Eur J Med Chem* 2009, **44:**165–178.

12. Shin HC, Song DW, Baek WK, Lee SR, Kwon TK, Lee J, Park SH, Jang BC, Park JW: **Anticancer activity and differentially expressed genes in head and neck cancer cells treated with a novel cyclin-dependent kinase inhibitor.** *Chemotherapy* 2009, **55:**353–362.

13. Papazisis KT, Geromichalos GD, Dimitriadis KA, Kortsaris AH: **Optimization of the sulforhodamine B colorimetric assay.** *J Immunol Methods* 1997, **208:**151–158.

14. Kalish LH, Kwong RA, Cole IE, Gallagher RM, Sutherland RL, Musgrove EA: **Deregulated cyclin D1 expression is associated with decreased efficacy of the selective epidermal growth factor receptor tyrosine kinase inhibitor gefitinib in head and neck squamous cell carcinoma cell lines.** *Clin Cancer Res* 2004, **10:**7764–7774.

15. Park HW, Song SY, Lee TJ, Jeong D, Lee TY: **Abrogation of the p16-retinoblastoma-cyclin D1 pathway in head and neck squamous cell carcinomas.** *Oncol Rep* 2007, **18:**267–272.

16. Åkervall J, Kurnit DM, Adams M, Zhu S, Fisher SG, Bradford CR, Carey TE: **Overexpression of cyclin D1 correlates with sensitivity to cisplatin in squamous cell carcinoma cell lines of the head and neck.** *Acta Otolaryngol (Stockh)* 2004, **124:**851–857.

17

The evolution of Taiwan's National Health Insurance drug reimbursement scheme

Jason C Hsu[1*] and Christine Y Lu[2]

Abstract

Background: The rapid growth of health care expenditures, especially pharmaceutical spending, is a challenge for many countries. To control increasing pharmaceutical expenditures and to enhance rational use of drugs, Taiwan's National Health Insurance drug reimbursement system has evolved over time since its introduction in 1995. This study reviewed Taiwan's drug reimbursement scheme: its development and evolution in the last two decades, and implications and impacts of recent policies for drug pricing. We also provide recommendations for possible improvement.

Methods: We conducted a review of Taiwan's National Health Insurance drug reimbursement scheme. We focused on three major components of the scheme: (i) the scope of drug coverage; (ii) pricing system for pharmaceuticals under the scheme; and (iii) adjustment of drug reimbursement prices. We reviewed the literature and public policy documents.

Results: The National Health Insurance delisted 176 and another 240 behind-the-counter products (e.g., antacids, vitamins) between 2005 and 2006 to reduce pharmaceutical expenditures. For the pricing of pharmaceuticals, policy evolution can be divided into four phases since 1995; the present system emphasizes stakeholder engagement, health technology assessment, domestic R&D, and improving quality of products. To close the gap between drug reimbursement prices and procurement prices, eight rounds of drug price surveys and adjustments have been implemented since 2000.

Conclusions: Taiwan's National Health Insurance drug reimbursement scheme has evolved substantially over time to provide more equitable and affordable access to prescription medicines. However, more work is still needed as irrational difference in reimbursement and procurement prices persists and the total expenditure of the drug reimbursement scheme continues to increase at unsustainable rates.

Keywords: Universal health coverage, Drug policy, Reimbursement, Medicines coverage, National Health Insurance, Taiwan

Introduction

Access to health care, including 'essential' medicines, is regarded as a human right by the International Covenant on Economic, Social and Cultural Rights [1]. The vast majority of people and governments around the world generally support the implementation of national health insurance. Many economically developed countries have implemented national health insurance that aims to provide its members with satisfactory care services to achieve "health for all" [2]. However, many healthcare systems have sometimes achieved poor performance given the resources spent and/or are still undergoing reform.

In Taiwan, the National Health Insurance (NHI) is a compulsory social insurance system in which the coverage rate of its 23 million residents is as high as 99% currently. Since the introduction in August 1995, the National Health Insurance has gained public recognition as Taiwan becomes comparable with neighboring countries (like Japan, South Korea and Singapore) in terms of quality of care, healthcare cost control, drug spending growth, and public satisfaction [3]. However, concerns have been raised about its financial sustainability.

* Correspondence: jasonhsuharvard@gmail.com
[1]School of Pharmacy and Institute of Clinical Pharmacy and Pharmaceutical Sciences, College of Medicine, National Cheng Kung University, No.1, Daxue Rd., East Dist., Tainan City 70101, Taiwan R.O.C
Full list of author information is available at the end of the article

Around the world, countries generally adopt a pluralistic system of healthcare coverage that maximizes consumer choice (e.g., USA) or a predominantly single, universal scheme for healthcare coverage that maximizes equity and the prospects for cost control. Taiwan adopts the single system model. The National Health Insurance is contracted with public, private, and corporate healthcare institutions, which provide a range of covered healthcare services, including prescription drugs. The National Health Insurance Administration (NHIA; formerly known as the Bureau of NHI, the name was changed in 2013), set up by the government, reimburses the contracted institutions for the services provided.

The rapid growth of healthcare costs is a challenge faced by all countries, especially the growth of pharmaceutical costs, which is even more evident [4,5]. The total drug expenditure of Taiwan's National Health Insurance was about US$2,133 million in 1997, and it increased by around US$173 million each year. In 2012, pharmaceutical expenditures reached US$4,733 million, which accounted for 25.1% of the total healthcare expenditure (Figure 1) [3]. The main causes of rising healthcare costs and pharmaceutical expenditures include the aging population, the increasing number of patients with chronic diseases, increasing drug prices, larger drug usages, and the availability of new, more expensive drugs [6-8].

To control growing pharmaceutical expenditures, the NHIA implemented multiple policies for prescription drug reimbursement. The purpose of this study was to review and summarize the evolution of Taiwan's drug reimbursement scheme over the last two decades, including its development and major changes for drug pricing, and implications and impacts of its recent policies. We also highlighted possible policy-induced problems that need to be addressed. Finally, we provide some recommendations for how Taiwan's drug reimbursement scheme can continue to evolve to ensure the goals of financial sustainability and rational use of medicines [9].

Method

We conducted a review of Taiwan's National Health Insurance drug reimbursement scheme. We focused on policies implemented by the NHIA over the last two decades. We reviewed policies that targeted different issues: (1) the scope of drug coverage, (2) the pricing system for pharmaceuticals under the scheme, and (3) adjustments of drug reimbursement prices. Similar to many countries, medicines are classified into three categories in Taiwan: (a) prescription drugs, (b) drugs designated by physicians or pharmacists, which can be purchased at pharmacies without prescriptions (e.g., antihistamines, antitussive agents) – generally known as behind-the-counter or pharmacist only drugs, and (c) over-the-counter (OTC) medications.

We collected and reviewed historical archives including official documents, books, published articles, research projects, conference records, websites, newspapers, speeches etc. After reviewing abovementioned materials relating to the drug reimbursement scheme, we also examined policy implementation and policy changes, summarized the known impacts of the policies, and highlighted possible policy-induced problems that need to be addressed for system improvement.

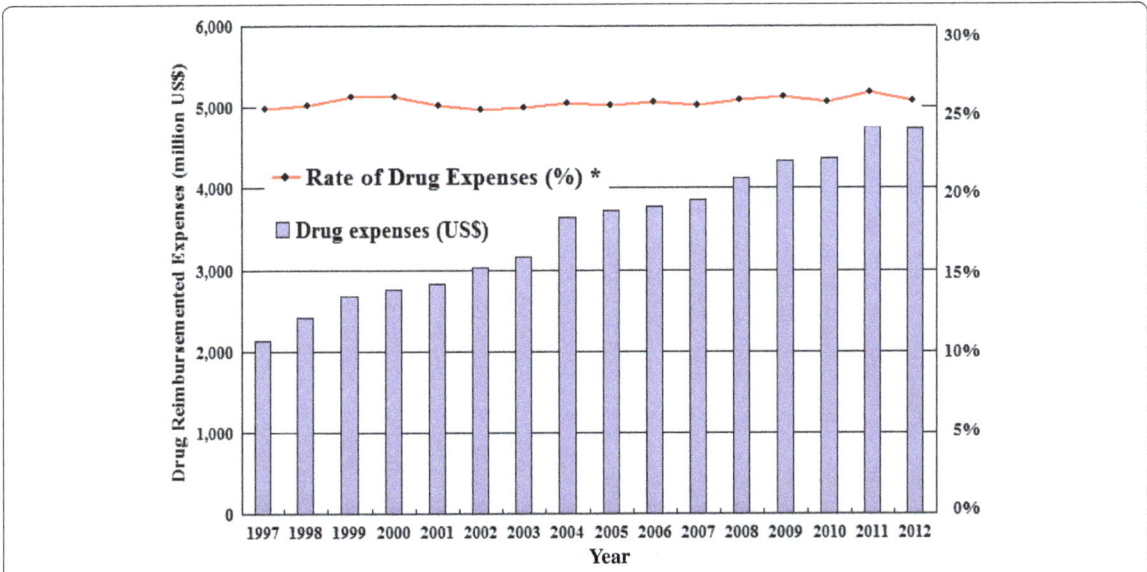

Figure 1 The evolution of drug reimbursement expenses. *Rate of Drug Expenses (%): proportion of drug expenditure of total health care costs.

Results

NHIA policies over the last two decades largely targeted prescription drugs and behind-the-counter drugs.

Policies governing the scope of drug coverage

According to Article 51 in the National Health Insurance Act (amended in 2011) [10], the NHIA does not reimburse the following: (1) medicines that are approved by the Taiwan Food and Drug Administration (Taiwan FDA) but are not used for disease treatment, such as contraceptive, hair tonic, dark spots detergent, smoking cessation patches; (2) some vaccines (e.g., quadrivalent Human papillomavirus types vaccine); (3) over-the-counter drugs and non-prescription drugs which should be used under the guidance of a physician or pharmacist (also called the behind-the-counter drugs); (4) drugs for human-subject clinical trials; (5) drugs which are deemed by the National Health Insurance as not essential for medical treatment (e.g. dentures, artificial eyes, spectacles, hearing aids, wheelchairs, canes, and other treatment equipment) or not cost-effective; (6) drugs which do not conform to the indication that stipulated in the approved indication for licensing and/or the "Reimbursement Restriction" enacted by the National Health Insurance. However, in special cases, an application for prior authorization can be made to the National Health Insurance, and the drug will be reimbursed if authorization is given; and (7) any other drug which the NHIA publicly announces that it will not be reimbursed [11].

Behind-the-counter drugs were covered by the former Civil Servant Insurance and Labor Insurance and in the early years of the National Health Insurance. The NHIA reviewed and reduced the scope of coverage of behind-the-counter drugs over time [11]. Some behind-the-counter drugs were delisted to meet the priorities of the National Health Insurance, in accordance with Article 51 of the National Health Insurance Act, and more generally, to establish patient expectations and the culture of rational use of medicines and basic self-healthcare. This change also intended to reduce costs of the National Health Insurance as well as making better use of its resources for treatment of major diseases.

This delisting of behind-the-counter drugs also benefited consumers who needed such products for treatment of minor illnesses (e.g., headache, cold). They can save time and related expenses when they choose to purchase medicines at pharmacies instead of visiting physicians at primary care clinics or hospitals. For example, a patient's out-of-pocket costs are less if s/he chooses to purchase medicines for headache from pharmacies (only US$3) compared with visiting a physician which requires physician visit copays (US$5).

In total, the National Health Insurance delisted 176 (e.g., some antacids) and 240 (e.g., some vitamins, electrolytes) behind-the-counter products in 2005 and 2006 respectively. However, there was considerable resistance from both physicians and patients; thus, no further behind-the-counter drugs were delisted. Currently, there are still around 1400 behind-the-counter products reimbursed by NHIA (e.g., gastrointestinal drugs, antihistamines, antitussive agents) [3]. However, delisting in the future is likely under the pressure to contain costs.

The pricing system for pharmaceuticals under the drug reimbursement scheme

The pricing system under the drug reimbursement scheme of the National Health Insurance can be divided into four phases over time: (1) internal audit price (1995/3-1997/3); (2) uniform pricing (1997/4-1999/2); (3) Pharmaceutical benefit scheme (1999/3-2012/12); and (4) Pharmaceutical benefits and reimbursement schedule (after 2013/1), which are described as below and summarized in Figure 2.

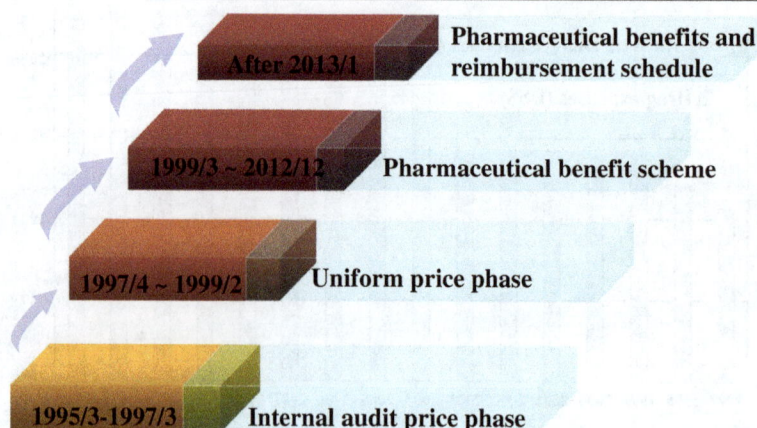

Figure 2 The evolution of drug pricing of the drug reimbursement scheme under Taiwan's National Health Insurance.

Prior to the implementation of the National Health Insurance in 1995 in Taiwan, about 50% of the population was insured under the Civil Servant Insurance, Labor Insurance, and Farmer's Health Insurance. At the time, pharmaceutical companies were allowed free pricing, and they were subject to hospitals' pharmaceutical tender and negotiation to determine the price of drugs in hospitals. Hospitals would bill the insurers. The insurers would then reimburse individual hospitals by an approach known as "transaction cost-plus". For drug reimbursements, the joint bid price would be paid to public hospitals while to this price plus 10-20% would be paid to private hospitals. Profits were usually used to pay for drug warehouse management, dispensing and other expenses. High-level hospitals tended to use more expensive, brand-name drugs or imported drugs because of profits from pharmaceutical sales. At the time of public bidding in public hospitals, manufacturers were reluctant to cut prices, resulting in high tender prices. Prescription drugs were paid out-of-pocket in primary care settings because most patients were not insured under the Government Employee's Insurance, Laborer Insurance, or Farmer's Health Insurance. As a result, patients were sensitive to drug prices; many would choose domestic, generic drugs over the more expensive, brand-name drugs or imported drugs.

At the early stage of the National Health Insurance (1995–1997), the NHIA released the "National Health Insurance Drug Items Table" that listed products being covered, and drugs were reimbursed through the "internal audit pricing" approach. However, the internal audit pricing system was unclear, and the price of imported generic drugs was relatively high due to a lack of international drug price comparison. These led to substantial variations in drug prices between domestic drugs and drugs by international manufacturers [12]. Hospitals generally adopted the "fee for service" approach for drug reimbursements while primary care clinics adopted the "fixed fees by days of supply" approach (e.g., one-day supply of any medications received a reimbursement of NT$35, regardless therapeutic indication and actual procurement price; two-day supply was NT$70; and three-day supply was NT$100). The following 'consequences' were observed: (1) primary care clinics tended to reduce drug costs and were reluctant to release prescriptions to patients so patients had to obtain drugs at the clinics (resulting in the phenomenon of "next-door pharmacy", which had negative impacts on the separation of drug prescribing and dispensing); (2) some patients were transferred to higher level hospitals in order to obtain drugs of higher prices and/or for longer supplies; and (3) use of drugs of higher prices in primary care clinics was subsequently reduced [13,14].

During 1997–1999, the NHIA invited the pharmaceutical industry to engage in the development of pricing guidance for drugs covered under the NHI ("National Health Insurance drug pricing principles"). The goals were to lower drug prices, control the growth of drug prices, reduce the prices of brand-name drugs and generic drugs, encourage the use of generic drugs, and protect the domestic generic drug market. The pricing guidance governed drug pricing by a drug classification system: (1) new drugs: the NHIA invited the medical and pharmaceutical experts to engage in the review and approval process; (2) the compound and special specification drugs: paid the same minimum price as other drugs of the same composition; (3) brand-name drugs: brand-name drugs were subdivided into two categories: ones that have no bioavailability/bioequivalence (BA/BE) generic drugs as alternatives in the market, and others that have BA/BE generic drugs as alternatives. Drugs of the former category were priced according to the international drugs with average market prices; while the price of the latter category must not exceed 85% of the average market price of international drugs; (4) the price of BA/BE generic drugs must not exceed the price of brand-name drugs; and (5) the price of non-BA/BE generic drugs must not exceed 80% of the price of brand-name drugs. From then on, drugs covered by the National Health Insurance were uniformly priced.

During 1999–2012, the NHIA attempted to address the problem of differences between drug procurement and reimbursement prices. To determine the market drug price difference, the NHIA required hospitals and manufacturers to provide the actual transaction prices and trading volumes. However, many hospitals and manufacturers resisted such investigation or supplied false declarations about prices, and the drug price gap remained a serious problem. The NHIA therefore announced the "Pharmaceutical Benefits Scheme" in March 1999 to govern the listing of drugs, the pricing of pharmaceuticals, and the adjustment of drug reimbursement prices. It also set the target to reduce the gap in drug prices to less than 15% within five years. Moreover, NHIA announced in April 1999 that drug price surveys for NHI reimbursed drugs were to be conducted every 1–2 years. Since then, the NHIA has implemented eight drug price surveys; new drug reimbursement prices were announced and implemented respectively on April 1st, 2000, April 1st, 2001, March 1st, 2003, September 1st, 2005, November 1st, 2006, October 1st, 2009, November 1st, 2011 and May 1st, 2014 (Table 1) [15]. Adjustments of drug prices are discussed in detail in the next section.

The "Pharmaceutical Benefit Scheme" was replaced by "Pharmaceutical benefits and reimbursement schedule" on January 1st, 2013. Compared with "Pharmaceutical Benefit Scheme", the present new scheme emphasizes

Table 1 List of drug price surveys and adjustments

Order	Date	Estimated cost-savings (million US$)
1st	April 1st, 2000	16.67
2nd	April 1st, 2001	153.33
3rd	March 1st, 2003	190.00
4th	September 1st, 2005	81.00
5th	November 1st, 2006	500.00
6th	October 1st, 2009	195.67
7th	November 1st, 2011	–
8th	May 1st, 2014	–

Resource: Huang [15].

stakeholder engagement (including the insurer and the relevant authorities, experts and scholars, the insured, employers, health care service providers, etc.) to discuss and design the listing of drugs and reimbursement prices for specific products. Further, health technology assessment (considering human health, medical ethics, cost-effectiveness of products, and financial sustainability of the NHI) was required for new drugs prior to listing in the National Health Insurance under this new phase. In 2007, the Center for Drug Evaluation (CDE) was created to conduct health technology assessment (HTA), that is, assessment of comparative efficacy, cost-effectiveness, and budget impact of new drugs. The CDE only provides HTA reports to the NHIA, it is not involved in pricing. The NHIA considers HTA evidence as part of the information used for listing and reimbursement decisions [16].

The adjustment of drug reimbursement prices

To ensure reasonable drug prices and close the gap between procurement and insurer reimbursement prices for prescription drugs, Taiwan made multiple efforts. Because institutions procure large quantities of medicines, procurement prices are typically lower than the amount reimbursed by the NHIA and the differences constitutes a profit for hospitals [17]. To assess procurement prices, the NHIA conducted surveys to obtain drug wholesale prices from pharmaceutical companies and procurement prices from hospitals since 1999 [18]. Reimbursements were adjusted if there was a difference of 30% or more between the average procurement price and the NHI reimbursed price. Prices were subsequently monitored and adjusted every two years for patented products, for products whose patent right has expired for more than five years, and for products that have no patent right. These drugs are further divided into the following two categories: (1) drugs from original R&D pharmaceutical companies, drugs of which the process of pharmaceutical form complies with "The Pharmaceutical Inspection Convention and Pharmaceutical Inspection Co-operation Scheme - Good manufacturing practice (PIC/S GMP)" requirements, BA/BE generic drugs, drugs approved to by the US

FDA and/or The European Medicines Agency for marketing, controlled items of BE generic drugs; (2) common generic drugs which do not fall into the first category [11].

Studies have been conducted to examine effects of drug reimbursement price reductions in Taiwan. Lee et al. [19] assessed the effects of six drug price policies and found that they reduced pharmaceutical expenditures, especially for outpatient medications and for hospitals (compared with clinics) [19]. Chen et al. [17] showed that reimbursement price reductions for targeted cardiovascular medications reduced the daily medical use and expenditures, but did not affect non-targeted products [17]. Chu et al. [20] studied price reductions for antihypertensive drugs. They suggested that reimbursement price adjustments may have created an incentive for physicians to prescribe drugs with higher profit margins, and to increase prescription duration or the number of drug items per prescription [20]. Hsiao et al. [21] did not find strong associations between reimbursement price adjustments and drug utilization and expenditures during 2001–2004. Chu et al. [22] studied effects of reimbursement price adjustments on outpatient hypertension treatments among the elderly. They found that the average cost per prescription increased slightly, and that physicians tended to prescribe drugs whose prices were not reduced instead of those subject to price reductions. Findings by Hsu et al. [18] indicated that prescribing shifted from targeted to non-targeted products [18]. Overall, these studies suggest shifts in use from targeted to non-targeted products to maintain profits from drug price gaps but whether they reduced pharmaceutical expenditures is unclear.

Discussion

The study provides a review of the development and evolution of Taiwan's universal drug reimbursement scheme under its National Health Insurance. We highlighted major policy changes for drug pricing over the last two decades and their known impacts and implications. It is important to note that many policy changes (e.g., delisting of behind-the-counter products, introduction of HTA) remain to be evaluated for their impacts on medication use, drug prices, quality of care, and pharmaceutical expenditures.

With the goal to reduce pharmaceutical expenditures to the government, about 400 behind-the-counter products were delisted from Taiwan's national Drug Reimbursement Scheme. This coverage change also aimed to establish patient expectations and the culture of rational use of medicines and basic self-healthcare for minor illnesses such as headache or cold. This is not surprising; many national drug coverage schemes do not reimburse or reimburse only selected few behind-the-counter products, e.g., Australia's Pharmaceutical Benefits Scheme. Misuse, under-use or over-use of behind-the-counter drugs are possible unintended consequences. Inappropriate consumer self-medication may lead to subsequent medication-related adverse health outcomes (e.g., medication error or poisoning), or negative health outcomes if appropriate treatment was delayed or not used, which may lead to subsequent increase in healthcare costs. It is important that delisting of behind-the-counter medications is accompanied by appropriate educational programs directed to consumers and pharmacists to ensure rational use of medicines. Taiwan may learn from Australia, which has worldly recognized multifaceted programs to improve rational use of medicines [23].

To ensure reasonable drug prices and close the gap between procurement and insurer reimbursement prices for prescription drugs, Taiwan and other countries (e.g., China) [24] have made multiple efforts. We highlighted how the pricing system under Taiwan's Drug Reimbursement Scheme has evolved over time. While the gap between drug procurement and reimbursement prices has narrowed, price difference persists. For instance, there are substantial price difference between drug reimbursements and claims made by primary care clinics for prescription drugs that use the "fixed fees by days of supply" approach mentioned above.

Whether drug price adjustments achieved the intended cost-savings is unclear. Despite several waves of drug price adjustments to close the gap between procurement and reimbursement prices, the total pharmaceutical expenditures is still on the rise (average yearly growth rate for pharmaceutical expenditures from 1997 to 2012 is 8.13%). Reasons for such growth include: (1) adjustments of drug reimbursement prices only reduce the prices of targeted products, not the volume of use; (2) off-label use: it has not been estimated how much expenditures are attributed to use of prescription medications outside approved indications under the Drug Reimbursement Scheme; reimbursed indications are largely based on clinical treatment guidelines, Taiwan FDA approved indications and specification made by NHIA or medical associations; (3) drug waste (unnecessary use and stockpiling of medications): this issue is particularly common for behind-the-counter drugs (e.g., antacid agents and vitamins), which led to delisting of some products by the NHI; however, delisting was opposed by many physicians and patients; and (4) the availability of innovative, expensive drugs such as cancer targeted therapies: the NHI created the HTA body to assess the cost-effectiveness of new drugs to inform decisions about reimbursement.

We recommend that capitation/case payment models [25], diagnosis related groups (DRGs) [26-28] and pay for performance [29,30] are some possible alternative approaches, that have been used by other countries and show promise in controlling total pharmaceutical expenditures without substantially reducing the quality of health care.

Health Technology Assessment is increasingly adopted for making drug reimbursement decisions throughout the Asia-Pacific markets. Apart from Taiwan, countries in this region with established HTA system include Australia, New Zealand, South Korea, and Thailand [31,32]. Economic evaluation should not only inform the decision of reimbursement but also used to negotiate prices with manufacturers. In addition, many countries (including countries in Asia-Pacific markets such as Australia, South Korea) are adopting risk-sharing agreements for funding high-cost innovative drugs such as adalimumab and imatinib. Risk-sharing agreements are typically between a payer and a pharmaceutical company in which the partners negotiate the price of a product and/or the overall spending depending on volumes sold, clinical outcomes achieved or patient populations who receive the drug [33-35]. The intent is that companies share the financial risk of payers to reimburse the drug, and pay for the drug when an agreed volume or budget is exceeded, or intended clinical outcomes are not achieved. Taiwan could learn lessons from neighboring countries adopting HTA and risk-sharing agreements to address the challenge of high-cost medicines.

Conclusion

Taiwan's Drug Reimbursement Scheme under its universal National Health Insurance has come a long way over the last two decades. It is highly regarded particularly on the basis of comprehensive drug coverage, minimal patient cost burden, and timely access to new medicines. The NHI implemented multiple policy changes to enhance rational use of drugs and to contain increasing pharmaceutical expenditures. However, while the data are limited, there were opposition from consumers and physicians for some of the changes. Many policy changes remain to be evaluated for their impacts on medication use, quality of care, and pharmaceutical expenditures. Further policy changes may be needed and these should be developed in light of lessons learned by other countries that are also facing similar challenges. Stakeholders (i.e., patients, clinicians, government, industry) need to work closely together to continue to improve rational use of drugs, the quality of healthcare, and the financial sustainability of the National Health Insurance. Evidence-informed policy changes with appropriate stakeholder engagement will be important for optimal patient outcomes.

Abbreviations
R&D: Research and development; NHI: National Health Insurance; NHIA: The National Health Insurance Administration; OTC: Over-the-counter; Taiwan FDA: Taiwan Food and Drug Administration; BA/BE: Bioavailability/bioequivalence; CDE: Center for Drug Evaluation; PIC/S GMP: The Pharmaceutical Inspection Convention and Pharmaceutical Inspection Co-operation Scheme - Good manufacturing practice; DRGs: Diagnosis related groups; HTA: Health technology assessment.

Competing interests

The authors declare that they have no competing interests.

Authors' contributions

JCH designed the study, collected data, performed analysis, and drafted the manuscript. CYL reviewed all data and revised the manuscript critically for intellectual content. Both authors approved the final version for submission.

Acknowledgements

Dr. Hsu conducted part of this work as a research fellow in the Harvard Medical School Fellowship in Pharmaceutical Policy Research.

Author details

[1]School of Pharmacy and Institute of Clinical Pharmacy and Pharmaceutical Sciences, College of Medicine, National Cheng Kung University, No.1, Daxue Rd., East Dist., Tainan City 70101, Taiwan R.O.C. [2]Department of Population Medicine, Harvard Medical School and Harvard Pilgrim Health Care Institute, Boston, MA, USA.

References

1. Hogerzeil H: Access to essential medicines as a human right. World Health Organisation: Essential Drugs Monitor 2003, (33):25–26. http://apps.who.int/medicinedocs/en/d/Js4941e/5.html.
2. Gil-Gonzalez D, Carrasco-Portino M, Vives-Cases C, Agudelo-Suarez AA, Castejon Bolea R, Ronda-Perez E: Is health a right for all? An umbrella review of the barriers to health care access faced by migrants. Ethn Health 2014, 13:1–19.
3. National Health Insurance Administration. Website. http://www.nhi.gov.tw/english/index.aspx.
4. Mullins CD, Wang J, Palumbo FB, Stuart B: The impact of pipeline drugs on drug spending growth. Health Aff (Millwood) 2001, 20(5):210–215.
5. Berndt ER: Pharmaceuticals in U.S. health care: determinants of quantity and price. J Econ Perspect 2002, 16(4):45–66.
6. Levit K, Smith C, Cowan C, Sensenig A, Catlin A: Health spending rebound continues in 2002. Health Aff (Millwood) 2004, 23(1):147–159.
7. Hsieh CR, Sloan FA: Adoption of pharmaceutical innovation and the growth of drug expenditure in Taiwan: is it cost effective? Value Health 2008, 11(2):334–344.
8. Yang CL, Chao HL, Huang WY, Lin WD, Huang KH, Lai MS: National Health Insurance. Taiwan: Wagner Co Ltd; 2012.
9. Huang SK, Tsai SL, Hsu MT: Ensuring the sustainability of the Taiwan National Health Insurance. J Formos Med Assoc 2014, 113(1):1–2.
10. National Health Insurance Act. Website http://mohwlaw.mohw.gov.tw/Chi/EngContent.asp?msgid=279&KeyWord=%A5%FE%A5%C1%B0%B7%B1d%ABO%C0I%AAk.
11. National Health Insurance Administration: The National Health Insurance Pharmaceutical Benefits and Reimbursement Schedule. Taiwan: National Health Insurance Administration; 2014. http://law.moj.gov.tw/Eng/LawClass/LawContent.aspx?PCODE=L0060035.
12. Huang CM: The Reform Strategy of NHI drug Expenditure Rationalization. Taiwan: The Bureau of National Health Insurance; 1998.
13. Cheng C, Hsieh CR: Economic analysis of NHI pharmaceutical policies and drug expenditures. Socioecon Law Inst Rev 2005, 35:1–42.
14. Cheng C: An Analysisi of NHI Drug Policies and Pharmaceutical Expenditures. Taiwan: Chang Gung University; 2003.
15. Huang HH, Shen MC, Liu HS: National Health Insurance. Taiwan: Wu-nan Book Inc; 2012.
16. Yang BM: The future of health technology assessment in healthcare decision making in Asia. Pharmacoeconomics 2009, 27(11):891–901.
17. Chen CL, Chen L, Yang WC: The influences of Taiwan's generic grouping price policy on drug prices and expenditures: evidence from analysing the consumption of the three most-used classes of cardiovascular drugs. BMC Public Health 2008, 8:118.
18. Hsu JC, Lu CY, Wagner AK, Chan KA, Lai MS, Ross-Degnan D: Impacts of drug reimbursement reductions on utilization and expenditures of oral antidiabetic medications in Taiwan: an interrupted time series study. Health Policy 2014, 116(2–3):196–205.
19. Lee YC, Yang MC, Huang YT, Liu CH, Chen SB: Impacts of cost containment strategies on pharmaceutical expenditures of the National Health Insurance in Taiwan, 1996–2003. Pharmacoeconomics 2006, 24(9):891–902.
20. Chu HL, Liu SZ, Romeis JC: Changes in prescribing behaviors after implementing drug reimbursement rate reduction policy in Taiwan: implications for the medicare system. J Health Care Finance 2008, 34(3):45–54.
21. Hsiao FY, Tsai YW, Huang WF: Price regulation, new entry, and information shock on pharmaceutical market in Taiwan: a nationwide data-based study from 2001 to 2004. BMC Health Serv Res 2010, 10:218.
22. Chu HL, Liu SZ, Romeis JC: Assessing the effects of drug price reduction policies on older people in Taiwan. Health Serv Manage Res 2011, 24(1):1–7.
23. Weekes LM, Mackson JM, Fitzgerald M, Phillips SR: National Prescribing Service: creating an implementation arm for national medicines policy. Br J Clin Pharmacol 2005, 59(1):112–116.
24. Lu CY, Ross-Degnan D, Stephens P, Liu BAW: Changes in use of antidiabetic medications following price regulations in China. J Pharm Health Serv Res 2013, 4:3–11.
25. Jirawattanapisal T, Kingkaew P, Lee TJ, Yang MC: Evidence-based decision-making in Asia-Pacific with rapidly changing health-care systems: Thailand, South Korea, and Taiwan. Value Health 2009, 12(Suppl 3):S4–S11.
26. Yan YH, Chen Y, Kung CM, Peng LJ: Continuous quality improvement of nursing care: case study of a clinical pathway revision for cardiac catheterization. J Nurs Res 2011, 19(3):181–189.
27. Schmid A, Cacace M, Gotze R, Rothgang H: Explaining health care system change: problem pressure and the emergence of "hybrid" health care systems. J Health Polit Policy Law 2010, 35(4):455–486.
28. Busato A, von Below G: The implementation of DRG-based hospital reimbursement in Switzerland: A population-based perspective. Health Res Policy Syst 2010, 8:31.
29. Chen PC, Lee YC, Kuo RN: Differences in patient reports on the quality of care in a diabetes pay-for-performance program between 1 year enrolled and newly enrolled patients. Int J Qual Health Care 2012, 24(2):189–196.
30. Cheng SH, Lee TT, Chen CC: A longitudinal examination of a pay-for-performance program for diabetes care: evidence from a natural experiment. Med Care 2012, 50(2):109–116.
31. Sivalal S: Health technology assessment in the Asia Pacific region. Int J Technol Assess Health Care 2009, 25(Suppl 1):196–201.
32. Kamae I: Value-based approaches to healthcare systems and pharmacoeconomics requirements in Asia: South Korea, Taiwan, Thailand and Japan. Pharmacoeconomics 2010, 28(10):831–838.
33. Lu C, Lupton C, Rakowsky S, Ross-Degnan D, Wagner A: Patient access schemes in asia-pacific markets: current experience and future potential. J Pharm Policy Pract 2014. in press.
34. Lu CY, Williams K, Day R, March L, Sansom L, Bertouch J: Access to high cost drugs in Australia. BMJ 2004, 329(7463):415–416.
35. Hall WD, Ward R, Liauw WS, Lu CY, Brien JA: Tailoring access to high cost, genetically targeted drugs. Med J Aust 2005, 182(12):607–608.

18

Cost-effectiveness and cost-utility analysis of OTC use of simvastatin 10 mg for the primary prevention of myocardial infarction in Iranian men

Mohammadreza Amirsadri* ⑩ and Abbas Hassani

Abstract

Background: Several clinical trials and meta-analyses have shown the advantageous effects of statins in populations with different levels of cardiovascular disease (CVD) risk. Considering the increasing cardiovascular risk among the Iranian population, the cost-effectiveness of the use of simvastatin 10 mg, as an Over-The-Counter (OTC) drug, for the primary prevention of myocardial infarction (MI) was evaluated in this modeling study, from the payer's perspective. The target population is a hypothetical cohort of 45-year CVD healthy men with an average (15 %) 10-year CVD risk.

Methods: A semi-Markov model with a life-long time horizon was developed to evaluate the Cost-Utility-Analysis (CUA) and Cost-Effectiveness-Analysis (CEA) of the use of OTC simvastatin 10 mg compared to no-drug therapy. Two measures of benefits were used in the model; Quality-Adjusted-Life-Years (QALYs) for the CUA and Life-Years-Gained (LYG) for the CEA. To examine the robustness of the results, one-way sensitivity analysis and probabilistic sensitivity analysis were applied to the model.

Results: For the base-case scenario with a discount rate of 0 % the estimated ICERs were 1113 USD/QALY and 935USD/LYG per patient (using governmental tariffs).
No threshold has been determined in Iran for the cost-effectiveness of health-related interventions. However, according to the recommendation of WHO, this intervention can be considered highly cost-effective as its ICER is far less than the reported GDP per capita for Iran by World bank in 2013 ($4763).

Conclusions: This modeling study showed that the use of an OTC low dose statin (simvastatin 10 mg) for the primary prevention of myocardial infarction (MI) in 45-year men with a 10-year CVD risk of 15 % could be considered highly cost-effective in Iran, as it meets the WHO threshold of the annual GDP per capita ($4763).

Keywords: Cost-effectiveness, Cost-utility, myocardial infarction, Markov model, Primary prevention, Simvastatin, Over-the-counter

Background

Chronic non-communicable diseases (NCDs) are universally recognized as the major causes of death and disability [1]. In 2008 around 48 % of NCD-related deaths were reported to be due to cardiovascular diseases (CVDs). It is predicted that by 2020, CVDs will be responsible for three-quarters of all deaths in countries with low- and middle-income [2].

Cardiovascular diseases are the most preventable causes of death in both developed and developing countries. The majority of CVD conditions with modifiable risk factors such as hypertension, dyslipidemia, obesity and diabetes are preventable or controllable [3]. Several clinical trials and meta-analyses have shown the advantageous effects of statins for the primary prevention of CVDs among populations with different levels of CVD risk [4]. Statins are a class of pharmaceuticals used to lower LDL-

* Correspondence: amirsadri@pharm.mui.ac.ir
Department of Clinical Pharmacy and Pharmacy Practice, Faculty of Pharmacy and Pharmaceutical Sciences, Isfahan University of Medical Sciences, Isfahan, Iran

cholesterol levels by inhibiting of the enzyme HMG-COA reductase [5]. Statins, independent of their lipid-lowering effect, may also improve endothelial function, inhibit inflammatory responses, stabilize atherosclerotic plaques and show vasculo-protective actions [6]. The indication for the use of statins also have been suggested for patients with even low normal LDL cholesterol levels in hopes of favorably altering the incidence of CVDs [7, 8].

To decrease the risk of a first major CVD event in people who are at moderate risk, the UK medicines and healthcare products regulatory agency reclassified simvastatin 10 mg (Zocor Heart-Pro) as an over the counter(OTC) medicine in 2004. The target population includes men aged 55 or more, men aged 45 to 54 years with one or more risk factor, and women aged 55 or more with one or more risk factor [9].

With respect to the increasing prevalence of CVDs among the Iranian population and its accrued costs, the cost-effectiveness and cost-utility of the use of 10 mg simvastatin among 45-year Iranian men with an average (15 %) 10-year CVD risk from the perspective of payer were estimated in this study [10].

Methods

The population of this study includes a hypothetical cohort of CVD-healthy men aged 45 with a 10-year CVD risk of 15 %.

For chronic disease with recurrent events like as CVD, particularly when the risk of the disease progression persists indefinitely, Markov modeling is generally the preferred choice. Markov models with the transition probabilities which change with respect to time are named semi-Markov models [11].

A semi-Markov model was developed to evaluate the cost-effectiveness and cost-utility of the use of OTC simvastatin10mg (a low dose statin) for the primary prevention of myocardial infarction (MI) compared to no drug-therapy.

The main measured consequences were LYG for the CEA and QALY for the CUA.

Life-years-gained is a measure of the benefits from use of an intervention in terms of increased average life expectancy or delay of death in the population when compared with the alternative intervention [12].

Quality-adjusted-life-year is used to illustrate the outcomes of health care programs through adjusting the life years gained by an estimate of utility generally measured using a preference based method [13]. QALYs gained with treatment therefore incorporate benefits in both quantity and quality of life.

The choice of cycle length depends upon the interventions of interest as well as the type of disease [14]. For models with life-long time horizon and relatively rare events the cycle length can be one year [15]. Majority of modeling studies on CVD adopted a cycle length of one

year [16]. The current model assumes Markov cycles of one year and consists of 5 different health states including: healthy, non-fatal MI (first year), post-MI, fatal-MI and death due to any reason other than MI (to prevent double counting). As in the following years after an acute (first year) MI, both the treatment costs and the probability of a recurrent MI are different from the first year; separated health states for this were considered in the model (Fig. 1).

In this model, each individual starts as a CVD-healthy person. A healthy person might develop a non-fatal MI, die from a fatal MI, or die for any reason other than MI. Otherwise he would be transferred to the next cycle as a healthy person. If a patient develops a non-fatal MI, the patient might experience a new non-fatal MI, die due to a fatal MI or die for other reasons. If none of these happened, the patient would be transferred to the next cycle with a history of MI (post-MI) with the probabilities and costs related to this health state (which are different from the first-year MI). Possible transitions from post-MI to other health states are similar to those of non-fatal MI.

Once patients experience an MI event, they would receive a POM (Prescription-Only-Medicine) statin (atorvastatin 10 mg) in both intervention and no-intervention groups for life time.

The time horizon of an economic evaluation should be long enough to be able to capture both the major costs and the major future outcomes of treatment including the benefits, potential side effects, morbidity and mortality. Therefore in many cases a patient's life time is the preferred time horizon for the study [14, 17].

Like as many economic evaluation studies on CVD, this model would be continued until 100 year of age (when most of the cohort have died) or death [16]. However, due to the nature of Markov models, some

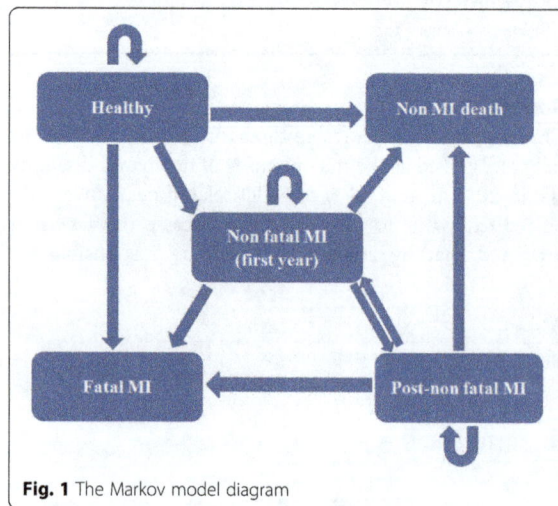

Fig. 1 The Markov model diagram

Table 1 Relative risks for the use of statins

The RR[a] for the use of simvastatin 10 mg	
healthy to non-fatal MI	0.752
healthy to fatal MI	0.813
The RR[b] for the use of atorvastatin 10 mg	
healthy to non-fatal MI	0.656
healthy to fatal MI	0.740

[a]RR = Relative risk, [b]data sourced from reference 16

proportion of the cohort remain alive, regardless of how high the applied mortality rates are [18].

For the base-case, a moderate 10-year total CVD risk of 15 % was taken into account. As the CVD risk rises with age, an annual increase of 0.03 % in CVD risk was considered in the model [16]. The proportions of fatal and non-fatal MI events among total CVD events were sourced from the Isfahan Cohort Study (ICS) [19]. Different scenarios were evaluated in this modeling study. For consistency with national studies, a second scenario was evaluated in which the probabilities of fatal and non-fatal MI, independent of base-line CVD risk, were sourced from the ICS population.

As people aged 70 or more could be considered at high risk of CVD, in a third scenario, a POM statin (atorvastatin 10 mg) was prescribed from 70 years of age for the primary prevention, in both intervention and no-intervention groups [20].

Three different scenarios of discounting were also considered in this study including: no discounting (0 %), a discount rate of 3 % for both costs and effects (following recommendations of the WHO-CHOICE) [21] and a discount rate of 7.2 % for costs and 3 % for effects, according to a domestic study [22].

Input parameters, including transition probabilities, relative risks related to treatment with statins and the related sources of data are illustrated in Tables 1 and 2.

To calculate QALYs, a utility weights of 0.76 for MI [16] and 0.88 for post-MI [23] were applied to the model. To account for diminishing in health with age, age-related utility weights were also applied to the

model. These utility weights were taken from the Ward et al. study on statins in 2007 [16].

This study was conducted from the payer's perspective. Direct costs including drug acquisition costs, laboratory tests, para-clinical examinations, physician's visits and hospitalization costs were taken into account. Considering the selected perspective, indirect costs were not investigated in this study. The costs were expressed in USD, considering an exchange rate of 26,912 Iranian Rials for each USD. The applied exchange rate was the monthly average (from 22.11.2014 to 22.12.2014) reported by the central bank of Iran [24].

To estimate the unit costs of treatment, we sought expert clinical advice from the cardiologists of Isfahan University of Medical Sciences teaching hospitals (Alzahra hospital and Chamran hospital). The treatment tariffs were sourced from the last published tariff books by the Iranian Ministry of Health and Medical Education. Also, in different scenarios, two separated series of tariffs for private and governmental sections were taken into account [25]. The acquisition cost of each OTC simvastatin 10 mg tablet (1,100 Rials = 0.041 USD) sourced from the Food and Drug Organization [26].

For those who received POM statin (atorvastatin 10 mg) for the primary prevention from 70 years of age, 4 annual general practitioner visits and two sets of liver function enzyme tests (SGOT and SGPT) were taken into account.

Table 3 shows the treatment costs used in the model.

We examined the effect of changing several different parameters in one-way (univariate) sensitivity analyses, for the base-case scenario. Results from the one-way sensitivity analyses are presented as Tornado charts.

Also parameter uncertainty was dealt with by probabilistic sensitivity analysis for the base-case scenario, using Monte Carlo simulation with 10,000 iterations for each evaluation. For each iteration, a value of each input variable was selected randomly from its distribution (lognormal distribution for relative risks and costs and beta distribution for transition probabilities) [27]. The parameters that we varied in the probabilistic sensitivity analysis (PSA) included relative risks of the

Table 2 The transition probabilities applied in the model

TP/age	45-49	50-54	55-59	60-64	65-69	70-74	75-79	80-84	85-100	Reference
MI To MI	0.1280	0.1280	0.1152	0.1152	0.1019	0.1019	0.0874	0.0874	0.0711	[16]
MI To FMI	0.0224	0.0348	0.0348	0.0700	0.0700	0.1054	0.1054	0.1270	0.1270	[34–37]
Post-MI To MI	0.0162	0.0162	0.0179	0.0179	0.0185	0.0185	0.0178	0.0178	0.0160	[16]
Post-MI To FMI	0.0052	0.0052	0.0092	0.0092	0.0152	0.0152	0.0235	0.0235	0.0340	[16, 38]
Non MI death	0.0028	0.0043	0.0056	0.0084	0.0131	0.0213	0.0426	0.0705	0.1143	[39, 40]
Healthy To MI (ICS)	0.0031	0.0031	0.0044	0.0044	0.0094	0.0094	0.0061	0.0061	0.0061	[19]
Healthy To FMI (ICS)	0.0015	0.0015	0.0050	0.0050	0.0082	0.0082	0.0080	0.0080	0.0080	[19]

TP = transition probability, MI = non-fatal myocardial infarction in first year, FMI = fatal myocardial infarction, Post-MI = subsequent years of non-fatal myocardial infarction, ICS = Isfahan Cohort Study

Table 3 The treatment costs for the first year and following years of MI. The costs in this table were obtained from references 32 & 33

	Governmental					Private				
		MI (first year)		Post- MI			MI (first year)		Post-MI	
	Cost ($)	Number of cost units	Total costs ($)	Number of cost units	Total costs ($)	Cost ($)	Number of cost units	Total costs ($)	Number of cost units	Total costs ($)
CCU hospitalization fee (per day)	77.59	2	155.17	-	-	230.75	2	461.50	-	-
General care units hospitalization fee (per day)	60.87	2	121.73	-	-	180.59	2	361.18	-	-
Consultant visit fee	3.72	7	26.01	2	7.43	9.66	7	67.63	2	19.32
General practitioner visit fee	2.97	3	8.92	4	11.89	6.13	3	18.39	4	24.52
-Para-clinical examinations:										
Electrocardiogram	3.27	9	29.43	2	6.54	7.43	9	66.88	2	14.86
Echocardiography	35.97	1	35.97	-	-	81.75	1	81.75	-	-
Exercise tolerance test	18.64	1	18.64	-	-	42.36	1	42.36	-	-
-Medical laboratory tests:										
Lab. patient admission fee	0.45	3	1.34	2	0.89	0.97	3	2.90	2	1.93
Lab. service fee	0.00	3	0.00	2	0.00	0.74	3	2.23	2	1.49
CBC Dif.	0.74	3	2.23	2	1.49	2.01	3	6.02	2	4.01
BUN	0.41	3	1.23	2	0.82	0.89	3	2.68	2	1.78
Cr	0.52	3	1.56	2	1.04	1.08	3	3.23	2	2.16
Na	0.59	3	1.78	2	1.19	1.30	3	3.90	2	2.60
K	0.59	3	1.78	2	1.19	1.30	3	3.90	2	2.60
BS	0.45	3	1.34	2	0.89	0.97	3	2.90	2	1.93
TG	0.71	3	2.12	2	1.41	1.56	3	4.68	2	3.12
Cholesterol	0.52	3	1.56	2	1.04	1.11	3	3.34	2	2.23
PT INR	0.93	1	0.93	-	-	1.82	1	1.82		
PTT	0.93	1	0.93	-	-	1.82	1	1.82	-	-
Troponin	2.45	2	4.90	-	-	8.62	2	17.24	-	-
LDH	1.86	1	1.86	-	-	4.35	1	4.35	-	-
CPK	2.49	1	2.49	-	-	5.39	1	5.39	-	-
SGOT	0.63	3	1.90	2	1.26	1.45	3	4.35	2	2.90
SGPT	0.63	3	1.90	2	1.26	1.45	3	4.35	2	2.90
ESR	0.26	1	0.26	-	-	0.56	1	0.56	-	-
-Pharmaceuticals:										
ASA 80	0.01	365	3.66	365	3.66	0.01	365	3.66	365	3.66
Clopidogrel	0.29	365	105.79	-	-	0.29	365	105.79	-	-
Metoprolol	0.01	365	4.61	365	4.61	0.01	365	4.61	365	4.61
Enoxaparin	3.72	1	3.72	-	-	3.72	1	3.72	-	-
Atorvastatin10	0.03	365	11.94	365	11.94	0.03	365	11.94	365	11.94
Ranitidine	0.02	30	0.60	-	-	0.02	30	0.60	-	-
Oxazepam	0.01	4	0.04	-	-	0.01	4	0.04	-	-
Captopril	0.01	4	0.05	-	-	0.01	4	0.05	-	-
Streptokinase	9.29	1	9.29	-	-	9.29	1	9.29	-	-
Drug dispensing fee	0.20	6	1.18	6	1.18	0.59	6	3.57	6	3.57
Total			566.85		59.74			1318.62		112.14

Table 4 Final results of different scenarios

Discount rate	Scenario	Cost (USD/Patient)				Effect (Per Patient)				Incremental results (Per Patient)			
		Governmental tariffs		Private tariffs		QALY		LYG		Inc-Cost/QALY		Inc-Cost/LYG	
		No-drug therapy	OTC statin	No-drug therapy	OTC statin	No-drug therapy	OTC statin	No-drug therapy	OTC statin	Governmental tariffs	Private tariffs	Governmental tariffs	Private tariffs
0 %	Base-case	214.70	652.05	445.21	830.02	26.37	26.77	33.82	34.29	1113.40	979.65	935.12	822.79
	ICS	261.18	676.05	543.45	896.28	25.84	26.31	33.13	33.69	884.99	752.65	736.79	626.62
	POM statin from 70	463.59	768.23	835.25	1107.22	26.50	26.80	33.98	34.34	1001.43	894.04	863.83	771.19
3 %	Base-case	110.71	384.95	231.85	477.97	16.56	16.74	20.71	20.91	1567.74	1407.00	1374.03	1233.16
	ICS	128.68	394.62	270.32	504.34	16.37	16.57	20.46	20.70	1309.20	1152.07	1131.89	996.04
	POM statin from 70	204.12	428.42	378.37	581.72	16.60	16.75	20.76	20.93	1526.75	1384.16	1369.28	1241.40
7.2 % for costs & 3 % for effects	Base-case	54.91	227.23	116.64	274.35	16.56	16.74	20.71	20.91	985.12	901.62	863.40	790.21
	ICS	59.31	229.65	126.25	281.06	16.37	16.57	20.46	20.70	838.56	762.14	724.99	658.92
	POM statin from 70	81.14	239.40	157.83	303.41	16.60	16.75	20.76	20.93	1077.21	990.87	966.11	888.68

use of statins for myocardial infarction (±10 %), secondary MI transition probabilities (±10 %), OTC statin tablet cost (±25 %), total MI and post-MI treatment costs (±20 %). Results from the PSA are presented as scatter plots of incremental cost-effectiveness ratios for QALY and LYG.

Results

Different scenarios were evaluated in this study including the base-case, ICS scenario, in which the primary transition probabilities were sourced from the ICS study, and a scenario in which patients in both groups received a POM statin for the primary prevention from 70 years of age. Also three different discount rates and two types of tariffs (governmental and private) were examined for each scenario. Table 4 shows the obtained results for these scenarios.

Figures 2, 3, 4 and 5 illustrate the Tornado charts for the one-way sensitivity analyses. The evaluated data and the examined range for each of them are shown in the

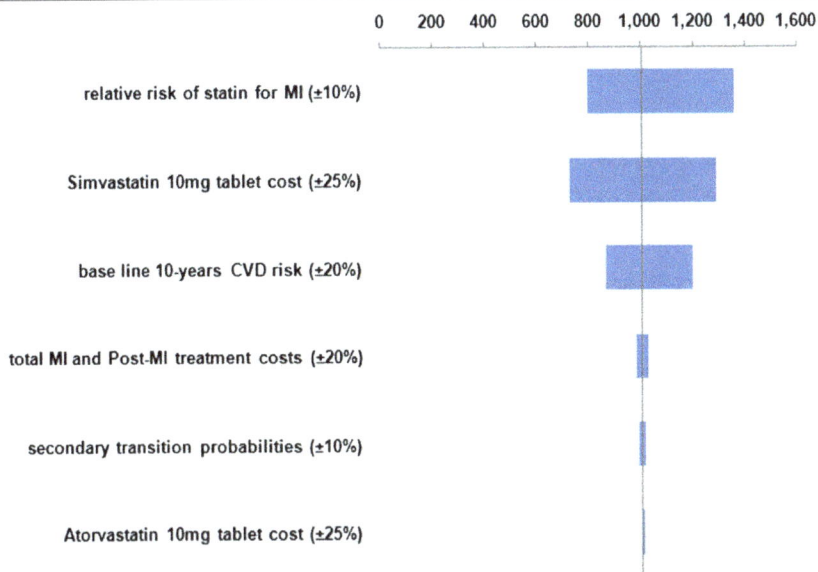

Fig. 2 Tornado chart for Incremental cost/QALY per patient (governmental tariffs)

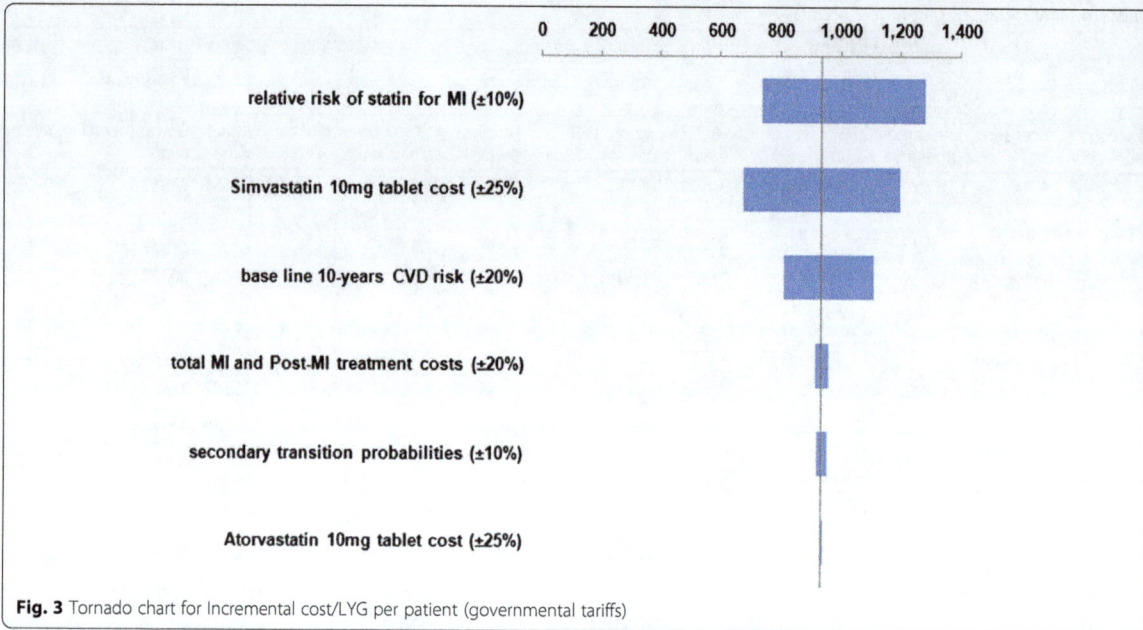

Fig. 3 Tornado chart for Incremental cost/LYG per patient (governmental tariffs)

charts. The Tornado charts show that the incremental-cost-effectiveness-ratios (ICERs) most affected by the relative risk of the use of statin and the cost of the OTC statin tablets.

Figures 6 and 7 for the probabilistic sensitivity analysis show that the use of OTC simvastatin 10 mg, compared with no-drug therapy for the primary prevention in 45-year men with a CVD 10-risk of 15 %, resulted in higher costs and more LYG and QALYs gained in all of the simulations. According to the probabilistic sensitivity analysis, estimated incremental cost per QALY gained and incremental cost per LYG are $1138 (95 % confidence interval [CI]: $797-$1595) and $960 (95 % confidence interval [CI]: $663-$1363), respectively. In addition, all the points comparing OTC simvastatin 10 mg with no-drug therapy for the primary prevention fell below the recommended threshold of WHO of GDP per capita (the reported GDP per capita by World bank for Iran in 2013

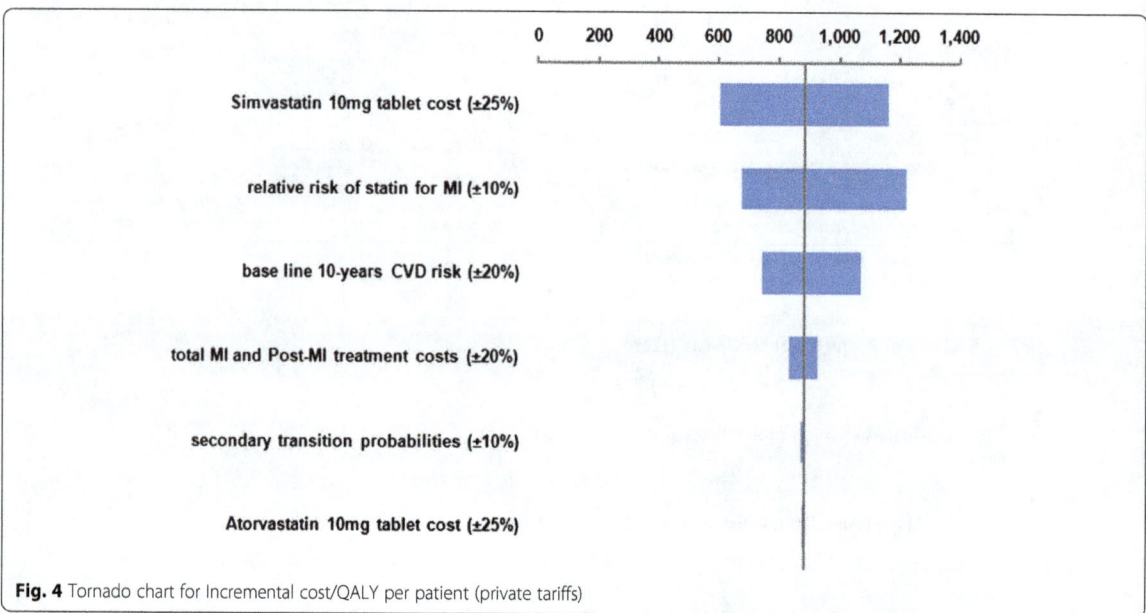

Fig. 4 Tornado chart for Incremental cost/QALY per patient (private tariffs)

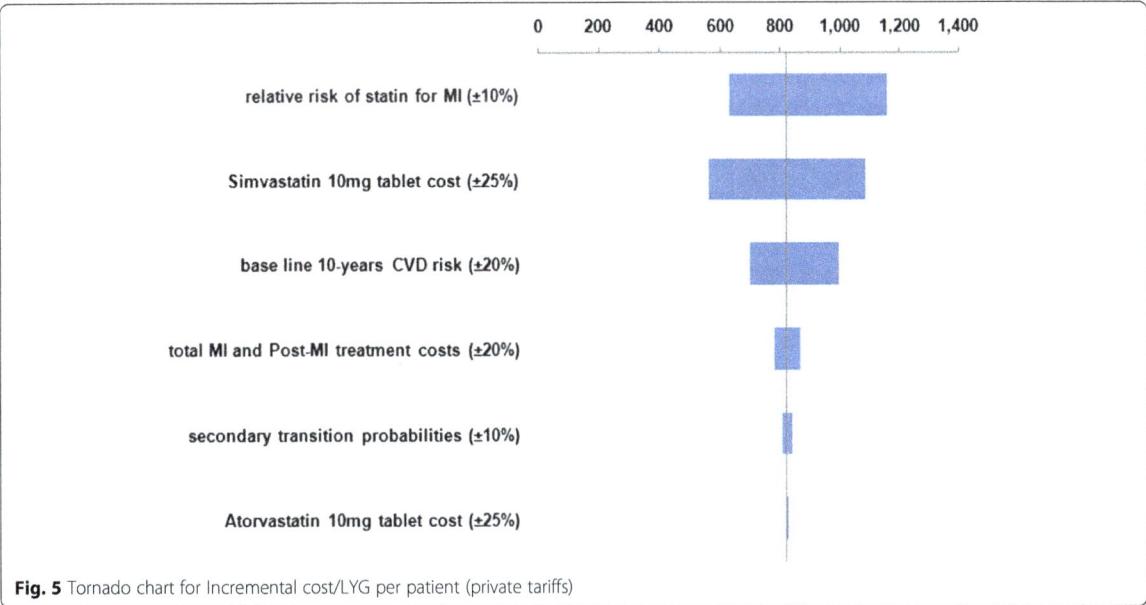

Fig. 5 Tornado chart for Incremental cost/LYG per patient (private tariffs)

($4763)) which means the intervention is highly cost-effective [28].

A cost-effectiveness acceptability curve (CEAC) illustrates the probability that an intervention is more cost-effective compared with the alternative intervention(s) over a range of ceiling values (λ), representing the willingness to pay (WTP) for an additional unit of effectiveness (such as $/QALY) [29, 30].

Figure 8 shows the CEAC for the base-case scenario, based on the QALY values for OTC statin therapy when compared to no-drug therapy.

This figure represents the traditional 'textbook' case of a CEAC in which OTC statin therapy is both more costly and more effective than no-drug therapy. As none of the pairs represent cost-saving the CEAC cuts the Y-axis at zero. Also as the whole density involves health gains the CEAC asymptotes to 1 [31].

A cross-over in acceptability between treatments is seen at a WTP of $240/QALY. This shows that the probability of no-drug therapy being more cost-effective than OTC statin therapy for the primary prevention of CVD is higher only if the WTP is less than this amount.

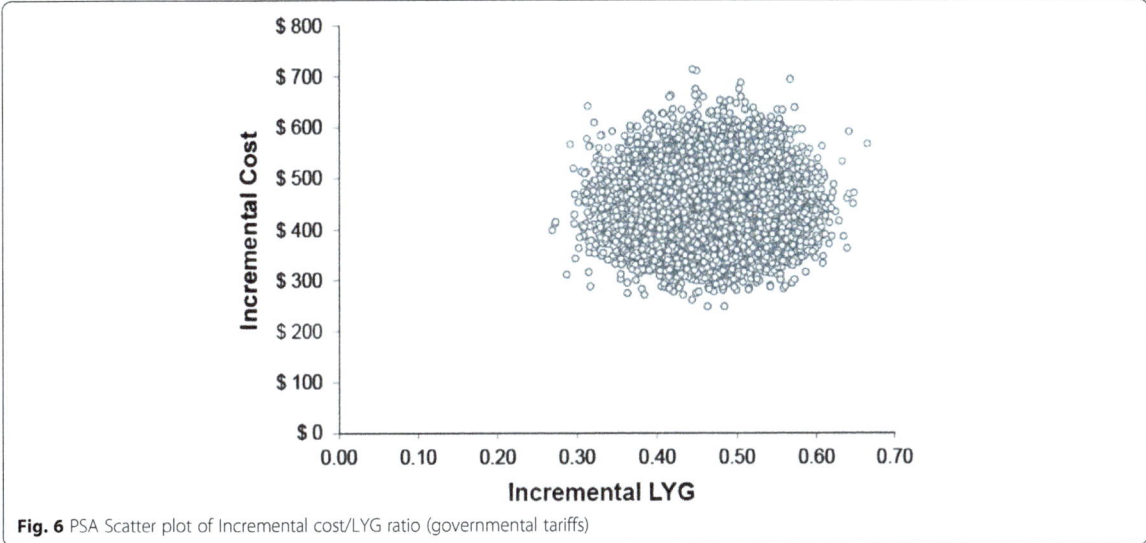

Fig. 6 PSA Scatter plot of Incremental cost/LYG ratio (governmental tariffs)

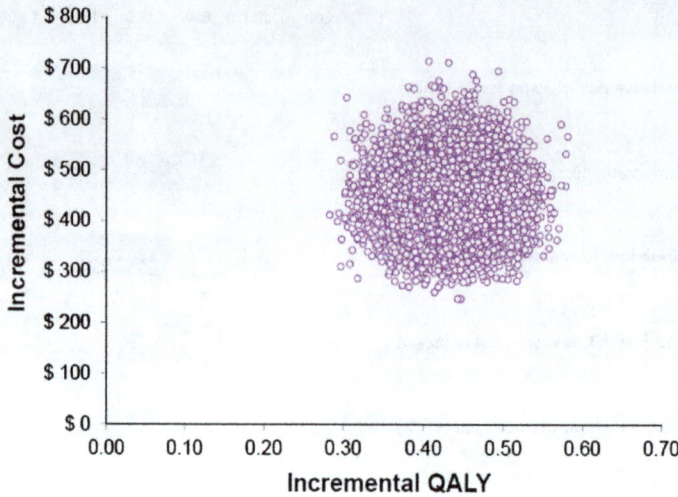

Fig. 7 PSA Scatter plot of Incremental cost/QALY ratio (governmental tariffs)

Discussion

There is extensive literature regarding the usefulness of the use of statins for the primary prevention of CVD. Considering the increasing risk of MI in the Iranian population, for the first time, we evaluated the cost-utility and cost-effectiveness of the use of an OTC low dose statin (simvastatin 10 mg) for the primary prevention of MI, among middle aged Iranian men with an average 10-year CVD risk.

We found that for the base-case scenario, simvastatin 10 mg had a cost-utility of $1113 per additional QALY ($979 with private tariffs) and a cost-effectiveness of $935 per additional LYG ($823 with private tariffs) for the primary prevention of MI in 45-year-old men with a 15 % 10-year CVD risk.

Although the total cost for health service is higher in private sector, the difference between intervention and no-intervention groups in private sector is less than the same difference in public sector.

The performed scenario analyses produced incremental costs of no more than $1568 per additional outcome per patient.

The results of PSA and one-way sensitivity analyses showed the robustness of our results.

We did not find any other study for the cost-effectiveness of the use of OTC statins in Iran. The results of our study is consistent with a previously published modeling study estimated an incremental QALYs of 0.06 (with a discount rate of 5 %) for the use of simvastatin 10 mg for primary prevention in a male

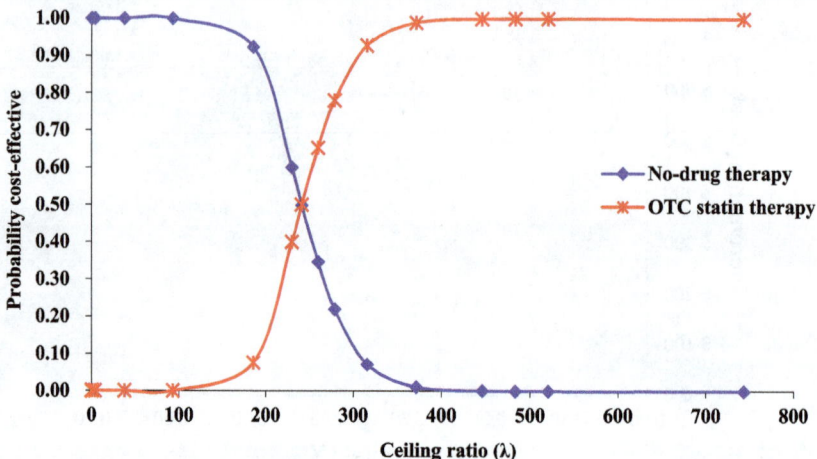

Fig. 8 CEAC for the base-case scenario (governmental tariffs)

patient with 15 % 10-year CVD risk. This study differs from ours in discounting rate, considered health states and treatment pathways [32].

No threshold has been determined in Iran for the cost-effectiveness of health-related interventions. However, considering the 2013 reported GDP per capita for Iran by World Bank ($4763) [28], the estimated ICERs of this study show that the evaluated intervention can be considered highly cost-effective according to WHO recommendations [33].

This analysis has several limitations. We adopted a payer's perspective and considered only direct medical costs due to limited data on indirect costs, as well as the existence of differences among patients in their socio-economic status and health insurance coverage. We did not model cardiovascular events other than MI and patients with cardiovascular risk factors such as hypertension or diabetes. Although we discounted the results in different scenarios, the effect of inflation was not taken into account. We also did not have male-specific data on costs. Due to the limitation of access to imported branded statins, only domestic generic statin costs were considered in the model. However, our model's use of probabilities varying with age, made it more realistic, although much more complex. We also attempted to deal with uncertainties by performing one-way and probabilistic sensitivity analyses and performing different scenarios.

As a final point, we believe that our modeling study has important implications for decision-makers in health practice and policy, particularly in Iran.

Competing interests
The authors declare that they have no competing interests.

Authors' contributions
MA made design of the study and the model, supervised whole study, contributed in acquisition and reviewing of data and interpretation of the results, revised the paper critically for important intellectual content, AH contributed in performing the model, acquisition and analysis of data, and drafting the article. All authors approved final version for submission.

Acknowledgement
The authors would like to thank Dr. Alireza Khosravi and Dr. Kian Heshmat for their expert opinions in estimating the treatment costs of this modeling study.

References
1. Thavendiranathan P, Bagai A, Brookhart MA, Choudhry NK. Primary prevention of cardiovascular diseases with statin therapy: a meta-analysis of randomized controlled trials. Arch Intern Med. 2006;166(21):2307–13.
2. Alwan A. Global status report on non-communicable diseases 2010. Geneva: World Health Organization (WHO); 2011.
3. Awad A, Al-Nafisi H. Public knowledge of cardiovascular disease and its risk factors in Kuwait: a cross-sectional survey. BMC public health. 2014;14(1):1131.
4. Reiner Ž. Statins in the primary prevention of cardiovascular disease. Nat Rev Cardiol. 2013;10(8):453–64.
5. Pichandi S, Pasupathi P, Rao YY, Farook J, Ambika A, Ponnusha BS. The role of statin drugs in combating cardiovascular diseases–A review. Int J Cur Sci Res. 2011;1(2):47–56.
6. Mason JC. Statins and their role in vascular protection. Clin Sci. 2003;105(3):251–66.
7. Karalis DG. Intensive lowering of low-density lipoprotein cholesterol levels for primary prevention of coronary artery disease. Mayo Clin Proc. 2009;84(4):345–52.
8. Michos ED, Blumenthal RS. Prevalence of low low-density lipoprotein cholesterol with elevated high sensitivity C-reactive protein in the US implications of the JUPITER (Justification for the Use of Statins in Primary Prevention: An Intervention Trial Evaluating Rosuvastatin) study. J Am Coll Cardiol. 2009;53(11):931–5.
9. Nash DB, Nash SA. Reclassification of simvastatin to over-the-counter status in the United Kingdom: a primary prevention strategy. Am J Cardiol. 2004;94(9):35–9.
10. Aghaeishahsavari M, Noroozianavval M, Veisi P, Parizad R, Samadikhah J. Cardiovascular disease risk factors in patients with confirmed cardiovascular disease. Saudi Med J. 2006;27(9):1358–61.
11. Cooper K, Brailsford S, Davies R. Choice of modelling technique for evaluating health care interventions. J Oper Res Soc. 2007;58(2):168–76.
12. Preedy VR, Watson RR. Handbook of disease burdens and quality of life measures. New York: Springer; 2010.
13. Berger ML, Bingefors K, Hedblom EC, Pashos C, Torrance GW. Health Care Cost, Quality and Outcomes, International Society for Pharmacoeconomics and Outcomes. New Jersey: Research Press; 2003.
14. Drummond M, Sculpher M, Torrance G, O'Brien B, Stoddart G. Economic evaluation using decision analytic modelling. Methods for the economic evaluation of health care programmes. 3rd ed. New York: Oxford University Press; 2005.
15. Sonnenberg FA, Beck JR. Markov models in medical decision making a practical guide. Med Decis Making. 1993;13(4):322–38.
16. Ward S, Jones ML, Pandor A, Holmes M, Ara R, Ryan A, Yeo W, Payne N. A systematic review and economic evaluation of statins for the prevention of coronary events. HTA. 2007; 11(14). http://dx.doi.org/10.3310/hta11140.
17. Evans C, Tavakoli M, Crawford B. Use of quality adjusted life years and life years gained as benchmarks in economic evaluations: a critical appraisal. Health Care Manag Sci. 2004;7(1):43–9.
18. National Collaborating Centre for Chronic Conditions. Hypertension: management in adults in primary care: pharmacological update. London: Royal College of Physicians; 2006.
19. NizalSarrafzadegan M, Sadeghi M, ShahramOveisgharan M, Marshall T. Incidence of cardiovascular diseases in an Iranian population: the Isfahan Cohort Study. Arch IranMed. 2013;16(3):138.
20. Greving J, Visseren F, de Wit G, Algra A. Statin treatment for primary prevention of vascular disease: whom to treat? Cost-effectiveness analysis. BMJ. 2011; doi:10.1136/bmj.d1672.
21. Edejer TT-T, Baltussen R, Adam T, Hutubessy R, Acharya A, Evans DB, et al. Making choice in health: WHO Guide to Cost-Effectiveness Analysis. Geneva: World Health Organization (WHO); 2003.
22. Abdoli G. Estimation of social discount rate for Iran. Eco Res Rev. 2009;10:135–56.
23. Smith SM, Campbell JD. Cost-effectiveness of renin-guided treatment of hypertension. Am J Hypertens. 2013;26(11):1303–10.
24. The Central Bank of Iran (CBI). Exchange Rates. 2015. http://www.cbi.ir/ExRates/rates_fa.aspx. Accessed 3 Jan 2015.
25. Ministry of Health and Medical Education. Tariff Book of Health Services. 2014. http://rvu.behdasht.gov.ir/index.aspx?fkeyid=&siteid=431&pageid=54142. Accessed 18 Oct 2014.
26. Isfahan University of Medical Sciences; Food and Drug Organization; Drugs price list. 2014. http://fdo.mui.ac.ir/index.php?option=com_content&view=category&layout=blog&id=245&Itemid=666. Accessed 17 Oct 2014.
27. Briggs A. Probabilistic analysis of cost-effectiveness models: statistical representation of parameter uncertainty. Value Health. 2005;8(1):1–2.
28. The World Bank; GDP per capita. 2014. http://data.worldbank.org/indicator/NY.GDP.PCAP.CD?display=default. Accessed 21 Jan 2015.
29. Claxton K, Sculpher M, McCabe C, Briggs A, Akehurst R, Buxton M, et al. Probabilistic sensitivity analysis for NICE technology assessment: not an optional extra. Health econ. 2005;14(4):339–47.
30. Briggs AH, Gray AM. Methods in health service research: Handling uncertainty in economic evaluations of healthcare interventions. BMJ. 1999;319(7210):635.
31. Fenwick E, O'Brien BJ, Briggs A. Cost-effectiveness acceptability curves–facts, fallacies and frequently asked questions. Health Econ. 2004;13(5):405–15.

32. Ribeiro RA, Duncan BB, Ziegelmann PK, Stella SF, Costa Vieira JL, Restelatto LF, Polanczyk CA. Cost-Effectiveness of High, Moderate and Low-Dose Statins in the Prevention of Vascular Events in the Brazilian Public Health System. Arq Bras Cardiol. 2014. doi:10.5935/abc.20140173

33. Marseille E., Larson B., Kazi D.S., Kahn J.G., Rosen S. Thresholds for the cost-effectiveness of interventions: alternative approaches. Bull World Health Organ. 2015;93:118–124. doi:2471/BLT.14.138206.

34. Hafshejani AM, Sarrafzadegan N, Attar Moghaddam HRB, Hosseini S, AsadiLari M. Predictive factors of survival in patients with an acute myocardial infarction among genders in Iran. J Isfahan Med Sch. 2012;30(209):1611–21.

35. Farkhani EM, Baneshi MR, Zolala F. Survival rate and its related factors in patients with acute myocardial infarction. Med J Mashhad Univ Med Sci. 2014;57(4):636–46.

36. Ghafarian SH, Javan AR, Hatamipoor E, Mousavizadeh A, Ghaedi H, Jabarinejad A, et al. Survival rate and its related factors in patients with acute myocardial infarction. ArmaghanDanesh. 2006;11(1):93–104.

37. Amani F, Hajizadeh E, Hoseinian F. Survival rate in MI patients. Koomesh. 2008;9(2):131–8.

38. Soltanian AR, Mahjub H, Goudarzi S, Nabi-Pour I, Jamali M. 5 Years Survival Rate in Patients with Myocardial Infarction in Bushehr. Sci Hamadan Univ Med Sci. 2009;16(3):33–7.

39. Statistical center of Iran, Selected Findings of the 2011 National Population and Housing Census. http://www.amar.org.ir/Portals/1/Iran/census-2.pdf (2012). Accessed 22 May 2014.

40. Ministry of Interior; National organization for civil registration; Statistical year book 1390. http://www.sabteahval.ir (2011). Accessed 23 May 2014.

19

Effect of peptide length on the conjugation to the gold nanoparticle surface

Fatemeh Ramezani[1], Mostafa Habibi[2], Hashem Rafii-Tabar[1] and Massoud Amanlou[2*]

Abstract

Background: Gold nanoparticles now command a great deal of attention for medical applications. Despite the importance of nano-bio interfaces, interaction between peptides and proteins with gold surfaces is not still fully understood, especially in a molecular level.

Methods: In the present study computational simulation of adsorption of 20 amino acids, in three forms of mono-amino acid, homo di-peptide and homo tri-peptide, on the gold nanoparticles was performed by Gromacs using OPLSAA force field. The flexibility, stability, and size effect of the peptides on the gold nanoparticles were studied as well as the molecular structure of them.

Results: According to our results, adsorbed homo tri-peptides on the gold surface had more flexibility, more gyration, and the farthest distance from the GNP in comparison with homo di-peptides and mono-amino acids.

Conclusion: Our findings provide new insights into the precise control of interactions between amino acids anchored on the GNPs.

Keywords: Gold nanoparticles, Interface, Amino acid, Interaction, Molecular dynamic

Background

Both natural processes and biotechnological applications involve the interaction of polypeptides with solid surfaces. For example, the growth of hard tissue is regulated by protein-mineral interactions and the adhesion of organisms to solid supports depends on protein–surface interactions [1]. Gold nanoparticle (GNP) is one of nanomaterials attracted a great deal of attention in medical sciences because of their biocompatibility and ability to conjugate to organic compounds and bio-molecules which make them useful in biochemical sensing and detection [2]. Besides, amino acids are used in bio-functionalization of GNPs as protective layers and they are used for assemble of GNPs [3].

The interface between GNP and amino acids is an important issue in bio-catalysis and biosensor designing [4,5]. Despite the critical importance of nano-bio interfaces,

the mechanism of binding of proteins and peptides to surfaces is not still fully understood, especially in a molecular level [1]. While finding actual experimental data for describing and visualizing protein/surface conjugates is difficult, molecular dynamic simulations open a new way to a better understanding of structure and dynamics of even individual atoms [6,7].

In 2007, with the help of molecular dynamic (MD) simulations and COMPASS force field, Zhen Xu et al. showed histidine and histidine containing peptide adsorption behavior on gold surface [5]. In 2010, using GOLP force field, amino acids conformation on the gold surface was founded by Martin Hoefling et al. [7] and also in 2011; they showed the interaction of beta-sheet peptides with a gold surface and found that adsorption occurs in a stepwise mechanism [8].

In 2012, using MD simulation, Lee and Ytreberg explored effect of the GNP conjugation on six different peptides [6]. They showed peptides dynamic and structure depends on the amino acids sequence. In the last paper our group compared 20 natural amino acids interaction

* Correspondence: amanlou@tums.ac.ir
[2]Department of Medicinal Chemistry, Faculty of Pharmacy and Pharmaceutical Sciences Research Center, Tehran University of Medical Sciences, Tehran, Iran
Full list of author information is available at the end of the article

with gold nanoparticle by molecular dynamic [9]. Next, we continue to understand the impact of peptide lengths on their adsorption, their flexibility and stability while interacting with GNPs from the molecular level point of view. We compared homo mono, di and tri- amino acids adsorption on the gold nanoparticle surface. Tri-peptides serve as model systems for understanding the so-called random-coil state of peptides and proteins [10].

Methods

20 different systems were used for this study (Table 1). Each system contains one kind of amino acid in mono, homo di-, and tri-peptides forms (Figure 1): $3 \times 3 \times 3$ nm^3 cubic shape GNP (111) was built of 2048 atoms by Hyperchem 8.0.3 software. GNP kept its cubic shape after 10 ns simulation time. In a previous study by our group, the effect of the size of nanoparticle was examined and it was found that the cubic nanoparticle size makes no difference on the interaction of amino acids [9]. So in this study GNP size was considered 3 nm.

Peptides and GNP were solvated in a 50 Å^3 length cubic water box. The distance between the peptides and the box edge was 9 Å. Then each system was ionized with 0.15 mol/l ion concentration using a mixture of Na$^+$ and Cl$^-$ ions such that each system had zero net charge. All simulation conditions were set, (normal saline, pH = 7.4, Temperature = 27°C), and kept constant during the simulation.

All simulations were performed in TIP3P water model [11,12]. During the simulation, periodic boundary conditions were applied in all three dimensions. All simulations were performed using Gromacs 4.6.3 software package [13] and OPLSAA force field [14,15]. Despite the perfect force fields such as Sutton-Chen are used for simulation of metals but it was not appropriate for investigating the interaction of metal with peptides. Among several force fields for peptide-gold interactions that have been reported in the literature (e.g. [16-18]) we used OPLSAA force field and gold atom parameters were taken from Hendrik Heinz et al. where $r_0 = 2.951$ Å and $\varepsilon_0 = 5.29$ kcal/mol [19]. As can be find in Hendrik Heinz results, these parameters can be implemented in the OPLS-AA force field and applied to the simulation of

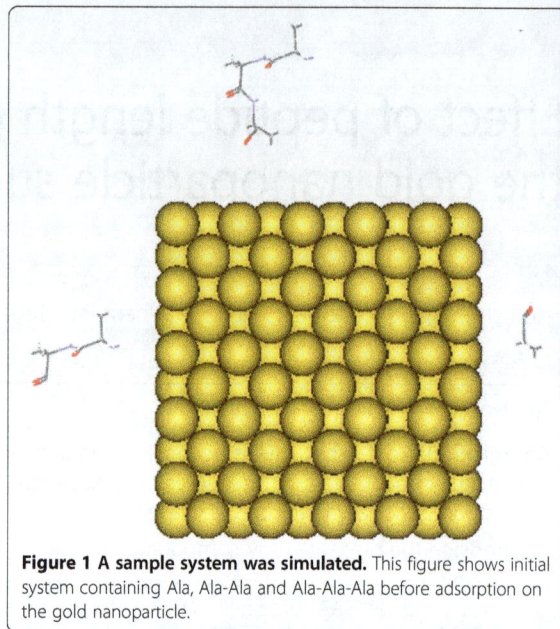

Figure 1 A sample system was simulated. This figure shows initial system containing Ala, Ala-Ala and Ala-Ala-Ala before adsorption on the gold nanoparticle.

GNPs and their interfaces with water, biopolymers, organic, and inorganic molecules. Using these parameters, we can consider all gold atoms in a dynamic mode [19]. This LJ models for fcc metals can be implemented in force fields such as AMBER, CHARMM, COMPASS, CVFF, OPLS-AA, PCFF, and applied to the simulation of metals and their interfaces with water, biopolymers, organic molecules, and inorganic components. This LJ models for fcc metals are typically an order of magnitude more accurate than previous LJ parameters due to the physical interpretation of the quantities r_0 and ε_0 in terms of the metal density and the surface tension of the {111} crystal face under standard conditions [19]. During the simulation, center of mass position is fixed.

Discovery Studio 2.1 [20] was used for the preparation of snapshots. Minimization was performed for 100 ps and followed by a 1.0 ns of dynamic simulation in the NPT ensemble and an 8.0 ns dynamic simulation in the NVT ensemble at T = 300 °K. A Nose'-Hoover thermostat was utilized for simulation processes to enforce the

Table 1 Amino acid sequences were considered for simulation in this study

1. Ala, Ala-Ala, Ala-Ala-Ala	2. Val, Val-Val, Val-Val-Val	3. Asp, Asp-Asp, Asp-Asp-Asp
4. Gly, Gly-Gly, Gly-Gly-Gly	5. Ser, Ser-Ser, Ser-Ser-Ser	6. Asn, Asn-Asn, Asn-Asn-Asn
7. Thr, Thr-Thr, Thr-Thr-Thr	8. Pro, Pro-Pro, Pro-Pro-Pro	9. Lys, Lys-Lys, Lys-Lys-Lys
10. Gln, Gln-Gln, Gln-Gln-Gln	11. His, His-His, His-His-His	12. Trp, Trp-Trp, Trp-Trp-Trp
13. Arg, Arg-Arg, Arg-Arg-Arg	14. Phe, Phe-Phe, Phe-Phe-Phe	15. Cys, Cys-Cys, Cys-Cys-Cys
16. Leu, Leu-Leu, Leu-Leu-Leu	17. Tyr, Tyr-Tyr, Tyr-Tyr-Tyr	18. Ile, Ile-Ile, Ile-Ile-Ile
19. Glu, Glu-Glu, Glu-Glu-Glu	20. Met, Met-Met, Met-Met-Met	

desired temperatures [21]. The LINKS algorithm was implemented to allow 8×10^{-4} ps time step [22]. The long-range electrostatic interactions were accounted for using the Ewald method with a real-space cut-off of 12 Å. Vander Waals interactions were cut off at 12 Å with a switching function between 10 and 12 Å.

Results and discussion
Root mean square deviation (RMSD)
Root mean square deviation (RMSD) (Eq. (1)) showed the calculated system equilibrations as follows [23]:

$$RMSD(t_1, t_2) = \left[\frac{1}{N} \sum_{i=1}^{N} m_i \| r_i(t_1) - r_i(t_2) \| \right]^{\frac{1}{2}} \quad (1)$$

Where N is the number of target molecules; and ri (t) is the position of molecule i at time t. The analysis of the RMSD graph of alpha carbons during the adsorption of amino acids on the GNP showed that all systems were stable after 2 ns (Additional file 1: Figure S1). This indicated that systems remained stable during the simulation. In Ser and Tyr, the hydroxyl group of side chain and in His and Pro, the ring of side chains constantly fluctuated on the surface of GNP which caused RMSD value increased related to the other amino acids. Only His homo di-peptide placed farther than its homo tri-peptides.

In the last paper published by our group we showed mono amino acids conformations after adsorption on the GNP surface [9]. Our results for Met, Cys, Pro, Phe, Gly and Leu were matched with the experimental results reported by Podstawka et al. In the current work we found di and tri- amino acids conformation after adsorption on the gold surface. These results and comparison with conformation of mono-amino acids were shown in Additional file 2. Our results for Met, Cys, Pro, Phe, Gly di-peptide interactions with gold atoms are also consistent with the experimental results reported by Podstawka et al. [24]. According to the experimental results Met-Met and Cys-Cys interaction with GNP is through sulphur atom that is near to our results. According to the Additional file 2, Gly-Gly adsorption was through –COOH group that is accordance with experimental results. In our simulation results and Podstawka experimental results Phe-Phe, aromatic rings had a main role in adsorption on the gold surface.

In all amino acids except Pro, interacting group with GNP in homo mono-, di-, and tri-peptides didn't change. Pro interaction in mono-amino acid and homo di-peptide is through N atom. But according to our result by increasing the length of prolin to homo tri-peptide, spatial limitation of left-handed 3(1)-helix conformation of tri-prolin didn't allow the N atoms to come near the GNPs surface.

Flexibility of peptides after adsorption on the GNP
Atomic fluctuations were studied using the root-mean square fluctuations (RMSF) analysis [19]. Additional file 2 indicates the last frame of adsorption of peptides on the GNP and the RMSF per residue of homo mono-, di-, and tri-peptides. Almost in all systems, fluctuations of homo tri- peptides were more than homo di-peptides and fluctuations of homo di-peptides were more pronounced than mono-amino acids. Therefore it can be concluded that increasing the peptide length increases the fluctuation. The exception is homo tri-peptide of Arg, Asp and Cys that has lower fluctuation than its homo di-peptide and mono-amino acid. The comparison of the 20 systems revealed that homo tri-peptides with aromatic rings which include Tyr, Phe, Trp have more and Pro has the lowest fluctuations than the other amino acids. Rigidity of the poly-proline reduces the degrees of freedom [25]. In outcome, increasing the aromatic rings in the structure of peptides increases the fluctuation of peptides on the GNP surface.

Compactness of peptides
In order to have a rough measure of the compactness of a structure, we calculated the radius of gyration as follows (Eq. (2)):

$$R_g = \left(\frac{\sum i \| r_i \|^2 m_i}{\sum i \, m_i} \right)^{\frac{1}{2}} \quad (2)$$

Where m_i is the mass of atom i; and r_i is the position of atom i about the centre of mass of the molecule.

Additional file 3 displays the time evolution of radius of gyration (Rg) for homo mono-, di-, and tri-peptides. According to the Rg trajectory and the comparison between the 20 systems, amino acids were divided into three groups. The first group includes Trp, Phe, Tyr, Arg, and Lys which have the most compactness. The second group encompasses Asp, Glu, Met, Leu, His, and Gln. The third, finally, includes Val, Ala, Gly, Asn, Thr, Ser, Pro, Ile, and Cys that have the lowest compactness than two other groups. Among all the amino acids, Arg had the most compactness which may be due to its more linear structure compared to other homo tri-peptides.

Distance of peptides from the GNP
Calculating and comparing peptides center of mass distances from the center of mass of GNP showed homo tri-peptides that have more flexibility on the GNP, fall farthest away from the nanoparticles. Most of homo di-peptides were also farther than mono-amino acids than the GNP (Additional file 1: Figure S2).

Conclusions

Amino acids are used for, both in functionalizing of GNPs and in cross-linking of amino acid capped GNPs [26]. Because of the importance of studying the interface between amino acids and GNP, in this study, 20 common amino acid interactions with GNP were performed by a computational simulation. In this paper, we have considered a square-shaped gold nanoparticle. Certainly the interaction of amino acids with surface and the defects on the GNP are different, but the aim of this study was to evaluate the effect of the peptide length from one to three amino acids on their binding to the GNP surface.

Lee and Ytreberg showed presence of GNP alter both the peptide structures and dynamics, and that the magnitude of the effect depends on the peptide sequence [6]. Conjugated peptides typically have decreased conformational flexibility, and the amount of decrease depends on the amino acid sequence. In this study we showed that GNP effects in addition to sequencing, it also depends on the length of the peptides. Homo tri-peptides that were adsorbed on the GNP surface have more flexibility, further radius of gyration, and fall in the farthest distance from the GNP, compared with homo mono and di-peptides.

Aromatic rings in amino acids made them more fluctuating on the GNP surface. These results can be used in amino acids usage as a linker on the GNPs.

These findings improve nanofabrication methods for immobilization of amino acids and proteins on the GNP at molecular precision to control both lateral and perpendicular orientations of peptides, the size, and the kind of amino acids on the GNP.

Additional files

Additional file 1: Due to the large number of figures in the manuscript, RMSD of amino acids and their distance from the gold surface has been shown in Additional file 1.

Additional file 2: Amino acids last snapshot and RMSF. This figure indicates peptides last frame snapshots (left column), root mean square fluctuations (RMSF) per atom about the time-averaged structure (right column) for mono-amino acids (black line), homo di-peptides (green line) and homo tri-peptides (red line).

Additional file 3: Amino acids radius of gyration. Graphs indicate Rg-time of mono-amino acids (black line), dipeptides (green line) and tripeptides (red line) on the GNP. In the images can be seen in all amino acids, with increasing the peptide lengths, they were farther away from the gold surface.

Competing interests

The authors declare that they have no competing interests.

Authors' contributions

All authors contributed to the design of study. FR and MH performed all computational experiments, data analyzes and write the manuscript. MA is responsible for the study registration and financial support. The guidance of the HR was used in understanding of the basic physical concepts. All authors read and approved the final version.

Acknowledgements

This paper is part of a Pharm. D. thesis by Mostafa Habibi and PhD thesis in nanomedicine by Fatemeh Ramezani. This study was supported by a grant from the Research Council of Tehran University of Medical Sciences.

Author details

[1]Department of Medical Physics and Biomedical Engineering, Shahid Beheshti University of Medical Sciences, Tehran, Iran. [2]Department of Medicinal Chemistry, Faculty of Pharmacy and Pharmaceutical Sciences Research Center, Tehran University of Medical Sciences, Tehran, Iran.

References

1. Cohavi O, Reichmann D, Abramovich R, Tesler A, Bellapadrona G, Kokh DB, et al. A quantitative, real-time assessment of binding of peptides and proteins to gold surfaces. Chem Eur J. 2011;17:1327–36.
2. Rai S, Kumar S, Singh H. A theoretical study on interaction of proline with gold cluster. Mater Sci. 2012;35:291–5.
3. Majzik A, Fülöp L, Csapó E, Bogár F, Martinek T, Penke B, et al. Functionalization of gold nanoparticles with amino acid, beta-amyloid peptides and fragment. Colloids Surf B. 2010;81:235–41.
4. Kumara S, Ganesan S. Preparation and characterization of gold nanoparticles with different capping agent preparation and characterization of gold nanoparticles with different capping agents. Int J Green Nanotechnol. 2011;3:47–55.
5. Xu Z, Yuan S, Yan H, Liu C. Adsorption of histidine and histidine-containing peptides on Au (1 1 1): a molecular dynamics study. Colloids Surf A Physicochem Eng Aspects. 2011;380:135–42.
6. Lee K, Ytreberg F. Effect of gold nanoparticle conjugation on peptide dynamics and structure. Entropy. 2012;14:630–41.
7. Hoefling M, Iori F, Corni S, Gottschalk K. The conformations of amino acids on a gold (111) surface. Chem Phys Chem. 2010;11:1763–7.
8. Hoefling M, Monti S, Corni S, Gottschalk K. Interaction of b-Sheet Folds with a Gold Surface. PLoS ONE. 2011;7:e20925.
9. Ramezani F, Amanlou M, Rafii-Tabar H. Comparison of amino acids interaction with gold nanoparticle. Amino Acids. 2014;46:911–20.
10. Schweitzer-Stenner R, Eker F, Perez A, Griebenow K, Cao X, Nafie L. The structure of tri-proline in water probed by polarized Raman, Fourier transform infrared, vibrational circular dichroism, and electric ultraviolet circular dichroism spectroscopy. Biopolymers. 2003;71:558–68.
11. Mark P, Nilsson L. Structure and Dynamics of the TIP3P, SPC, and SPC/E Water Models at 298 K. J Phys Chem A. 2001;105:9954–60.
12. Guillot B. A reappraisal of what we have learnt during three decades of computer simulations on water. J Mol Liq. 2002;101:219–60.
13. Spoel D, Lindahl E, Hess B, Groenhof G, Mark A, Berendsen H. GROMACS: fast, flexible, and free. J Comput Chem. 2005;26:1701–18.
14. Kahn K, Bruice T. Parameterization of OPLS-AA force field for the conformational analysis of macro cyclic polypeptides. J Comput Chem. 2002;23:977–96.
15. Jorgensen W, Tirado-Rives J. The OPLS force field for proteins. Energy minimizations for crystals of cyclic peptides and crambin. J Am Chem Soc. 1998;110:1657–66.
16. Verde A, Acres J, Maranas J. Investigating the specificity of peptide adsorption on gold using molecular dynamics simulations. Biomacromolecules. 2009;10:2118–28.
17. Miao L, Seminario J. Molecular dynamics simulations of the vibrational signature transfer from a glycine peptide chain to nanosized gold clusters. J Phys Chem C. 2007;111:8366–71.
18. Iori F, Felice R, Molinari E, Corni S. GolP: an atomistic force-field to describe the interaction of proteins with Au (111) surfaces in water. J Comput Chem. 2009;30:1465–76.
19. Heinz H, Vaia R, Farmer B, Naik R. Accurate simulation of surfaces and interfaces of face-centered cubic metals using 12–6 and 9–6 Lennard-Jones potentials. J Phys Chem C. 2008;112:17281–90.
20. Accelrys Software Inc.: Discovery Studio Modeling Environment, Release 4.0, San Diego: Accelrys Software Inc., 2013.
21. Hunenberger P. Thermostat algorithms for molecular dynamics simulations. Adv Polymer Sci. 2005;173:105–49.

22. Hess B, Bekker H, Berendsen H, Fraaije J. LINCS: a linear constraint solver for molecular simulations. J Comp Chem. 1997;18:1463–72.

23. Yang Z, Zhao Y. Adsorption of His-tagged peptide to Ni, Cu and Au (1 0 0) surfaces: molecular dynamics simulation. Eng Anal Bound Elem. 2007;31:402–9.

24. Podstawka E, Ozaki Y, Proniewicz LM. Part III: surface-enhanced Raman scattering of amino acids and their homodipeptide monolayers deposited onto colloidal gold surface. Appl Spectrosc. 2005;59:1516–26.

25. Kay B, Williamson M, Sudol M. The importance of being proline: the interaction of proline-rich motifs in signaling proteins with their cognate domains. The FASEB J. 2000;14:231–41.

26. Brevern A, Bornot A, Craveur P, Etchebest C, Gelly J. Flexibility and local structure prediction from sequence. Nucleic Acids Res. 2012;40:W317–22.

20

Synthesis, HIV-1 RT inhibitory, antibacterial, antifungal and binding mode studies of some novel N-substituted 5-benzylidine-2,4-thiazolidinediones

Radhe Shyam Bahare[1*], Swastika Ganguly[1], Kiattawee Choowongkomon[2] and Supaporn Seetaha[2]

Abstract

Background: Structural modifications of thiazolidinediones at 3rd and 5th position have exhibited significant biological activities. In view of the facts, and based on *in silico* studies carried out on thiazolidine-2,4-diones as HIV-1- RT inhibitors, a novel series of 2,4-thiazolidinedione analogs have been designed and synthesized.

Methods: Title compounds were prepared by the reported method. Conformations of the structures were assigned on the basis of results of different spectral data. The assay of HIV-1 RT was done as reported by Silprasit *et al.* Antimicrobial activity was determined by two fold serial dilution method. Docking study was performed for the highest active compounds by using Glide 5.0.

Results: The newly synthesized compounds were evaluated for their HIV-1 RT inhibitory activity. Among the synthesized compounds, compound **24** showed significant HIV-1 RT inhibitory activity with 73% of inhibition with an IC_{50} value of 1.31 μM. Compound **10** showed highest activity against all the bacterial strains. A molecular modeling study was carried out in order to investigate the possible interactions of the highest active compounds **24**, **10** and **4** with the non nucleoside inhibitory binding pocket(NNIBP) of RT, active site of GlcN-6-P synthase and cytochrome P450 14-α-sterol demethylase from *Candida albicans* (*Candida* P450DM) as the target receptors respectively using the Extra Precision (XP) mode of Glide software.

Conclusion: A series of novel substituted 2-(5-benzylidene-2,4-dioxothiazolidin-3-yl)-N-(phenyl)propanamides (**4–31**) have been synthesized and evaluated for their HIV-1 RT inhibitory activity, antibacterial and antifungal activities. Some of the compounds have shown significant activity. Molecular docking studies showed very good interaction.

Keywords: Antibacterial, Antifungal, Docking, HIV-1 RT inhibitory activity, Thiazolidinediones, Synthesis

Background

The thiazolidinedione scaffold has been identified to play an essential role in medicinal chemistry [1,2]. Compounds containing the thiazolidinedione moiety have been found to exhibit a wide range of biological activities viz., antihyperglycemic [3], anti-inflammatory [4], antimalarial [5], antioxidant [6], antitumor [7], cytotoxic [8], antimicrobial [9], antiproliferative [10], MurD ligase inhibitor [11], monoamine oxidase B (MAO-B) inhibitor [12] neuroprotective [13], COX-2 inhibitor [14] and chemotherapeutic activities [15]. Recently, a novel series of thiazolidin-4-ones

have emerged as selective NNRTIs [16]. However not much work has been reported on thiazolidine –2,4- diones as HIV-1-RT inhibitors.

HIV is the causative organism for AIDS and is continuously evolving and rapidly spreading throughout the world as a global infection. The HIV infection targets the monocytes expressing surface CD4 receptors and produces profound defects in cell-mediated immunity [17]. Overtime infection leads to severe depletion of CD4 T-lymphocytes (T-cells) resulting in opportunistic infections like tuberculosis (TB), fungal, viral, protozoal and neoplastic diseases and ultimately death [18].

Reverse transcription of the single-stranded (+) RNA genome into double-stranded DNA is an essential step in the HIV-1 replication life-cycle and requires the concerted

* Correspondence: radhe118@gmail.com
[1]Department of Pharmaceutical Sciences, Birla Institute of Technology, Mesra, Ranchi 835215, Jharkhand, India
Full list of author information is available at the end of the article

function of both the DNA polymerase and ribonuclease H (RNase H) active sites of HIV-1 reverse transcriptase (RT). Due to its essential role in HIV-1 replication, RT is a major target for anti-HIV drug development and two classes of inhibitors, (1) the nucleoside and nucleotide RT inhibitors and (2) the nonnucleoside RT inhibitors (NNRTIs) have been approved by the United States Food and Drug Administration (FDA) for the treatment of HIV-1 infection [19]. Though the NNRTIs are effective and generally well-tolerated in the majority of patients, treatment durability is limited by drug-related side effects and rapid emergence of resistance among HIV isolates. Thus, the therapeutic efficacy of NNRTIs is mainly restricted due to development of viral resistance to NNRTIs associated with mutations that include K103N, L100I and Y188L, and with the development of second generation NNRTIs, the search for a more suitable NNRTI, which blocks the replication of all existing resistant viral strains and retains potency for longer periods of time by modifying the existing drug classes or by incorporating appropriate substitutions in the newer chemical scaffolds, according to the pharmacophoric requirements using multi-disciplinary approaches is the call of the day.

With the advent of AIDS and as a result of promiscuous use of drug therapy, antibacterial cytotoxins, steroids, or due to underlying disease or medical manipulation the normal defenses conferred by the microbial flora breaks down resulting in the prevalence of opportunistic bacterial and fungal infections. Bacterial diseases such as tuberculosis, typhus, plague, diphtheria, typhoid fever, cholera, dysentery and pneumonia have taken a high toll on humanity [20]. Along with this prevalence of multi-drug resistant microbial pathogens as an important and challenging therapeutic problem and therefore a search for newer antibacterial agents is the call of the day [21].

Opportunistic fungal infections have emerged as important causes of morbidity and mortality in immunocompromised patients and such infections include candidiasis, aspergillosis and mucormycosis [22]. A dramatic increase in invasive fungal infections over the past decade has been observed [23]. To overcome these problems, the development of new and safe antifungal agents with higher selectivity and lower toxicity is urgently required.

Glucosamine-6-phosphate synthase (GlcN-6-P synthase, L-glutamine:D-fructose-6P amidotransferase), is a new target for antibacterials [24] and antifungals [25]. GlcN-6-P synthase catalyzes the first step in hexosamine metabolism, converting fructose 6-phosphate into glucosamine 6-phosphate (GlcN6P) in the presence of glutamine. The reaction catalyzed by GlcN-6-P synthase is irreversible, and is therefore considered as a committed step. The end product of the pathway, N-acetyl glucosamine, is an essential building block of bacterial and fungal cell walls.

Recent modeling studies report that azoles may be acting as antimicrobials by inhibition of GlcN-6-P synthase [24].

The fungal cell wall, a structure essential to fungi and lacking in mammalian cells, is an obvious target for antifungal agents. Its major macromolecular components are chitin, ß-glucan, and mannoproteins [26]. In fungi, lanosterol 14-α-demethylase, a member of the cytochrome P450 superfamily, is an essential requirement for fungal viability. Azoles inhibit fungal cytochrome P-450 14-α-demethylase (DM) which is responsible for the conversion of lanosterol to ergosterol leading to the depletion of ergosterol in the fungal cell membrane [27-29]. Thus cytochrome P-450DM plays a key role in fungal sterol biosynthetic pathways, and this has been an important target for design of potent antifungals [30].

Structural modifications of thiazolidinediones at 3rd and 5th position have exhibited significant biological activities [31]. In view of the mentioned above facts, and based on *in silico* studies carried out on thiazolidine 2,4-diones as HIV-1- RT inhibitors [32], a novel series of 2,4-thiazolidinedione analogs have been designed based on the pharmacophoric model of NNRTIs 18 with the thiazolidinedione moiety attached to the propionamide moiety ($-CH_2-CH_2-CO-NH-$) constituting the "body (hydrophilic)" flanked by aryl rings (hydrophobic) linked to the 3rd and 5th position of the thiazolidinedione ring and to that of substituted aromatic amines as the "wings" to enhance the hydrophobicity of the molecules (Figure 1).

Herein we wish to report the synthesis of newer thiazolidine-2,4- diones, which have been evaluated for anti-HIV, antibacterial and antifungal activities. Binding mode analyses for the compounds with the highest HIV-1- RT inhibitory activity, antibacterial and antifungal activities have been carried out to understand the pharmacophoric features responsible for these activities.

Experimental
Materials
Synthetic studies

All reagents were purchased from commercial suppliers like Sigma Aldrich, Merck India Ltd., Himedia and Rankem chemicals. All reagents were GR or AR grade and were used without purification. The purity and homogeneity of the compounds were assessed by the TLC performed on Merck silica gel 60 F_{254} aluminium sheets using chloroform: methanol (9:1) as eluents. Iodine chamber and Shimadzu (UV-254) spectrometer were used for visualization of TLC spots. Ashless Whatmann No.1 filter paper was used for vacuum filtration. Melting points were determined on an SRS Opti-melting point automatic apparatus and were uncorrected. Elemental data of C, H and N were within ±0.4% of the theortical value as determined by Perkin Elmer Model 240 analyzer. IR spectra (KBr disc/or pallets) were recorded on SHIAMADZU FT/IR 8400 and

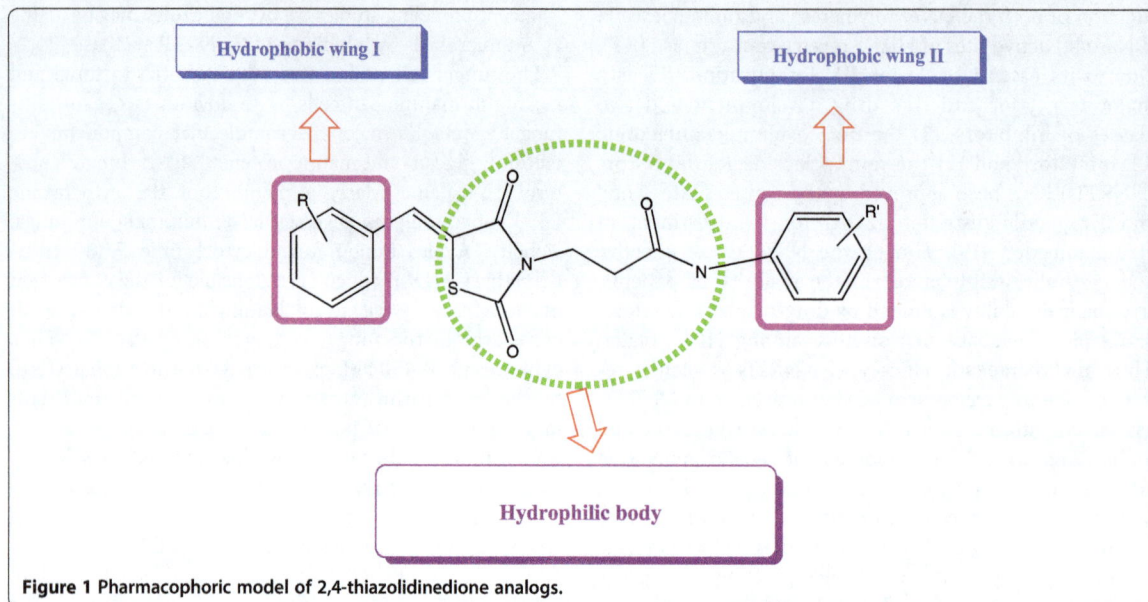

Figure 1 Pharmacophoric model of 2,4-thiazolidinedione analogs.

were reported in cm.$^{-1}$ ^{1}H-NMR and ^{13}C NMR spectra were respectively recorded at 400 and 100 MHz with BRUKER Advance Digital Spectrophotometer. Chemical shifts are expressed in δ-values (ppm) relative to TMS as an internal standard, using DMSO-d$_6$. Chemical shifts are expressed in δ-values (ppm) relative to TMS as an internal standard, using DMSO-d$_6$ and Mass spectra were recorded with a AZILANT Q-TOF Micromass LC-MS by using (ESI+).

Methods

General Procedure for the preparation of compounds (4–31)

Compounds 4–31 were synthesized as per the reported procedure [33]. Substituted 5-benzylidene-2,4-thiazolidinediones (2a-l) (0.01 mol) and the corresponding 3-chloro-N-phenylpropanamides (3a-l) (0.01 mol) were dissolved in 20 ml of acetonitrile. 0.02 mol of triethylamine was added dropwise to this solution with stirring. The reaction mixture was refluxed for 12 h, evaporated in rotary evaporator, cooled and poured into crushed ice and then basified with solid potassium carbonate. The resulting precipitate was filtered, washed with water (3 × 100 ml) and further washed with n-hexane (3 × 20 ml). The solid residue obtained was recrystallized from methanol to yield the desired compounds.

Thiazolidine-2,4-dione (1)
IR (KBr) cm^{-1}: 3132 (NH stretching), 1741, 1681, 1586 (C = O), ^{1}H-NMR (DMSO-d$_6$, 400 MHz): 12.50 (s; 1H; NH), 4.39 (2H, s, CH$_2$).
5-(benzylidene) thiazolidine-2,4-dione (2)

IR (KBr) cm^{-1}: 3146 (NH stretching), 3039 (Ar-CH stretching), 2789 (C-CH stretching), 1741, 1693 (C = O stretching).
^{1}H-NMR (DMSO-d$_6$, 400 MHz): 9.94 (s; 1H; NH), 8.11 (s; 1H; C = CH), 8.09-6.91 (m, 5H, Ar-H).
2-chloro-N-phenylpropionamide (3)
IR (KBr) cm^{-1}: 3138 (NH stretching), 1689 (C = O stretching), 1303 (C-CN stretching), ^{1}H-NMR (DMSO-d$_6$, 400 MHz): 8.60 (s; 1H; NH), 8.12-7.24 (5H, m, Ar-H), 4.82 (q; 1H; CH- CH$_3$),1.58 (s; 3H; CH-CH$_3$).
3-(5-benzylidene-2,4-dioxothiazolidin-3-yl)-N-(3-hydroxyphenyl)propanamide (4)
IR (KBr) cm^{-1}: 3353 (OH stretching), 3153 (NH stretching), 1741,1676, 1648 (C = O stretching), 1329 (C-N aliphatic stretching), ^{1}H-NMR (DMSO-d$_6$, 400 MHz): 10.39 (s; 1H; 3''OH), 9.83(s; 1H; NH), 7.80 (s;1H; C = CH), 7.51-6.85(m; 9H; Ar-H), 3.93 (t; 2H; N-CH$_2$-CH$_2$-CO), 2.66 (t; 2H; N-CH$_2$-CH$_2$-CO), ^{13}C NMR(δ)DMSO-d$_6$: 167.0, 166.0, 164.5 (C = O), 149.1 (C, Ar), 140.0 (C, Ar), 136.0 (=CH-), 135.1 (C, Ar), 130.0 (CH, Ar), 129.2 (2C, CH, Ar), 128.5 (2C, CH, Ar), 128.1, 124.3 (CH, Ar), 121.5 (C-5 TZD), 119.8 (CH, Ar), 117.1 (CH, Ar), 41.5 (CH$_2$-CH$_2$), 31.2 (CH$_2$-CH$_2$), MS (ESI+) m/z 369.0 (M+).
3-(5-(3-hydroxybenzylidene)-2,4-dioxothiazolidin-3-yl)-N-phenylpropanamide (5)
IR (KBr) cm^{-1}: 3363 (OH stretching), 3153 (NH stretching), 3045, 2962 (Ar-CH stretching), 1676, 1648, 1640 (C = O stretching), ^{1}H-NMR (DMSO-d$_6$, 400 MHz): 10.02 (s; 1H; 3'OH), 9.84 (s; 1H; NH), 7.80 (s; 1H; C = CH), 7.51-6.85 (m; 9H; Ar-H), 3.93 (t; 2H;

N-CH_2-CH_2-CO), 2.63 (t; 2H; N-CH_2-CH_2-CO), MS (ESI+) m/z 369.0 (M+).

3-(5-(2-fluorobenzylidene)-2,4-dioxothiazolidin-3-yl)-N-phenylpropanamide (6)

IR (KBr) cm^{-1}: 3313 (NH stretching), 3051, 2929 (Ar-CH stretching), 1753, 1687, 1661 (C = O stretching), 1136 (C-F stretching), ^{1}H-NMR (DMSO-d_6, 400 MHz): 10.03 (s; 1H; NH), 7.88 (s; 1H; C = CH), 7.58-6.98 (m; 9H; Ar-H), 3.93 (t; 2H; N-CH_2-CH_2-CO), 2.66 (t; 2H; N-CH_2-CH_2-CO), MS (ESI+) m/z 371.0 (M+).

3-(5-(3-hydroxybenzylidene)-2,4-dioxothiazolidin-3-yl)-N-(3-hydroxyphenyl)propanamide (7)

IR(KBr) cm^{-1}: 3525, 3416 (OH stretching), 3232 (NH stretching), 3053, 2947 (Ar-CH stretching),1722, 1664, 1652 (C = O stretching), ^{1}H-NMR (DMSO-d_6, 400 MHz): 10.00 (s;1H; NH), 9.79 (s; 1H; 3'OH), 9.78 (s; 1H; 3''OH), 7.80 (s; 1H; C = CH), 7.51-6.85 (m; 8H; Ar-H), 3.90 (t; 2H; N-CH_2-CH_2-CO), 2.63 (t; 2H; N-CH_2-CH_2-CO), MS (ESI+) m/z 385.1 (M+).

3-(5-benzylidene-2,4-dioxothiazolidin-3-yl)-N-(2-chlorophenyl)propanamide (8)

IR (KBr) cm^{-1}: 3306 (NH stretching), 1743, 1683, 1649 (C = O stretching), 821 (C-Cl stretching), ^{1}H-NMR (DMSO-d_6, 400 MHz): 10.02 (s; 1H; NH), 8.01(s; 1H; C = CH), 7.91 -7.32 (m; 9H; Ar-H), 3.93(t; 2H; N-CH_2-CH_2-CO), 2.63 (t; 2H; N-CH_2-CH_2-CO), MS (ESI+) m/z 386.0 (M+).

3-(5-(2,4-dimethylbenzylidene)-2,4-dioxothiazolidin-3-yl)-N-p-tolylpropanamide (9)

IR (KBr) cm^{-1}: 3386 (NH stretching), 2935, 2852 (C-CH_3 stretching), 1747, 1703, 1685 (C = O stretching), ^{1}H-NMR (DMSO-d_6, 400 MHz): 10.05 (s; 1H; NH), 8.06 (s; 1H; C = CH), 8.02-7.20 (m; 7H; Ar-H), 3.33 (t; 2H; N-CH_2-CH_2-CO), 2.66 (t; 2H; N-CH_2-CH_2-CO), 2.30 (s; 6H; 4',4''CH_3), 2.24 (s; 3H; 4''CH_3), MS (ESI+) m/z 395.2 (M+).

3-(5-(2,5-dimethylbenzylidene)-2,4-dioxothiazolidin-3-yl)-N-(2-hydroxyphenyl)propanamide (10)

IR (KBr) cm^{-1}: 3389 (OH stretching), 3198 (NH stretching), 2995, 2885 (C-CH_3 stretching) 1668, 1646, 1640 (C = O stretching),^{1}H-NMR (DMSO-d_6, 400 MHz): 10.20 (s; 1H; OH), 10.11 (s; 1H; NH), 7.90 (s; 1H; C = CH), 7.61-7.29 (m; 7H; Ar-H), 3.93 (t; 2H; N-CH_2-CH_2-CO), 2.70 (t; 2H; CH_2), 2.45 (s; 3H; 2' CH_3), 2.24 (s; 3H; 5'CH_3), ^{13}C NMR(δ)DMSO-d_6: 166.7, 166.4, 164.5 (C = O), 148.1 (C, Ar), 135.8, 134.7, 133.0 (C, Ar), 132.8 (=CH-), 130.2, 129.0, 127.2, 125.4 (CH, Ar), 122.2 (CH, Ar), 121.5 (C-5 TZD), 120.2, 119.2 (CH, Ar), 116.0 (CH, Ar), 121.0, 119.4 (C-CH_3), 41.5 (CH_2-CH_2), 31.2 (CH_2-CH_2), MS (ESI+) m/z 397.2 (M+).

3-(5-(2,4-dimethylbenzylidene)-2,4-dioxothiazolidin-3-yl)-N-(2-hydroxyphenyl)propanamide (11)

IR (KBr) cm^{-1}: 3404 (OH stretching), 3136 (NH stretching), 2742 (C-CH_3 stretching), 1734, 1681, 1641

(C = O stretching), 665 (C-S stretching), ^{1}H-NMR (DMSO-d_6, 400 MHz): 10.15 (s; 1H; 2'OH), 10.03 (s; 1H; NH), 8.06 (s; 1H; C = CH), 8.03 -7.20 (m; 7H; Ar-H), 3.92 (t; 2H; N-CH_2-CH_2-CO), 2.66 (s; tH; CH_2), 2.29 (s; 3H; 2'CH_3), 2.23 (s; 3H; 4'CH_3), MS (ESI+) m/z 397.2 (M+).

3-(5-(3,5-dimethylbenzylidene)-2,4-dioxothiazolidin-3-yl)-N-(2-hydroxyphenyl)propanamide (12)

IR (KBr) cm^{-1}: 3304 (OH stretching), 3203 (NH stretching), 2980 (C-CH_3 stretching), 1658, 1650, 1642 (C = O stretching), 690 (C-S stretching), ^{1}H-NMR (DMSO-d_6, 400 MHz): 10.20 (s; 1H; 2''OH), 10.11 (s; 1H; NH), 7.90 (s; 1H; C = CH), 7.61-7.27 (m; 7H; Ar-H), 3.90 (t; 2H; N-CH_2-CH_2-CO), 2.63 (s; tH; CH_2), 2.24-2.27 (s; 6H; 2'5'CH_3), MS (ESI+) m/z 397.0 (M+).

3-(5-(2,4-dihydroxybenzylidene)-2,4-dioxothiazolidin-3-yl)-N-(2-hydroxyphenyl)propanamide (13)

IR (KBr) cm^{-1}: 3657, 3566, 3412 (OH stretching), 3390 (NH stretching), 3087, 3032 (Ar-CH stretching), 1687, 1669, 1656 (C = O stretching), ^{1}H-NMR (DMSO-d_6, 400 MHz): 12.44 (s; 1H; 2''OH), 10.70 (s; 1H; 2'OH), 10.01 (s; 1H; 4'OH), 9.98 (s; 1H; NH), 8.01 (s; 1H; C = CH), 8.03-7.24 (m; 7H; Ar-H), 3.98 (t; 2H; N-CH_2-CH_2-CO), 2.23 (t; 2H; 2 CH_2), MS (ESI+) m/z 401.2 (M+).

3-(5-benzylidene-2,4-dioxothiazolidin-3-yl)-N-(2-chloro-4-methylphenyl)propanamide (14)

IR (KBr) cm^{-1}: 3281 (NH stretching), 1664, 1650 (C = O stretching), 1329 (C-N aromatic stretching), 783 (C-Cl stretching), ^{1}H-NMR (DMSO-d_6, 400 MHz): 10.17 (s; 1H; NH), 7.93 (s; 1H; C = CH), 7.64 -6.44 (m; 8H; Ar-H), 2.66-3.96 (t; 2H; N-CH_2-CH_2-CO), 2.31 (t; 2H; N-CH_2-CH_2-CO), 2.26 (s; 3H; 4''CH_3), MS (ESI+) m/z 401.5 (M+).

3-(5-benzylidene-2,4-dioxothiazolidin-3-yl)-N-(4-chloro-3-methylphenyl)propanamide (15)

IR (KBr) cm^{-1}: 3283 (NH stretching), 1684, 1654, 1609 (C = O stretching), 1305 (C-N aromatic stretching), 761 (C-Cl stretching), ^{1}H-NMR (DMSO-d_6, 400 MHz): 10.19 (s; 1H; NH), 7.93 (s; 1H; C = CH), 7.93-6.23 (m; 8H; Ar-H), 2.67-3.95 (t; 2H; N-CH_2-CH_2-CO), 2.30 (s; 3H; 4''CH_3), 2.27 (t; 2H; N-CH_2-CH_2-CO), MS (ESI+) m/z 401.3 (M+).

3-(5-(2-chlorobenzylidene)-2,4-dioxothiazolidin-3-yl)-N-p-tolylpropanamide (16)

IR (KBr) cm^{-1}: 3215 (NH stretching) 1666, 1655, 1645 (C = O stretching), 717 (C-Cl stretching),^{1}H-NMR (DMSO-d_6, 400 MHz): 10.02 (s; 1H; NH), 7.88 (s; 1H; C = CH), 7.58 -7.23 (m; 8H; Ar-H), 3.94 (t; 2H; N-CH_2-CH_2-CO), 2.67 (t; 2H; N-CH_2-CH_2-CO), 2.30 (s; 3H; 4''CH_3), MS (ESI+) m/z 401.3 (M+).

3-(5-(2,3,4-trihydroxybenzylidene)2,4-dioxothiazolidin-3-yl)-N-p-tolylpropanamide (17)

IR(KBr)cm^{-1}: 3649, 3629, 3595 (OH-stretching), 3312 (NH-stretching), 2869 (C-CH_3 stretching), 1745,

1683,1656 (C = O stretching), ^{1}H-NMR (DMSO-d$_6$, 400 MHz): 14.09 (s; 1H; 2'OH), 10.09 (s; 1H; 3'OH), 9.50 (s; 1H; 4'OH), 9.31 (s;1H; NH), 8.06(s;1H; C = CH), 8.04 -7.20 (m; 6H; Ar-H), 3.84 (t; 2H; N-CH$_2$-CH$_2$-CO), 2.39 (s; 3H; 4''CH$_3$), 2.33 (t; 2H; N-CH$_2$-CH$_2$-CO), MS (ESI+) m/z 415.3 (M+).

3-(5-(3-hydroxybenzylidene)-2,4-dioxothiazolidin-3-yl)-N-(2-chloro-5-methylphenyl)- propanamide (18)
IR (KBr) cm^{-1}: 3308 (OH stretching), 3223 (NH stretching), 3057, 2960 (Ar-CH stretching), 2924, 2854 (C-CH$_3$ stretching), 1691,1656, 1646 (C = O stretching), 752 (C-Cl stretching), ^{1}H-NMR (DMSO-d$_6$, 400 MHz): 10.19 (s; 1H; 3'OH), 10.11 (s; 1H; NH), 7.93 (s; 1H; C = CH), 7.64-6.23 (m; 7H; Ar-H), 3.96-2.66 (t; 2H; N-CH$_2$-CH$_2$-CO), 2.30 (s; 3H; 5''CH$_3$), 2.27 (t; 2H; N-CH$_2$-CH$_2$-CO), MS (ESI+) m/z 417.2 (M+).

3-(5-(2-fluorobenzylidene)-2,4-dioxothiazolidin-3-yl)-N-(2-chloro-4-methylphenyl)- propanamide (19)
IR (KBr) cm^{-1}: 3306 (NH stretching), 2926, 2856 (C-CH$_3$ stretching), 1743, 1693, 1654 (C = O stretching), 1282 (C-F stretching), 754 (C-Cl stretching), ^{1}H-NMR (DMSO-d$_6$, 400 MHz): 10.02 (s; 1H; NH), 7.88 (s; 1H; C = CH), 7.58-7.23 (m; 7H; Ar-H), 3.99 ((t; 2H; N-CH$_2$-CH$_2$-CO), 2.60 (t; 2H; N-CH$_2$-CH$_2$-CO), 2.28 (s; 3H; 4''CH$_3$), MS (ESI+) m/z 419.2 (M+).

3-(5-(3,5-dimethylbenzylidene)-2,4-dioxothiazolidin-3-yl)-N-(2-chloro-4-methylphenyl)- propanamide (20)
IR (KBr) cm^{-1}: 3267 (NH stretching), 3039 (Ar-CH stretching), 2916, 2858 (C-CH$_3$ stretching), 1681, 1651,1644 (C = O stretching), 742 (C-Cl stretching) ^{1}H-NMR (DMSO-d$_6$, 400 MHz): 10.07 (s; 1H; NH), 8.04 (s; 1H; C = CH), 7.84-7.20 (m; 6H; Ar-H), 3.92 (t; 2H; N-CH$_2$-CH$_2$-CO), 2.66 (t; 2H; N-CH$_2$-CH$_2$-CO), 2.30 (s; 6H; CH$_3$), 2.24 (s; 3H; 4'CH$_3$).

3-(5-(2-chlorobenzylidene)-2,4-dioxothiazolidin-3-yl)-N-(4-nitrophenyl)propanamide (21)
IR (KBr) cm^{-1}: 3145 (NH stretching), 1685, 1657, 1644 (C = O stretching), 1311 (C-NO$_2$ stretching), 776 (C-Cl stretching),^{1}H-NMR (DMSO-d$_6$, 400 MHz): 10.39 (s; 1H; NH), 8.01(s;1H; =CH), 7.91-7.32 (m; 8H; Ar-H), 3.91 (t; 2H; N-CH$_2$-CH$_2$-CO), 2.72 (t; 2H; N-CH$_2$-CH$_2$-CO), MS (ESI+) m/z 432.8 (M+).

3-(5-(2-chlorobenzylidene)-2,4-dioxothiazolidin-3-yl)-N-(2-nitrophenyl)propanamide (22)
IR (KBr) cm^{-1}: 3306 (NH stretching), 1743, 1693, 1612 (C = O stretching), 1342 (C-NO$_2$ stretching), 754 (C-Cl stretching), ^{1}H-NMR (DMSO-d$_6$, 400 MHz): 10.00 (s; 1H; NH), 7.80 (s; 1H;C = CH), 7.51-6.85 (m; 8H; Ar-H), 3.90 (t; 2H; N-CH$_2$-CH$_2$-CO), 2.63 (t; 2H; N-CH$_2$-CH$_2$-CO).

3-(5-(4-chlorobenzylidene)-2,4-dioxothiazolidin-3-yl)-N-(2-nitrophenyl)propanamide (23)
IR (KBr) cm^{-1}: 3267 (NH stretching), 1702, 1664, 1650 (C = O stretching), 1373 (C-NO$_2$ stretching), 752 (C-Cl stretching), ^{1}H-NMR (DMSO-d$_6$, 400 MHz): 10.00 (s; 1H; NH), 7.80 (s; 1H; C = CH), 7.51 -6.87 (m; 8H; Ar-H), 3.90 (t; 2H; N-CH$_2$-CH$_2$-CO), 2.63 (t; 2H; N-CH$_2$-CH$_2$-CO).

3-(5-(2,3,4-trihydroxybenzylidene)-2,4-dioxothiazolidin-3-yl)-N-(2-mercaptophenyl) propanamide (24)
IR (KBr) cm^{-1}: 3649, 3629, 3587(OH stretching), 3312 (NH stretching) 2975, 2931 (Ar-CH stretching), 2896 (C-CH$_3$ stretching), 2546 (SH-stretching), 1688, 1647, 1638 (C = O stretching), ^{1}H-NMR (DMSO-d$_6$, 400 MHz): 13.96 (s; 1H; 2'OH), 10.09 (s; 1H; 3'OH), 9.50 (s; 1H; 4'OH), 9.31 (s;1H; NH), 8.01 (s;1H; C = CH), 7.90-7.18 (m; 6H; Ar-H), 3.84 (t; 2H; N-CH$_2$-CH$_2$-CO), 3.49 (s; 1H; 2''SH), 2.30 (t; 2H; N-CH$_2$-CH$_2$-CO), ^{13}CNMR(δ)DMSO-d$_6$: 167.2, 165.5, 164.5 (C = O), 148.2, 145.2, 142.1, 136.0 (C, Ar), 136.1 (=CH-), 130.2, 129.0, 125.8 (CH, Ar), 124.3 (C, Ar), 123.6, 123.0 (CH, Ar), 121.5 (C-5 TZD), 110.1, (C, Ar), 109.3 (CH, Ar), 41.5 (CH$_2$-CH$_2$), 31.2 (CH$_2$-CH$_2$), MS (ESI+) m/z 432.8 (M+).

3-(5-(2,4-dihydroxybenzylidene)-2,4-dioxothiazolidin-3-yl)-N-(3-chloro-2-methylphenyl)propanamide (25)
IR (KBr) cm^{-1}: 3630, 3444 (OH stretching), 3273 (NH stretching), 3053(Ar-CH stretching), 2793 (C-CH$_3$ stretching), 1730, 1674, 1648 (C = O stretching), 792 (C-Cl stretching), ^{1}H-NMR (DMSO-d$_6$, 400 MHz): 10.51 (s; 1H; 2'OH), 10.19 (s; 1H; 4'OH), 9.69 (s; 1H; NH), 8.09 (s; 1H; C = CH), 7.41-7.16 (m; 6H; Ar-H), 3.95 (t; 2H; N-CH$_2$-CH$_2$-CO), 2.68 (t; 2H; N-CH$_2$-CH$_2$-CO), 2.19 (s; 3H; 2''CH$_3$), MS (ESI+) m/z 432.9 (M+).

3-(5-(4-chlorobenzylidene)-2,4-dioxothiazolidin-3-yl)-N-(2-chloro-4-methylphenyl)propanamide (26)
IR (KBr) cm^{-1}: 3198 (NH stretching), 2918, 2848 (C-CH$_3$ stretching), 1750, 1672, 1658 (C = O stretching), 1307 (C-N aromatic stretching), 748 (C-Cl stretching), ^{1}H-NMR (DMSO-d$_6$, 400 MHz): 9.65 (s; 1H; NH), 7.94 (s; 1H; C = CH), 7.90 -6.53 (m; 7H; Ar-H), 3.94-3.91 (t; 2H; N-CH$_2$-CH$_2$-CO), 2.70-2.76 (t; 2H; N-CH$_2$-CH$_2$-CO), 2.32 (s; 3H; CH$_3$), ^{13}C NMR(δ)DMSO-d$_6$: 167.6, 165.8, 164.5 (C = O), 135.7 (=CH-), 135.6, 133.0, 131.9, 132.0, 131.0 (C, Ar), 130.0 (3C, CH, Ar) 127.8, (3C, CH, Ar), 124.2 (CH, Ar), 121.5 (C-5 TZD), 113.1, (C, Ar), 112.2, 109.5, 103.7 (CH, Ar), 41.5 (CH$_2$-CH$_2$), 31.2 (CH$_2$-CH$_2$), 20.7 (CH$_3$), MS (ESI+) m/z 436.2 (M+).

3-(5-(4-chlorobenzylidene)-2,4-dioxothiazolidin-3-yl)-N-(2-chloro-5-methylphenyl)propanamide (27)
IR (KBr) cm^{-1}: 3273 (NH stretching), 1739, 1670, 1652 (C = O stretching), 808 (C-Cl stretching), ^{1}H-NMR (DMSO-d$_6$, 400 MHz): 9.64 (s; 1H; NH), 7.95 (s; 1H; C = CH), 7.62 -6.20 (m; 7H; Ar-H), 3.94-3.20 (t; 2H; N-CH$_2$-CH$_2$-CO), 2.76-2.32 (t; 2H; N-CH$_2$-CH$_2$-CO), 2.23 (s; 3H; 5''CH$_3$), MS (ESI+) m/z 435.9 (M+).

3-(5-(2-bromobenzylidene)-2,4-dioxothiazolidin-3-yl)-N-(2-hydroxyphenyl)propanamide (28)

IR (KBr) cm^{-1}: 3411 (OH stretching), 3372 (NH stretching), 1688, 1669, 1646 (C = O stretching), 668 (C-Br stretching), ^{1}H-NMR (DMSO-d$_6$, 400 MHz): 9.97 (s; 1H; 2''OH), 9.84 (s; 1H; NH), 7.80 (s; 1H; C = CH), 7.51-6.85 (m; 8H; Ar-H), 3.91 (t; 2H; N-CH$_2$-CH$_2$-CO), 2.64 (t; 2H; N-CH$_2$-CH$_2$-CO), ^{13}CNMR(δ) DMSO-d$_6$: 167.2, 165.2, 164.5 (C = O), 148.9, 138.1, 135.3 (=CH-), 135.1 (C, Ar), 132.3, 130.1, 128.1, 127.1, 127.0 (CH, Ar), 121.5 (C-5 TZD), 113.0, (C, Ar), 112.9, 109.5, 104.8 (CH, Ar), 41.5 (CH$_2$-CH$_2$), 31.2 (CH$_2$-CH$_2$), MS (ESI+) m/z 448.0.

3-(5-(2-bromobenzylidene)-2,4-dioxothiazolidin-3-yl)-N-(3-hydroxyphenyl)propanamide (29)

IR (KBr) cm^{-1}: 3444 (OH stretching), 3315 (NH stretching), 1752, 1680, 1650 (C = O stretching), 680 (C-Br stretching), ^{1}H-NMR (DMSO-d$_6$, 400 MHz): 9.84 (s; 1H; OH), 9.61 (s; 1H; NH), 7.81 (s; 1H; C = CH), 7.52-6.86 (m; 8H; Ar-H), 3.91 (t; 2H; N-CH$_2$-CH$_2$-CO), 2.64 (t; 2H; N-CH$_2$-CH$_2$-CO), MS (ESI+) m/z 448.2 (M+).

3-(5-(2-bromobenzylidene)-2,4-dioxothiazolidin-3-yl)-N-(4-nitrophenyl)propanamide (30)

IR (KBr) cm^{-1}: 3207 (NH stretching), 1710, 1685, 1658 (C = O stretching), 1319 (C-NO$_2$ stretching), 750 (C-Br stretching), ^{1}H-NMR (DMSO-d$_6$, 400 MHz): 9.73 (s; 1H; NH), 8.12 (s; 1H; C = CH), 8.09 -7.53 (m; 8H; Ar-H), 3.83 ((t; 2H; N-CH$_2$-CH$_2$-CO), 2.20 (t; 2H; N-CH$_2$-CH$_2$-CO).

3-(5-(3-bromobenzylidene)-2,4-dioxothiazolidin-3-yl)-N-(4-chloro-3-methylphenyl) propanamide (31)

IR (KBr) cm^{-1}: 3284 (NH stretching), 3014, 2922 (C-CH$_3$ stretching) 1702, 1676, 1652 (C = O stretching), 779 (C-Br Stretching), 675 (C-Br stretching), ^{1}H-NMR (DMSO-d$_6$, 400 MHz): 10.11 (s; 1H; NH), 7.90 (s; 1H; C = CH), 7.61 -7.29 (m; 7H; Ar-H), 3.90 (t; 2H; N-CH$_2$-CH$_2$-CO), 2.64 (t; 2H; N-CH$_2$-CH$_2$-CO), 2.45 (s; 3H; 3'' CH$_3$), MS (ESI+) m/z 480.2 (M+).

Biological assays

The standard strains were procured from Institute of Microbial Technology, Chandigarh and National Chemical Laboratory, Pune. Antimicrobial activity was determined by two fold serial dilution method [34] in duplicates against pathogenic microorganisms Gram-positive bacteria: *Staphylococcus aureus* (NCIM 2122), *Bacillus subtilis* (MTCC 121), Gram-negative bacteria: *Escherichia coli* (MTCC118), *Pseudomonas aeruginosa* (MTCC 647), *Salmonella typhi* (NCIM 2501), *Klebsiella pneumonia* (MTCC 3384) and fungus *Candida albicans* (MTCC 227), *Aspergillus niger* (NCIM 1056). Test compounds were dissolved in 10% DMSO, to produce a 2000 µg/ml stock solution. These test tubes were serially diluted to give a concentration of 100, 50, 25, 12.5, 6.25, 3.125, 1.56, and 0.78 µg/mL. MHB (Mueller-Hinton Broth) was used for bacteria and SDB (Sabouraud Dextrose Broth) was used

for fungus. The cell density of each inoculum was adjusted in sterile water of a 0.5 McFarland standard. A final concentration of ~10^7 CFU/mL and ~10^6 CFU/mL was obtained for bacteria and fungus, respectively. Microbial inocula were added to the twofold diluted samples. The test tubes were incubated 18–24 h at 37° C ±1°C for bacteria and 2–5 days at 25°C ±1°C for fungus. Ciprofloxacin and fluconazole were used as standard drugs. The highest dilution of the test compound that completely inhibited the growth of test organism was considered as the MIC value of the test compound and was expressed in µg/ml.

HIV-1 reverse transcriptase inhibition assay

The assay of HIV-1 RT was done as reported by Silprasit *et al.* [35]. All reagents used were provided in the EnzChek® Reverse Transcriptase Assay Kit (Molecular Probes, USA). A mixture of 5 µL of 1 mg/mL 350 bases-poly(rA) ribonucleotide template and 5 µL of 50 µg/mL oligo d(T)$_{16}$ primer in a nuclease-free microcentrifuge tube were incubated at room temperature (25°C) for 1 hour to allow the primer/template annealing. The primer/template was prepared by 200-fold dilution in polymerization buffer. The primer/template was aliquoted and kept at –20°C until used. Five microliter of 8 µM stock purified HIV-1 reverse transcriptase was aliquoted and kept at –80°C until used. The working enzyme was diluted to 400 nM with 50 mM Tris–HCl, 20% glycerol, 2 mM DTT, pH 7.5.

The assays were performed in a total volume 15 µL of the polymerization reaction. The reaction containing 3 µl of 400 nM recombinant HIV-1 RT (the final concentration is 80 nM), 2 µL of TE buffer (10 mM Tris–HCl at pH 7.5) were added and gently mixed on ice prior. The polymerization reaction was initiated by the addition of 10 µL of the primer/template and incubated at room temperature for 30 minutes. After the reactions reached the desired incubation time, 5 µL of 0.2 M EDTA was added to stop the polymerization reaction (RTControl). The blank reaction was prepared by mixing 5 µL of 0.2 M EDTA with enzyme before adding primer/template (RTBlank). After termination of the reactions, the plate was gently shaken and incubated at room temperature for 3 min to allow the formation of a stable heteroduplex DNA/RNA complex, followed by addition of 180 µL of PicoGreen reagent diluted 700-fold with TE buffer for each well, making the final volume 200 µL and incubation at room temperature in the dark for 3 min, during which PicoGreen binds to double-stranded DNA and RNA-DNA hybrids, was followed by measurement of fluorescence with a fluorometer (excitation 485 nm; emission 535 nm).

To test the inhibition efficiency of the compounds, all the compounds were dissolved in dimethyl sulfoxide (DMSO) to make a 20 mM stock solution. Ten micromolar working solution of each inhibitor was further diluted by 10 mM

Tris–HCl, pH 7.5 containing 50% DMSO. Two microliter of each inhibitor and 3 µL of 400 nM recombinant HIV-1 RT were added and gently mixed on ice prior. The reaction was initiated by the addition of 10 µL of the primer/template and incubated at room temperature for 30 minutes. After the reactions reached the desired incubation time, 5 µL of 0.2 M EDTA was added to stop the polymerization reaction. The relative inhibitory effect of HIV-1 RT activity was compared by using percent inhibition, which was calculated via the following eq (1):

$$\% \text{ relative inhibition} = \frac{\left[\left(RT_{Control} - RT_{Background}\right) - \left(RT_{Sample} - RT_{Background}\right)\right]}{\left[\left(RT_{Control} - RT_{Background}\right)\right]} \times 100$$

$$(1)$$

Determination of the IC_{50} inhibition value

Determination of the IC_{50} was done by adding 2 µL of each two-fold serial dilution of inhibitors. Two microliters of each test compound was diluted serially 2-fold. Then, 2 µL of 30 ng/µL purified HIV-1 RT was added and mixed. A volume of 4 µL of the template/primer polymerization buffer was added into each well. The mixtures were incubated at 37°C for 10 min. The reactions were stopped with 5 µL of 200 mM EDTA and immediately incubated on ice for 30 min. The activity was determined by the PicoGreen–fluorometric method. The reaction was repeated three times and were determined using Graph pad Prism4 version with a non-linear regression model.

Computational method with Glide 5.0

Docking study was performed for the highest active compounds by using Glide 5.0 (Schrodinger) [36] installed in a single machine running on a 3.4 GHz Pentium 4 processor with 1GB RAM and 160 GB Hard Disk with Red Hat Linux Enterprise version 5.0 as the operating system.

Protein structure preparation

The X-ray crystallographic structure of (PDB code 1RT2, 2VF5 and 1EA1) was obtained from Brookhaven Protein Data Bank (RCSB) [37]. All water molecules were removed from the complex, and the protein was minimized using the protein preparation wizard. Partial atomic charges were assigned according to the OPLS_AA force field. A radius of 10 Å was selected for active site cavity during receptor grid generation for 2VF5. After assigning charge and protonation state finally refinement (energy minimization) was done using MM3 force field runs.

Crystallographic structure of the complex between cytochrome P450 14-R-sterol demethylase from *Mycobacterium tuberculosis* (*Mycobacterium* P450DM) and fluconazole

was present in the Protein Data Bank with the ID 1EA1 [38]. The high homology existing between these two analogous enzymes [39] suggested building a simple model consisting of the crystallographic structure of the complex 1EA1 in which the residues that are arranged in a range of 7 Å from fluconazole, were substituted with those of *Candida* P450DM according to reported method [33]. Only 12 substitutions were made by replacement of the residues Pro77, Phe78, Met79, Arg96, Met99, Leu100, Phe255, Ala256, His258, Ile322, Ile323 and Leu324 by Lys77, His78, Leu79, Leu96, Lys99, Phe100, Met255, Gly256, Gln258, His322, Ser323 and Ile324, which were thought to be necessary for the ligand-receptor interaction. The complex between the chimeric enzyme thus obtained and was then minimized.

Ligand structure preparation

All the compounds used in the docking study with Glide were built within maestro by using build module of Schrodinger Suite 2008. These structures were geometry optimized by using the Optimized Potentials for Liquid Simulations-2005 (OPLS_2005) force field with the steepest descent protocol followed by truncated Newton conjugate gradient protocol. Partial atomic charges were computed using the OPLS_2005 force field.

Docking protocol and their validation

All docking calculations were then performed using the "Extra Precision" (XP) mode of Glide Program 5.0. A grid was prepared with the center defined by the co-crystallized ligand. During the docking process, initially Glide performed a complete systematic search of the conformational, orientational and positional space of the docked ligand and eliminated unwanted conformations using scoring followed by energy optimization. Finally the conformations were further refined via Monte Carlo sampling of pose conformation. Predicting the binding affinity and rank-ordering ligands in database screens was implemented by modified and expanded version of the Glide scoring function. The most suitable method of evaluating the accuracy of a docking procedure is to determine how closely the lowest energy pose predicted by the scoring function resembles an experimental binding mode as determined by X-ray crystallography. Docking validation was performed with an obtained RMSD value of 0.370 Å for 1RT2, 1.674 Å for 2VF5 and 2.094 Å for 1EA1 ensuring precision and reproducibility of the docking process.

Results and discussion

Chemistry

An attempt has been made to incorporate aryl groups in the 3rd and 5th position of the thiazolidinedione structure according to Scheme 1. In the first step the cyclization of

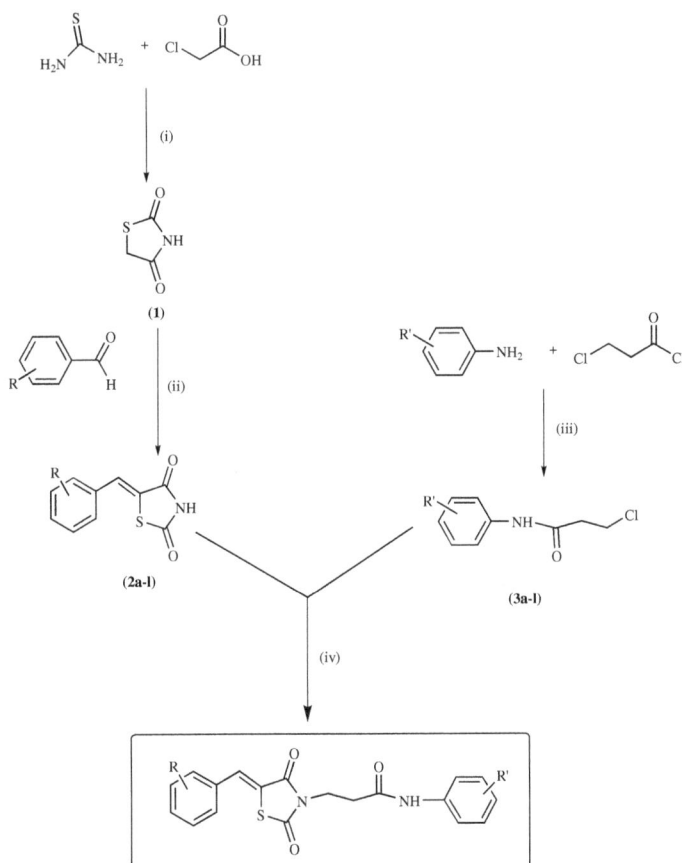

Scheme 1 Reagents and conditions: (i) Water, Conc. HCl, reflux 10-12 h (ii) ethanol, piperidine, reflu 4 h (iii) Glacial acetic acid (GAA), 0-5°C, 0.5 h, 4rt, stirring (iv) CH3CN, triethylamine, reflux 12h. General scheme for the synthesis of compounds (4–31).

chloroacetic acid was carried out with equilmolar amounts of thiourea and chloroacetic acid, and then hydrolysed with 2 N HCl to afford 2,4-thiazolidinedione (**1**). Knoevenagel condensation of 2,4-thiazolidinedione and appropriate aryl aldehydes was carried out in ethanol under reflux conditions containing catalytic amount of piperidine, as base, to form the corresponding substituted 5-benzylidene-2,4-thiazolidinediones (**2**) [33]. *N*-chloro-3-(phenylamino)propanamides (**3**) were prepared by the reported method [40]. Substituted *N*-chloro-3-(phenylamino)propanamides (**3**) were thus prepared by reacting appropriate aryl amines with 3-chloropropionyl chloride in the presence of glacial acetic acid in cold condition. The substituted 5-benzylidene-2,4-thiazolidinediones (**2**) were condensed with substituted *N*-chloro-3-(phenylamino)propanamides (**3**) in the presence of triethylamine using acetonitrile as the solvent to get substituted 3-(5-benzylidene-2,4-dioxothiazolidin-3-yl)-*N*-phenylpropanamides **4–31**.

The physical data are given in Table 1. FTIR, ^{1}H-NMR and mass spectral data for all the synthesized compounds

are given in the above experimental protocols. The IR spectrum of all the final compounds exhibited very similar features and showed the expected bands for the characteristic groups present in the compounds such as N-H stretching in the range of 3390–3136 cm^{-1} and C = O stretching in the range of 1750–1645 cm^{-1} to confirm the presence of thiazolidinedione ring system. ^{1}H NMR showed a characteristic singlet peak assigned to a δ value in the range of 10.39-9.31 thus confirming the presence of NH proton of thiazolidinedione scaffold in compounds **4–31**. The methylenic (C = CH) protons of compounds **4–31** were seen as a singlet between 8.12-7.80 δppm while aromatic protons appeared as multiple peaks within the range 8.04-6.20 δ ppm. Characteristic triplet of 2 protons was assigned at δ ranging 3.99-2.66 to the methylenic protons of N-CH$_2$-CH$_2$-CO. Similarly; a triplet of 2 protons was assigned to the methylenic protons of N-CH$_2$-CH$_2$-CO observed at δ ranging 2.76-2.20 for all the compounds **4–31**. The ^{13}C NMR depicted the peaks of thiazolidine-2,4-dione (TZD) nucleus within the range δ 166.2-164.3 (thiazolidine-

Table 1 Physical data of synthesized compounds (4–31)

Comp. no.	R	R'	Mol. formula	Yield (%)	M.P. (°C)	M.W.	Elemental analysis calculated/found		
							C	H	N
4	H	3-OH	$C_{19}H_{16}N_2O_4S$	57	289	368.41	61.94	4.38	7.60
							61.90	4.34	7.55
5	3-OH	H	$C_{19}H_{16}N_2O_4S$	55	243	368.41	61.94	4.38	7.60
							61.90	4.36	7.66
6	2-F	H	$C_{19}H_{14}ClFN_2O_3S$	52	186	370.40	56.37	3.49	6.92
							56.33	3.44	6.88
6	2-F	H	$C_{19}H_{14}ClFN_2O_3S$	52	186	370.40	56.37	3.49	6.92
							56.33	3.44	6.88
7	3-OH	3-OH	$C_{19}H_{16}N_2O_5S$	58	129	348.41	59.37	4.20	7.29
							59.32	4.16	7.24
8	H	Cl	$C_{19}H_{15}ClN_2O_3S$	55	183	386.85	58.99	3.91	7.24
							58.55	3.89	7.26
9	2,4-CH$_3$	4-CH$_3$	$C_{22}H_{22}N_2O_3S$	62	284	394.49	66.98	5.62	7.10
							66.95	5.56	7.05
10	2,5-CH$_3$	2-OH	$C_{21}H_{20}N_2O_4S$	64	302	396.46	63.62	5.08	7.07
							63.58	5.11	7.10
11	2,4-CH$_3$	2-OH	$C_{21}H_{20}N_2O_4S$	58	189	396.46	63.62	5.08	7.07
							63.58	5.11	7.11
12	3,5-CH$_3$	2-OH	$C_{21}H_{20}N_2O_4S$	56	293	396.46	63.62	5.08	7.07
							63.59	5.06	7.02
13	2,4-OH	2-OH	$C_{19}H_{16}N_2O_6S$	52	243	400.41	56.99	4.03	7.00
							56.95	4.00	7.03
14	H	2-Cl, 4-CH$_3$	$C_{20}H_{17}ClN_2O_3S$	58	109	400.88	59.92	4.27	6.99
							59.88	4.24	6.95
15	H	4-Cl, 3-CH$_3$	$C_{20}H_{17}ClN_2O_3S$	56	113	400.88	59.92	4.27	6.99
							59.88	4.24	6.95
16	2-Cl	4-CH$_3$	$C_{20}H_{17}ClN_2O_3S$	68	279	400.88	59.92	4.27	6.99
							59.95	4.24	6.96
17	2,3,4-OH	4-CH$_3$	$C_{20}H_{18}N_2O_6S$	44	253	414.43	57.96	4.38	6.76
							59.95	4.42	6.72
18	3-OH	2-Cl,5-CH$_3$	$C_{20}H_{17}ClN_2O_4S$	66	173	416.88	57.62	4.11	6.72
							57.59	4.08	6.70
19	2-F	2-Cl,4-CH$_3$	$C_{20}H_{16}ClFN_2O_3S$	60	175	418.87	57.35	3.85	6.69
							57.30	3.81	6.66
20	3,5-CH$_3$	2-Cl,4-CH$_3$	$C_{22}H_{21}ClN_2O_3S$	55	308	428.93	61.60	4.93	6.53
							61.56	4.88	6.49
21	2-Cl	4-NO$_2$	$C_{19}H_{14}ClN_3O_5S$	58	282	431.85	52.84	3.27	9.73
							52.86	3.21	9.69
22	2-Cl	2-NO$_2$	$C_{19}H_{14}ClN_3O_5S$	66	174	431.85	52.84	3.27	9.73
							52.86	3.21	9.69
23	4-Cl	2-NO$_2$	$C_{19}H_{14}ClN_3O_5S$	52	240	431.85	52.84	3.27	9.73
							52.86	3.22	9.70

Table 1 Physical data of synthesized compounds (4–31) (Continued)

24	2,3,4-OH	2-SH	$C_{19}H_{16}N_2O_6S_2$	53	119	432.47	52.77	3.73	6.48
							52.74	3.68	6.44
25	2,4-OH	3-Cl,2-CH$_3$	$C_{20}H_{17}ClN_2O_5S$	50	78	432.88	55.49	3.96	6.47
							55.45	3.94	6.42
26	4-Cl	4-Cl,3-CH$_3$	$C_{20}H_{16}Cl_2N_2O_3S$	70	302	435.32	46.62	3.13	5.44
							46.58	3.08	5.40
27	4-Cl	2-Cl,5-CH$_3$	$C_{20}H_{16}Cl_2N_2O_3S$	65	158	435.32	46.62	3.13	5.44
							46.58	3.08	5.40
28	2-Br	2-OH	$C_{19}H_{15}BrN_2O_4S$	52	113	447.30	51.02	3.38	6.26
							51.10	3.40	6.30
29	2-Br	3-OH	$C_{19}H_{15}BrN_2O_4S$	58	237	447.30	51.02	3.38	6.26
							51.10	3.40	6.30
30	2-Br	2-NO$_2$	$C_{19}H_{14}BrN_3O_5S$	62	297	476.66	47.91	2.96	8.82
							47.88	2.94	8.85
31	3-Br	4-Cl,3-CH$_3$	$C_{20}H_{16}BrClN_2O_3S$	67	309	479.77	50.07	3.36	5.84
							50.11	3.31	5.80

2,4-dione -C = O). ^{13}C NMR spectrum showed signals for thiazolidine-2,4-dione-C-5 atom at δ 121.5.

Biological activity

All the synthesized compounds were also evaluated for *in vitro* antibacterial activity against Gram-positive bacteria: *Staphylococcus aureus* (NCIM 2122), *Bacillus subtilis* (MTCC 121), Gram-negative bacteria: *Escherichia coli* (MTCC118), *Pseudomonas aeruginosa* (MTCC 647), *Salmonella typhi* (NCIM 2501), *Klebsiella pneumonia* (MTCC 3384) and fungus *Candida albicans* (MTCC 227), *Aspergillus niger* (NCIM 1056), by using the two-fold serial dilution technique and the results are summarized in Table 2. Ciprofloxacin was used as the standard for antibacterial activity and fluconazole was used as the standard for antifungal activity.

Compound **10** showed highest activity against all the bacterial strains. Compound **4** and **10** showed highest activity against *E. coli* while compound **24** exhibited moderate activity against the same bacterial strain while exhibited weak activity against all the other bacterial strains. Compound **5** and **7** exhibited highest activity against *B. subtilis and K. pneumoniae* respectively while compound **17** exhibited moderate activity against all the three bacterial strains *B. subtilis*, *E. coli* and *S. typhi*. Compound **8** exhibited moderate activity against *S. aureus*. However, all these compounds exhibited activity less than that of standard drug ciprofloxacin. Rest of the compounds showed mild to moderate activity against all other bacterial strains.

Compound **4** exhibited excellent activity against the fungal strains *C. albicans* and *A. niger*. In fact, the activity was higher than that of standard fluconazole. Compound **7, 8, 15, 19, 21, 24** and **27** also exhibited very high activity against both the fungal strains comparable to the standard drug. Compounds **5, 10, 11, 18** and **28** exhibited significant activity against *C. albicans* while showing moderate activity against *A. niger*. All other compounds showed moderate to weak antifungal activity against both the fungal strains.

The introduction of phenyl groups substituted at different positions with electronegative groups such as chloro, hydroxyl and nitro enhances the antimicrobial activity, particularly evident in case of antifungal activity. However, the introduction of one methyl group does not have much influence in the increase or decrease of antifungal activity as in case of compounds **19** and **27**. The introduction of two methyl groups in the phenyl ring directly substituted at the 5th position of the thiazolidine – 2,4-dione nucleus results in slight decrease in the antifungal activity but increases antibacterial activity as is evident from the activity of compound **10**.

The newly synthesized compounds were evaluated for their HIV-1 RT inhibitory activity. Percentage of inhibition has given in Table 3. Among the synthesized compounds, compound **24** showed significant HIV-1 RT inhibitory activity with 73% of inhibition with an IC$_{50}$ value of 1.31 μM. Compound **23** also showed 58% inhibition, however its IC$_{50}$ value was negligent. Rest of compounds showed weak activity.

From the results of HIV-1-RT inhibitory activity, it is evident that compound **24** with hydroxyl groups substituted at 2, 3 and 4 positions of the phenyl ring attached at the 5th position of the thiazolidinedione ring with a linker

Table 2 In *vitro* antibacterial and antifungal activity data of test compounds: 4-31

Minimum inhibitory concentration MIC (µg/mL)

Comp. code	S a	B.s	E.c	P.a	S.t	K.P	C.a	A.n
4	50	25	6.25	50	50	50	3.12	6.25
5	50	6.25	25	25	50	50	12.5	25
6	100	50	50	100	100	50	25	50
7	25	50	50	50	25	6.25	6.25	12.5
8	12.5	25	25	50	25	50	12.5	6.25
9	100	100	100	100	50	100	50	50
10	3.12	6.25	6.25	6.25	6.25	6.25	12.5	25
11	25	50	100	100	25	100	12.5	25
12	50	25	25	50	50	25	25	50
13	25	25	50	25	50	50	50	25
14	50	50	25	50	50	50	25	25
15	25	50	12.5	50	50	100	12.5	25
16	100	50	100	100	100	100	>100	>100
17	50	12.5	12.5	50	12.5	25	50	50
18	50	100	50	100	100	100	12.5	25
19	25	50	25	100	50	25	12.5	12.5
20	>100	>100	>100	>100	>100	>100	>100	>100
21	50	25	50	50	50	25	6.25	12.5
22	50	50	50	50	50	50	25	25
23	50	50	50	50	50	50	50	25
24	100	100	6.25	100	100	12.5	12.5	12.5
25	100	100	50	100	50	50	50	50
26	50	50	25	50	50	50	25	25
27	25	25	12.5	50	25	50	6.25	12.5
28	50	50	50	100	50	100	12.5	25
29	25	25	25	100	25	100	25	12.5
30	50	100	50	100	100	>100	25	12.5
31	>100	>100	>100	>100	>100	>100	>100	>100
*CIP.	0.78	0.78	0.78	0.78	0.78	0.78	-	-
*FLU.	-	-	-	-	-	-	12.5	12.5

S.a: *Staphylococcus aureus*, B.s:*Bacillus subtilis*, E.c:*Escherichia coli*, P.a: *Pseudomonas aeruginosa*, S.t: *Salmonella typhi*, K.p: *Klebsiella pneumonia*, C.a: *Candida albicans*, A.n: *Aspergillus niger*.
*CIP: Ciprofloxacin, *FLU: Fluconazole.
Experiments in duplicates.

Table 3 HIV-RT inhibitory activity

Comp. code	% inhibition
4	26.2
5	15.7
6	42
7	17.7
8	31
9	27
10	13.8
11	25.8
12	23.5
13	31.8
14	16.2
15	26
16	11
17	23
18	34
19	41.2
20	18.8
21	34
22	24
23	58
24*	73
25	34
26	23
27	34
28	6.5
29	24.5
30	14.1
31	10
Efavirenz*	98

IC_{50} (µM) of compound 24 is1.31 & efavirenz 0.0717, concentration used was 1 µM, experiments in duplicates.

Binding mode analysis

With the aim of rationalizing the biological data obtained and considering the best obtained *in vitro* results for the compounds **4–31**, a molecular modeling study was carried out in order to investigate the possible interactions of the highest active compounds **24, 10** and **4** with the non nucleoside inhibitory binding pocket (NNIBP) of RT, active site of GlcN-6-P synthase and cytochrome P450 14-α-sterol demethylase from *Candida albicans* (*Candida* P450DM) as the target receptors respectively using the Extra Precision (XP) mode of Glide software [36].

To validate the Glide software, firstly the interaction between TNK651 and HIV-1 RT was modeled. Superimposition of the experimental bound (co-crystallized)

group CH_2CH_2CONH at the N-3 position linked to a second phenyl ring substituted with a 2-mercapto group positively influenced the activity.

According to the above obtained data, we found that compounds **4–31** exhibited promising antimicrobial activities. In case of HIV-1-RT inhibitory activity, only compound **24** was found to be significantly active while the others exhibited weak non-nucleoside reverse transcriptase activity.

conformation of TNK651 [41] and that predicted by Glide are shown in Figure 2a. Glide successfully reproduced the experimental binding conformations of TNK 651 in the NNRTI-binding pocket of HIV-1 RT with an acceptable root-mean-square deviation (RMSD) of 2.4 Å. Visual inspection was then performed on the resulting docking solutions of the compound **24** to analyze the binding mode and key protein ligand interactions and was compared with that of the experimentally determined binding mode and interactions of the bound ligand TNK-651 and the standard efavirenz. The key interactions were mainly hydrogen bonding interactions with Lys103 and Lys101 respectively. The carbonyl oxygen at position 4 in the thiazolidinedione moiety forms a strong H-bond interaction with the NH terminal group of Lys103.Another strong H-bond interaction of the hydroxyl group at the ortho position of the first phenyl ring with one of carbonyl oxygen atoms of Lys101 was observed. The phenyl ring in the 2, 3, 4-trihydroxybenzaldehyde moiety along with the thiazolidinedione moiety was oriented in the bigger hydrophobic pocket formed by Phe227, Pro225 Leu234 Tyr181, Tyr188, Leu100 and Val179 while the CH_2CH_2CONH linker showed favorable interaction with the amino acid residues Tyr318, Pro236 and Val106. Docking score of the compound **24** (Glide XP score-11.30) was lower than the bound ligand TNK-651 (Glide XP score-13.29) but comparable to that of standard efavirenz (Glide XP score-11.33) .Possible interactions for the reference ligand TNK-651, efavirenz and compound **24** have been shown in Figure 2a,b and c respectively.

The active site of GlcN-6-P synthase (PDB code 2VF5) consists of 16 amino acid residues as Glu488, Ser303, Ala602 Ser347, Ser349, Gln348, Thr302, Thr352, Val605, Ala400, Cys300, Val399, Leu601, Leu484, Ser401 and Lys603 as shown in Figure 2d. Figure 2d and f shows the docked poses of the reference ligand and of highest active compound **10** respectively. The binding mode of GlcN-6-P synthase (2VF5) with its bound inhibitor glucosamine-6-Phosphate (Figure 2d) shows 9 hydrogen bonds with residues Glu488, Ser303, Ala602, Ser347, Ser349, Gln384, Thr302, Thr352, hydrophobic interactions with Val605, Ala400, Cys300, Val399, Leu601, Leu484 and electrostatic interactions with Ser401 and Lys603 with a docking score – 7.16. Docking validation was performed with an RMSD value of 1.674 Å ensuring precision and reproducibility of the docking process. The docked pose of active compound **10** (Glide XP score –4.89) has been depicted in Figure 2f. It was interesting to note that three important hydrogen bonds are formed by compound **10**. The hydroxyl group on the benzylidene moiety forms a hydrogen bond with the carbonyl oxygen of Thr302. The NH in the CH_2CH_2CONH linker forms a strong hydrogen bond with the carbonyl oxygen of Val399. Another strong

H-bond is evident between the carbonyl oxygen of thiazolidinedione with the NH terminal group of Ala602. The 2-hydroxyphenyl group makes favorable interaction with the side chain of Ala 400. The thiazolidinedione ring shows favorably oriented towards the residues Leu601, Cys300, Val605 and Ala353. The linker (CH_2CH_2CONH) shows favorable interactions with Leu484.

As the target enzyme *Candida* P450DM is a membrane-bound enzyme, it is difficult to crystallize by X-ray analysis; therefore, no experimental data has been available for the structure of this enzyme. However, the crystallographic structure of the complex between cytochrome P450 14-α-sterol demethylase from *Mycobacterium tuberculosis* (*Mycobacterium* P450DM) and fluconazole is present in the Protein Data Bank with the ID 1EA1. A perusal of the literature showed that high homology exists between the two analogous enzymes, *Candida* P450DM and *Mycobacterium* P450DM [42].

A chimeric enzyme of *Candida* P450DM complexed with fluconazole was modeled following the procedure of Rosello *et al.* [42]. Fluconazole maintained practically the same orientation as in 1EA1 with a docking score of –6.01. In fluconazole, interaction of triazole ring with heme is co-ordination of N atom with Fe atom of heme, while another triazole ring also forms π– π stacking interactions with Tyr78 and His78. The diflurophenyl group also forms π–π stacking interactions with Phe100. Phenyl ring shows hydrophobic interactions with amino acid residues Leu79, Leu96, Phe83, Met255, Ala256, Leu321 and Val 434. Docking validation was performed with RMSD value of 2.094 Å ensuring precision and reproducibility of the docking process (Figure 2e).

To illustrate the binding mode of the newly synthesized compounds in the active site of chimeric 1EA1, the docked pose of the highest active compound **4** (Glide XP score –8.13) has been analysed as follows (Figure 2g). The key interactions are mainly hydrogen bonding interactions. The hydroxyl group on the benzylidene moiety forms a hydrogen bond with Hie392. The CO in the CH_2CH_2CONH linker forms a strong coordinate bond with Hem460. The aromatic ring forms π–π stacking interactions with Phe83 residue. The thiazolidinedione ring is oriented in the hydrophobic pocket formed by Tyr181, Phe100, Met255, Val395 and Leu79. Both phenyl rings attached to the thiazolidinedione nucleus makes favorable interactions with the side chains of Leu96, Al173, Tyr76, Cys394, Phe387, Ile324, Ala389 and Leu321.

These docking results demonstrate that hydrogen bond interactions, hydrophobic interactions and the coordinate bond with the Hem residue in 1EA1 are very important for binding of compound **4** with the active site residues and may be responsible for the very high antifungal activity as shown by compound **4**.

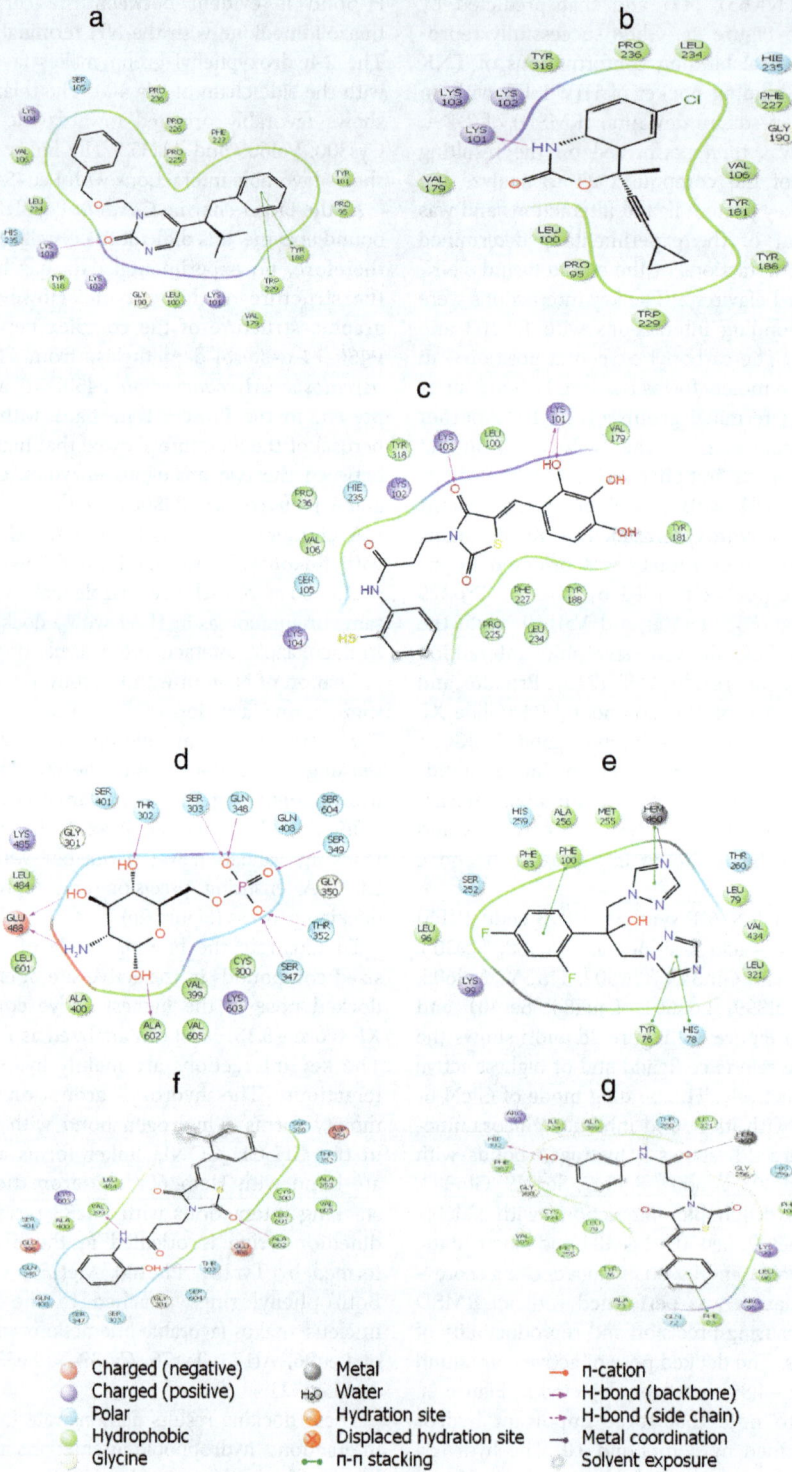

Figure 2 2D sketch views. Binding mode of **a)** Ref. ligand (TNK-651) **b)** efavirenz **c)** compound 24 into the NNIBP of 1RT2 **d)** Glucosamine-6-Phosphate (2VF5) **e)** Ref ligand fluconazole (chimeric 1EA1) and compounds **f)** 10 in the active site of 2VF5 **g)** 4 in the active site of chimeric 1EA1.

Conclusion

In the present study, a series of thiazolidinedione analogs have been synthesized and their structures have been characterized by IR, NMR and mass spectroscopy. All the newly synthesized compounds were tested for HIV-1- RT inhibitory activity by microplate assay method and for antimicrobial activity by two fold serial dilution method. From the modeling studies as well as from the SAR, electronegative groups substituted at various positions of the phenyl rings with a thiazolidinedione scaffold may be responsible for the very high HIV-1-RT inhibitory activity of compound 24. In case of antibacterial activity the methyl groups substituted in the phenyl group attached to the 5th position of the thiazolidinedione ring system plays a significant role while in case of antifungal activity the electronegative groups, particularly hydroxyl groups substituted in the various positions of both the phenyl groups are responsible for enhanced antifungal activity. The study encourages us to consider a new molecular skeleton of thiazolidinediones substituted at the 3rd and 5th position by aryl groups with adequate spacers may be identified as a potential lead compound for the development of ant-HIV agents with the ability to combat opportunistic bacterial and fungal infections.

Abbreviations

Å: Angstrom; AIDS: Acquired Immuno Deficiency Syndrome; AR: Analytical reagent; °C: Degree centigrade; DMSO: Dimethyl sulfoxide; CD4: Cluster of differentiation 4; CFU: Colony forming unit; GHz: Giga hertz; GR: Guaranteed reagent; h: Hour; Hz: Hertz; HIV: Human Immuno Deficiency Virus; HIV-1: Human Immuno Deficiency Virus Type-1; ^{1}H NMR: Proton Nuclear Magnetic Resonance; IR: Infrared; IC$_{50}$: 50% Inhibitory Concentration; MS: Mass Spectroscopy; MTCC: Microbial Type Culture Collection; NCIM: National Collection of Industrial Microorganisms; NNRTIs: Non Nucleoside Reverse Transcriptase Inhibitors; OPLS: Optimized potentials for liquid simulations; PDB: Protein Data Bank; RMSD: Root mean square deviation; RT: Reverse transcriptase; SAR: Structure activity relationship; XP: Extra precision.

Competing interests

The authors declare that they have no competing interests.

Authors' contributions

SG: Design of target compounds, supervision of the synthetic part and manuscript preparation. RSB: Synthesis of target compounds and performed the biological tests. KC and SS: Collaboration in identifying of the structures of target compounds for anti-HIV activity. All authors read and approved the final manuscript.

Acknowledgements

The authors acknowledge the University Grants Commission for providing financial support in the form of a Major Research Project. One of the authors (RSB) gratefully acknowledges University Grants Commission-Basic Science Research (UGC-BSR) for award of fellowship during the work.

Author details

[1]Department of Pharmaceutical Sciences, Birla Institute of Technology, Mesra, Ranchi 835215, Jharkhand, India. [2]Department of Biochemistry, Faculty of Science, Kasetsart University, Bangkean, Bangkok 10900, Thailand.

References

1. Patel D, Kumari P, Patel N. Synthesis of 3-{4-[4-dimethylamino-6-(4-methyl-2-oxo-2H-chromen-7-yloxy)-[1,3,5]triazin-2-ylamino]-phenyl}-2-phenyl-5-(4-pyridin-2-yl-piperazin-1-ylmethyl)-thiazolidin-4-one and their biological evaluation. Med Chem Res. 2012;21(10):2926–94.
2. Shiradkar MR, Ghodake M, Bothara KG, Bhandari SB, Nikalje A, Akula KC, et al. Synthesis and anticonvulsant activity of clubbed thiazolidinone–barbituric acid and thiazolidinone–triazole derivatives. ARKIVOC. 2007;XIV:58.
3. Lohray BB, Bhushan V, Rao BP, Madhavan GR, Murali N, Rao KN, et al. Novel euglycemic and hypolipidemic agents. 1. J Med Chem. 1998;41:1619–30.
4. Prabhakar C, Madhusudhan G, Sahadev K, Maheedhara Reddy C, Sarma M, Reddy GO, et al. Synthesis and biological activity of novel thiazolidinediones. Bioorg Med Chem Lett. 1998;8:2725–30.
5. Sunduru N, Srivastava K, Rajakumar S, Puri S, Saxena J, Chauhan P. Synthesis of novel thiourea, thiazolidinedione and thioparabanic acid derivatives of 4-aminoquinoline as potent antimalarials. Bioorg Med Chem Lett. 2009;19:2570–3.
6. Reddy KA, Lohray B, Bhushan V, Reddy AS, Kishore PH, Rao VV, et al. Novel euglycemic and hypolipidemic agents: Part-2 antioxidant moiety as structural motif. Bioorg Med Chem Lett. 1998;8:999–1002.
7. Hafez HN, El-Gazzar A-R. Synthesis and antitumor activity of substituted triazolo [4, 3-a] pyrimidin-6-sulfonamide with an incorporated thiazolidinone moiety. Bioorg Med Chem Lett. 2009;19:4143–7.
8. Patil V, Tilekar K, Mehendale-Munj S, Mohan R, Ramaa C. Synthesis and primary cytotoxicity evaluation of new 5-benzylidene-2, 4-thiazolidinedione derivatives. Eur J Med Chem. 2010;45:4539–44.
9. Bonde CG, Gaikwad NJ. Synthesis and preliminary evaluation of some pyrazine containing thiazolines and thiazolidinones as antimicrobial agents. Bioorg Med Chem. 2004;12:2151–61.
10. Amarnath N, Guo Y, Harbinski F, Fan YH, Chen H, Luus L, et al. Novel arylsulfoanilide-oxindole hybrid as an anticancer agent that inhibits translation initiation. J Med Chem. 2004;47(21):4979–82.
11. Tomasic T, Zidar N, Mueller-Premru M, Kikelj D, Masic LP. Synthesis and antibacterial activity of 5- ylidenethiazolidin-4-ones and 5-benzylidene-4,6-pyrimidinediones. Eur J Med Chem. 2010;45(4):1667–72.
12. Carroll RT, Dluzen DE, Stinnett H, Awale PS, Funk MO, Geldenhuys WJ. Structure–activity relationship and docking studies of thiazolidinedione-type compounds with monoamine oxidase B. Bioorg Med Chem Lett. 2011;21:4798–803.
13. Youssef AM, Sydney White M, Villanueva EB, El-Ashmawy IM, Klegeris A. Synthesis and biological evaluation of novel pyrazolyl-2, 4-thiazolidinediones as anti-inflammatory and neuroprotective agents. Bioorg Med Chem. 2010;18:2019–28.
14. Ali AM, Saber GE, Mahfouz NM, El-Gendy MA, Radwan AA, Hamid MA. Synthesis and three-dimensional qualitative structure selectivity relationship of 3, 5-disubstituted-2, 4-thiazolidinedione derivatives as COX2 inhibitors. Arch Pharm Res. 2007;30:1186–204.
15. Malik S, Choudhary A, Bahare RS. Synthesis of some novel substituted arylidene and substituted benzylthiazolidine-2, 4-dione analogues as chemotherapeutic agents. Asian J Chem. 2011;23:5547–8.
16. Barreca ML, Balzarini J, Chimirri A, Clercq ED, Luca LD, Höltje HD, et al. Design, Synthesis, Structure Activity Relationships, and Molecular Modeling Studies of 2,3-Diaryl-1,3-thiazolidin-4-ones as Potent Anti-HIV Agents. J Med Chem. 2002;45(24):5410–3.
17. Zhang GH, Wang Q, Chen JJ, Zhang XM, Tam SC, Zheng YT, et al. The anti-HIV-1 effect of scutellarin. Biochem Biophys Res Commun. 2005;334:812–6.
18. Sriram D, Bal TR, Yogeeswari P. Design, synthesis and biological evaluation of novel non-nucleoside HIV-1 reverse transcriptase inhibitors with broad-spectrum chemotherapeutic properties. Bioorg Med Chem. 2004;12(22):5865–73.
19. Ganguly S, Murugesan S, Prasanthi N, Alptürk O, Herman B, Cremer NS. Synthesis and Anti-HIV-1 Activity of a Novel Series of Aminoimidazole Analogs. Lett Drug Des Discov. 2010;7(5):318–23.
20. Dündar B, Özgen OB, Menteşe A, Altanlar N, Atli N, Kendi E, et al. Synthesis and antimicrobial activity of some thiazolyl thiazolidine-2, 4-dione derivatives. Bioorg Med Chem. 2007;15(18):6012–7.
21. Chopra I, Schofield C, Everett M, Neill AO, Miller K, Wilcox M, et al. Treatment of health-care- associated infections caused by Gram-negative bacteria: a consensus statement. Lancet Infect Dis. 2008;8(2):133–9.
22. Beale JM, Block J. Organic Medicinal & Pharmaceutical Chemistry. Philadelphia: Lippincott Williams & Wilkins; 2010.

23. Edmond MB, Wallace SE, McClish DK, Pfaller MA, Jones RN, Wenzel RP. Nosocomial blood stream infections in United States hospitals: a three-year analysis. Clin Infect Dis. 1999;29(2):239–44.

24. Vijesh AM, Isloor AM, Telkar S, Fun HK. Molecular docking studies of some new imidazole derivatives for antimicrobial properties. Arabean J Chem. 2013;6:197–204.

25. Chmara H, Andruszkiewicz R, Borowski E. Inactivation of glucosamine-6-phosphatesynthetase from Salmonella typhimurium LT2 SL 1027 by N-beta-fumarylcarboxyamido-l-2,3-diamino-propionic acid. Biochem Biophys Res Commun. 1984;120:865–72.

26. Sangamwar AT, Deshpande UD, Pekamwar SS. Antifungals: need to search for a new molecular target. Indian J Pharm Sci. 2008;70(4):423–30.

27. Georgopapadakou NH, Walsh TJ. Antifungal agents: chemotherapeutic targets and immunologic strategies. Antimicrob Agents Chemother. 1996;40(2):279.

28. Perfect JR. Molecular targets for new antifungal drugs. Can J Bot. 1995;73(S1):1187–91.

29. Groll AH, De Lucca AJ, Walsh TJ. Emerging targets for the development of novel antifungal therapeutics. Trends Microbiol. 1998;6(3):117–24.

30. Sangshetti JN, Lokwani DK, Sarkate AP, Shinde DB. Synthesis, Antifungal Activity, and Docking Study of Some New 1, 2, 4-triazole Analogs. Chem Biol Drug Des. 2011;78(5):800–9.

31. Prakash O, Aneja DK, Arora S, Sharma C, Aneja KR. Synthesis and antimircrobial activities of some new 5-(3- aryl)-phenyl-1H-pyrazol-4-yl) methylene)-3-phenylthiazolidin-2,4-diones. Med Chem Res. 2012;21:10–5.

32. Ganguly S, Bahare RS. Molecular docking studies of novel thiazolidinedione analogs as HIV-1-RT inhibitors. Med Chem Res. 2013;22(7):3350–63.

33. Sachan N, Kadam SS, Kulkarni VM. Synthesis and antihyperglycemic activity and QSAR of 5-benzylidine2,4- thiazolidinediones. Indian J Hetrocycl Chem. 2007;7:57.

34. NCCLS. Method for dilution antimicrobial susceptibility tests for bacteria that grow aerobically, 5th ed. Approved standard M7: A5. Villanova, PA: NCCLS; 2000.

35. Silprasit K, Thammaporn R, Tecchasakul S, Hannongbua S, Choowongkomon K. Simple and rapid determination of the enzyme kinetics of HIV-1 reverse transcriptase and anti-HIV-1 agents by a fluorescence based method. J Virol Methods. 2011;117:381–7.

36. Glide 5.0, Schrödinger, Inc. New York, U.S.A; 2008, www.schrodinger.com.

37. Ganguly S, Bahare RS. Comparative molecular docking studies of novel 3, 5-disubstituted. Med Chem Res. 2014;23:1300–8.

38. Podust LM, Stojan J, Poulos TL, Waterman MR. Substrate recognition sites in 14α-sterol Demethylase from comparative analysis of amino acid sequences and X-ray structure of Mycobacterium tuberculosis CYP51. Proc Natl Acad Sci U S A. 2001;98:3068–73.

39. Podust LM, Stojan J, Poulos TL, Waterman MR, Stojan J, Poulos TL, et al. Substrate recognition sites in 14α-sterol demethylase from comparative analysis of amino acid sequences and X-ray structure of Mycobacterium tuberculosis CYP51. J Inorg Biochem. 2001;87(4):227–35.

40. Murugesan S, Ganguly S, Maga G. Synthesis, evaluation and molecular modelling studies of some novel 3-(3, 4- dihydroisoquinolin-2(1H)-yl)-N-(substitutedphenyl) propanamides as HIV-1 non-nucleoside reverse transcriptase inhibitors. J Chem Sci. 2010;122:169–76.

41. Hopkins AL, Ren J, Esnouf RM, Willcox BE, Jones EY, Ross C, et al. Complexes of HIV-1 reverse transcriptase with inhibitors of the HEPT series reveal conformational changes relevant to the design of potent non-nucleoside inhibitors. J Med Chem. 1996;39(8):589–1600.

42. Rosell A, Bertini S, Lapucci A, Macchia M, Martinelli A, Rapposelli S, et al. Synthesis, antifungal activity, and molecular modeling studies of new inverted oxime ethers of oxiconazole. J Med Chem. 2002;45(22):4903–12.

21

Zinc and diabetes mellitus: understanding molecular mechanisms and clinical implications

Priyanga Ranasinghe[1][*] [iD], Shehani Pigera[1], Priyadarshani Galappatthy[1], Prasad Katulanda[2] and Godwin R. Constantine[2]

Abstract

Background: Diabetes mellitus is a leading cause of morbidity and mortality worldwide. Studies have shown that Zinc has numerous beneficial effects in both type-1 and type-2 diabetes. We aim to evaluate the literature on the mechanisms and molecular level effects of Zinc on glycaemic control, β-cell function, pathogenesis of diabetes and its complications.

Methods: A review of published studies reporting mechanisms of action of Zinc in diabetes was undertaken in PubMed and SciVerse Scopus medical databases using the following search terms in article title, abstract or keywords; ("Zinc" or "Zn") and ("mechanism" or "mechanism of action" or "action" or "effect" or "pathogenesis" or "pathology" or "physiology" or "metabolism") and ("diabetes" or "prediabetes" or "sugar" or "glucose" or "insulin").

Results: The literature search identified the following number of articles in the two databases; PubMed ($n = 1799$) and SciVerse Scopus ($n = 1879$). After removing duplicates the total number of articles included in the present review is 111. Our results show that Zinc plays an important role in β-cell function, insulin action, glucose homeostasis and the pathogenesis of diabetes and its complications.

Conclusion: Numerous *in-vitro* and *in-vivo* studies have shown that Zinc has beneficial effects in both type-1 and type-2 diabetes. However further randomized double-blinded placebo-controlled clinical trials conducted for an adequate duration, are required to establish therapeutic safety in humans.

Introduction

Diabetes mellitus is a leading cause of morbidity and mortality worldwide, with an estimated 387 million adults being affected in year 2014, a figure which is expected to increase by nearly 40 % by year 2035 [1]. Ninety to ninety five percent of those with the disease have type-2 diabetes. In a patho-physiologic sense, type-2 diabetes is a multi-organ, multi-factorial condition characterized primarily by insulin resistance, hyper insulinaemia and β-cell dysfunction, which ultimately leads to β-cell failure [2]. Type-1 diabetes has historically been most prevalent in populations of European origin, and the latest edition of the Diabetes Atlas estimates that 490,100 children below the age of 15 years are living with type-1 diabetes [1]. Currently 77 % of those with diabetes live in low- and middle-income countries of the African, Asian, and South American regions [1, 3, 4]. In 2014, diabetes was responsible for 4.9 million deaths worldwide and at least US$ 612 billion in global healthcare expenditures (11 % of the total global healthcare expenditures in adults) [1]. Recent cost estimates, include those for Brazil (US$ 3.9 billion), Argentina (US$ 0.8 billion) and Mexico (US$ 2.0 billion) [5]. Each of these is an annual figure and is rising as diabetes prevalence increases. Overall, direct health care costs of diabetes ranges from 2.5 to 15 % annual health care budgets, depending on local diabetes prevalence and the sophistication of the treatment available [5]. Diabetes is also associated with a host of potentially disabling macro- and micro-vascular complications. Hence, there is also a much larger burden in the form of lost productivity as a result of restricted daily activity. This rapidly increasing prevalence is attributable to population growth, aging, urbanization, unhealthy dietary habits, increasing prevalence of obesity and physical inactivity [6].

* Correspondence: priyanga.ranasinghe@gmail.com
[1]Department of Pharmacology, Faculty of Medicine, University of Colombo, Colombo, Sri Lanka
Full list of author information is available at the end of the article

Although comprehensive diabetes management guidelines are readily available, even in developed countries like the US 30–50 % adults with diabetes do not meet individualized targets for glycaemic, blood pressure, or lipid control [7]. Reasons for failure to achieve glycaemic control includes the progression of underlying β-cell dysfunction, incomplete adherence to treatment (often due to adverse effects of medication) and reluctance of clinicians to intensify therapy [8]. Anti-diabetic agents currently in use can directly or indirectly enhance the functioning of β-cells. However, reducing the decline and the eventual failure of β-cells is crucial in preventing type-2 diabetes in those at risk and halting disease progression in the affected patients [8]. The increasing worldwide prevalence of type-2 diabetes and the progressive loss of metabolic control in patients are clear demonstrations that the current therapeutic strategies aimed at protecting the β-cells are largely inadequate. Hence there is an urgent need for anti-diabetic agents targeting the intimate mechanisms of β-cell damage and optimizing its function at cellular level.

Insulin, is stored as a hexamer containing two Zinc ions in β-cells of the pancreas and released into the portal venous system at the time of β-cell de-granulation [9]. In-vitro and in-vivo studies in animals and humans have shown that Zinc has numerous beneficial effects in both type-1 and type-2 diabetes [10–14]. A recent meta-analysis confirmed these findings, and concluded that Zinc supplementation in patients with diabetes improves glycaemic control and promotes healthy lipid parameters [15]. Hence, it is evident that Zinc has a promising potential as a novel therapeutic agent in diabetes. Studies have also shown that diabetes is commonly accompanied by hypozincemia and hyperzincuria [16, 17]. Furthermore the high prevalence of Zinc deficiency in developing countries could be contributing towards driving the current diabetes epidemic encountered by them [4, 18]. Numerous research studies have been conducted to clarify the molecular mechanisms underlying the action of Zinc in diabetes. Understanding the molecular mechanisms of action of Zinc will help to further develop targeted therapy and guide future research. The present study aims to systematically evaluate the literature on the mechanisms and molecular level effects of Zinc on glycaemic control, β-cell function, pathogenesis of diabetes and its complications.

Methods

A systematic review of published studies reporting mechanisms of action of Zinc in diabetes was undertaken in accordance with the Preferred Reporting Items for Systematic reviews and Meta-Analyses (PRISMA) statement (Additional file 1).

Search strategy

A comprehensive search of the literature was conducted in the PubMed® (U.S. National Library of Medicine, USA) and SciVerse Scopus® (Elsevier Properties S.A, USA) databases for studies published before 31st July 2015. During the first stage the above databases were searched using the following search terms in article title, abstract or keywords; ("Zinc" or "Zn") and ("mechanism" or "mechanism of action" or "action" or "effect" or "pathogenesis" or "pathology" or "physiology" or "metabolism") and ("diabetes" or "prediabetes" or "sugar" or "glucose" or "insulin").

In the second stage the total hits obtained from searching these three databases were pooled together and duplicates were removed. This was followed by screening of the retrieved articles by reading the article title in the third and abstracts in fourth stage. In the fifth stage individual manuscripts were screened, and those not satisfying inclusion criteria (given below) were excluded. This search process was conducted independently by two reviewers (PR and SP) and the final group of articles to be included in the review was determined after an iterative consensus process.

Inclusion/exclusion criteria and data extraction

The following inclusion criteria were used; a) In-vitro or in-vivo studies reporting effect of Zinc on diabetes/prediabetes, evaluating effects of Zinc on sugar/glucose, insulin and/or related metabolic parameters, evaluating the effects of Zinc on pathogenesis and/or complication of diabetes b) Published in English, or with detailed summaries in English and c) Peer-reviewed fully published research papers. Conference proceedings, editorials, commentaries, review articles and book chapters/book reviews were excluded.

Data were extracted from the included studies by one reviewer using a standardized form and checked for accuracy by a second reviewer. The data extracted from each study were: a) study details (lead author, year published/year of survey, type of study—In-vitro/In-vivo), b) methods (study design, sample size, duration) and c) mechanism of action data. Discrepancies in the extracted data were resolved by discussion, with involvement of a third reviewer when necessary.

Results

The literature search using the above search criteria identified the following number of articles in the two databases; Medline® ($n = 1799$) and SciVerse Scopus® ($n = 1879$). After removing duplicates the total number of articles included in the present review is 111. The search strategy is summarized in Fig. 1.

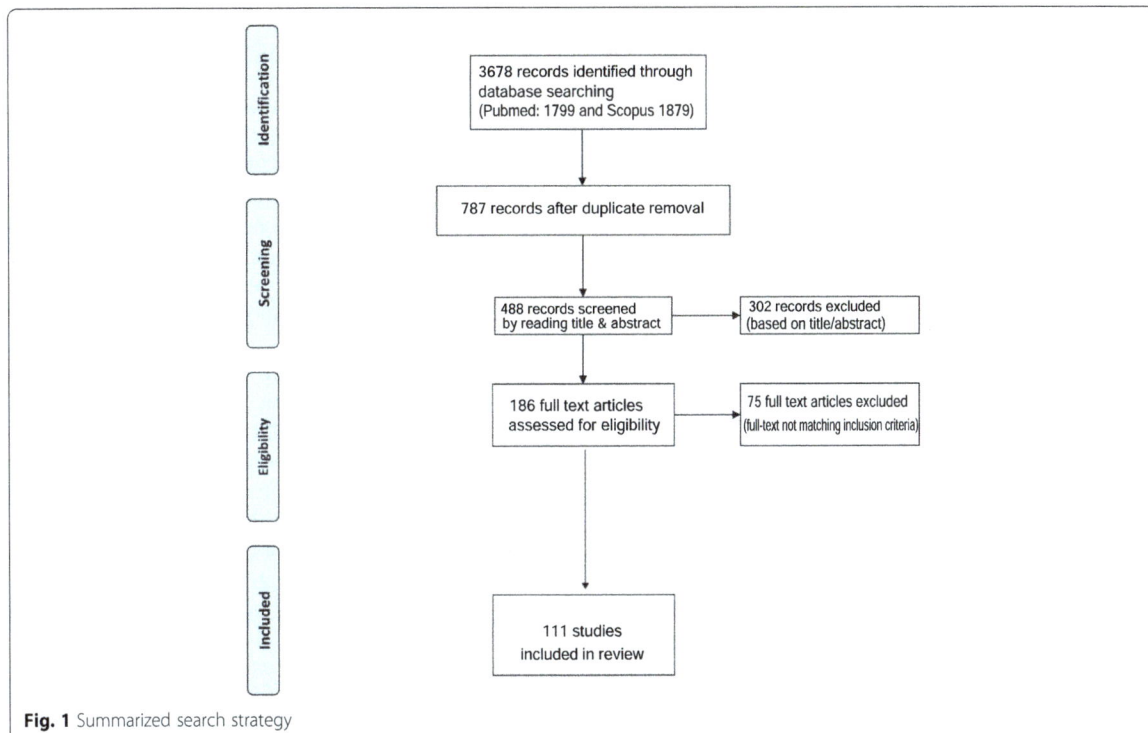

Fig. 1 Summarized search strategy

Anti-oxidant properties

Anti-oxidant properties of Zinc have been evaluated *in-vitro*, as well as *in-vivo* animal and human studies. Hypozincaemia and hyperzincuria is known to be present in patients with both type-1 and type-2 diabetes, and Zinc supplementation is known to be helpful in restoring plasma Zinc levels to normal [11, 19–21]. Plasma Thiobarbituric acid reactive substances (TBARS), a marker of oxidative stress is high in both type-1 and type-2 diabetic patients, and significantly decreased by supplementation of Zinc 30 mg/day for 3–6 months [11, 19]. Selenium-dependent glutathione peroxidase (Se-GPx), an anti-oxidant enzyme was also low at baseline in patients with type-1 diabetes, and was normalized after Zinc supplementation [11]. However, no significant difference in anti-oxidant metallo-enzyme activity was observed in patients with type-2 diabetes [19]. Plasma Zinc levels are known to be negatively correlated with the TBARS levels in both obese and non-obese patients with type-2 diabetes [22].

In animal models of insulin resistance, Zinc supplementation is known to enhance insulin sensitivity and antioxidant status [23, 24]. Furthermore, in diabetes induced animal models anti-oxidant enzymes catalase, GPx and super-oxide dismutase (SOD) are decreased than in normal animals [25–27]. Zinc supplementation in these animals restored the enzyme activity and increased glutathione synthesis [25–27]. Plasma malondialdehyde (MDA) levels, an index of lipid peroxidation was increased in

diabetic animals and significantly decreased following Zinc supplementation [26, 28]. When rats were simultaneously treated with a single injection of alloxan and $ZnCl_2$, the increase in blood glucose concentration induced by alloxan was significantly reduced at 24, 48, and 72 h post-treatment with $ZnCl_2$ [29]. $ZnCl_2$ injection also increased the retinal, pancreatic, and liver glutathione and reduced the TBARS content in comparison with the alloxan-treated group [29]. Zinc supplementation or injection is also known to cause a significant induction of anti-oxidant metallothionein (MT) protein synthesis in the pancreatic islets, kidneys, liver and heart of diabetes-induced animals [27, 28, 30–34].

A significant increase in cardiac morphological impairment, fibrosis, and dysfunction is seen in diabetic mice, which is reversed by Zinc [33]. Cultured cardiac cells that were directly exposed to high levels of glucose (HG) and free fatty acid (FFA), treatment that mimics diabetes, resulted in reduced cell survival rate, which was reversed by Zinc [33]. Furthermore, when MT expression was silenced with the use of MT small-interfering RNA, the preventive effect of pretreatment with Zinc was abolished [33]. Hence, the prevention of diabetic cardiomyopathy by Zinc supplementation is predominantly mediated by an increase in cardiac MT and the resultant anti-oxidant effects [33, 35]. Diabetes-induced renal oxidative damage, inflammation and up-regulated expression of pro-fibrosis mediators were also markedly attenuated by

Zinc supplementation, mediated via the expression of MT [27, 36]. *In-vivo* studies in diabetes induced rats have shown that Zinc has a protective effect against diabetes induced peripheral nerve damage by stimulating MT synthesis and reducing oxidative stress [37].

Diabetes induced a significant increase in aortic oxidative damage, inflammation, and remodeling in mice (increased fibrosis and wall thickness) [38]. Zinc treatment of these diabetic mice completely prevented the above pathogenic changes in the aorta, and also significantly up-regulated the expression and function of nuclear factor (erythroid-derived 2)-like 2 (Nrf2), a pivotal regulator of anti-oxidative mechanisms, and the expression of MT [38]. The same up-regulation of Nrf2 by Zinc has been demonstrated in human renal tubule cells *in-vitro* and mouse kidney *in-vivo* under the diabetic conditions [39]. In cultured renal tubular epithelial cells (NRK-52E), Zinc supplementation inhibited high glucose induced cell apoptosis by attenuating reactive oxygen species production, facilitated via Nrf2 up-regulation [40]. In postmenopausal women with type-2 diabetes Zinc supplementation increases TNF-α gene expression, suggesting a close interaction between Zinc homeostasis, oxidative stress and inflammation [41].

Effects on carbohydrate and lipid metabolism

Zinc is known to stimulate glycolysis and inhibit gluconeogenesis, an effect that is not overcome by the presence of glucagon [42–44]. *In-vitro* studies have demonstrated that Zinc increases the activity of glycolytic enzymes, phosphofructokinase (PFK) and pyruvate kinase (PK) in a concentration- and time-dependent manner [45, 46]. Lactate production which reflects the PFK activity, was increased by Zinc [46]. However, the effects of Zinc and insulin were not additive and Zinc pretreatment prevented the stimulation of glycolytic enzymes by insulin. Furthermore, in Zinc-treated cells a progressive activation of ERK2/MAPK1 (Mitogen-activated protein kinase-1) was observed [45]. However, a recent *in-vitro* study using hepatocytes has shown that at sub-lethal concentrations, ZnO nanoparticles increase both gluconeogenesis and glycogenolysis, contradicting the finding from the earlier studies given above [47].

Zinc is also known to be a concentration dependent reversible inhibitor of α-glucosidase activity in the intestines [48, 49]. Zinc binding to α-glucosidase directly induced tertiary structural changes, however the concentration required to induce structural changes was greater than that required to achieve inhibition [49]. In skeletal muscles Zinc-α2-glycoprotein stimulates the phosphorylation of AMP-activated protein kinase (AMPKα) and increases cellular GLUT4 protein [50]. This increase in the expression of the GLUT4 has also been observed in adipose tissue with resultant increase in glucose uptake [44, 51, 52].

Studies have also shown that whole body as well as adipose tissue specific insulin sensitivity was positively associated with Zinc-α2-glycoprotein expression in subcutaneous adipose tissue and that obesity related decrease in Zinc-α2-glycoprotein is selectively present in subcutaneous but not in visceral adipose tissue [53]. However, two recent studies have indicated that Zinc-α2-glycoprotein functions to inhibit insulin signaling and, in consequence, insulin-induced glucose uptake in adipocytes, whereas, Zinc Finger Protein 407 (ZFP407) is known to stimulate GLUT4 mRNA transcription in adipocytes, facilitating insulin-stimulated glucose uptake via GLUT4 [54, 55].

Zinc also enhanced glucose transport in adipocytes in a dose dependant manner, independent of insulin [43, 56–58]. Zinc was observed to stimulate the phosphorylation of the IR-ß (Insulin Receptor) subunit [52, 56]. Zinc also inhibits Glycogen synthase kinase-3 (GSK-3β), which is a phosphorylating and an inactivating agent of glycogen synthase, with resultant increase in glycogen synthesis [57]. Furthermore, Zinc-α2-glycoproteins increase the expression of the lipolytic enzymes, adipose triglyceride lipase and hormone-sensitive lipase in the white adipose tissue [51]. Incubation of adipocytes with Zinc, augmented lipogenesis and this lipogenic effect was 80 % of maximum insulin stimulation [43, 59]. In isolated rat liver membrane cells, Zinc alone stimulated lipogenesis in a dose-related manner [60].

Treatment of 3 T3-L1 adipocytes with Zinc-chelated vitamin C (ZnC) has been shown to promote adipogenesis, characterized by increased glycerol-3-phosphate dehydrogenase activity and intracellular lipid accumulation in 3 T3-L1 cells, associated with a pronounced up-regulation of the expression of glucose transporter type 4 (GLUT4) [61]. ZnC further increased the expression of peroxisome proliferator-activated receptor gamma (PPARγ) and CCAAT/enhancer-binding protein alpha, the key transcription factors of adipogenesis [61]. A decrease in insulin receptor binding has been observed in Zinc deficient rat adipocytes and addition of Zinc stimulates insulin binding in a dose-dependent manner [60, 62].

Islet cell function

In-vitro environments increasing the extracellular Zinc concentration is known to increase the free insulin concentration in the immediate vicinity of β-cells, mediated by enhanced Zinc-insulin dissociation [63]. However, glucose stimulated insulin secretion in β-cells of the pancreas is inhibited by Zinc, suggesting that co-secreted Zinc acts in an autocrine inhibitory modulator [64, 65]. In pancreatic β-cells of mice and clonal HIT-T15 β-cells, KCl and glucose induced an increase in free cytosolic Zinc levels, which facilitated the processing and/or storage of insulin [66, 67]. This is facilitated by an increase in the expression of cellular Zinc importers (Slc39a6, Slc39a7, and Slc39a8).

However, chronic increase in cytosolic Zinc levels following sustained hyperglycemia, as in diabetes may contribute towards β-cell dysfunction and death [66].

Human Islet Amyloid Polypeptide (hIAPP) (a polypeptide hormone secreted from pancreatic β-cells in response to glucose) and is cleared by the peptidases in the kidney. hIAPP is known to aggregate in the pancreas to form dense, insoluble extracellular fibrillar deposit, causing β-cell destruction in type-2 diabetes [68]. Zinc, significantly inhibits hIAPP amyloid fibrillogenesis at concentrations similar to those found *in-vivo* extracellular environments [68]. This probably explains the linkage between the mutations of SLC30A8 zinc transporter (Zinc Transporter 8 [ZnT8]), which transports Zinc into the secretory granules, and type-2 diabetes. In human pancreatic islet cells, ZnT8 is the key protein responsible for both intracellular Zinc accumulation in insulin-containing vesicles and regulation of insulin secretion [69–73]. ZnT8 down regulated cells show reduced insulin content and decreased insulin secretion in response to hyperglycemic stimuli [74]. However, absence of ZnT8 expression did not alter rates of insulin biosynthesis, insulin content and glucose metabolism, but contributed to the packaging efficiency of stored insulin [75–77]. When ZnT8 absent mice were fed a control diet, glucose tolerance and insulin sensitivity were normal. However, after high-fat diet feeding, these mice became glucose intolerant or diabetic, and islets became less responsive to glucose [75]. ZnT8 is down regulated on exposure to metabolic stress associated with diabetic and pre-diabetic states, suggesting that it might further contribute to progression of type-2 diabetes [78, 79]. In β-cell specific SLC30A8 deficiency (ZnT8 knockout mice) a low peripheral blood insulin levels was observed, due to a substantial amount of the insulin being degraded during its first passage through the liver [80]. This is possibly due to the low level of Zinc in the portal circulation co-secreted by β-cells, due to the absence of ZnT8 (reducing uptake of Zinc by β-cells), which leads to augmented hepatic insulin clearance. The ZnT8 is also downregulated in response to exposure of pancreatic β-cells to hypoxia, resulting in lowered cytosolic Zn^{2+} concentrations [81].

Pancreatic islet cells harvested from rats conditioned under intermittent hypoxia showed a significant reduction in Zinc Influx Transporter 8 (ZIP8) expression in the β-cell membrane, with resultant reduction in cellular Zinc concentration and insulin production [82]. ZIP6 and ZIP7 function as two important zinc influx transporters to regulate cytosolic Zinc concentrations and insulin secretion in β-cells and ZIP-6 is also capable of directly interacting with GLP-1R to facilitate the protective effect of GLP-1 on β-cell survival [83]. Zip4 protein is located in human pancreatic β-cells, is important for

the accumulation of Zinc in the cytosol and granules of β-cells [84]. Other Zinc transporters like ZnT3 and ZIP7 might also play a role in insulin secretion and glucose metabolism [85, 86].

L-type voltage-gated Ca^{2+} channels and TRMP3 (transient receptor potential cation channel subfamily M member 3) are also in part responsible for Zinc transport into β-cells, which is also dependent upon the metabolic status of the cell [87, 88]. Culture of rat pancreatic islets in either low or high vs. intermediate glucose concentrations triggers early mitochondrial oxidative stress and late β-cell apoptosis with loss of glucose stimulated insulin secretion [89]. $ZnCl_2$ reduces mitochondrial oxidative stress and rat β-cell apoptosis under these culture conditions [89]. ZnO nanoparticles at dose of 70 ng/mL improved viability and function of pancreatic islets, by reducing oxidative stress and preventing cells from entering the apoptotic phase [90]. It is well known that Reactive Oxygen Species (ROS) can cause pancreatic β-cell death. This occurs due to the activation of Transient Receptor Potential Melastatin2 (TRPM2) channels by ROS. TRPM2 causes Ca^{2+} influx into the β-cells causing release of lysosomal Zinc, which results in β-cell death [91]. The tumor suppressor gene ST18 is a neural Zinc finger transcription factor, expressed in pancreatic β-cells and is known to impair insulin secretion, induce β-cell apoptosis and curtail β-cell replication [92].

In glucagon producing α-cells of the pancreas Zinc accumulates under low and high glucose conditions through both Ca^{2+} channels and other Zinc transporting mechanisms, and the intracellular Zinc inhibits glucagon secretion [93]. Furthermore during hypoglycemia the principal signal that initiates glucagon secretion could be the detection by α-cells of a sudden decrease in Zinc paralleling the fall in insulin in the islet periportal circulation and this drop in concentration of Zinc, closes α-cell ion channels, promoting entry of calcium which stimulates glucagon secretion [94, 95].

Insulin-mimetic compounds

Zinc ions and its' complexes, have shown insulin-like action both *in-vitro* and *in-vivo* experiments (Table 1) [96–117]. *In-vitro*, Zinc complexes inhibit the release of FFA from cultured rat adipocytes [96–104, 106, 108, 110–112, 114, 116]. In cultured 3 T3-L1 adipocytes these Zinc complexes activates the insulin signaling cascade through Akt/PKB (protein-kinase B) phosphorylation resulting in GLUT4 translocation to the plasma membrane and enhanced cellular glucose uptake [105, 107, 113]. *In-vivo* type 2 diabetic KK-Ay mice, these complexes have demonstrated an ability to reduce blood glucose, HbA1c, triglycerides and total cholesterol [98, 100, 102, 104, 110–112, 116, 117]. They are also known to improve the glucose tolerance

Table 1 Summary of Zinc Insulin-mimetic compounds

Author, year	Zinc complexes evaluated	Study design	Main findings	Conclusion
Adachi, et al. 2004 [100]	Bis(maltolato)-zinc(II) [Zn(ma)₂]	*In vitro*—isolated rat adipocytes	*In-vitro*—Inhibitory activity on FFA release observed with Zn(alx)₂, Zn(ma)₂, Zn(ema)₂ and Zn(3 hp)₂; Zn(alx)₂ exhibited the highest; Zn(alx)₂ and Zn(ma)₂ induced a concentration dependent increase in glucose uptake	Significant insulin-mimetic properties were exhibited by Zn(alx)₂
	Bis(allixinato)-zinc(II) [Zn(alx)₂]	*In-vivo*—Type 2 diabetic KK-Aʸ mice (i.p. injections for 14 days); Zn(alx)₂ was compared with that of Zn(ma)₂		
	Bis(3-hydroxy-4-pyronato)-zinc(II) [Zn(3 hp)₂]			
	Ethyl maltol-zinc(II) [Zn(ema)₂]		*In-vivo*—Both complexes reduced BG, TG, leptin & insulin; HbA1c was lower with Zn(alx)₂ > Zn(ma)₂	
	Kojic acid-zinc(II) [Zn(ka)₂]			
Adachi, et al. 2007 [104]	Zinc(II)-N-acetyl-L-cysteine [Zn(NAC)]	*In-vitro*—Isolated rat adipocytes	*In-vitro*—A dose-dependent inhibitory effect on FFA release	Zn(NAC) improves insulin resistance and glucose tolerance; Low bioavailability with oral administration (22.3 %)
		In-vivo—Type 2 diabetic KK-Aʸ mice (i.p. injections for 28 days)	*In-vivo*—BG lowered to normal; BW, serum TG and FFA levels unchanged; TC reduced; Serum insulin and HbA1c reduced	
Basuki, et al. 2007 [105]	Bis(1-oxy-2-pyridine-thiolato)-zinc(II) [Zn(opt)₂]	*In-vitro*—3 T3-L1 adipocytes	Zn(opt)₂ induced concentration- and time-dependent Akt/PKB (protein-kinase B) phosphorylation and increased GLUT-4 levels in cell membrane	Zn(opt)₂ exhibited insulin-mimetic activity by activating insulin signalling cascade through Akt/PKB phosphorylation resulting in GLUT4 translocation
	Bis(picolinato)-zinc(II) [Zn(pa)₂]			
	Bis(aspirinato)-zinc(II) [Zn(asp)₂]			
	Bis(1-oxy-2-pyridonato)-zinc(II) [Zn(opd)₂]			
Fujimoto, et al. 2013 [116]	Di(2-selenopyridine-N-oxidato)zinc(II) [ZPS]	*In-vitro*—Isolated rat adipocytes	*In-vitro*—A dose-dependent inhibitory effect on FFA release	ZPS exhibits anti-diabetic activity, even at low doses.
		In-vivo—Type 2 diabetic KK-Aʸ mice (Oral for 28 days)	*In-vivo*—BG and HbA1c reduced; TG, TC, insulin, leptin and adiponectin levels unchanged	
Kadowaki, et al. 2013 [117]	Zinc-3,4-heptanedione-bis(N⁴-methylthiosemicarbazonato) (Zn-HTSM)	*In-vivo*—Type 2 diabetic KK-Aʸ mice (Oral for 14 days)	*In-vivo*—BG lowered to normal; Serum leptin reduced; improved glucose tolerance with OGTT; Serum insulin and adiponectin unchanged	Zn-HTMS has anti-diabetic activity and also acts on leptin metabolism
Karmaker, et al. 2009 [110]	Zinc(II)-Poly-γ-glutamic acid [Zn(γ-pga)]	*In-vitro*—Isolated rat adipocytes	*In-vitro*—A dose-dependent inhibitory effect on FFA release and enhanced glucose uptake	Significant insulin-mimetic properties were exhibited by Zn(γ-pga) complex
		In-vivo—Type 2 diabetic KK-Aʸ mice (Oral for 30 days)	*In-vivo*—BG lowered to normal; HbA1c and insulin reduced; improved glucose tolerance with OGTT; TC and TG unchanged;	
Kojima, et al. 2005 [102]	Zinc(II)-6-ethylpicolinate [Zn(6epa)₂]	*In-vitro*—Isolated rat adipocytes	*In-vitro*—A dose-dependent inhibitory effect on FFA release	Significant insulin-mimetic properties were exhibited by Zn(6epa)₂
		In-vivo—Type 2 diabetic KK-Aʸ mice (i.p. injections for 14 days)	*In-vivo*—BG lowered to normal; serum TG and TC unchanged; TC reduced; Serum HbA1c reduced	
Matsumoto, et al. 2011 [111]	Zn(II)-ascorbic acid [Zn(VC)₂]	*In-vitro*—Isolated rat adipocytes	*In-vitro*—Inhibitory activity on FFA release; highest activity Zn(VC)₂	A Zn(II) complex with VU or VC showed preventive effects on metabolic syndrome in Fructose Fed Rats
	Zn(II)-methylmethionine sulfonium [Zn(VU)₂)]	*In-vivo*—Fructose fed rats (oral, 4 weeks)	*In-vivo*—Zn(VU)₂ Significantly reduced mesenteric adipocytes and BG; TC and TG unchanged;	
	Zn(II)-L-carnitine [Zn(Car)₂]			

Table 1 Summary of Zinc Insulin-mimetic compounds *(Continued)*

Moniz, et al. 2011 [112]	Zinc(II) complexes of 3-hydroxy-4-pyridinones	*In-vitro*—Isolated rat adipocytes	*In-vitro*—Inhibitory activity on FFA release	Zinc(II)-3-hydroxy-4-pyridinones showed insulin-mimetic properties
		In-vivo—STZ induced diabetic rats (i.p injections for 33 hrs)	*In-vivo*—BG lowered	
Naito, et al. 2011 [113]	Di(hinokitiolato)-zinc(II) [Zn(hnk)$_2$]	*In-vitro*—3 T3-L1 adipocytes	Zn(hnk)$_2$ induced dose dependant AKT/PKB phosphorylation, stimulated GSK3β in a dose-dependent manner and enhanced glucose uptake	Zn(hnk)$_2$ showed insulin-mimetic properties by inducing insulin signalling pathways
	Di(tropolonato)-zinc(II) [Zn(trp)$_2$]			
Nakayama, et al. 2008 [107]	Bis(allixinato)-zinc(II) [Zn(alx)$_2$]	*In-vitro*—3 T3-L1 adipocytes	Both complexes induced concentration- and time-dependent Akt/PKB (protein-kinase B) phosphorylation and increased GLUT-4 levels in cell membrane; They also inhibited FFA release	Zn(alx)$_2$ and Zn(tanm)$_2$ activated the Akt/PKB-mediated insulin-signalling pathway and improved utilization and lipid metabolism
	Bis(thioallixin-N-methyl)-zinc(II) [Zn(tanm)$_2$]			
Nishide, et al. 2008 [108]	Bis(pyrrole-2-carboxylato)-zinc(II) [Zn(pc)$_2$]	*In-vitro*—Isolated rat adipocytes	*In-vitro*—Inhibitory activity on FFA release seen with all complexes; Zn(ta)$_2$ showed highest activity	Significant insulin-mimetic properties were exhibited by Zn(ta)$_2$
	Bis(α-furonic acidato)-zinc(II) [Zn(fa)$_2$]			
	Bis(thiophene-2-carboxylato)-zinc(II) [Zn(tc)$_2$]			
	Bis(thiophene-2-acetato)-zinc(II) [Zn(ta)$_2$]			
Rasheed, et al. 2008 [109]	Zinc (II) glibrnclamide [Zn(II)–GBA]	*In-vivo*—Alloxan treated diabetic rabbits (oral, single dose)	The Zn(II)—GBA showed a faster on set of action with prolonged duration compared to the standard drug(GBA)	The Zn(II)—GBA complex showed significant hypoglycaemic activity
Ueda, et al. 2002 [98]	Zinc(II)-2-picolinamide [Zn(pa-a)$_2$]	*In-vitro*—Isolated rat adipocytes	*In-vitro*—A dose-dependent inhibitory effect on FFA release	Significant insulin-mimetic properties were exhibited by Zn(pa-a)^2 and Zn(6mpa-ma)$_2$
	Zinc(II)-6-methyl-2-picolinmethylamide [Zn(6mpa-ma)$_2$]	*In-vivo*—Type 2 diabetic KK-A^y mice (i.p. injections for 14 days)	*In-vivo*—BG and HbA1c lowered; TC unchanged;	
Vijayaraghavan, et al. 2012 [115]	Zinc-3-hydroxy flavone [Zn-flavonol]	*In-vivo*—STZ induced diabetic rats (Oral, 30 days)	At 5, 10, 20 and 50 mg/kg/day, Zn-flavonol complex exhibited significant hypoglycaemic activity; HbA1c, glucose and insulin levels were restored to near normal	Zn-flavonol complex has significant anti-hyperglycemic activity
Yoshikawa, et al. 2001 [96]	Bis(maltolato)-zinc(II) [Zn(ma)$_2$]	*In-vitro*—Isolated rat adipocytes	*In-vitro*—A dose-dependent inhibitory effect on FFA release; Combination of insulin and Zn(ma)$_2$ further enhanced inhibitory effect than insulin or Zn(ma)$_2$ alone	Zn(ma)$_2$ improves insulin resistance and glucose tolerance
		In-vivo—Type 2 diabetic KK-A^y mice (i.p. injections for 14 days)		
			In-vivo—BG lowered to normal; serum TG and insulin reduced; FFA unchanged	
Yoshikawa, et al. 2001 [97]	Zinc (II) complexes of α-amino acids (L- and D- Asn, Pro, Thr, Val, Gly, Asp, Ala, Gln and His)	*In-vitro*—Isolated rat adipocytes	*In-vitro*—Only Zinc(II) complexes with lower over-all stability constants showed insulin-mimetic activity	There is an interrelationship between the stability constants and the insulin-mimetic activity of zinc(II) complexes
		In-vivo—Type 2 diabetic KK-A^y mice (i.p. injections for 14 days) (Only [Zn(L-Thr)$_2$(H$_2$O)$_2$])	*In-vivo*—BG lowered to normal; improved glucose tolerance with OGTT	
Yoshikawa, et al. 2003 [99]	Bis(l-carnitinato)-zinc(II) [Zn(car)$_2$]	*In-vitro*—Isolated rat adipocytes	*In-vitro*—A dose-dependent inhibitory effect on FFA release	Zn(car)$_2$ improves insulin resistance and glucose tolerance

Table 1 Summary of Zinc Insulin-mimetic compounds *(Continued)*

		In-vivo—Type 2 diabetic KK-A^y mice (oral for 16 days)	In-vivo—BG lowered; improved glucose tolerance with OGTT	
Yoshikawa, et al. 2004 [101]	Bis(picolinato)-zinc(II) [Zn(pa)$_2$] Bis(maltolato)-zinc(II) [Zn(ma)$_2$] Bis(threoninato)-zinc(II) [ZT]	In-vitro—Isolated rat adipocytes	In-vitro—All 3 complexes inhibited FFA release and increased GLUT 4 levels	The complexes exhibited insulin-mimetic activity by activating insulin signalling and enhancing GLUT4 translocation
Yoshikawa, et al. 2005 [103]	Zinc-2-aminomethyl-pyridine [Zn(2-ampy)$_2$] Zinc-1,5,9-Triazanonane [Zn(1,5,9-TN)] Zinc-1,5,8,12-tetraazadodecane [Zn(1,5,8,12-TD)]	In-vitro—Isolated rat adipocytes In-vivo—Type 2 diabetic KK-A^y mice (i.p. injections for 14 days) (Zn(2-ampy)$_2$ only)	In-vitro—All 3 complexes inhibited FFA release [Zn (2-ampy)$_2$ and Zn(1,5,9-TN) > Zn(1,5,8,12-TD)] In-vivo—BG and HbA1c lowered; improved glucose tolerance with OGTT;	Zn(2-ampy)$_2$ improves insulin resistance and glucose tolerance
Yoshikawa, et al. 2007 [107]	Zinc dimethyldithiocarbamic acid [Zn(dmd)$_2$] Zinc diethyldithiocarbamic acid [Zn(ded)$_2$] Zinc pyrrolidine-N-dithiocarbamic acid [Zn(pdc)$_2$] Zinc N-ethyl-N-phenyldithio carbamate [Zn(epd)$_2$]	In-vitro—Isolated rat adipocytes In-vivo—Type 2 diabetic KK-A^y mice (oral for 25 days) (Zn(pdc)$_2$ only)	In-vitro—Zn(pdc)$_2$ was most effective in inhibiting FFA and enhancing glucose-uptake In-vivo—BG, insulin, HbA1c, TG, leptin and systolic BP reduced;	Zn(pdc)$_2$ complex improves hyperglycemia and insulin resistance
Yoshikawa, et al. 2011 [114]	Bis(aspirinato)-zinc(II) [Zn(asp)$_2$]	In-vitro—Isolated rat adipocytes In-vivo—Type 2 diabetic KK-A^y mice (i.p. injections for 14 days and oral for 24 days)	In-vitro—No effect In-vivo—BG lowered; improved glucose tolerance with OGTT;	Zn(asp)$_2$ improves insulin resistance and glucose tolerance

BG blood glucose; *BP* blood pressure; *FFA* free fatty acid; *GBA* glibenclamide; *GLUT* glucose transporter; *OGTT* oral glucose tolerance test; *TC* total cholesterol; *TG* triglycerides

as demonstrated by Oral Glucose Tolerance Testing (OGTT) [96, 99, 103, 110, 114, 117].

In addition to Zinc containing complexes, Zinc Oxide nanoparticles (ZnO) are known to posses anti-diabetic activity. ZnO nanoparticles induce a significant reduction in blood glucose, elevates serum insulin levels and glucokinase activity, whilst stimulating a higher expression of insulin, insulin receptor, GLUT-2 and glucokinase genes in STZ induced (Type-1) diabetic rats [118]. Blood glucose level is also reduced in Type-2 diabetic rats administered ZnO nanoparticles, with improved glucose tolerance and a 70 % increase in serum insulin levels [119]. In addition a significant lowering of circulating triglycerides and free fatty acids was also observed suggesting a beneficial effect of ZnO on lipid metabolism [119].

Other effects

In STZ-diabetes induced mice, Zinc supplementation has shown to increase the serum leptin concentration [120]. However, this finding has been contradicted by several other studies [100, 106, 121]. Hence, although it is evident that Zinc has an effect on leptin levels, the exact relationship and mechanisms are yet to be determined. *In-vitro*, ZnCl$_2$ is known to stimulate the trans-differentiation of human heptoma (HpG2) cells into pancreatic-like cells, with increased expression of amylase and insulin mRNAs over 1000 and 10 000 fold respectively [122]. Zinc is also known to activate C-peptide, with resultant increased energy utilization in red cells leading to release of ATP, which in turn stimulates NO production in platelets and endothelium causing reduction in platelet activity [123].

Zinc supplementation has been shown to prevent bone loss in chronic T1DM rats by stimulating expression of the mineralizing phenotype in osteoblasts and reducing expression of the resorptive phenotype in osteoclasts, achieved by osteocalcin up-regulation and RANKL, OPG, COL1A, and MMP-9 protein down-regulation

[124]. Furthermore, *in-vitro* Zinc inhibited advanced glycation end product (AGE)-induced MC3T3-E1 cell (mouse osteoblasts) apoptosis by attenuating the production of reactive oxygen species, inhibiting caspase-3 and caspase-9 activation, and inhibiting the release of cytochrome c from between the mitochondria and the cytosol [125]. Zinc significantly inhibited AGE formation of albumin *in-vitro* and reduced secondary and tertiary structural modifications of albumin and may have in controlling/preventing AGEs-mediated diabetic pathological conditions *in vivo* [126, 127].

Discussion

Numerous *in-vitro* and *in-vivo* studies have shown that Zinc has beneficial effects in both type-1 and type-2 diabetes. A finding which has been confirmed by a recent meta-analysis, where Zinc supplementation resulted in improved glycaemic control [15]. It is evident from the findings of the present systematic review, that Zinc plays an important role in β-cell function, insulin action, glucose homeostasis and the pathogenesis of diabetes and its complications.

Our results clearly show that Zinc has anti-oxidant properties and that Zinc supplementation reduces oxidative stress. Zinc supplementation enhances the activity and levels of key anti-oxidant enzymes and proteins, whilst significantly reducing lipid peroxidation. Some of these effects are brought on by interactions at nuclear level, by stimulation of nuclear factors like Nrf2 [38]. It is well known that oxidative stress is high in both type-1 and type-2 diabetic patients, as evident by elevated TBARS levels in the plasma [11, 19]. This contributes towards further β-cell dysfunction, with resultant deterioration of glycaemic control. Oxidative stress also plays a pivotal role in the pathogenesis of both micro- and macro-vascular complications of diabetes [128]. The resultant increase in the production of ROSs is responsible for the activation of five major pathways involved in the pathogenesis of diabetes complications [128]. Increased formation of AGEs, and the increased expression of the receptor for AGEs and its activating ligands is one such primary pathway responsible for the pathogenesis of diabetes related complications [128]. Both *in-vitro* and *in-vivo* Zinc significantly inhibited the formation of AGEs. Hence, by alleviating the oxidative stress associated with diabetes and by reducing the formation of AGEs, Zinc supplementation could delay the progression of diabetes and also delay/prevent the numerous micro- and macro-vascular complications associated with diabetes.

Furthermore, our results show that Zinc plays an important role in glucose and lipid metabolism. Zinc reduces glucose absorption and synthesis, whilst promoting glucose metabolism and storage. This is primarily via the enhanced activity of key enzymes involved in these metabolic processes, such as α-glucosidase, PFK, PK and glycogen synthase. Its insulinomimetic action possibly mediated via Zinc-α2-glycoporteins increases cellular GLUT4 levels in skeletal muscles and adipose tissue facilitating glucose absorption. Zinc-α2-glycoprotein is gaining increasing recognition as a marker of insulin resistance in type-2 diabetes. Zinc-α2-glycoproteins are also involved in lipid metabolism, affecting the expression of several lipolytic enzymes at hepatic and adipose tissue level. Two recent meta-analyses have shown that Zinc supplementation reduces Fasting Blood Glucose, 2 h Post Prandial Blood Glucose and HbA1c in patients with diabetes, as well as reducing total cholesterol, LDL cholesterol and triglycerides in both patients with and without diabetes [15, 129]. The above molecular/enzymatic level mechanisms probably explain the beneficial effects of Zinc supplementation on glycaemic control and lipids observed in humans.

Zinc also plays an important role in the normal functioning of the islet cells of the pancreas. β-cells and their granules are extremely rich in Zinc. Zinc Transporters (ZnTs) transport zinc from the cytoplasm to extracellular spaces or to intra-cytoplasmic vacuoles, such as secretory granules, while the ZIPs are thought to increase cytoplasmic zinc [130]. Insulin production and efficient packaging into vesicles is closely linked with the transport of Zinc in to the β-cells and subsequent concentration inside vesicles mediated by the Zinc transporter ZnT8, a product of the SLC30A8 gene, specifically expressed in the β-cells of the pancreas [131]. Alterations and/or variations in the activity of ZnT8 is associated with impaired glucose induced insulin response, which promotes progression from glucose intolerance to type-2 diabetes in susceptible individuals [131]. ZnT8 has also been identified as a novel target auto-antigen in patients with type-1 diabetes and hence has diagnostic implications [132]. Auto-antibodies to ZnT8 (ZnT8A) are detected in 50–60 % of Japanese patients with acute-onset and 20 % with slow-onset type-1 diabetes [132]. Hence, it is evident that ZnT8 is a key mediator in the pathogenesis of both type-1 and type-2 diabetes. In addition to ZnT8, altered activity of many other Zinc transporters and Zinc influx proteins (ZIP 6, 7, 8) have been implicated in the pathogenesis of diabetes. Zinc is also an important mediator of α-cell function, as it inhibits glucagon secretion [93]. Identification and characterization of these ZnTs and ZIPs will help in the development of novel therapies for diabetes targeting these molecules and to develop new methods to protect β-cell mass and function, in both type-1 and type-2 diabetes.

Patients' adherence to present therapeutic regimes for diabetes treatment are poor, resulting in unsatisfactory diabetes control [133]. Regime complexity, hypoglycaemia and other side-effects, lack of confidence in immediate or future benefits and patients' education/beliefs are among the common reasons identified that limits adherence [134–137]. Inadequacies in current treatments has resulted in 2 to 3.6 million people in USA relying on alternative therapies for management diabetes [138]. In addition current treatment modalities are not very efficacious in preventing and/or delaying the progression of β-cell dysfunction and ultimate β-cell failure in patients with type-2 diabetes. The development of new compounds for treating diabetes is currently important to reduce the need for insulin injection in diabetic patients and to replace the clinically used synthetic therapeutics, which has several severe side effects [139].

Zinc ions and its' numerous complexes, have shown insulin-like action both *in-vitro* and *in-vivo* [71–90]. Zinc complexes activate the insulin signaling cascade via Akt/PKB, which resultant increase in cellular GLUT4 and enhanced cellular glucose uptake. In animal models of type-2 diabetes these complexes have shown a significant ability to reduce blood glucose, HbA1c, serum insulin, triglycerides and total cholesterol, whilst improving glucose tolerance. On the basis of these findings and observations, it is evident that Zinc complexes have promise as a novel therapeutic modality that mimics the action of insulin [139]. However, presently the findings are only from *in-vitro* and *in-vivo* animal studies, there is a paucity of data from randomized controlled trials in humans. It is necessary to identify few efficacious compounds, with the least amounts of toxicity and for those complexes to be carefully evaluated in humans. The fruitful outcome of such trials may offer a novel and effective oral medication with better anti-diabetic in place of insulin [140].

Conclusion

Numerous *in-vitro* and *in-vivo* studies have shown that Zinc has beneficial effects in both type-1 and type-2 diabetes. It is evident from the findings of the present systematic review, that Zinc plays an important role in β-cell function, insulin action, glucose homeostasis and the pathogenesis of diabetes and its complications. However further randomized double-blinded placebo-controlled clinical trials conducted for an adequate duration, are required to establish therapeutic efficacy and safety in humans.

Additional file

Additional file 1: PRISMA 2009 Checklist. (DOC 64 kb)

Competing interest
The authors declare that they have no competing interests.

Authors' contributions
PR and SP substantially contributed to the general idea and design of the study. PR and SP were involved in data collection. PR, PK, PG and GRC

planned data analysis. PR and SP drafted the manuscript. All authors have read and consented to the manuscript.

Author details
[1]Department of Pharmacology, Faculty of Medicine, University of Colombo, Colombo, Sri Lanka. [2]Diabetes Research Unit, Department of Clinical Medicine, Faculty of Medicine, University of Colombo, Colombo, Sri Lanka.

References
1. IDF Diabetes Atlas - The Economic Impacts of Diabetes. [http://www.diabetesatlas.com/content/economic-impacts-diabetes]
2. Stumvoll M, Goldstein BJ, van Haeften TW. Type 2 diabetes: principles of pathogenesis and therapy. Lancet. 2005;365(9467):1333–46.
3. Wild S, Roglic G, Green A, Sicree R, King H. Global prevalence of diabetes: estimates for the year 2000 and projections for 2030. Diabetes Care. 2004;27(5):1047–53.
4. WHO Diabetes Fact Sheet. [http://www.who.int/mediacentre/factsheets/fs312/en/index.html]
5. Diabetes: the cost of diabetes [http://www.who.int/mediacentre/factsheets/fs236/en/]
6. Stuckler D. Population Causes and Consequences of Leading Chronic Diseases: A Comparative Analysis of Prevailing Explanations. The Milbank Quarterly. 2008;86(2):273–326.
7. Ali MK, Bullard KM, Saaddine JB, Cowie CC, Imperatore G, Gregg EW. Achievement of goals in U.S. diabetes care 1999–2010. N Engl J Med. 2013;368(17):1613–24.
8. Khunti K, Davies M. Glycaemic goals in patients with type 2 diabetes: current status, challenges and recent advances. Diabetes Obes Metab. 2010;12(6):474–84.
9. Dodson G, Steiner D. The role of assembly in insulin's biosynthesis. Curr Opin Struct Biol. 1998;8(2):189–94.
10. Simon SF, Taylor CG. Dietary zinc supplementation attenuates hyperglycemia in db/db mice. Exp Biol Med (Maywood). 2001;226(1):43–51.
11. Faure P, Benhamou PY, Perard A, Halimi S, Roussel AM. Lipid peroxidation in insulin-dependent diabetic patients with early retina degenerative lesions: effects of an oral zinc supplementation. Eur J Clin Nutr. 1995;49(4):282–8.
12. Shidfar F, Aghasi M, Vafa M, Heydari I, Hosseini S, Shidfar S. Effects of combination of zinc and vitamin A supplementation on serum fasting blood sugar, insulin, apoprotein B and apoprotein A-I in patients with type i diabetes. Int J Food Sci Nutr. 2010;61(2):182–91.
13. Afkhami-Ardekani M, Karimi M, Mohammadi SM, Nourani F. Effect of zinc sulfate supplementation on lipid and glucose in type 2 diabetic patients. Pak J Nutr. 2008;7(4):550–3.
14. Al-Maroof RA, Al-Sharbatti SS. Serum zinc levels in diabetic patients and effect of zinc supplementation on glycemic control of type 2 diabetics. Saudi Med J. 2006;27(3):344–50.
15. Jayawardena R, Ranasinghe P, Galappatthy P, Malkanthi R, Constantine G, Katulanda P. Effects of zinc supplementation on diabetes mellitus: a systematic review and meta-analysis. Diabetol Metab Syndr. 2012;4(1):13.
16. Garg VK, Gupta R, Goyal RK. Hypozincemia in diabetes mellitus. J Assoc Physicians India. 1994;42(9):720–1.
17. Pidduck HG, Wren PJ, Evans DA. Hyperzincuria of diabetes mellitus and possible genetical implications of this observation. Diabetes. 1970;19(4):240–7.
18. Black RE. Zinc deficiency, infectious disease and mortality in the developing world. J Nutr. 2003;133(5 Suppl 1):1485S–9S.
19. Anderson RA, Roussel AM, Zouari N, Mahjoub S, Matheau JM, Kerkeni A. Potential antioxidant effects of zinc and chromium supplementation in people with type 2 diabetes mellitus. J Am Coll Nutr. 2001;20(3):212–8.
20. Blostein-Fujii A, DiSilvestro RA, Frid D, Katz C, Malarkey W. Short-term zinc supplementation in women with non-insulin-dependent diabetes mellitus: effects on plasma 5'-nucleotidase activities, insulin-like growth factor I concentrations, and lipoprotein oxidation rates in vitro. Am J Clin Nutr. 1997;66(3):639–42.
21. Pathak A, Sharma V, Kumar S, Dhawan DK. Supplementation of zinc mitigates the altered uptake and turnover of 65Zn in liver and whole body of diabetic rats. Biometals. 2011;24(6):1027–34.

22. Konukoglu D, Turhan MS, Ercan M, Serin O. Relationship between plasma leptin and zinc levels and the effect of insulin and oxidative stress on leptin levels in obese diabetic patients. J Nutr Biochem. 2004;15(12):757–60.

23. Faure P, Barclay D, Joyeux-Faure M, Halimi S. Comparison of the effects of zinc alone and zinc associated with selenium and vitamin E on insulin sensitivity and oxidative stress in high-fructose-fed rats. J Trace Elem Med Biol. 2007;21(2):113–9.

24. Vijayaraghavan K, Iyyampillai S, Subramanian SP. Antioxidant potential of zinc-flavonol complex studied in streptozotocin-diabetic rats. J Diabetes. 2013;5(2):149–56.

25. Bădescu M, Păduraru I, Colev V, Saramet A, Bohotin C, Bădescu L. The relation zinc-lipidic peroxidation in experimental diabetes mellitus. Rom J Physiol. 1993;30(3–4):167–71.

26. Duzguner V, Kaya S. Effect of zinc on the lipid peroxidation and the antioxidant defense systems of the alloxan-induced diabetic rabbits. Free Radic Biol Med. 2007;42(10):1481–6.

27. Tang Y, Yang Q, Lu J, Zhang X, Suen D, Tan Y, et al. Zinc supplementation partially prevents renal pathological changes in diabetic rats. J Nutr Biochem. 2010;21(3):237–46.

28. Wang X, Li H, Fan Z, Liu Y. Effect of zinc supplementation on type 2 diabetes parameters and liver metallothionein expressions in Wistar rats. J Physiol Biochem. 2012;68(4):563–72.

29. Moustafa SA. Zinc might protect oxidative changes in the retina and pancreas at the early stage of diabetic rats. Toxicol Appl Pharmacol. 2004;201(2):149–55.

30. Ohly P, Dohle C, Abel J, Seissler J, Gleichmann H. Zinc sulphate induces metallothionein in pancreatic islets of mice and protects against diabetes induced by multiple low doses of streptozotocin. Diabetologia. 2000;43(8):1020–30.

31. Özcelik D, Nazıroglu M, Tunçdemir M, Çelik Ö, Öztürk M, Flores-Arce MF. Zinc supplementation attenuates metallothionein and oxidative stress changes in kidney of streptozotocin-induced diabetic rats. Biol Trace Elem Res. 2012;150(1–3):342–9.

32. Zimny S, Gogolin F, Abel J, Gleichmann H. Metallothionein in isolated pancreatic islets of mice: induction by zinc and streptozotocin, a naturally occurring diabetogen. Arch Toxicol. 1993;67(1):61–5.

33. Wang J, Song Y, Elsherif L, Song Z, Zhou G, Prabhu SD, et al. Cardiac metallothionein induction plays the major role in the prevention of diabetic cardiomyopathy by zinc supplementation. Circulation. 2006;113(4):544–54.

34. Liang T, Zhang Q, Sun W, Xin Y, Zhang Z, Tan Y, et al. Zinc treatment prevents type 1 diabetes-induced hepatic oxidative damage, endoplasmic reticulum stress, and cell death, and even prevents possible steatohepatitis in the OVE26 mouse model: Important role of metallothionein. Toxicol Lett. 2015;233(2):114–24.

35. Lu Y, Liu Y, Li H, Wang X, Wu W, Gao L. Effect and mechanisms of zinc supplementation in protecting against diabetic cardiomyopathy in a rat model of type 2 diabetes. Bosn J Basic Med Sci. 2015;15(1):14–20.

36. Zhang X, Liang D, Chi ZH, Chu Q, Zhao C, Ma RZ, et al. Effect of zinc on high glucose-induced epithelial-to-mesenchymal transition in renal tubular epithelial cells. Int J Mol Med. 2015;35(6):1747–54.

37. Liu F, Ma F, Kong G, Wu K, Deng Z, Wang H. Zinc supplementation alleviates diabetic peripheral neuropathy by inhibiting oxidative stress and upregulating metallothionein in peripheral nerves of diabetic rats. Biol Trace Elem Res. 2014;158(2):211–8.

38. Miao X, Wang Y, Sun J, Sun W, Tan Y, Cai L, et al. Zinc protects against diabetes-induced pathogenic changes in the aorta: Roles of metallothionein and nuclear factor (erythroid-derived 2)-like 2. Cardiovasc Diabetol. 2013;12:54.

39. Li B, Cui W, Tan Y, Luo P, Chen Q, Zhang C, et al. Zinc is essential for the transcription function of Nrf2 in human renal tubule cells in vitro and mouse kidney in vivo under the diabetic condition. J Cell Mol Med. 2014;18(5):895–906.

40. Zhang X, Zhao Y, Chu Q, Wang ZY, Li H, Chi ZH. Zinc modulates high glucose-induced apoptosis by suppressing oxidative stress in renal tubular epithelial cells. Biol Trace Elem Res. 2014;158(2):259–67.

41. Chu A, Foster M, Hancock D, Bell-Anderson K, Petocz P, Samman S. TNF-alpha gene expression is increased following zinc supplementation in type 2 diabetes mellitus. Genes & nutrition. 2015;10(1):440.

42. Brand IA, Kleineke J. Intracellular zinc movement and its effect on the carbohydrate metabolism of isolated rat hepatocytes. J Biol Chem. 1996;271(4):1941–9.

43. Shisheva A, Gefel D, Shechter Y. Insulinlike effects of zinc ion in vitro and in vivo. Preferential effects on desensitized adipocytes and induction of normoglycemia in streptozocin-induced rats. Diabetes. 1992;41(8):982–8.

44. May JM, Contoreggi CS. The mechanism of the insulin-like effects of ionic zinc. J Biol Chem. 1982;257(8):4362–8.

45. Canesi L, Betti M, Ciacci C, Gallo G. Insulin-like effect of zinc in mytilus digestive gland cells: modulation of tyrosine kinase-mediated cell signaling. Gen Comp Endocrinol. 2001;122(1):60–6.

46. Tamaki N, Ikeda T, Funatsuka A. Zinc as activating cation for muscle glycolysis. J Nutr Sci Vitaminol. 1983;29(6):655–62.

47. Filippi C, Pryde A, Cowan P, Lee T, Hayes P, Donaldson K, et al. Toxicology of ZnO and TiO2 nanoparticles on hepatocytes: impact on metabolism and bioenergetics. Nanotoxicology. 2015;9(1):126–34.

48. Yoshikawa Y, Hirata R, Yasui H, Sakurai H. Alpha-glucosidase inhibitory effect of anti-diabetic metal ions and their complexes. Biochimie. 2009;91(10):1339–41.

49. Zeng YF, Lee J, Si YX, Yan L, Kim TR, Qian GY, et al. Inhibitory effect of Zn2+ on α-glucosidase: Inhibition kinetics and molecular dynamics simulation. Process Biochem. 2012;47(12):2510–7.

50. Eckardt K, Schober A, Platzbecker B, Mracek T, Bing C, Trayhurn P, et al. The adipokine zinc-α2-glycoprotein activates AMP kinase in human primary skeletal muscle cells. Arch Physiol Biochem. 2011;117(2):88–93.

51. Russell ST, Tisdale MJ. Studies on the anti-obesity activity of zinc-α 2-glycoprotein in the rat. Int J Obes (Lond). 2011;35(5):658–65.

52. Miranda ER, Dey CS. Effect of chromium and zinc on insulin signaling in skeletal muscle cells. Biol Trace Elem Res. 2004;101(1):19–36.

53. Balaz M, Vician M, Janakova Z, Kurdiova T, Surova M, Imrich R, et al. Subcutaneous adipose tissue zinc-alpha2-glycoprotein is associated with adipose tissue and whole-body insulin sensitivity. Obesity (Silver Spring, Md). 2014;22(8):1821–9.

54. Ceperuelo-Mallafre V, Ejarque M, Duran X, Pachon G, Vazquez-Carballo A, Roche K, et al. Zinc-alpha2-glycoprotein modulates AKT-dependent insulin signaling in human adipocytes by activation of the PP2A phosphatase. PLoS One. 2015;10(6):e0129644.

55. Buchner DA, Charrier A, Srinivasan E, Wang L, Paulsen MT, Ljungman M, et al. Zinc finger protein 407 (ZFP407) regulates insulin-stimulated glucose uptake and glucose transporter 4 (Glut4) mRNA. J Biol Chem. 2015;290(10):6376–86.

56. Tang X, Shay NF. Zinc has an insulin-like effect on glucose transport mediated by phosphoinositol-3-kinase and Akt in 3 T3-L1 fibroblasts and adipocytes. J Nutr. 2001;131(5):1414–20.

57. Ilouz R, Kaidanovich O, Gurwitz D, Eldar-Finkelman H. Inhibition of glycogen synthase kinase-3beta by bivalent zinc ions: insight into the insulin-mimetic action of zinc. Biochem Biophys Res Commun. 2002;295(1):102–6.

58. Ezaki O. IIb group metal ions (Zn2+, Cd2+, Hg2+) stimulate glucose transport activity by post-insulin receptor kinase mechanism in rat adipocytes. J Biol Chem. 1989;264(27):16118–22.

59. Coulston L, Dandona P. Insulin-like effect of zinc on adipocytes. Diabetes. 1980;29(8):665–7.

60. Herington AC. Effect of zinc on insulin binding to rat adipocytes and hepatic membranes and to human placental membranes and IM-9 lymphocytes. Horm Metab Res. 1985;17(7):328–32.

61. Ghosh C, Yang SH, Kim JG, Jeon TI, Yoon BH, Lee JY, et al. Zinc-chelated vitamin C stimulates adipogenesis of 3 T3-L1 cells. Asian-Australas J Anim Sci. 2013;26(8):1189–96.

62. Gomot MJ, Faure P, Roussel AM, Coudray C, Osman M, Favier A. Effect of acute zinc deficiency on insulin receptor binding in rat adipocytes. Biol Trace Elem Res. 1992;32:331–5.

63. Aspinwall CA, Brooks SA, Kennedy RT, Lakey JR. Effects of intravesicular H+ and extracellular H+ and Zn2+ on insulin secretion in pancreatic beta cells. J Biol Chem. 1997;272(50):31308–14.

64. Slepchenko KG, James CB, Li YV. Inhibitory effect of zinc on glucose-stimulated zinc/insulin secretion in an insulin-secreting beta-cell line. Exp Physiol. 2013;98(8):1301–11.

65. Slepchenko KG, Daniels NA, Guo A, Li YV. Autocrine effect of Zn on the glucose-stimulated insulin secretion. Endocrine. 2015;50:110–22.

66. Bellomo EA, Meur G, Rutter GA. Glucose regulates free cytosolic Zn2+ concentration, Slc39 (ZiP), and metallothionein gene expression in primary pancreatic islet β-cells. J Biol Chem. 2011;286(29):25778–89.

67. Slepchenko KG, Li YV. Rising intracellular zinc by membrane depolarization and glucose in insulin-secreting clonal HIT-T15 beta cells. Exp Diabetes Res. 2012;2012:190309–9.

68. Brender JR, Hartman K, Nanga RPR, Popovych N, De La Salud BR, Vivekanandan S, et al. Role of zinc in human islet amyloid polypeptide aggregation. J Am Chem Soc. 2010;132(26):8973–83.

69. Chimienti F, Devergnas S, Pattou F, Schult F, Garcia-Cuenca R, Vandewalle B, et al. In vivo expression and functional characterization of the zinc transporter ZnT8 in glucose-induced insulin secretion. J Cell Sci. 2006;119(20):4199–206.

70. Chimienti F, Devergnas S, Favier A, Seve M. Identification and cloning of a beta-cell-specific zinc transporter, ZnT-8, localized into insulin secretory granules. Diabetes. 2004;53(9):2330–7.

71. Chimienti F, Favier A, Seve M. ZnT-8, a pancreatic beta-cell-specific zinc transporter. Biometals. 2005;18(4):313–7.

72. Wijesekara N, Dai FF, Hardy AB, Giglou PR, Bhattacharjee A, Koshkin V, et al. Beta cell-specific Znt8 deletion in mice causes marked defects in insulin processing, crystallisation and secretion. Diabetologia. 2010;53(8):1656–68.

73. Nicolson TJ, Bellomo EA, Wijesekara N, Loder MK, Baldwin JM, Gyulkhandanyan AV, et al. Insulin storage and glucose homeostasis in mice null for the granule zinc transporter ZnT8 and studies of the type 2 diabetes-associated variants. Diabetes. 2009;58(9):2070–83.

74. Fu Y, Tian W, Pratt EB, Dirling LB, Shyng S-L, Meshul CK, et al. Down-regulation of ZnT8 expression in INS-1 rat pancreatic beta cells reduces insulin content and glucose-inducible insulin secretion. PLoS One. 2009;4(5):e5679–9.

75. Lemaire K, Ravier MA, Schraenen A, Creemers JWM, Van de Plas R, Granvik M, et al. Insulin crystallization depends on zinc transporter ZnT8 expression, but is not required for normal glucose homeostasis in mice. Proc Natl Acad Sci U S A. 2009;106(35):14872–7.

76. Pound LD, Sarkar SA, Benninger RKP, Wang Y, Suwanichkul A, Shadoan MK, et al. Deletion of the mouse Slc30a8 gene encoding zinc transporter-8 results in impaired insulin secretion. Biochem J. 2009;421(3):371–6.

77. Pound LD, Sarkar SA, Ustione A, Dadi PK, Shadoan MK, Lee CE, et al. The physiological effects of deleting the mouse SLC30A8 gene encoding zinc transporter-8 are influenced by gender and genetic background. PLoS One. 2012;7(7):e40972–2.

78. Lefebvre B, Vandewalle B, Balavoine AS, Queniat G, Moerman E, Vantyghem MC, et al. Regulation and functional effects of ZNT8 in human pancreatic islets. J Endocrinol. 2012;214(2):225–32.

79. Liu B-Y, Jiang Y, Lu Z, Li S, Lu D, Chen B. Down-regulation of zinc transporter 8 in the pancreas of db/db mice is rescued by Exendin-4 administration. Mol Med Rep. 2011;4(1):47–52.

80. Tamaki M, Fujitani Y, Hara A, Uchida T, Tamura Y, Takeno K, et al. The diabetes-susceptible gene SLC30A8/ZnT8 regulates hepatic insulin clearance. J Clin Invest. 2013;123(10):4513–24.

81. Gerber PA, Bellomo EA, Hodson DJ, Meur G, Solomou A, Mitchell RK, et al. Hypoxia lowers SLC30A8/ZnT8 expression and free cytosolic Zn2+ in pancreatic beta cells. Diabetologia. 2014;57(8):1635–44.

82. Pae EK, Kim G. Insulin production hampered by intermittent hypoxia via impaired zinc homeostasis. PLoS One. 2014;9(2):e90192.

83. Liu Y, Batchuluun B, Ho L, Zhu D, Prentice KJ, Bhattacharjee A, et al. Characterization of zinc influx transporters (ZIPS) in pancreatic beta cells: roles in regulating cytosolic zinc homeostasis and insulin secretion. J Biol Chem. 2015;290(30):18757–69.

84. Hardy AB, Prentice KJ, Froese S, Liu Y, Andrews GK, Wheeler MB. Zip4 mediated zinc influx stimulates insulin secretion in pancreatic beta cells. PLoS One. 2015;10(3):e0119136.

85. Smidt K, Jessen N, Petersen AB, Larsen A, Magnusson M, Jeppesen JB, et al. SLC30A3 responds to glucose- and zinc variations in beta-cells and is critical for insulin production and in vivo glucose-metabolism during beta-cell stress. PLoS One. 2009;4(5):e5684–4.

86. Myers SA, Nield A, Chew GS, Myers MA. The zinc transporter, Slc39a7 (Zip7) is implicated in glycaemic control in skeletal muscle cells. PLoS One. 2013;8(11):e79316.

87. Gyulkhandanyan AV, Lee SC, Bikopoulos G, Dai F, Wheeler MB. The Zn2+−transporting pathways in pancreatic β-cells: A role for the L-type voltage-gated Ca2+ channel. J Biol Chem. 2006;281(14):9361–72.

88. Wagner TFJ, Drews A, Loch S, Mohr F, Philipp SE, Lambert S, et al. TRPM3 channels provide a regulated influx pathway for zinc in pancreatic beta cells. Pflugers Arch. 2010;460(4):755–65.

89. Duprez J, Roma LP, Close A-F, Jonas J-C. Protective antioxidant and antiapoptotic effects of ZnCl2 in rat pancreatic islets cultured in low and high glucose concentrations. PLoS One. 2012;7(10):e46831–1.

90. Shoae-Hagh P, Rahimifard M, Navaei-Nigjeh M, Baeeri M, Gholami M, Mohammadirad A, et al. Zinc oxide nanoparticles reduce apoptosis and oxidative stress values in isolated rat pancreatic islets. Biol Trace Elem Res. 2014;162(1–3):262–9.

91. Manna PT, Munsey TS, Abuarab N, Li F, Asipu A, Howell G, et al. TRPM2-mediated intracellular Zn2+ release triggers pancreatic beta-cell death. Biochem J. 2015;466(3):537–46.

92. Henry C, Close AF, Buteau J. A critical role for the neural zinc factor ST18 in pancreatic beta-cell apoptosis. J Biol Chem. 2014;289(12):8413–9.

93. Gyulkhandanyan AV, Lu H, Lee SC, Bhattacharjee A, Wijesekara N, Fox JEM, et al. Investigation of transport mechanisms and regulation of intracellular Zn2+ in pancreatic alpha-cells. J Biol Chem. 2008;283(15):10184–97.

94. Zhou H, Zhang T, Harmon JS, Bryan J, Robertson RP. Zinc, not insulin, regulates the rat alpha-cell response to hypoglycemia in vivo. Diabetes. 2007;56(4):1107–12.

95. Slucca M, Harmon JS, Oseid EA, Bryan J, Robertson RP. ATP-sensitive K+ channel mediates the zinc switch-off signal for glucagon response during glucose deprivation. Diabetes. 2010;59(1):128–34.

96. Yoshikawa Y, Ueda E, Miyake H, Sakurai H, Kojima Y. Insulinomimetic bis(maltolato)zinc(II) complex: blood glucose normalizing effect in KK-A(y) mice with type 2 diabetes mellitus. Biochem Biophys Res Commun. 2001;281(5):1190–3.

97. Yoshikawa Y, Ueda E, Suzuki Y, Yanagihara N, Sakurai H, Kojima Y. New insulinomimetic zinc(II) complexes of alpha-amino acids and their derivatives with Zn(N2O2) coordination mode. Chem Pharm Bull. 2001;49(5):652–4.

98. Ueda E, Yoshikawa Y, Ishino Y, Sakurai H, Kojima Y. Potential insulinomimetic agents of zinc(II) complexes with picolinamide derivatives: preparations of complexes, in vitro and in vivo studies. Chem Pharm Bull. 2002;50(3):337–40.

99. Yoshikawa Y, Ueda E, Sakurai H, Kojima Y. Anti-diabetes effect of Zn(II)/carnitine complex by oral administration. Chem Pharm Bull. 2003;51(2):230–1.

100. Adachi Y, Yoshida J, Kodera Y, Kato A, Yoshikawa Y, Kojima Y, et al. A new insulin-mimetic bis(allixinato)zinc(II) complex: structure-activity relationship of zinc(II) complexes. J Biol Inorg Chem. 2004;9(7):885–93.

101. Yoshikawa Y, Ueda E, Kojima Y, Sakurai H. The action mechanism of zinc(II) complexes with insulinomimetic activity in rat adipocytes. Life Sci. 2004;75(6):741–51.

102. Kojima Y, Yoshikawa Y, Ueda E, Kishimoto N, Tadokoro M, Sakurai H. Synthesis, structure, and in vitro and in vivo insulinomimetic activities of the zinc(II)-6-ethylpicolinate complex. Bull Chem Soc Jpn. 2005;78(3):451–5.

103. Yoshikawa Y, Kondo M, Sakurai H, Kojima Y. A family of insulinomimetic zinc(II) complexes of amino ligands with Zn(Nn) (n = 3 and 4) coordination modes. J Inorg Biochem. 2005;99(7):1497–503.

104. Adachi Y, Yoshikawa Y, Sakurai H. Antidiabetic zinc(II)-N-acetyl-L-cysteine complex: evaluations of in vitro insulinomimetic and in vivo blood glucose-lowering activities. Biofactors (Oxford, England). 2007;29(4):213–23.

105. Basuki W, Hiromura M, Sakurai H. Insulinomimetic Zn complex (Zn(opt)2) enhances insulin signaling pathway in 3 T3-L1 adipocytes. J Inorg Biochem. 2007;101(4):692–9.

106. Yoshikawa Y, Adachi Y, Sakurai H. A new type of orally active anti-diabetic Zn(II)-dithiocarbamate complex. Life Sci. 2007;80(8):759–66.

107. Nakayama A, Hiromura M, Adachi Y, Sakurai H. Molecular mechanism of Antidiabetic zinc-allixin complexes: regulations of glucose utilization and lipid metabolism. J Biol Inorg Chem. 2008;13(5):675–84.

108. Nishide M, Yoshikawa Y, Yoshikawa EU, Matsumoto K, Sakurai H, Kajiwara NM. Insulinomimetic Zn(II) complexes as evaluated by both glucose-uptake activity and inhibition of free fatty acids release in isolated rat adipocytes. Chem Pharm Bull. 2008;56(8):1181–3.

109. Rasheed K, Tariq MI, Munir C, Hussain I, Siddiqui HL. Synthesis, characterization and hypoglycemic activity of Zn(II), Cd(II) and Hg(II) complexes with glibenclamide. Chem Pharm Bull. 2008;56(2):168–72.

110. Karmaker S, Saha TK, Yoshikawa Y, Sakurai H. A zinc(II)/poly(γ-glutamic acid) complex as an oral therapeutic for the treatment of type-2 diabetic KKAy mice. Macromol Biosci. 2009;9(3):279–86.

111. Matsumoto K, Motoyasu N, Sera K, Fujii T, Yoshikawa Y, Yasui H, et al. Effects of Zn(II) complex with vitamins C and U, and carnitine on metabolic syndrome model rats. Metallomics. 2011;3(7):683–5.

112. Moniz T, Amorim MJ, Ferreira R, Nunes A, Silva A, Queirós C, et al. Investigation of the insulin-like properties of zinc(II) complexes of 3-hydroxy-4-pyridinones: identification of a compound with glucose lowering effect in STZ-induced type I diabetic animals. J Inorg Biochem. 2011;105(12):1675–82.

113. Naito Y, Yoshikawa Y, Yasui H. Cellular mechanism of zinchinokitiol complexes in diabetes mellitus. Bull Chem Soc Jpn. 2011;84(3):298–305.

114. Yoshikawa Y, Adachi Y, Yasui H, Hattori M, Sakurai H. Oral administration of Bis(aspirinato)zinc(II) complex ameliorates hyperglycemia and metabolic syndrome-like disorders in spontaneously diabetic KK-A(y) mice: structure-activity relationship on zinc-salicylate complexes. Chem Pharm Bull. 2011;59(8):972–7.

115. Vijayaraghavan K, Iyyam Pillai S, Subramanian SP. Design, synthesis and characterization of zinc-3 hydroxy flavone, a novel zinc metallo complex for the treatment of experimental diabetes in rats. Eur J Pharmacol. 2012;680(1–3):122–9.

116. Fujimoto S, Yasui H, Yoshikawa Y. Development of a novel antidiabetic zinc complex with an organoselenium ligand at the lowest dosage in KK-A(y) mice. J Inorg Biochem. 2013;121:10–5.

117. Kadowaki S, Munekane M, Kitamura Y, Hiromura M, Kamino S, Yoshikawa Y, et al. Development of new zinc dithiosemicarbazone complex for use as oral antidiabetic agent. Biol Trace Elem Res. 2013;154(1):111–9.

118. Alkaladi A, Abdelazim AM, Afifi M. Antidiabetic activity of zinc oxide and silver nanoparticles on streptozotocin-induced diabetic rats. Int J Mol Sci. 2014;15(2):2015–23.

119. Umrani RD, Paknikar KM. Zinc oxide nanoparticles show antidiabetic activity in streptozotocin-induced Type 1 and 2 diabetic rats. Nanomedicine (Lond). 2014;9(1):89–104.

120. Chen MD, Song YM, Lin PY. Zinc effects on hyperglycemia and hypoleptinemia in streptozotocin-induced diabetic mice. Horm Metab Res. 2000;32(3):107–9.

121. Liu MJ, Bao S, Bolin ER, Burris DL, Xu X, Sun Q, et al. Zinc deficiency augments leptin production and exacerbates macrophage infiltration into adipose tissue in mice fed a high-fat diet. J Nutr. 2013;143(7):1036–45.

122. Kanoh Y, Tomotsune D, Shirasawa S, Yoshie S, Ichikawa H, Yokoyama T, et al. In vitro transdifferentiation of HepG2 cells to pancreatic-like cells by CCl4, D-galactosamine, and ZnCl2. Pancreas. 2011;40(8):1245–52.

123. Meyer JA, Subasinghe W, Sima AAF, Keltner Z, Reid GE, Daleke D, et al. Zinc-activated C-peptide resistance to the type 2 diabetic erythrocyte is associated with hyperglycemia-induced phosphatidylserine externalization and reversed by metformin. Mol Biosyst. 2009;5(10):1157–62.

124. Bortolin RH, da Graca Azevedo Abreu BJ, Abbott Galvao Ururahy M, de Souza KS C, Bezerra JF, Loureiro MB, et al. Protection against T1DM-induced bone loss by zinc supplementation: biomechanical, histomorphometric, and molecular analyses in STZ-induced diabetic rats. PLoS One. 2015;10(5):e0125349.

125. Xiong M, Liu L, Liu Z, Gao H. Inhibitory effect of zinc on the advanced glycation end product-induced apoptosis of mouse osteoblastic cells. Molecular medicine reports 2015. 10.3892/mmr.2015.4088.

126. Tupe R, Kulkarni A, Adeshara K, Sankhe N, Shaikh S, Dalal S, et al. Zinc inhibits glycation induced structural, functional modifications in albumin and protects erythrocytes from glycated albumin toxicity. Int J Biol Macromol. 2015;79:601–10.

127. Baraka-Vidot J, Navarra G, Leone M, Bourdon E, Militello V, Rondeau P. Deciphering metal-induced oxidative damages on glycated albumin structure and function. Biochim Biophys Acta. 2014;1840(6):1712–24.

128. Giacco F, Brownlee M. Oxidative stress and diabetic complications. Circ Res. 2010;107(9):1058–70.

129. Ranasinghe P, Wathurapatha WS, Ishara MH, Jayawardana R, Galappatthy P, Katulanda P, et al. Effects of Zinc supplementation on serum lipids: a systematic review and meta-analysis. Nutr Metab. 2015;12:26.

130. Rungby J. Zinc, zinc transporters and diabetes. Diabetologia. 2010;53(8):1549–51.

131. Chistiakov DA, Voronova NV. Zn2 + –transporter-8: A dual role in diabetes. Biofactors. 2009;35(4):356–63.

132. Kawasaki E. ZnT8 and type 1 diabetes. Endocr J. 2012;59(7):531–7.

133. Cramer JA. A systematic review of adherence with medications for diabetes. Diabetes Care. 2004;27(5):1218–24.

134. Alvarez Guisasola F, Tofe Povedano S, Krishnarajah G, Lyu R, Mavros P, Yin D. Hypoglycaemic symptoms, treatment satisfaction, adherence and their associations with glycaemic goal in patients with type 2 diabetes mellitus: findings from the Real-Life Effectiveness and Care Patterns of Diabetes Management (RECAP-DM) Study. Diabetes Obes Metab. 2008;10 Suppl 1:25–32.

135. Odegard PS, Capoccia K. Medication taking and diabetes: a systematic review of the literature. Diabetes Educ. 2007;33(6):1014–29. discussion 1030–1011.

136. Grant RW, Devita NG, Singer DE, Meigs JB. Polypharmacy and medication adherence in patients with type 2 diabetes. Diabetes Care. 2003;26(5):1408–12.

137. Bailey CJ, Kodack M. Patient adherence to medication requirements for therapy of type 2 diabetes. Int J Clin Pract. 2011;65(3):314–22.

138. Dham S, Shah V, Hirsch S, Banerji MA. The role of complementary and alternative medicine in diabetes. Curr Diab Rep. 2006;6(3):251–8.

139. Sakurai H, Adachi Y. The pharmacology of the insulinomimetic effect of zinc complexes. Biometals. 2005;18(4):319–23.

140. Sakurai H, Katoh A, Kiss T, Jakusch T, Hattori M. Metallo-allixinate complexes with anti-diabetic and anti-metabolic syndrome activities. Metallomics. 2010;2(10):670–82.

22

Determination of stress-induced degradation products of cetirizine dihydrochloride by a stability-indicating RP-HPLC method

Paloma Flórez Borges[1,2*†], Pilar Pérez Lozano[1†], Encarna García Montoya[1†], Montserrat Miñarro[1†], Josep R Ticó[1†], Enric Jo[2†] and Josep M Suñe Negre[1†]

Abstract

Background: A new, simple and accurate stability-indicating reverse phase high performance liquid chromatography method was developed and validated during the early stage of drug development of an oral lyophilizate dosage form of cetirizine dihydrochloride.

Methods: For RP-HPLC analysis it was used an Eclipse XDB C8 column 150 mm × 4.6 mm, 5 μm (Agilent columns, Barcelona, Spain) as the stationary phase with a mobile phase consisted of a mixture of 0.2 M K_2HPO4 pH 7.00 and acetonitrile (65:35, v/v) at a flow rate of 1 mL min^{-1}. Detection was performed at 230 nm using diode array detector. The method was validated in accordance with ICH guidelines with respect to linearity, accuracy, precision, specificity, limit of detection and quantification.

Results: The method results in excellent separation between the drug substance and its stress-induced degradation products. The peak purity factor is >950 for the drug substance after all types of stress, which confirms the complete separation of the drug substance peak from its stress induced degradation products.
Regression analysis showed $r^2 > 0.999$ for cetirizine dihydrochloride in the concentration range of 650 μg mL^{-1} to 350 μg mL^{-1} for drug substance assay and a $r^2 > 0.999$ in the concentration range of 0.25 μg mL^{-1} to 5 μg mL^{-1} for degradation products. The method presents a limit of detection of 0.056 μg mL^{-1} and a limit of quantification of 0.25 μg mL^{-1}. The obtained results for precision and accuracy for drug substance and degradation products are within the specifications established for the validation of the method.

Conclusions: The proposed stability-indicating method developed in the early phase of drug development proved to be a simple, sensitive, accurate, precise, reproducible and therefore useful for the following stages of the cetirizine dihydrochloride oral lyophilizate dosage form development.

Background

In the early stage of drug development, forced degradation studies are used to facilitate the development of an analytical methodology, in order to obtain a better understanding of the drug substance (DS) studied and the final drug product (DP) stability, providing data regarding degradation pathways and degradation products (DE) [1]. Such studies are needed to assure that all

the regulatory requirements of a drug are fulfilled, such as the identification of possible DE, degradation pathways and intrinsic stability of the drug molecule. Part of the study is the development and validation of the stability indicating analytical method involved [2,3]. The overall objective of this work is to develop a new formulation with the drug substance ($C_{21}H_{27}Cl_3N_2O_3$) cetirizine dihydrocloride (CTZ; the dihydrochloride of a 2-[4-chlorobenzhydryl) piperazin-1-yl] ethoxyacetic acid). CTZ is a non-sedative H_1 antihistaminic drug, a piperazine derivative and metabolite of hydroxyzine (Figure 1) [4]. CTZ presents an increased degree of polarity, which makes it less capable of crossing the blood brain barrier, hence reducing the sedative side effects in comparison

---

* Correspondence: pflorezb@gmail.com
†Equal contributors
[1]Pharmacy and Pharmaceutical Technology Department, Faculty of Pharmacy, University of Barcelona, Avda Joan XXIII s/n 08028, Barcelona, Spain
[2]Reig Jofre Group, c. Gran Capitá 6 08970, Sant Joan Despi, Barcelona, Spain

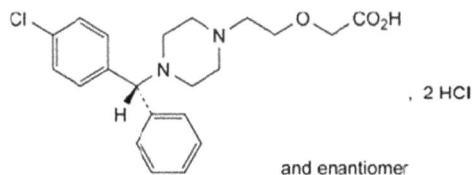

Cetirizini dihydrochloridum

, 2 HCl

and enantiomer

$C_{21}H_{27}Cl_3N_2O_3$
[83881-52-1]

M_r 461.8

Figure 1 Chemical structure of cetirizine dihydrochloride. Ph. Eur. 7th Edition 2014 (8.0).

with first generation antihistamines, such as diphenhydramine and hydroxyzine [5-7]. CTZ is administrated generally in tablets and liquid forms orally to promote the relief of symptoms related to allergic rhinitis, chronic idiopathic urticaria and other rashes [8,9].

This new formulation consists of an oral lyophilized dosage form, whose aim is to facilitate swallowing (in the case of patients with dysphagia, such as children and elderly, for instance), easy to administer, effective, safe and stable over time.

Several HPLC methods have been reported in literature for the determination of CTZ alone [10-13] and also determining CTZ simultaneously with other drug substances, as in multicomponents preparations [14-16]. In order to develop a new chromatographic method for the determination and quantification of CTZ and its DE generated after a forced degradation study, several chromatographic methods for CTZ were investigated in the literature. Among them, was the Ph. Eur. method for CTZ [17]. However, the latter was discarded due to the use of a normal phase chromatographic column and mobile phase that used much organic solvent (acetonitrile, not very cost-effective). Also, the Ph. Eur. method presents a very acid mobile phase pH (pH <0.5), which is known to diminish the life span of the chromatographic column [18]. Also, some chromatographic analytical methods [12,13] used chromatographic columns of reverse phase, usually C18 and C8. Depending on the type of separation pursued (as for instance, CTZ combined with another DS), isocratic or gradient methods were used, and also mobile phases with ionic pairing. We have developed a reverse-phase high performance liquid chromatography (RP-HPLC) method by studying the effect of the stationary phase (C18 or C8 analytical columns) on peak resolution, the influence of pH -mobile phase- when adjusting the desired retention time (t_R) for the DS. Plus, by using a reverse-phase column, we reduced the amount of organic solvent (acetonitrile) used for the

identification of the DS, in comparison to the analytical method validated by Ph. Eur. [17], which uses a normal phase chromatographic column, requiring more organic solvent due to its characteristics [18-25]. Therefore the aim of this study is to determine all possible DE generated under stress conditions, by developing and validating a stability-indicating RP-HPLC method for cetirizine dihydrochloride in the early stage of drug development of an oral lyophilizate.

Methods

Chemicals and reagents

All chemicals were analytical grade and used as received. All solutions were prepared in Milli-Q deionized water from a Milli Q gradient A10 water purification system (Molsheim, France). CTZ bulk powder (Cetirizine dihydrochloride, Ph. Eur) was purchased from Jubilant Lifesciences Ltd (Mysore, India) and kindly provided by Reig Jofre Group (Barcelona, Spain). HPLC grade acetonitrile was obtained from Panreac (Barcelona, Spain). Ortho-phosphoric acid 85% was purchased from Panreac (Barcelona, Spain). Potassium phosphate dibasic Ph. Eur. (K_2HPO_4) was purchased from Fagron (Terrassa, Spain). Hydrochloric acid 37%, sodium hydroxide and hydrogen peroxide (H_2O_2) at 33% were purchased from Panreac (Barcelona, Spain).

Equipment and chromatographic conditions

Samples were analyzed on Dionex Ultimate 3000 HPLC Thermo Fisher Scientific (California, USA), equipped with data system Chromeleon version 6.8 SP2 Build 2284, with degasifier SR3000, LPG-3400 quaternary pump, injector WPS3000, oven 6P TCC-3100, UV–vis detector PDA-3000. For initial development studies it was used an analytical chromatographic column Kromasyl 100-5C18 150 mm × 4.6 mm, 5 μm particle size (Tecnokroma Akzonobel, Terrasa, Spain). For final development and method validation, it was used an analytical chromatographic column Eclipse XDB-C8 150 mm × 4.6 mm, 5 μm particle size (Agilent columns, Barcelona, Spain). An isocratic mobile phase consisting of acetonitrile and 0.2 M potassium phosphate dibasic Ph. Eur. buffer solution at pH 7.00 (35:65 v/v) was used, and the analysis was carried out at a flow rate of 1 mL min $^{-1}$. All determinations were performed at 30°C. The injection volume was 25 μL. The detector was set at λ 230 nm. The peak homogeneity was expressed in terms of peak purity factor and was obtained directly from spectral analysis report using the above mentioned software. Other apparatus included a Crison micropH 2002 pH

meter (Barcelona, Spain) and Heraeus oven T5028 for thermal degradation (dry heat at 105°C) (Hanaus, Germany).

Forced degradation studies and preparation of samples
The forced degradation studies were carried out by preparing several standard solutions of CTZ at 500 μg mL $^{-1}$, for each degradation study. Each sample was analyzed according to the previous procedures described under the proposed analytical method. In order to determine whether the analytical method is suitable to be a stability-indicating

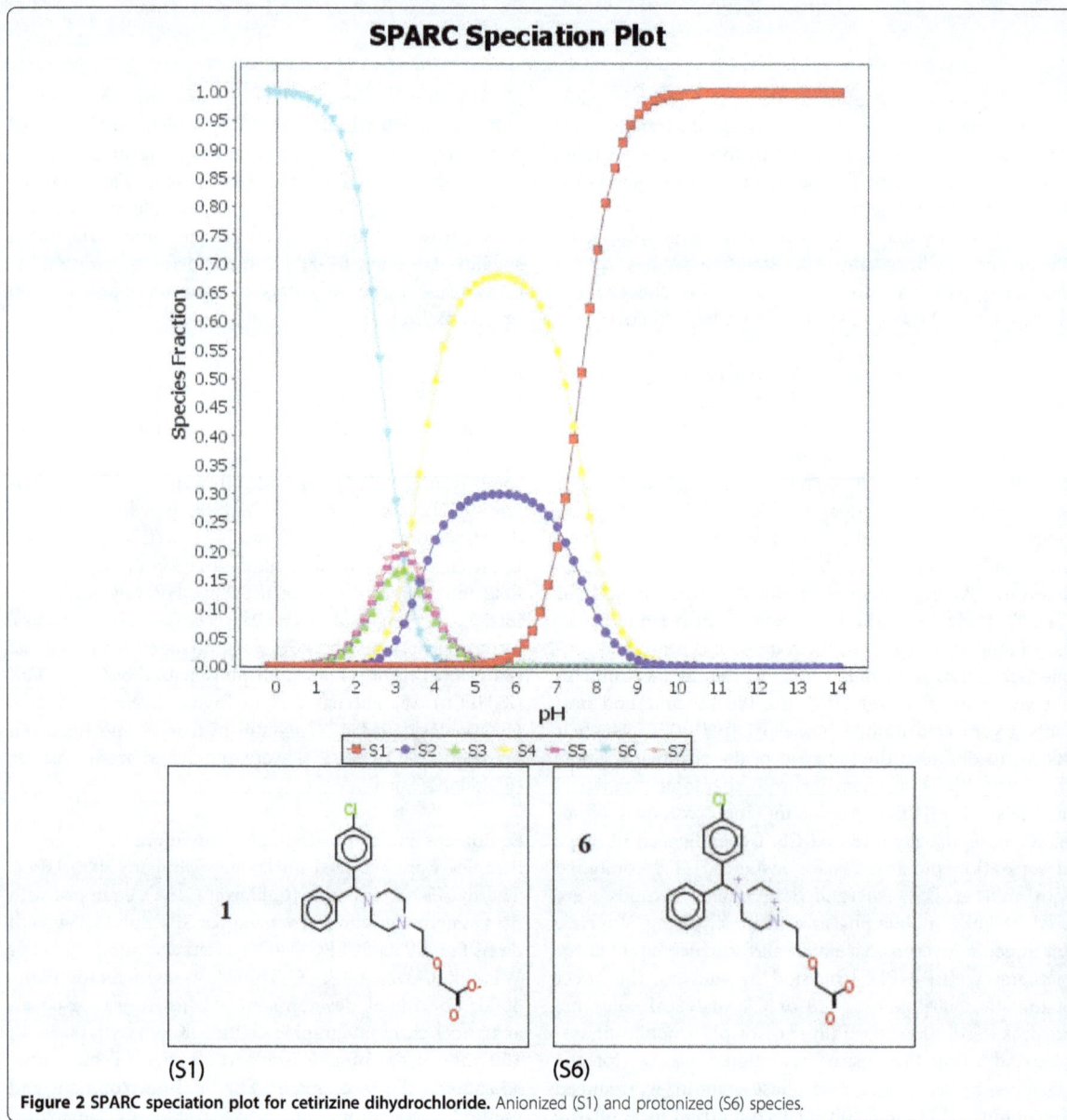

Figure 2 SPARC speciation plot for cetirizine dihydrochloride. Anionized (S1) and protonized (S6) species.

assay, forced degradation studies under different conditions were carried out according to the following procedure:

a) Acid and basic hydrolysis: 5 mg of bulk powder was treated with 5 mL of 0.1 M HCl and 0.1 M NaOH. The flasks were placed in a dry air oven at 105°C. Another 5 mg of bulk powder was also treated with 5 mL of 0.1 M HCl and 0.1 M NaOH at room temperature, for 24 hours.

b) Oxidation with H_2O_2 at 33%: 5 mg of bulk powder was exposed to 5 mL of hydrogen peroxide at 33% (W/v). The vial was kept at room temperature for 24 hours.

c) Infrared (IR) and Ultraviolet (UV) light: 5 mg of bulk powder was exposed under an infrared lamp and another 5 mg of bulk powder was exposed under an ultraviolet lamp, for 24 hours.

d) Humidity HR 79%: the 5 mg bulk powder sample was placed inside a humidifier with HR 79%, for 24 hours.

e) Heat at 105°C: 5 mg of bulk powder sample was placed inside a 105°C dry air oven for 24 hours.

f) Shed sunlight for 15 days: 5 mg of bulk powder was kept in a vial for 15 days, at room temperature and exposed to direct sunlight.

Once the stress conditions were complete, 10 mL of 0.2 M phosphate buffer (pH 7.00) was added to the samples in order to achieve the standard solution concentration of 500 μm mL-1. Moreover, all the solutions and blanks were filtered with a 0.45 μm syringe filtration disk PVDF. Results were compiled in terms of relative retention times (rtR) found during the analysis.

Validation of the analytical method

In order to validate the RP-HPLC method developed, ICHQ2B guideline recommendations were followed, in terms of selectivity, linearity, range, accuracy, precision, limit of detection (LOD) and limit of quantification (LOQ) [26]. In order to fulfill ICH specifications in terms of linearity and range for the analytical method (content uniformity and assay of DS and finished product), a linear range within 70-130% was studied, by analyzing a series of three replicates, i.e., three independent sets (k = 3), each with seven different concentrations (n = 6): 350 μg ml^{-1} - 650 μg ml^{-1}, considering 500 μg ml^{-1} as 100% (standard solution), in order to provide information on the variation in peak area values between samples of the same concentration. For evaluation of the precision estimates, repeatability and intermediate precision were performed at three concentration levels (650, 500 and 350 μg ml^{-1}, corresponding to 130, 100 and 70%), and 10 injections of each sample (K = 10), per day. Mean average, standard deviation (SD) and relative standard deviation (RSD) of t_R and the peak area achieved individually of day 1 and 2 were calculated. After the HPLC analysis, the response factor (RF) was calculated between the response (Y) and concentration achieved (X), as Y/X. Therefore, mean average, SD and RSD were calculated using the response factors obtained with an Excel 2007 spread sheet. The response factors results must comply with a RSD ± 2%. For accuracy the concentration found expressed by function of repeatability of the standard

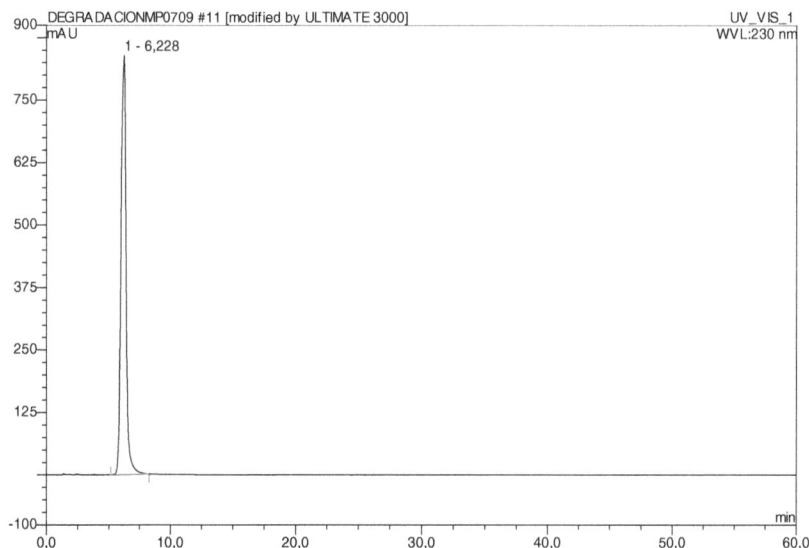

Figure 3 Cetirizine dihydrochloride under normal conditions.

Table 1 Summary of product degradation peaks in relative retention time (rt$_R$)

Stress conditions	rt$_R$ (min)								CTZ								
Humidity HR79%									1.00								
Acid hydrolysis *RT			0.51				0.81	0.87	1.00								
Acid hydrolysis at 105°C	0.46		0.50		0.64			0.87	1.00						5.00		
Ultraviolet light (UV)			0.52	0.59			0.81		1.00		2.00			4.30			
Infrared light (IR)			0.51	0.60	0.66		0.81		1.00								
Basic hydrolysis *RT			0.53				0.81	0.87	1.00								
Basic hydrolysis at 105°C	0.46	0.48	0.51	0.58		0.71		0.86	1.00	1.60	2.00	2.80	3.40		5.00		9.10
Dry heat at 105°C			0.50			0.72	0.80	0.90	1.00					4.30	5.00		
Shed sunlight 15 days				0.60					1.00								
H$_2$O$_2$ at 33%			0.51						1.00	1.90	2.60			4.40		5.70	
Normal conditions									1.00								

*RT: Room temperature.

solution, relative error in percentage and the percentage of recovery, with mean average, SD and RSD deviation of each of the three concentrations studied (650, 500 and 350 μg ml^{-1}, was considered of three replicates) were calculated. For the DS, 98-102% percentage of recovery was considered as being acceptable [27].

For the determination and quantification of the DE, linearity, precision, accuracy and LOD and LOQ were calculated. In order to carry out this validation, further dilutions from a stock solution of 500 μg ml^{-1} with the specified mobile phase were carried out in order to achieve the correspondent concentrations: 5 μg mL^{-1}, 2.5 μg mL^{-1}, 1.25 μg mL^{-1}, 0.5 μg mL^{-1}, 0.25 μg mL^{-1}, 0.125 μg mL^{-1}. A total of seven independent calibration curves, i.e., seven replicates (k = 7) were prepared. The LOD and LOQ were calculated by the ratio between the standard deviation of y-intercepts of regression lines of the seven calibration curves mentioned before by averaging the slopes of calibration curve multiplied by 3.3 and

10, respectively [26,27]. Each serial dilution (k = 7) was analyzed, with n = 6 (level of concentrations).

In terms of relative error and percentage of recovery three concentrations (5, 1.25 and 0.25 μg mL^{-1}) from the range of DE were evaluated. All the solutions prepared were filtered with a 0.45 μm syringe filtration disk PVDF to the vials for injection in the HPLC system.

Results and discussion

HPLC method development

As an early stage study of drug development, our goal was to acknowledge all possible DE generated under stress conditions for CTZ. The information acquired in the early stage of the study will lead us to a better understanding of the DS itself and also the possible DE that we may find during the next step of the oral lyophilized development study. Therefore it was not our objective the development of a fast analytical method for the DS per se, but actually the development of an analytical

Table 2 Peak purity determination by diode-array UV–vis spectra of CTZ and stress studies results

Forced degradation conditions	[a]Peak purity index match	Decomposition (%)	Extent of decomposition
Humidity HR79%	952	0	None
Acid hydrolysis *RT	990	0	None
Acid hydrolysis at 105°C	998	19	Substantial
Ultraviolet light (UV)	962	9	Substantial
Infrared light (IR)	962	8	Substantial
Basic hydrolysis *RT	972	0	None
Basic hydrolysis at 105°C	986	15	Substantial
Dry heat at 105°C	953	3	Substantial
Shed sunlight 15 days	996	10	Substantial
Oxidative medium *RT	998	79	Substantial
CTZ (phosphate buffer solution)	990	0	Normal conditions

[a]indicates the value for peak purity index match of CTZ above 950, considering 1000 as 100% match; *RT: Room temperature.

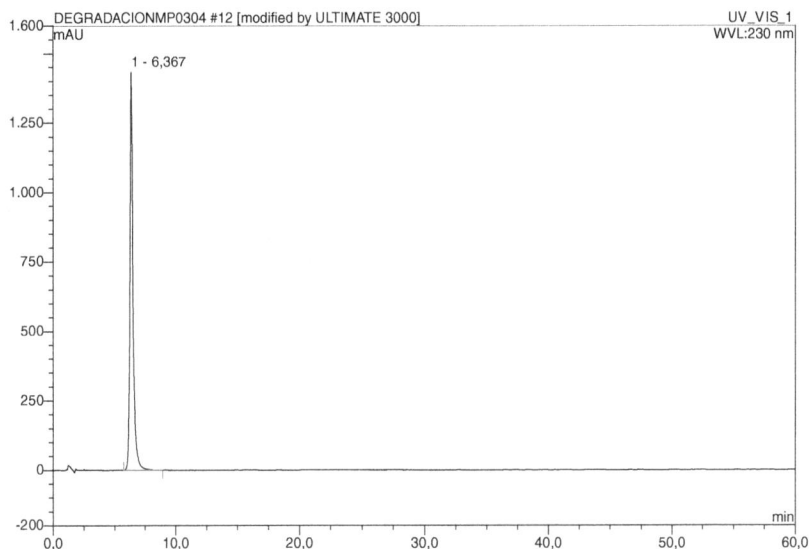

Figure 4 Cetirizine dihydrochloride under humidity HR79%.

method that could detect a complete profile of DE for this DS, leaving for the following studies of drug development the aim of reducing run time, for instance.

CTZ is freely soluble in water, and practically insoluble in acetone and metilen chlorate [17]. Considering its hydrophilic nature, reverse phase columns were chosen in order to investigate the chromatographic profile with two types of packing material for stationary phases: C18 (more hydrophobic, octadecylsilyl), and C8 (intermediate hydrophobicity, octylsilyl). We also studied the molecule of CTZ using the physicochemical calculator SPARC (Sparc Performs Automated Reasoning in Chemistry) developed by the United States Environmental Protection Agency (EPA) for the purpose of predicting which pH would suit best for CTZ ionization [28]. The speciation plot for CTZ (Figure 2) shows that pH3 is not recommended for the ionization of CTZ due to the existence of six different species of ionized CTZ with no clear definition among them, whereas at pH2 we can find the protonated CTZ (S6) and at pH7 the anionized

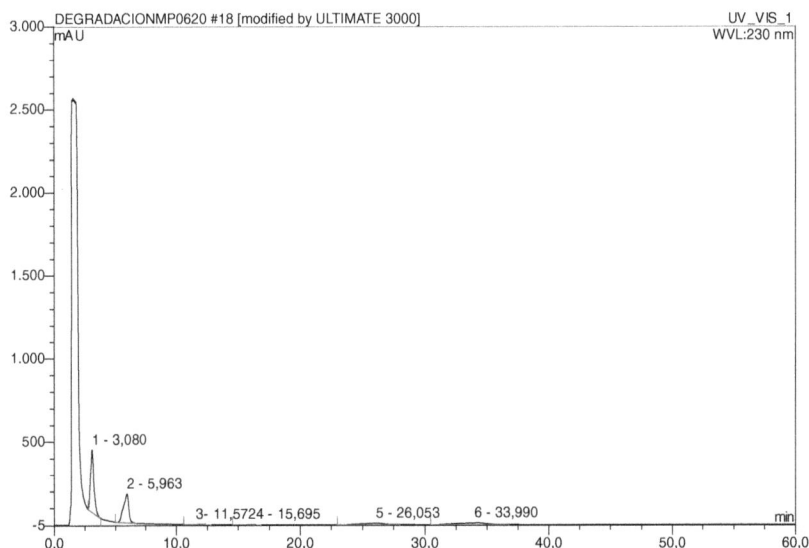

Figure 5 Cetirizine dihydrochloride under H_2O_2 at 33%.

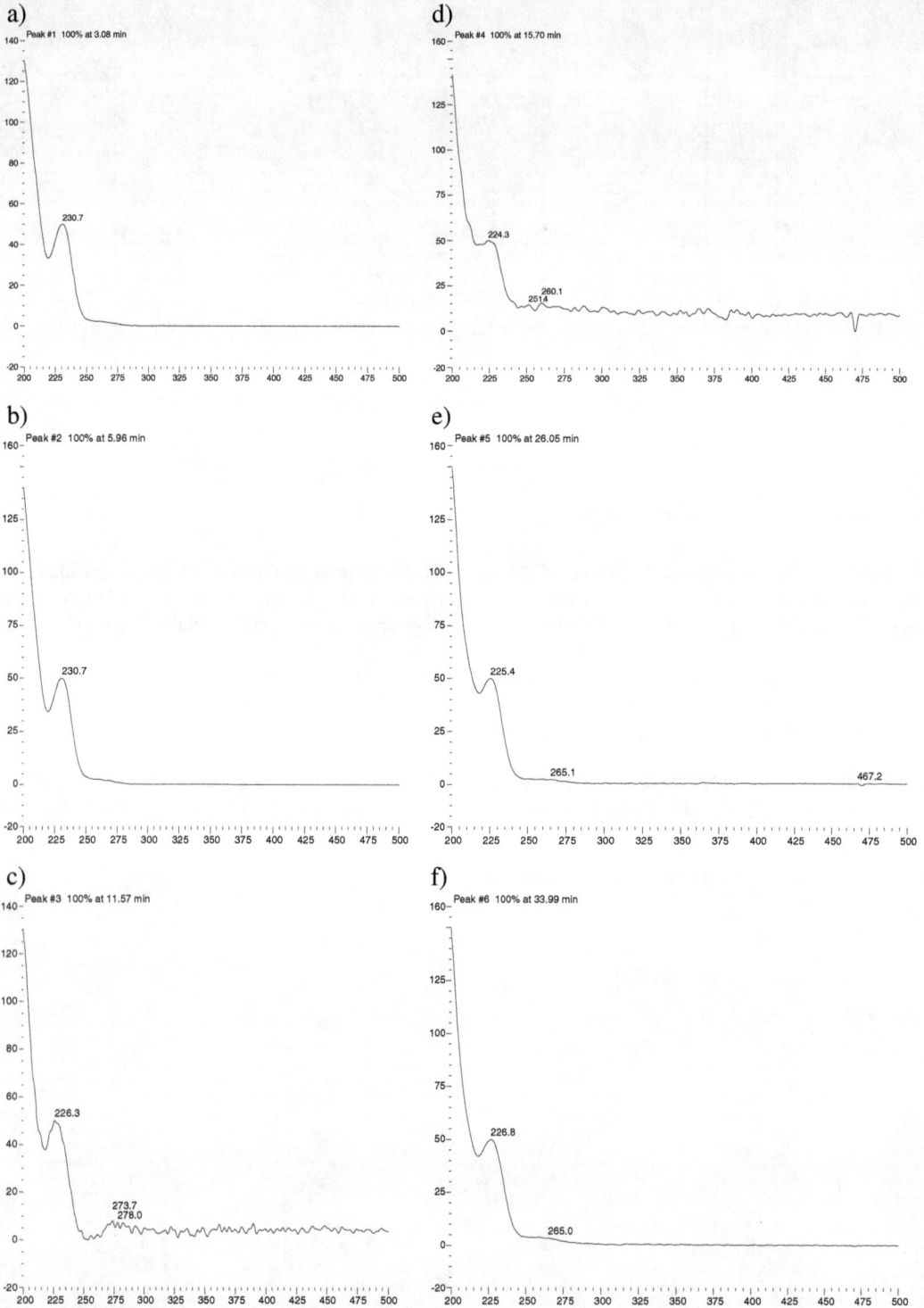

Figure 6 Chromatographic spectra of cetirizine dihydrochloride (b) and its degradation products (a, c, d, e and f) under H_2O_2 at 33%, in nm.

Table 3 Repeatability and intermediate precision according to retention time (t_R) and peak area for CTZ assay

Day	t_R				Peak area		
	$\mu g\ mL^{-1}$	Mean average $\pm$ [a]SD (min) [b]K = 10		[c]RSD (%)	Mean average $\pm$ [a]SD (mAU.min) [b]K = 10		[c]RSD (%)
1	650	5.79 ± 0.0274		0.4747	512.54 ± 1.7865		0.5365
	500	5.79 ± 0.0327		0.5646	399.69 ± 1.9090		0.4777
	350	5.80 ± 0.0228		0.3929	281.21 ± 1.7867		0.6353
2	650	5.77 ± 0.0195		0.3384	511.75 ± 2.2059		0.4310
	500	5.78 ± 0.0149		0.2584	399.54 ± 1.5972		0.3997
	350	5.80 ± 0.0248		0.4279	281.63 ± 1.0483		0.3722

[a]SD (Standard deviation); [b]K (number of injections); [c]RSD (Relative standard deviation).

CTZ (S1) (Figure 3). The pKa values estimated for CTZ are: 2.7 (pKa1), 3.6 (pKa2) and 7.6 (pKa 3) [29]. However, due to the finding of chromatographic methods that used buffer solutions at pH3 or around 3 (2.8, 3.5, for instance) we decided to considered pH3 in our study [10-12,14]. During the preliminary studies of the analytical method development, we have combined different proportions of acetonitrile and aqueous solution at pH3 (MilliQ water acidified at pH3 with orto-phosphoric acid 85%). The preliminary studies were carried out by the injection of a 500 $\mu g\ mL^{-1}$ solution of CTZ, using a C18 analytical chromatographic column, flow rate of mobile phase of 1 mL min $^{-1}$, an injection volume of 25 μL, oven temperature of 30°C, 230 nm of wavelength, in isocratic mode. The effects of the optimum eluent composition were studied, obtaining a retention time (t_R) of eight minutes for CTZ with a 35:65 (v/v) of acetonitrile and aqueous solution at pH3. Also, we tried to adjust the mobile phase –studying the effect of the proportion between the organic solvent and buffer solution pH– in order to achieve a t_R of approximately 6–7 for CTZ. To diminish the t_R, we finally tried to use a buffer solution of 0.2 M K$_2$HPO$_4$ pH7. We observed that maintaining the same proportions of organic solvent and buffer solution, but changing the pH from 3 to 7, using potassium phosphate dibasic buffer solution at 0.2 M

solution at pH7, we achieved a t_R of 5–6 minutes. However, CTZ peak shape presented tail broadening. Therefore, in order to avoid using ion pair to improve peak resolution, we have changed the analytical chromatographic column C18 (Kromasyl 100–5 C18) to a C8 (Eclipse XDB C8), and tested with the same conditions as before: acetonitrile and phosphate buffer solution pH 7 (35:65, respectively), injection volume 25 μL, flow rate 1 mL min $^{-1}$, temperature 30°C, 230 nm of wavelength. This resulted in eliminating tail broadening. Having determined the eluent proportions of the isocratic mobile phase and the pH of the aqueous solution as pH7, obtaining the desired t_R, we have established the stability-indicating method to carry out the forced degradation studies.

Results of forced degradation study

CTZ was degraded up to 19% under acid hydrolysis at 105°C, presenting five degradation peaks. Under basic hydrolysis at 105°C, CTZ was degraded up to 15%, presenting twelve degradation peaks, followed by shed sun light (10%, one degradation peak), UV (9%, four degradation peaks), IR (8%, four degradation peaks) and dry heat at 105°C (3%, 6 degradation peaks). CTZ under photolytic stress -shed sunlight during 15 days, IR and UV light- presented degradation peaks with two, four

Table 4 Concentrations found, relative error in percentage, percentage of recovery and estimates for CTZ assay

[a]Theoretical concentration ($\mu g\ mL^{-1}$)	Concentration found ($\mu g\ mL^{-1}$)	Relative error%	[b]Recovery%	Mean recovery	[c]SD of recovery
650	641.29	1.25	98.75	98.66	0.09
650	641.27	1.36	98.65		
650	640.67	1.45	98.56		
500	500.96	0.19	100.19	100.49	0.57
500	500.71	0.14	100.14		
500	505.80	1.14	101.16		
350	352.16	0.61	100.61	100.95	0.43
350	352.77	0.78	100.79		
350	355.05	1.42	101.44		

[a]650 $\mu g\ mL^{-1}$ = 130%, 500 $\mu g\ mL^{-1}$ = 100%, 350 $\mu g\ mL^{-1}$ = 70%; [b]recovery limits (98-102%); [c]SD (Standard deviation).

Table 5 Mean average, standard deviation (SD) and relative standard deviation (RSD%) of peak area mAU (5 – 0.125 μ mL^{-1})

Theoretical concentration (μg mL^{-1})	Mean concentration average ± [a] SD (μg mL^{-1}) ([b] k = 7)	[c]RSD (%)
5.000	4.0495 ± 0.1040	2.5701
2.500	2.0121 ± 0.0251	1.2502
1.250	1.0012 ± 0.0326	3.2622
0.500	0.4021 ± 0.0327	8.1334
0.250	0.1818 ± 0.0111	6.1605

[a]SD (Standard deviation); [b]k (number of replicates); [c]RSD (relative standard deviation).

and five peaks, respectively (Table 1). CTZ presented DE peaks under acid (three DE peaks) and basic hydrolysis at room temperature (three DE peaks). However, degradation was not substantial in both cases (Table 2). Comparing the chromatographic profile of CTZ dissolved in buffer solution (Figure 3) with no stress conditions (normal conditions) with CTZ under Humidity HR79% (Figure 4), it is observed that CTZ showed no substantial degradation under Humidity HR79%, presenting a similar chromatographic profile with CTZ dissolved in buffer solution at the same concentration. Under oxidative stress, CTZ presented 79% of degradation, showing five degradation peaks (Figure 5) and in Figure 6 it can be visualized by the chromatographic spectra of each DE and CTZ. Furthermore, the peak purity value for CTZ under oxidative stress was of 998 (considering 1000 as 100% match), indicating a homogenous peak (Table 2). However, in the beginning of the elution process, the diode-array assay detects DE higher that its threshold, demonstrating a possible saturation of the chromatographic column with H_2O_2 at 33%. There is also the hypothesis that 79% of decomposition can also be the result of the degradation of DE, which would generate more DE, due to the exposure of CTZ during 24 hours under oxidative condition. This leads to the conclusion that may be necessary to change the oxidative stress condition procedure, by reducing the concentration of peroxide (33%) or reducing the time of exposure of the DS with H_2O_2 (24 hours), or both. Satisfactory results were obtained studying the peak purity

Table 6 Relative error (%) and percentage of recovery

Concentration (μg mL^{-1})	Mean concentration found (μg mL^{-1}) ([a]k = 7)	[b]Relative error% (mean)	[c]Mean Recovery%	[d]SD of recovery%
5	5.000	0.620	100.070	0.74
1.25	1.248	3.310	99.840	4.10
0.25	0.235	9.390	94.210	10.00

[a]k = 7 (number of replicates); [b]mean relative error% ; [c]mean recovery%; [d]standard deviation.

index for CTZ under stress conditions, which confirms the high specificity of the analytical method for CTZ (Table 2).

Method validation
The developed method was validated using ICH guidelines [26]. Validation parameters included linearity, precision, accuracy, precision, and specificity, LOD and LOQ [26,27].

Assay for drug substance method
Linearity for CTZ assay was verified by triplicate analysis of seven different concentrations, i.e., three sets of 130-70% range of CTZ. As a result, the linear regression equation was found to be Y = 769.56 X + 14.573 (r^2 = 0.9994, k = 3 (number of replicates), n = 7 (level of concentrations), 650 μg mL^{-1} to 350 μg mL^{-1}) for CTZ. In which, Y was the dependent variable, X was independent variable, 769.56 was the slope and which showed change in dependent (Y) variable per unit change in independent (X) variable; 14.573 was the Y-intercept i.e., the value of Y variable when X = 0.

As for the analytical method precision (Table 3), three concentration levels (650, 500 and 350 μg ml^{-1}, corresponding to 130, 100 and 70%), and 10 injections of each sample, per day were prepared. The results have shown the repeatability and intermediate precision presenting a RSD inferior to 2.7% according to AOAC [27] (1.43% and 1.03%, respectively). In terms of accuracy, according to the obtained results (Table 4), the percentage of recovery ranges from 98.56 to 101.44, from being within the limits established according to AOAC [27] (98-102%), which indicates the accuracy of the method for CTZ.

It was studied seven independent sets of dilutions, i.e., seven replicates (k =7), each set with six different concentrations (n = 6) in the range of 5–0.125 μg mL^{-1}. Calculating LOD and LOQ by the ratio between the SD of y-intercepts of regression lines of the seven serial dilutions of six different concentrations mentioned before by averaging the slopes of calibration curve multiplied by 3.3 and 10, respectively, the analytical method presented a LOD of 0.056 μg mL^{-1} and a LOQ of 0.17 μg mL^{-1}. However, it was demonstrated that the LOQ value of 0.17 μg mL^{-1} was not lineal. Therefore, taken into account the range defined in ICH guidelines to the DE, for linearity reasons it was considered the range around a suggested (probable) limit [26]. Therefore, the linearity should be established from the LOQ to 120%. So a new LOQ (SD (μg mL^{-1}) = 0.0111, RSD (%) = 6.1605) was established (0.25 μg mL^{-1}). The linear regression equation was found to be Y = 0.8125X-0.014 (r^2 = 0.9999, n = 5 (level of concentrations), k = 7 (number of replicates), 0.25-5 μg mL^{-1}) (Table 5).

In reference to the results of the analytical method validation, in both Table 5 (repeatability) and Table 6 (recovery), the RSD and the range complies with RSD permitted (2.7%) and the range (90-110%) according to AOAC [27], assuring the applicability of the developed analytical method for the determination and quantification of DE.

Conclusions

A new and simple RP-HPLC method was developed for the determination of CTZ and its DE during the early stage of drug development of an oral lyophilized dosage form. The proposed method was demonstrated to be linear, precise, accurate and specific, based on method validation. Satisfactory results were obtained in separating the peak of CTZ from the DE produced by forced degradation. Plus, it is a cost-effective method that requires a simple mobile phase (phosphate buffer solution and acetonitrile, 65:35 v/v) and also does not require the use of ion pairing, which can result in difficulty in recovering initial column properties. It was also able to separate with good specificity the DS peak from the entire DE generated during the stress condition study, which help us in the next step of the drug development of the oral lyophilizate, by adapting the validated method considering further aspects, such as the interactions between CTZ and the excipients chosen for the final medicinal product. The proposed analytical method proved to be stability-indicating and therefore useful in the following stages of drug development.

Abbreviations

DS: Drug substance; DP: Drug product; DE: Degradation products; CTZ: Cetirizine dihydrochloride; RP-HPLC: Reverse phase high performance liquid chromatography; t_R: Retention time; rt_R: Relative retention time; LOD: Limit of detection; LOQ: Limit of quantification; IR: Infrared light; UV: Ultraviolet light.

Competing interests

The authors declare that they have no competing interests.

Authors' contributions

PFB, PPL and EGM: participate in method development and optimization, perform the experiments for forced degradation studies and method validation, collect experimental data and write the manuscript. JMSN and EJ: propose and supervise the implementation of various experiments and revised the manuscript. JRT and MM: revised data and supervised the manuscript. All authors read and approved the final manuscript.

References

1. Ahuja S: Overview of HPLC Method Development for Pharmaceuticals. In *HPLC Method Development for Pharmaceuticals*. Edited by Ahuja S, Rasmussen HT. Amsterdam: Academic Press; 2007:1–17.
2. Rasmussen HT, Swinney KA, Gaiki S: HPLC Method Development in Early Phase Pharmaceutical Development. In *HPLC Method Development for Pharmaceuticals*. Edited by Ahuja S, Rasmussen HT. Amsterdam: Academic Press; 2007:353–371.
3. Alsante KM, Ando A, Brown R, Ensing J, Hatajik TD, Kong W, Tsuda Y: The role of degradant profiling in active pharmaceutical ingredients and drug products. *Adv Drug Deliv Rev* 2007, 59(1):29–37.
4. Sweetman SC: Martindale: the complete drug reference: [https://www.medicinescomplete.com/mc/martindale/current/]
5. Simons FER: Advances in H1-antihistamines. *N Engl J Med* 2004, 351:2203–2217.
6. Atkins PC, Zweiman B, Moskowitz A, von Allmen C, Ciliberti M: Cellular inflammatory responses and mediator release during early developing late-phase allergic cutaneous inflammatory responses: effects of cetirizine. *J Allergy Clin Immunol* 1997, 99:806–811.
7. Walsh GM, Annunziato L, Frossard N, Knol K, Levander S, Nicolas JM, Tagliatela M, Tharp MD, Tillemant JP, Tillemant H: New insights into the second generation antihistamines. *Drugs* 2001, 61:207–236.
8. Ortonne JP: Urticaria and its subtypes: the role of second-generation antihistamines. *Eur J Intern Med* 2012, 23:26–30.
9. Komarow HD, Metcalfe DD: Office-based management of urticaria. *Am J Med* 2008, 121:379–384.
10. Kim CK, Yeong KJ, Ban E, Hyun MJ, Kim JK, Jin SE, Park JS: Narrow-bore high performance liquid chromatographic method for the determination of cetirizine in human plasma using column switching. *J Pharm Biomed Anal* 2005, 37:603–609.
11. Zaater MF, Tahboub YR, Najib NM: RP-LC method for the determination of cetirizine in serum. *J Pharm Biomed Anal* 2000, 22:739–744.
12. El Walily AFM, Korany MA, El Gindy A, Bedair MF: Spectrophotometric and high performance liquid chromatographic determination of cetirizine dihydrochloride in pharmaceutical tablets. *J Pharm Biomed Anal* 1998, 17:435–442.
13. Macek J, Ptáček P, Klíma J: Determination of cetirizine in human plasma by high-performance liquid chromatography. *J Chromatogr B* 1999, 736:231–235.
14. Dharuman J, Vashudevan M, Ajithlal T: High performance liquid chromatographic method for the determination of cetirizine and ambroxol in human plasma and urine— a boxcar approach. *J Chromatogr B* 2011, 879:2624–2631.
15. Likar MD, Mansour HL, Harwood JW: Development and validation of a dissolution test for a once-a-day combination tablet of immediate-release cetirizine dihydrochloride and extended-release pseudoephedrine hydrochloride. *J Pharm Biomed Anal* 2005, 39:543–551.
16. Hadad GM, Emara S, Mahmoud WMM: Development and validation of a stability-indicating RP-HPLC method for the determination of paracetamol with dantrolene or/and cetirizine and pseudoephedrine in two pharmaceutical dosage forms. *Talanta* 2009, 79:1360–1367.
17. European Pharmacopoeia 7th Edition 2014 (8.0): [http://online6.edqm.eu/ep801/]
18. Jaber AMY, Al Sherife HA, Al Omari MM, Badwan AA: Determination of cetirizine dihydrochloride, related impurities and preservatives in oral solution and tablet dosage forms using HPLC. *J Pharm Biomed Anal* 2004, 36:341–350.
19. Karakuş S, Küçükgüzel I, Küçükgüzel SG: Development and validation of a rapid RP-HPLC method for the determination of cetirizine or fexofenadine with pseudoephedrine in binary pharmaceutical dosage forms. *J Pharm Biomed Anal* 2008, 46:295–302.
20. Neue UD, Alden BA, Grover R, Grumbach ES, Iraneta PC, Méndez A: HPLC Columns and Packings. In HPLC Method Development for Pharmaceuticals. In *HPLC Method Development for Pharmaceuticals*. Edited by Ahuja S, Rasmussen HT. Amsterdam: Academic Press; 2007:45–83.
21. Visky D: Column Characterization and Selection. In *HPLC Method Development for Pharmaceuticals*, Volume 8. Edited by Ahuja S, Rasmussen HT. Amsterdam: Academic Press; 2007:85–109.
22. Bosch E, Espinosa S, Rosés M: Retention of ionizable compounds on high-performance liquid chromatography III. Variation of pK values of acids and pH values of buffers in acetonitrile-water mobile phases. *J Chromatogr A* 1998, 824:137–146.
23. Bosch E, Espinosa S, Rosés M: Retention of ionizable compounds in high-performance liquid chromatography IX. Modelling retention in reversed-phase liquid chromatography as a function of pH and solvent composition with acetonitrile-water mobile phases. *J Chromatogr A* 2002, 947:47–58.
24. Espinosa S, Bosch E, Rosés M: Retention of ionizable compounds in high-performance liquid chromatography 14. Acid–base pK values in acetonitrile–water mobile phases. *J Chromatogr A* 2002, 964:55–66.
25. Agrafiotou P, Ràfols C, Castells C, Bosch E, Rosés M: Simultaneous effect of pH, temperature and mobile phase composition in the chromatographic retention of ionizable compounds. *J Chromatogr A* 2011, 1218:4995–5009.

26. International Conference on Harmonization, ICH Q2B: Validation of Analytical Procedures: Terms and Definitions. Step 5 (1996) [http://www. ich.org/products/guidelines/quality/article/quality-guidelines.html]

27. Official methods of analysis of AOAC [http://www.eoma.aoac.org/]

28. Sparc Performs Automated Reasoning in Chemistry [http://archemcalc.com/ sparc]

29. Pubchem Open chemistry database [http://pubchem.ncbi.nlm.nih.gov/ compound/2678?from=summary#section=Top]

23

A novel approach for inventory problem in the pharmaceutical supply chain

Gökçe Candan[*] and Harun Reşit Yazgan

Abstract

Background: In pharmaceutical enterprises, keeping up with global market conditions is possible with properly selected supply chain management policies. Generally; demand-driven classical supply chain model is used in the pharmaceutical industry. In this study, a new mathematical model is developed to solve an inventory problem in the pharmaceutical supply chain.

Method: Unlike the studies in literature, the "shelf life and product transition times" constraints are considered, simultaneously, first time in the pharmaceutical production inventory problem. The problem is formulated as a mixed-integer linear programming (MILP) model with a hybrid time representation. The objective is to maximize total net profit. Effectiveness of the proposed model is illustrated considering a classical and a vendor managed inventory (VMI) supply chain on an experimental study.

Results: To show the effectiveness of the model, an experimental study is performed; which contains 2 different supply chain policy (Classical and VMI), 24 and 30 months planning horizon, 10 and 15 different cephalosporin products. Finally the mathematical model is compared to another model in literature and the results show that proposed model is superior.

Conclusion: This study suggest a novel approach for solving pharmaceutical inventory problem. The developed model is maximizing total net profit while determining optimal production plan under shelf life and product transition constraints in the pharmaceutical industry. And we believe that the proposed model is much more closed to real life unlike the other studies in literature.

Keywords: Pharmaceutical supply chain, Shelf life, MILP, Vendor managed inventory

Background

Pharmaceutical industry applies a supply chain policy that allows the continuation of a wide variety of materials with large quantities in a very fast flow. Within pharmaceutical supply chains, the product variety is a huge problem to manage within short time windows. Nevertheless, depending on the medicine drugs, amounts can be a big problem to trade with costs. In here, the requirements of small batches are particularly hard to handle. The production of pharmaceutical products has two stages as primary and secondary level. Primary production includes the production of basic molecules active components or pharmaceutical active ingredients. The secondary production also includes the processes of being formulated of these active components and the delivery to the customers. Many operations in pharmaceutical production occur in bulks called charge. Quality control also takes place with monitoring each charge. On the production line, cleaning is a matter in the case of product change (transition) and this situation is to prevent the contamination of different products. Besides, raw materials and products have a certain shelf life. All these constraints are reducing the efficiency in the pharmaceutical industry. Shelf life controls are performed for raw materials by subjecting to retest procedure at certain intervals. During retest, raw materials are kept in quarantine; they are not definitely included in the production line and if test results indicate that the raw materials can already be used, they are taken from the quarantine and transferred to production stores. In shelf life control for the products, expiration date is printed on the packaging while the

* Correspondence: gcandan@sakarya.edu.tr
Industrial Engineering Department, Sakarya University, 54187 Sakarya, Turkey

product is on production line and the expiry date starts from the date of production.

Compared with supply chain of other products, pharmaceutical supply chain is very complex. The factors such as long set-up times, resource-intensive operations, short shelf life and high production of waste make the pharmaceutical supply chain different from other sectors. Pharmaceutical production is demand managed. Firms rarely deliver the product to pharmacy or patient; instead of this, they deliver products to the consumer through wholesalers (pharmaceutical warehouses).

In such a different featured sector to maintain a presence in the market despite all these constraints is possible with correctly selected supply chain management policies. To adapt to changing market conditions, sustainable supply chain policy and to compete in global market, the pharmaceutical supply chain should be carried out by mathematical models based on scientific formulas determined with correct strategies [27]. In planning, the importance of inventory management has also great importance. Considering countless complications, it is very difficult to obtain optimal schedules. However, mathematical models help to take right decisions.

For an optimal production plan in the pharmaceutical industry, cleaning and preparation times (these occur on product transition times), facility maintenance times, testing and the production of new chemicals, resource allocations, manpower utilization and inventory management must be decided and planned in an integrated way. This case requires a production planning strategy evaluating operational configurations with repeated consultations with several departments, process constraints, statistical combinations and business scenarios. The production must be planned at certain time intervals and in accordance with a hierarchical approach [11]. In planning, the importance of inventory management has also great importance. Also to compete in pharmaceutical production in the global market, it is required to develop effective inventory control policies. Companies want to meet customer demands at the highest levels and prefer product storage to avoid falling below a safety stock level. In this way, high amount of inventory cost occurs. While reducing the inventory level for minimizing costs, firms cannot meet the demands, delivery dates delays, and there are some decreases in service levels [30].

With the latest developments in information technologies, the fast and easy internet networks are used to make the information sharing easier and increase security across the supply network. Accordingly, VMI defined as "cooperation with a customer and a supplier to optimize an inventory management for least-cost on both companies" began to be used. With this model, the supplier takes responsibility for the operational management of inventory with agreed performance targets. These performance targets

are continuously monitored and updated to ensure continuous improvement [12]. In order to optimize supply chain performance, the manufacturer takes the responsibility of distributor's inventory levels. Distributor also shares the demand forecast and sales data as well as inventory data. Manufacturer manages the distributor's inventory with this data. The manufacturer is responsible for determining the order quantities and time in this model [31].

In this study, in cephalosporin department of a factory making secondary pharmaceutical production, a mixed integer mathematical model is developed to obtain the best production plan while maximizing the total net profit in long term. Especially the presence of constraints related to "shelf life, product transition times that are ignored in many studies about pharmaceutical production is also added to the model and an experimental study is implemented. The proposed mathematical model is applied on two different types of supply chain (classical supply chain and vendor managed inventory) and the results of both methods are compared in terms of the total supply chain cost. In addition, the proposed model is also compared with another model from literature to illustrate effectiveness of model.

Literature review

Planning and scheduling problems have been the subject of innumerable studies in the mathematical programming literature. Various types' industrial sectors are considered with different time representations in these studies. But some studies cover various industrial sectors for planning and scheduling problem like Fleischmann and Meyr [10]. Pharmaceutical production is a batch process and a type of chemical production. Chemical productions are made in multiproduct plants. The studies for planning and scheduling in multi-product plants are Oh and Karimi [28], Alle and Pinto [1], Dogan and Grossmann [9], Mendez and Cerda [25], Liu et al. [23], Chen et al. [6]. Some studies in literature have handled production and distribution planning together (Lee and Kim [21], Bilgen and Günther [4]).

Also in this part of the study, the studies in the literature related to administrative issues, planning, scheduling and the cost optimization in the pharmaceutical supply chain are listed. The studies about optimization in pharmaceutical supply chain with mathematical methods developed by using mixed integer programming, are as follows; Papageorgiou et al. [29] stduied to optimize the problems in strategic areas such as product development, promotion strategy, capacity planning and investment strategy using a mixed integer programming in the pharmaceutical supply chain. Maravelias and Grossmann [24] discussed simultaneous optimization problem for source constrained scheduling in pharmaceutical production. They proposed MILP that maximizes expected net present value in a multi-period problem. Sundaramoorthy and Karimi [35] developed a MILP including a flexible approach increasing demand meeting ratio against changing production plans in a pharmaceutical supply chain that is the outset of contract manufacturing and new production. Levis and Papageorgiou [22] proposed a mathematical model for long-term capacity planning in a multi-site pharmaceutical industry under uncertainty. The model is an improved version of the model previously proposed by Papageorgiou et al. [29]. All problems are formulated with two-stage MILP model. Then, they developed a hierarchical algorithm for solving large-scale problems. The accuracy of their proposed method was displayed by comparing with several examples. Kim [18] applied an integrated approach to the pharmaceutical supply chain in the health sector. The aim was to reduce holding cost and to optimize inventory costs. For this, VMI was applied to reduce total supply chain cost. Amaroa and Barbosa [2] developed a planning and scheduling approach in the management of reverse flow supply chain applied in a pharmaceutical company. In their study where optimal production plans were obtained, the economical profit of the model was analyzed separately in terms of supply chain operations and customer satisfaction. Lakhdar and Papageorgiou [19] submitted a mathematical programming approach for medium-term production planning under uncertainty in biopharmaceutical manufacturing. Uncertainty in the study is related to with the fermentation concentration ratio. All problems were discussed in the two-stage multi-scenario planning problem and an algorithm was proposed for the problems in larger size. Venditti [39] developed a heuristic algorithm for production planning in the pharmaceutical industry. Baboli et al. [3] studied pharmaceutical supply chain management with two separate approaches as centralized and decentralized using mathematical programming. They reached to the conclusion that the centralized method reduced the cost much more. Sousaa et al. [34] calculated the dynamic resource allocation problem in the pharmaceutical industry with the delivery costs and the different tax rates to maximize the net profit of the company. Susarla and Karimi [37] taken into account the sequence-dependent pattern change, resource using, maintenance schedules and security stocks using the mathematical model with considering integrated planning and resources in the pharmaceutical production facility. Susarla and Karimi [36] studied to optimize supply chain costs about integrated supply chain planning more than one production plant for pharmaceutical production activities. Kelle et al. [17] developed a solution with MILP for demand point in a hospital pharmaceutical supply chain organized

medication requirements plan. Chen et al. [7] used a simulation-based optimization technique while increasing customer service level and reducing supply chain costs of pharmaceutical clinical trials and they planned production and distribution activities with MILP. Kelle et al. [17] developed a strategic and tactical level of decision support models in their work related to pharmaceutical supply chain and inventory solutions in a hospital. Kabra et al. [14] planned multi-stage and multi-production processes in the biopharmaceutical production as long-term by using MILP.

The studies about administrative subjects that made extended literature survey in pharmaceutical supply chain can be listed as follows; Shah [32] determined the key issues and optimization strategies for pharmaceutical supply chain in the study to determine the pharmaceutical supply chain and optimization strategies. In the study, by mentioning all pharmaceutical processes, from raw material production until delivered to the customer were explained and made some suggestions about how to increase customer service level. Besides, Shah [32] analyzed all stages one by one ensuring added value to the pharmaceutical supply chain and emphasized the important matters. Yu et al. [40] conducted a study making an evaluation for current issues and health system reform about pharmaceutical supply chain in China. Jaberidoost et al. [13] studied revealing strategic risks of supply chain management in pharmaceutical industry and they mentioned different studies about this area. Narayana et al. [26] discussed the existing studies on the pharmaceutical supply chain in their study. They classified the studies in literature according to the countries, research methods, terminology and the level of analysis. They made evaluations about the future of the studies from the administrative perspective.

In addition the studies about the implementation of VMI model in the pharmaceutical industry are limited. These are; Danese [8] discussed the project of the implementation of VMI to the entire production and distribution facilities and expressed how to manage the entire supply chain with VMI model from one side, data networks established and data systems supporting them and the performances of them in detail. This VMI model as seen in the study was a model applicable to the entire pharmaceutical industry. Shen et al. [33] tried to identify economic production amount under minimum volume constraints in the production of perishable products such as pharmaceuticals that is important for public health. They developed an approach consists of a mathematical model and VMI which was more economic in in terms of total supply chain cost. Kannan et al. [15] proposed a model revealing the benefits of VMI in pharmaceutical industry. Kannan [16] tried to identify the most appropriate supply policy to stochastic demand environment depending on the time with VMI in pharmaceutical industry. All these studies summarized as seen in Table 1.

In this study, a new mathematical model is developed to solve an inventory problem in the pharmaceutical industry. The mathematical model contains shelf life and product transition constraints together and the model is much more dealing with real life constraints unlike the studies in literature. Besides, the model contains parameters about general supply chain parameters such as costs of production, inventory holding, transition, waste product and unmet demand penalty. There are a few articles about VMI method in pharmaceutical sector. The model applied to classical supply chain method and VMI, so this study is implemented VMI method and handled a new technic in pharmaceutical supply chain.

Methods
The problem and detailed mathematical formulation
The studies in the literature discuss a simplified model of production occurs in real life. In models, they take into account only materials and machinery as resources and mathematical models try to solve the model by making critical assumptions about the case such as transit or installation times of material transfers, human resources, waste storage and treatment capacity. These assumptions prevent to be applicable of the models established in practice. However, the studies should include more comprehensive models to completely adapt to real life. To make a decision by combining entire supply chain under unique plan in real life is very difficult in dynamic market and environment conditions. Some problems in literature (Shah [32], Yu et al. [40], Jaberidoost et al. [13], Narayana et al. [26]) are studied solution suggestions by taking into account the supply, production and distribution processes. However, simple and flexible models are ensuring rapid solution and being appropriate for the real life are much needed. Although it is generally ignored in literature, pharmaceutical raw material and end product have a definite expiry date and it cannot be used after the expiry date. If there is a presence of raw material and product inventory in warehouse, they are turned into waste product and they will reflect

to the supply chain as waste cost. For this reason, the raw materials and product expiry conditions must be taken into account.

In this study, a long-term planning model is developed in order to obtain the production plan that optimally fulfills a net profit objective. This criterion presents the trade between sales returns and costs issues. The main contribution of this study is to solve an inventory problem in the pharmaceutical industry by proposing a new mathematical model that contains shelf life and product transition constraints together. We believe that the proposed model is much more dealing with real life constraints unlike the studies in literature. Besides, the model contains general supply chain parameters such as costs of production, inventory holding, transition, waste product and unmet demand penalty.

A hybrid time representation is applied over a planning horizon, in which the months of the planning horizon are modeled and each month is represented by a continuous time formulation. The most effective characteristic of the problem is that, inventory amounts depend on the shelf life of the products. Also, transition conditions are handled that occur while switching from one product to another.

In the mathematical model, constraints about transitions are adopted from the models of Liu et al. [23]. However, being different from them in our model, inventory amounts changes depending on the shelf life of the product. And so; all inventory formulations are novel. The cost criterion subtracted from the total sales revenue in the objective function is novel in this model. Nomenclature of the proposed mathematical model is given at the Appendix 1. There is a little literature about VMI method in pharmaceutical sector. So this study is implemented VMI method and handled a new technic in pharmaceutical supply chain.

As close as a real life problem, a hypothetical problem is considered in cephalosporin department of a pharmaceutical factory. Our mathematical model is applied in order to obtain the best production plan while maximizing total net profit in long term. The efficiency of the model is shown on classical supply chain and VMI method.

Table 1 Studies about optimization in pharmaceutical industry

The subject of the study	Method	Authors
Planning, scheduling and cost optimization in pharmaceutical industry	Classical supply chain model	Papageorgiou et al. [29], Maravelias and Grossmann [24], Sundaramoorthy and Karimi [35], Levis and Papageorgiou [22], Shah [32], Lakhdar and Papageorgiou [19], Amaroa and Barbosa [2], Venditti [39] Yu et al. [40], Baboli et al. [3], Sousaa et al. [34], Susarla and Karimi [37], Susarla and Karimi [36], Kelle et al. [17], Chen et al. [7], Kabra et al. [14], Jaberidoost et al. [13], Narayana et al. [26]
	Vendor managed inventory model	Danese [8], Shen et al. [33], Kannan et al. [15], Kannan [16]

Objective function

The total net profit is maximized to obtain from sales revenue minus supply chain costs, involving the total, production cost, product transition costs, the unmet demand costs, inventory holding cost, product transportation cost and the cost of waste products.

$$\begin{aligned}
NP = &\sum_c\sum_i\sum_t PS_{ic} * S_{cit} - \sum_i\sum_t P_{it} * CP_i - \sum_i\sum_{j\neq i}\sum_t CC_{ij} \\
&* Z_{ijt} - \sum_i\sum_{j\neq i}\sum_{t\in T-\{1\}} CC_{ij} * ZF_{ijt} - \sum_c\sum_i\sum_t CUD_{ic} \\
&* UD_{cit} - \sum_i\sum_t CI_i * SM_{it} - \sum_c\sum_i\sum_t TC_i \\
&* S_{cit} - \sum_i\sum_t CW_i * W_{it}
\end{aligned} \tag{1}$$

Product assignment constraints

$$\sum_i F_{it} = 1 \qquad \forall\, t\in T \tag{2}$$

$$\sum_i L_{it} = 1 \qquad \forall\, t\in T \tag{3}$$

In each period one product is assigned as first or last product to be processed and these two equations show whether they are the first product or last product.

$$F_{it} \leq E_{it} \qquad \forall\, i\in I,\; t\in T \tag{4}$$

$$L_{it} \leq E_{it} \qquad \forall\, i\in I,\; t\in T \tag{5}$$

When the relevant product is not produced in this period, it assumes as $E_{it} = 0$.

Product transition constraints

$$\sum_{i\neq j} Z_{ijt} = E_{jt} - F_{jt} \qquad \forall\, i\in I,\; j\in J\; t\in T \tag{6}$$

$$\sum_{j\neq i} Z_{ijt} = E_{it} - L_{it} \qquad \forall\, i\in I,\; j\in J\; t\in T \tag{7}$$

While Z_{ijt} binary variables are representing the product transitions occurring in a period, ZF_{ijt} variable represents the product transition between two consecutive periods.

If there is a product transition within a period, they are the variables indicating that there will be no product before the first product produced and it is not the first product, other products will give priority to this product.

Similarly, if there is a product transition within a period, there will not be any product production after the last product produced and if it is not the last product, this product will be followed by the production of other products.

$$\sum_i ZF_{ijt} = F_{jt} \qquad \forall\, i\in I,\; j\in J\; t\in T-\{1\} \tag{8}$$

$$\sum_i ZF_{ijt} = L_{it-1} \qquad \forall\, i\in I,\; j\in J\; t\in T-\{1\} \tag{9}$$

If there is a product transition between two consecutive periods and if the production of a product begins in that period for the first time, there will certainly be a product transition a period before the relevant period. If a product is not the first or the last one processed, then there is not a changeover involving the product between two periods.

Travelling salesman problem formulation based subtour prevention constraints

$$\beta_{jt} - (\beta_{it} + 1) \geq -M * (1 - Z_{ijt}) \qquad \forall\, i\in I,\; j\in J,\; t\in T,\; j\neq i \tag{10}$$

$$\beta_{it} \leq M * E_{it} \qquad \forall\, i\in I,\; t\in T \tag{11}$$

β_{it} variable can be called as demand index or production row. The aim of writing these constraints is to determine row of the product in a period and to take the product transition cases under control.

If i^{th} product is produced before j^{th} product, production sequence number of ith product will be at least one more than j^{th} product.

If that product has never been produced, demand index will be zero.

These constraints are similar to the constraints preventing the sub-tours in classical Travelling Salesman problem (TSP) [23]. In TSP problem binary variables are used to represent transition one city to another. As similar in this model to maximize net profit there should be minimum number of transition in production sequence. And Z_{ijt} and ZF_{ijt} variables are added to model the product transition in a period and between t-1 and t periods respectively.

$$F_{it} \leq \beta_{it} \leq \sum_j E_{jt} \qquad \forall\, i\in I,\; t\in T \tag{12}$$

This constraint enables the demand index to take at least the value of 1 and to take value up to the maximum product number.

Timing constraints

$$\theta^L * E_{it} \leq O_{it} \leq \theta^U * E_{it} \qquad \forall\, i\in I,\; t\in T \tag{13}$$

For each product produced in a period, the highest and lowest time limits are given.

$$\sum_i O_{it} + \sum_i \left((Z_{ijt} + ZF_{ijt}) * TZ_{ijt}\right) \le \theta^U \quad \forall \; t \in T - \{1\} \quad (14)$$

$$\sum_i O_{it} + \sum_i (Z_{ijt} * TZ_{ijt}) \le \theta^U \quad \forall \; t \in \{1\} \quad (15)$$

The total of the production in a period and product transition times cannot exceed the existing time given for the shift.

Production constraints

$$P_{it} = rr_i * O_{it} \quad \forall \; i \in I , \; t \in T \quad (16)$$

The product amount produced in a period is as much as the multiplication of the production ratio and production time.

Demand constraints

$$UD_{cit} = RD_{cit} - S_{cit} \quad \forall \; c \in C, \; i \in I , \; t \in T \quad (17)$$

The amount of the unmet demand from a product is as much as the difference between the realized demand within that period and the product amount delivered to the customer (satisfied demand) within that period.

$$S_{cit} \le RD_{cit} \quad \forall \; c \in C, \; i \in I , \; t \in T \quad (18)$$

Sales amount may be lower than or equal to demand amount that was realized; in this model the unmet demands in a period are not delivered to the customer in the next period (no backlogs).

Shelf life and inventory constraints

$$SM_{it} = SM_{it-1} + P_{it} - \sum_c S_{cit} \quad if \; t < \alpha_i \; \forall \, i \in I , t \in T \quad (19)$$

$$SM_{it} = \sum_{t+1-\alpha_i}^{t-1} SM_{it-1} + P_{it} \quad if \; t \ge \alpha_i \quad \forall \, i \in I , t \in T \quad (20)$$

α_i is shelf life and depends on products characteristics and it is defined as an integer multiple of t.
Inventory quantity varies depending on the product shelf life. If the relevant time is lower than the product's shelf life, that is to say, if the product's term has

Table 2 Experimental set

Experiment No	Supply chain method	Planning horizon (months)	Product amounts
1	Classical supply chain	24	10
2	Classical supply chain	24	15
3	Classical supply chain	30	10
4	Classical supply chain	30	15
5	VMI	24	10
6	VMI	24	15
7	VMI	30	10
8	VMI	30	15

not been expired yet, the inventory amount of that product is as much as the difference of the sales amount within that period in the total of the stock amount transferred from the previous period and the product amount produced in that period.

$$W_{it} = \sum_{t=1}^{t-\alpha_i} SM_{it}, \; if \; t \ge \alpha_i \quad \forall \, i \in I , t \in T \quad (21)$$

But if the relevant time is longer than the product's shelf life, the products whose term is expired will be waste product.

$$W_{it} = 0 , \; if \; t < \alpha_i \quad (22)$$

Numerical investigation
Around the proposed mathematical model, our main research focus is addressed in numerical investigation and the following questions are answered:

- Does this mathematical model provide reasonable results for a long term planning horizon?
- Does the proposed mathematical model offer cost advantages?
- How does the proposed model run for different demand profiles and different numbers of products?
- Does this mathematical model run for different kind of supply chain methods?
- Which supply chain method is more profitable with this mathematical model?
- When compared other studies in literature, does this model provide advantage?

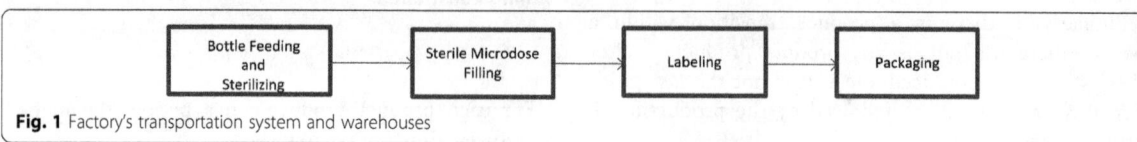

Bottle Feeding and Sterilizing → Sterile Microdose Filling → Labeling → Packaging

Fig. 1 Factory's transportation system and warehouses

To answer these questions, an experimental study is considered based on numerical experiments and comparisons. Experimental set is summarized in Table 2.

To illustrate the applicability of our mathematical model, we consider a hypothetical pharmaceutical plant. In this case, long term production scheduling problem in the pharmaceutical secondary production is discussed.

In the cephalosporin department of this factory, injectable beta-lactam products are manufactured. In a separate facility that is completely independent from non-beta - lactam production fields, micro powder refilling is conducted in aseptic conditions and the production conditions are provided to be monitored continuously via computer aided production systems.

In our study, it is aimed to satisfy the customer demands for 15 different products produced in cephalosporin department of the factory in 24 and 30 months period to find optimal production plan maximizing the total net profit and to show in which type of supply chain (classical or vendor managed).

We hypothesized that; the pharmaceutical factory has agreements with 5 pharmaceutical warehouses. In Fig. 1 factory's transportation system and warehouses scheme is given. The factory delivers the products to pharmaceutical stores and pharmaceutical stores deliver them to the pharmacies. Before the expiry, all the products that are not delivered to the consumer return to the factory and its disposal is carried out by the factory. In this way, it is seen that the production, delivery and waste product costs (disposal cost) belonging to the products whose

Table 3 Cephalosporin products

No	Active raw material
1	Ceftriaxone 1 g IM/IV
2	Cefotaxime 1 g IM/IV
3	Ceftizoxime 0,5 g IM/IV
4	Cefsulodin 1 g IM/IV
5	Cefoperazone 1 g IM/IV
6	Ceftazidime 0,5 g IM/IV
7	Moxalactam 1 g IM/IV
8	Cefuroxime 0,5 g IM/IV
9	Cephalothin 0,5 g IM/IV
10	Cephapyrine 1 g IM/IV
11	Cefdinir 0,5 g IM/IV
12	Cefprozil 1 g IM/IV
13	Ceftibuten 0,5 g IM/IV
14	Cefpodoxim Proxetil 0,5 g IM/IV
15	Cefaclor Monohydrate 1 g IM/IV

term is expired and that will be returned being sold, creates serious cost damages to the factory and a mathematical model is developed to minimize these costs and the model is compared by being applied in two separate types of supply chain. In this study, product name is not specified and 15 different products are named according to the active raw materials. These are shown in Table 3.

A work flow chart belonging to cephalosporin production site is seen above in the Fig. 2. As shown here, the

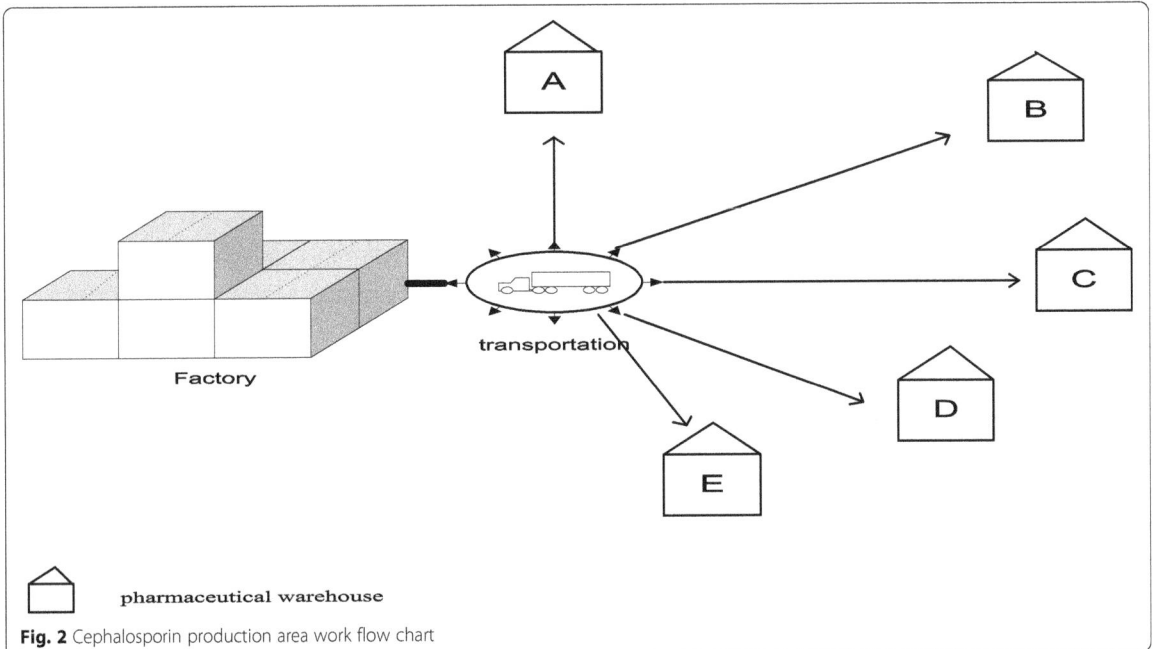

Fig. 2 Cephalosporin production area work flow chart

production is performed on a unique line. Filling machine is isolated from the production environment and in a sterile manner. The active material is loaded into the filling machine; these raw materials are again filled in pharmaceutical bottles in a sterilized way; the bottles filled are checked, labeled and boxed. The production and the expiry date determining the shelf life of the product are printed on the label and box when the product is on the line during relevant transitions.

Key model parameters
Demand types
Demand forecast was made while making production plan for the next two years. Forecasted demand and sales amounts were obtained from the real old data belonging to a real pharmaceutical company. The average of sales amounts (29000) can be seen to conform to normal distribution having standard deviation (10500).

Since normal probability distribution a widely known type, in many studies related to inventory management in supply chain that demand structure is in accordance with normal distribution (Lau et al. [20]).

$$FD_{it} = normal\ (29000, 10500) \qquad (23)$$

Equation 23 gives the distribution of forecasted demand amounts.

In current and proposed situation, the average of customer demands is 27500 and it is assumed to comply with the normal distribution, the standard deviation of which is 19000. The equation 24, gives the distribution of customer demands performed.

Table 5 Unit product transportation costs to warehouses

Pharmaceutical warehouses	Transportation costs for unit product
A	0,005
B	0,02
C	0,017
D	0,015
E	0,045

$$RD_{it} = normal\ (27500, 19000) \qquad (24)$$

Production capacity
In literature there are studies in accordance with uniform distributed production capacities [5, 38]. The aim of the manufacturers is always to satisfy the demand completely. Maximum production capacities are limited, but this capacity varies according to the events to occur during the processes (malfunction or periodic maintenances, or even stops).

The factory works 12 h a day. Total available processing time in a month is 264 h. Production capacity is up to maximum 4500 boxes of product/hour. But this capacity vary in real life because of deteriorations or stops in production lines. When it is statistically analyzed, the capacity of cephalosporin department production line is uniformly distributed in the range of (0, 4500).

Shelf life conditions
The shelf life of each product is fixed and it is 12 months. The products whose terms are expired cannot sold within this time period, it is assumed as waste products

Table 4 Unit costs and sales price data of products

Product no	Sales price ($)	Production cost ($)	Unmet demand cost ($)	Transition cost ($)
Product 1	7	1,2	0,2	TZij *10
Product 2	7	1,2	0,25	TZij *10
Product 3	7	1,16	0,18	TZij *10
Product 4	7	1,16	0,25	TZij *10
Product 5	7	1,2	0,2	TZij *10
Product 6	7	1,1	0,15	TZij *10
Product 7	7	1	0,15	TZij *10
Product 8	10	1,25	0,2	TZij *10
Product 9	10	1,2	0,18	TZij *10
Product 10	10	1,2	0,22	TZij *10
Product 11	10	1,16	0,25	TZij *10
Product 12	8	1,2	0,22	TZij *10
Product 13	8	1,16	0,25	TZij *10
Product 14	8	1,16	0,15	TZij *10
Product 15	8	1,2	0,22	TZij *10

Table 6 The transition time (hour) from i to j

i\j	1	2	3	4	5	6	7	8	9	10	11	12	13	14	15
1	0	10	7	8	7	9	8	12	10	8	7	6	9	7	10
2	12	0	10	6	12	9	7	8	8	12	9	8	8	8	9
3	8	6	0	7	11	8	10	8	9	6	8	9	7	8	8
4	8	9	7	0	12	10	8	9	9	6	7	10	8	9	6
5	6	12	8	12	0	7	11	14	7	9	6	7	11	8	10
6	14	10	6	14	12	0	10	9	12	6	9	9	7	7	9
7	10	8	11	8	9	7	0	8	7	9	8	11	7	9	8
8	7	11	7	9	12	6	8	0	9	7	8	10	9	12	6
9	9	12	8	12	12	8	7	9	0	10	9	8	7	9	8
10	6	8	10	11	7	9	8	8	10	0	6	9	8	10	8
11	11	6	9	7	6	11	8	10	6	9	0	11	7	8	10
12	8	11	8	9	7	8	6	11	7	9	8	0	6	11	7
13	10	8	7	9	8	11	8	9	10	7	8	10	0	8	9
14	9	7	9	12	8	12	12	8	7	9	8	9	8	0	7
15	8	7	9	8	7	11	8	10	9	6	11	8	10	7	0

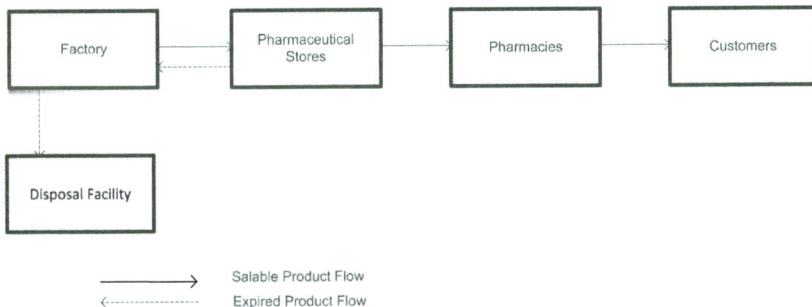

Fig. 3 Pharmaceutical supply chain processes

and the costs belonging to this reflect as waste product cost (ie. 0.125 $/unit).

Product transition conditions

Transition cost is proportional to transition times by a factor of 10.

Unit inventory holding cost data are the values such as 0.005 $/unit identified by the company for a package of product, unit sales price and rest of the other costs are given in Table 4.

Product transportation costs are varies to warehouses and given in Table 5.

The transition times from one product to another (cleaning and mold change) are variable and they are stated in Table 6 below.

Results

Details of experiments

In this part of study, some of the experimental results are given for comparison. Firstly Experiment Number 1 and 5's details are given and compared.

In Experiment 1; factory has a classical supply chain model and produced products transfer due to the orders from pharmaceutical stores and deliver to the end user from there. The products which are expired before sold from the factory to the pharmaceutical store are sent to

disposal facility. Besides, the products which is expired in the pharmaceutical store before sold to pharmacy, are sent to the producer company by the pharmaceutical stores and when these products are reached to the producer company, it is taken to "reject store" and it is delivered to the company for disposal facilities. During this returning process, all costs (transport + disposal costs) are subject to the company. A scheme of pharmaceutical supply chain processes can be seen in Fig. 3.

The above example is modeled using GAMS/CPLEX 12 for the MILP optimization. When the model is run, maximized total net profit is 42556741$ for 24 months with 10 products. The graphs including demand amounts, production amounts, stock amounts and unmet demand amounts belonging to the model are given in following Fig. 4.

Production schedule is given in Fig. 5. This figure shows how the transition times affects to the production sequence. It is hard to show all planning horizon (24 months) scheduling, so we illustrate for a part of two months planning time.

In Experiment 5, the inventory is vendor-managed. According to the agreement, pharmaceutical factory can see the inventory and sales information in the pharmaceutical stores online with the established information system. At the beginning, a production plan is created according to estimated demand amounts and with the

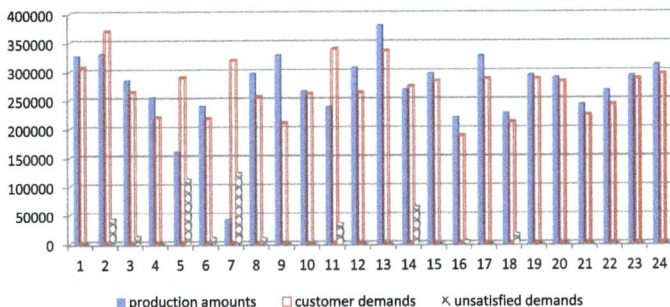

Fig. 4 The graph of production, demand and the unsatisfied demand for Experiment 1

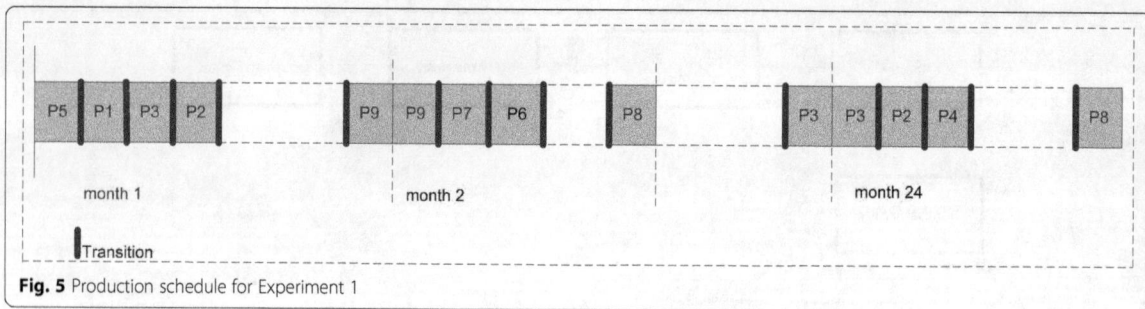

Fig. 5 Production schedule for Experiment 1

information obtained from pharmaceutical store, production plans are updated and within the framework of these plans, delivery plans will be made and the product will be delivered. The amounts and time information will be communicated with the store. For each product, the level of safety stocks in the store is determined and the stocks will be controlled continuously in order not to fall under safety stock levels in the store. Safety stock levels are given in Table 7. Equation 16 in Exp. 1 turns into the equation 25 in Exp.5.

$$P_{it} = FD_{cit} + SS_i - SM_{it-1} \quad \forall\, i \in I, t \in T \qquad (25)$$

$$S_{cit} = P_{it} \quad \forall\, c \in C,\ i \in I, t \in T \qquad (26)$$

In Experiment 5, each product is sold to pharmaceutical stores according to the agreement. For this reason, in addition to the equation 18 created for sales amounts, the equation 26 above should be added. According to

Table 7 Safety stock levels

Product	Product active item	Safety stock amount
Product 1	Ceftriaxone 1 g IM/IV	1000
Product 2	Cefotaxime 1 g IM/IV	2250
Product 3	Ceftizoxime 0.5 g IM/IV	350
Product 4	Cefsulodin 1 g IM/IV	500
Product 5	Cefoperazone 1 g IM/IV	175
Product 6	Ceftazidime 0.5 g IM/IV	1250
Product 7	Moxalactam 1 g IM/IV	350
Product 8	Cefuroxime 0.5 g IM/IV	175
Product 9	Cephalothin 0.5 g IM/IV	1450
Product 10	Cephapyrine 1 g IM/IV	1250
Product 11	Cefdinir 0,5 g IM/IV	250
Product 12	Cefprozil 1 g IM/IV	1000
Product 13	Ceftibuten 0,5 g IM/IV	750
Product 14	Cefpodoxim Proxetil 0,5 g IM/IV	700
Product 15	Cefaclor Monohydrate 1 g IM/IV	350

production plans, the products produced in the factory are directly sent to the pharmaceutical store. That is to say, sales amount is equal to the production amount. Then, the production plans are revised from month to month in the factory in accordance with the demands. Here, the aim is to prevent shortages and waste product costs and making the supply chain more profitable.

When the model is run, the maximized total net profit is 47389739 $ for 24 months with 10 products. The graphs including demand amounts, production amounts, stock amounts and unmet demand belonging to the Experiment 5 are given in Fig. 6.

The result of comparison for these two experiments is as follows in Table 8.

The mathematical model created to reveal the best production plan while minimizing supply chain costs and maximizing the total net profit. The model compared with two experiments. For the both situations, the common data and data distributions are used. Two different optimum results are obtained according to supply chain types. When these results are compared, sales revenue in Experiment 1 is less than in Experiment 5. The sales revenue difference between them is so much. Transition costs are also seen as more advantageous in Experiment 5. The unmet demand amounts are less in Experiment 5 and accordingly, its cost is lower. Production and transportation costs in Experiment 1 is less than Experiment 5. This is because the sales amounts are less than Experiment 5. Considering waste product costs, in Experiment 1, 1.72 % of the production is waste product and in Experiment 5, this rate is 0.03 %. So we can say, VMI is more advantageous in terms of waste product cost and wastage amounts. Because, the production plans advance in more controlled way in Experiment 5. A comparison of these experiments' expired product amounts can be seen in Fig. 7. When total net profit is compared, VMI is more profitable as much as 10.19 % than Classical Supply Chain. Finally, when two experiments are compared, VMI is much better in all costs except for production and transportation costs.

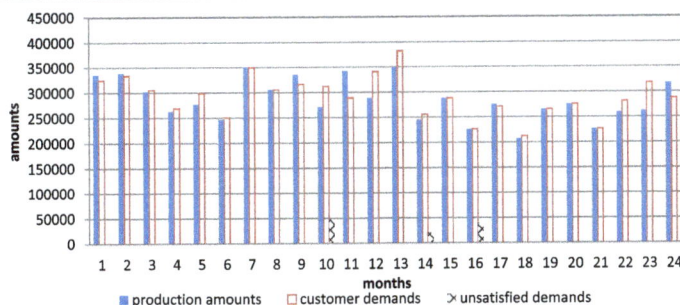

Fig. 6 The graph of production, demand and the unmet demand amounts for Experiment 5

The model is run for all experimental set and the total net profit for all the experiments are given below in Table 9.

As seen in Table 8, VMI Method is more profitable (nearly 8,8 %) than Classical Supply Chain method.

Production planning is a crucial issue in pharmaceutical supply chain in terms of meeting customer demands just in time. Because pharmaceuticals are perishable products, the shelf life constraints have to be considered while planning, scheduling and all supply chain activities are organized.

According to our limited knowledge, some pharmaceutical companies do not take into account the shelf life constraints during their planning processes. It is assumed that all produced items will be sold after reasonable waiting time in the inventory. In reality, in some cases, there can be long waiting time of products. So their perishing day of products can be very close to shelf life because of long waiting time. Although the long waited products are still considered as "inventory products" from the planner, they must be considered "wasted" instead of inventory product.

In this study we consider shelf life constraints and product transition constraints together. In terms of the

practical implications of this work in real pharmaceutical companies; the proposed model can be adapted to production planning activities in the pharmaceutical supply chain. Because; the model produces real time inventory information through the shelf life constraints and deals with "long waited (waste) and "inventory" products while the planning is done. This situation has a great opportunity to cope with wastage costs. The model balances the inventory levels, demands and lost sales. And also real time inventory information provides to reduce risks about market demands and efficient production scheduling activities. This helps to reduce all supply chain costs and the model offers a collaborative, planning and scheduling system to pharmaceutical companies while managing shelf life of products.

Discussion
Comparison with another model

In this part of study, the efficiency of our model is compared with Chen et al. [6] model. To make a comparison, the Chen et al. [6] mathematical model is modified. Modified and original model are given in Appendix 2 and Appendix 3 respectively.

The objective function of proposed model consists of production cost, product delivery cost and wastage cost and it is written as follow:

Table 8 Comparison of solution results for experiment 1 and 5 for 24 months with 10 products

		Exp. 1	Exp. 5
Revenue ($)			
	Sales revenue	50823262	55825164
Costs ($)			
	Production cost	8131853	8412132
	Transition cost	5030	4050
	Unmet demand cost	78908	4012
	Inventory holding cost	29963	7876
	Product transportation cost	6612	7028
	Disposal cost	14153	325
Total net profit ($)		42556741	47389739

$$NP = \sum_c \sum_i \sum_t PS_{ic} * S_{cit} - \sum_i \sum_t P_{it}$$
$$*CP_i - \sum_i \sum_{j \neq i} \sum_t CC_{ij} * Z_{ijt} - \sum_c \sum_i \sum_t CUD_{ic}$$
$$*UD_{cit} - \sum_i \sum_t CI_i * SM_{it} - \sum_c \sum_i \sum_t TC_{ic}$$
$$*S_{cit} - \sum_i \sum_t CW_i * W_{it}$$

There is no storage capacity limit, so the (C12.) constraint is removed from the model.

In addition, backlogs are not allowed, therefore we remove the constraint (C14) from the model. But we

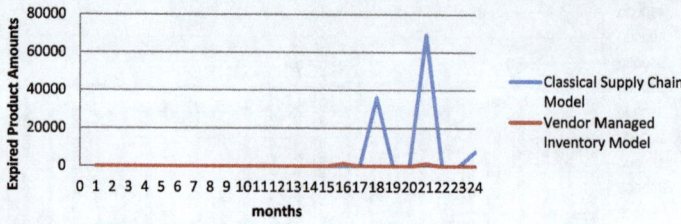

Fig. 7 Expired product amounts for Experiment 1 and 5

have to calculate unmet demand amount so a new constraint is added as given below:

$$UD_{cit} = RD_{cit} - S_{cit}$$

The stock amounts is written with considering shelf life conditions, the constraint (C13) as follow:

$$SM_{it} = SM_{it-1} + P_{it} - \sum_c S_{cit} \quad if \ t < \alpha_i \ \forall i \in I, t \in T$$

$$SM_{it} = \sum_{t+1-\alpha_i}^{t-1} SM_{it-1} + P_{it} \quad if \ t \geq \alpha_i \quad \forall i \in I, t \in T$$

Wastage cost is added to the model;

$$W_{it} = \sum_{t=1}^{t-\alpha_i} SM_{it}, \ if \quad t \geq \alpha_i \quad \forall i \in I, t \in T$$

$$W_{it} = 0 \ , \quad if \ t < \alpha_i$$

The model is run under 24 and 30 months production period, the CPU times were 856 and 4150 respectively.

The details of comparison of these models are given in Table 10.

Table 9 Solution results for all experimental set

Experiment no	Supply chain method	Planning horizon (months)	Product amounts	Total net profit ($)
1	Classical supply chain	24	10	42556741
2	Classical supply chain	24	15	61625811
3	Classical supply chain	30	10	52489164
4	Classical supply chain	30	15	72209637
5	VMI	24	10	47389739
6	VMI	24	15	66800579
7	VMI	30	10	55163846
8	VMI	30	15	79625469

Models were run for 24 and 30 months under classical supply chain. Sales revenues and inventory holding costs are more profitable in our model. And the total net profits are in average %0,8 much more in our model.

Conclusion

In this study, a new mathematical model was developed to solve inventory problem and maximizing total net profit while determining optimal production plan under shelf life and product transition constraints in the pharmaceutical industry. The proposed MILP model contains "shelf life and product transition times" constraints together and we believe that the proposed model has much more real life constraints unlike the other studies in literature. Besides, the model contains parameters such as costs of production, inventory holding, transition, transport, waste product and unmet demand penalty.

As we defined at literature review section of this study; VMI method is not often used in the literature of the pharmaceutical sector. So this study implemented VMI method and handled a new technic for the pharmaceutical supply chain.

To show the effectiveness of the model, an experimental study; which contains 2 different supply chain policy (Classical and VMI), 24 and 30 months planning horizon, 10 and 15 different cephalosporin products were chosen. The results illustrated that the VMI provided much better results in terms of total supply chain costs. Especially; the waste amount that was very important in pharmaceutical sector and the cost was reduced in the VMI. The waste product amounts were 1.72 and 0.03 % of the products in experiment 1 and experiment 5 respectively. In terms of total supply chain costs, 10.19 % of an advantage was gained by the proposed VMI model. As a result, we believe that the proposed model should be adapted in the pharmaceutical industry to reduce total supply chain cost. In addition that, the proposed model is compared with a recently published study in literature. And so the results are illustrated that the proposed model is better than the other.

Table 10 Comparison results for 24 months and 30 months

		24 moths		30 moths	
		Chen et.al.	The proposed	Chen et.al.	The proposed
Revenue ($)					
	Sales revenue	50313184	50823262	62491581	62888928
Costs ($)					
	Production cost	8118125	8131853	10172676	10308595
	Transition cost	4976	5030	6038	6325
	Unmet demand cost	67059	78908	8624	13653
	Inventory holding cost	30056,3	29963	36570	42703
	Product transportation cost	4590	6612	6038	8145
	Disposal cost	10048	14153	17560	20342
Total net profit ($)		42078328	42556741	52244073	52489164

Appendix 1
Nomenclature
Indices
i,j, products
c, customers
t, period

Sets
I, J, product set
C, customer set
T, periods set

Parameters
CP_i, unit production cost of i product
CUD_{ic}, unit unmet demand penalty cost of product i to customer c
CC_{ij}, product transition from product i to product j. (change and cleaning cost on the line while passing from product i to product j)
CI_i, unit inventory holding cost of product i
CW_i, unit waste product cost of product i
TC_{ic}, unit product delivery cost of product i to customer c
FD_{cit}, forecasted demand of customer c, from i th product, at period t
RD_{cit}, the demand amount realized by customer c, from i th product, at period t
M, large number
PS_{ic}, unit selling price product i to customer c
α_i, shelf life
Θ^L, the lowest production rate in a period
Θ^U, the highest production rate in a period
$TZ_{i,j}$, cleaning and mold changing time while passing from i product to j product
β_{it}, demand index
rr_i, production rate

Variables
E_{it} = 1, 0, product i produced in t period?

F_{it} = 1, 0, product i the first product in t period?
L_{it} = 1, 0, product i the last product in period t?
Z_{ijt} = 1, 0, product i produced before product j?
ZF_{ijt} =1,0 if there is any product transition between t-1 and t period?
P_{it}, the production amount from product i in period t
S_{cit}, sales amount from product i to customer c in period t
O_{it}, processing time for product i in period t
SM_{it}, inventory amount of product i in period t
SS_i, security stock amount of product i
UD_{cit}, unmet demand amount from product i to customer c in period t
W_{it}, waste product amount product i in period t
NP, total net profit

Appendix 2
Modified Chen et. al. model

$$NP = \sum_c \sum_i \sum_t PS_{ic} * S_{cit} - \sum_i \sum_t P_{it} * CP_i - \sum_i \sum_{j\neq i} \sum_t CC_{ij}$$
$$* Z_{ijt} - \sum_c \sum_i \sum_t CUD_{cit} * UD_{cit} - \sum_i \sum_t CI_i * SM_{it}$$
$$- \sum_c \sum_i \sum_t TC_{ic} * S_{cit} - \sum_i \sum_t CW_i * W_{it}$$

$$\sum_i y_{it} = 1$$

$$0 \leq O_{it} \leq \theta^U * y_{it}$$

$$\sum_i O_{it} \geq \theta^L * y_{it}$$

$$\sum_i O_{it} + \left(\sum_j TZ_{ji} * Z_{jit} \right) \leq \theta^U$$

$$\sum_j Z_{ijt} = y_{it-1} \qquad t \neq 1$$

$$\sum_i Z_{ijt} = y_{jt} \qquad t \neq 1$$

$$\sum_j Z_{ijt+1} = y_{it}$$

$$\sum_i Z_{ijt+1} = y_{it+1}$$

$$P_{it} = rr_i * O_{it}$$

$$SM_{it} = SM_{it-1} + P_{it} - \sum_c S_{cit} \quad if \ t < \alpha_i \ \forall i \in I, t \in T$$

$$UD_{cit} = RD_{cit} - S_{cit}$$

$$S_{cit} \leq RD_{cit}$$

$$SM_{it} = \sum_{t+1-\alpha_i}^{t-1} SM_{it-1} + P_{it} \quad if \quad t \geq \alpha_i \quad \forall i \in I, t \in T$$

$$W_{it} = \sum_{t=1}^{t-\alpha_i} SM_{it}, \quad if \quad t \geq \alpha_i \quad \forall i \in I, t \in T$$

$$W_{it} = 0, \ if \ t < \alpha_i$$

Appendix 3
The proposed model by Chen et. Al.

Nomenclature
Indices
c, customers
i,j, products
k, time slots
w, weeks

Sets
C, customers
I,J, products
Kw, time slots in week w
W, weeks

Parameters
CBci, backlog cost of product i to customer c
CIiw, inventory cost of product i in week w
CTij, transition cost of product i to product j
Dciw, demand of product i from customer c in week w
PSci, price of product i to customer c
ri, processing rate of product i
Vimax, maximum storage of product i
Vimin, minimum storage of product i
ΘL, lower bound for processing time
ΘU, upper bound for processing time
τij, changeover time from product i to product j

Variables
Pro, operating profit

Piw, production of product i in week w
Sciw, sales of product i to customer c in week w
Tkw, end time of slot k in week w
Viw, volume of product i in week w
Δciw, backlog of product i for customer c in week w
θikw, processing time of product i in slot during week w

Binary variables
Eiw, 1 if product i is produced in week w, 0 otherwise
yikw, 1 if product i is produced in time slot k during week w, 0 otherwise
Zijkw, 1 if product i (slot k-1) precedes product j (slot k) in week w, 0 otherwise

Mathematical formulation
Objective function

$$Pro = \sum_i \sum_w \left[\sum_c (PS_{ic} * S_{ciw} - CB_{ic} * \Delta_{ciw}) \right. \tag{C1}$$
$$\left. - \left(\sum_j \sum_k CT_{ij} * Z_{ijkw} + CI_{iw} * V_{iw} \right) \right]$$

Assignment constraints

$$\sum_i y_{ikw} = 1 \quad w \in W \tag{C2}$$

Timing constraints

$$T_{0w} = 0 \quad w \in W \tag{C3}$$

$$0 \leq \theta_{ikw} \leq \theta^U * y_{ikw} \qquad i \in I \ k \in K \ w \in W \tag{C4}$$

$$\sum_k \theta_{ikw} \geq \theta^L * E_{iw} \quad i \in I \ k \in K \ w \in W \tag{C5}$$

$$T_{kw} - T_{k-1\,w} = \sum_i \left(\theta_{ikw} + \sum_i \tau_{ji} * Z_{ijkw} \right) \quad \forall k \in K \ w \in W \tag{C6}$$

Transition constraints

$$\sum_j Z_{ijkw} = y_{ik-1w} \quad i \in I \ k \in K - \{1\} \ w \in W \tag{C7}$$

$$\sum_j Z_{ijkw} = y_{jkw} \quad j \in J \ k \in K - \{1\} \ w \in W \tag{C8}$$

$$\sum_j Z_{ij1w+1} = y_{jK_w} \quad i \in I \quad w \in W \tag{C9}$$

$$\sum_i Z_{ij1w+1} = y_{j1w+1} \quad j \in J \quad w \in W \qquad \text{(C10)}$$

Process and storage capacity constraints

$$P_{iw} = r_i * \sum_k \theta_{ikw} \quad i \in I \quad w \in W \qquad \text{(C11)}$$

$$V_i^{min} \leq V_{iw} \leq V_i^{max} \quad i \in I \quad w \in W \qquad \text{(C12)}$$

$$V_{iw} = V_{iw+1} + P_{iw} - \sum_c S_{ciw} \qquad \text{(C13)}$$

$$\Delta_{ciw} = \Delta_{ciw-1} + D_{ciw} - S_{ciw} \quad c \in C \quad i \in I \quad w \in W \qquad \text{(C14)}$$

Degeneracy prevention constraints

$$\sum_k y_{ikw} \leq E_{iw} + (K_w - 1) * y_{iK_w} \quad i \in I \quad w \in W \qquad \text{(C15)}$$

$$E_{iw} \geq y_{iK_w} \quad i \in I \quad w \in W \qquad \text{(C16)}$$

$$\sum_{j \neq i} \sum_k (Z_{ijkw} + Z_{jikw}) \leq 2 - y_{iK_w} \quad i \in I \quad w \in W \qquad \text{(C17)}$$

Competing interests

The authors declare that they have no competing interests.

Authors' contributions

GC; reviewed the literature section and developed the mathematical model and performed experiments and researched about pharmaceutical industry and draft the manuscript. HRY; studied about supply chain types. (VMI and Classical) and participated in manuscripts design and coordination. Both authors read and approved the final manuscript.

Acknowledgements

Authors thank to DARU journals' editors and reviewers.

References

1. Alle A, Pinto JM. Mixed-integer programming models for the scheduling and operational optimization of multiproduct continuous plants. Ind Eng Chem Res. 2002;41:2689–704.
2. Amaroa ACS, Barbosa APD. Planning and scheduling of industrial supply chains with reverse flows: a real pharmaceutical case study. Comput Chem Eng. 2008;32:2606–25.
3. Baboli A, Fondrevelle J, Moghaddam R, Mehrabi A. A replenishment policy based on joint optimization in a downstream pharmaceutical supply chain: centralized vs. decentralized replenishment. Int J Adv Manuf Technol. 2011; 57:367–78.
4. Bilgen B, Günther HO. Integrated production and distribution planning in the fast moving consumer goods industry: a block planning application. OR Spectrum. 2010;32:927–55.
5. Chandra P, Fisher ML. Coordination of production and distribution planning. Eur J Oper Res. 1994;72:503–17.
6. Chen P, Papageorgiou LG, Pinto JM. Medium-term planning of single-stage single-unit multiproduct plants using a hybrid discrete/continuous-time MILP model. Ind Eng Chem Res. 2008;47:1925–34.
7. Chen Y, Mockus L, Orcun S, Reklaitis GV. Simulation-optimization approach to clinical trial supply chain management with demand scenario forecast. Comput Chem Eng. 2012;40:82–96.
8. Danese P. Beyond vendor managed inventory: the GlaxoSmithKline case. Supply Chain Forum Int J. 2004;5(2):32–9.
9. Dogan ME, Grossmann IE. A decomposition method for the simultaneous planning and scheduling of single-stage continuous muliproduct plants. Ind Eng Chem Res. 2006;45:299–315.
10. Fleischmann B, Meyr H. The general lotsizing and scheduling problem. OR Spektrum. 1997;19:11–21.
11. Gaither N. Productions and operations management. California: Duxbury Press; 1996.
12. Hines P, Lamming R, Jones D, Cousins P, Rich N. Value stream management-strategy and excellence in the supply chain. London: Prentice Hall; 2000.
13. Jaberidoost M, Nikfar S, Abdollahias A, Dinarvand R. Pharmaceutical supply chain risks: a systematic review. DARU J Pharm Sci. 2013;21:69.
14. Kabra S, Shaik MA, Rathore AS. Multi-period scheduling of a multi-stage multi-product bio-pharmaceutical process. Comput Chem Eng. 2013;57:95–103.
15. Kannan G, Grigore MC, Devika K, Senthilkumar A. An analysis of the general benefits of a centralised VMI system based on the EOQ model. Int J Prod Res. 2013;51(1):172–88.
16. Kannan G. The optimal replenishment policy for time-varying stochastic demand under vendor managed inventory. Eur J Oper Res. 2015;242:402–23.
17. Kelle P, Woosleyb J, Schneider H. Pharmaceutical supply chain specifics and inventory solutions for a hospital case. Oper Res Health Care. 2012;1:54–63.
18. Kim D. An integrated supply chain management system: a case study in healthcare sector. E-Commerce Web Technol Proc Lect Notes Comput Sci. 2005;3590:218–27.
19. Lakhdar K, Papageorgiou LG. An iterative mixed integer optimisation approach for medium term planning of biopharmaceutical manufacture under uncertainty. Chem Eng Res Des. 2008;8(6):259–67.
20. Lau JSK, Huang GQ, Mak KL. Impact of information sharing on inventory replenishment in divergent supply chains. Int J Prod Res. 2004;42:919–41.
21. Lee H, Kim H. Optimal production-distribution planning in supply chain management using a hybrid simulation-analytic approach. In: Proceedings of the 2000 winter simulation conference. 2000.
22. Levis AA, Papageorgiou LG. A hierarchical solution approach for multi-site capacity planning under uncertainty in the pharmaceutical industry. Comput Chem Eng. 2004;28(5):707–25.
23. Liu S, Pinto JM, Papageorgiou LG. A TSP-based MILP model for medium-term planning of single-stage continuous multiproduct plants. Ind Eng Chem Res. 2008;47:7733–43.
24. Maravelias CT, Grossmann IE. Simultaneous planning for new product development and batch manufacturing facilities. Ind Eng Chem Res. 2001; 40:6147–64.
25. Mendez CA, Cerda J. An efficient MILP continuous-time formulation for short-term scheduling of multiproduct continuous facilities. Comput Chem Eng. 2002;26:687–95.
26. Narayana SA, Pati RK, Vrat P. Managerial research on the pharmaceutical supply chain – a critical review and some insights for future directions. J Purch Supply Manag. 2014;20:18–40.
27. Norman G. Production and operations management. California: Duxbury Press; 1996.
28. Oh HC, Karimi IA. Planning production on a single processor with sequence-dependent setups part 1: determination of campaigns. Comput Chem Eng. 2001;25:1021–30.
29. Papageorgiou LG, Rotstein GE, Shah N. Strategic supply chain optimization for the pharmaceutical industries. Ind Eng Chem Res. 2001;40:275–86.
30. Ru J. The Impacts of vendor managed inventory on supply chain performance in retail industry, PhD Thesis, University of Texas. 2010.
31. Salzarulo PA. Vendor managed inventory programs and their effect on supply chain performance, PhD Thesis, Indiana University. 2006.
32. Shah N. Pharmaceutical supply chains: key issues and strategies for optimisation. Comput Chem Eng. 2004;28(6-7):929–41.
33. Shen Z, Dessouky M, Ordonez F. Perishable inventory management system with a minimum volume constraint. J Oper Res Soc. 2011;62(12):2063–82.
34. Sousaa RT, Liu S, Papageorgiou LG, Shah N. Global supply chain planning for pharmaceuticals. Chem Eng Res Des. 2011;89:2396–409.
35. Sundaramoorthy A, Karimi IA. Planning in pharmaceutical supply chains with outsourcing and new product introductions. Ind Eng Chem Res. 2004; 43:8293–306.

36. Susarla N, Karimi IA. Integrated supply chain planning for multinational pharmaceutical enterprises. Comput Chem Eng. 2012;42:168–77.

37. Susarla N, Karimi IA. Integrated campaign planning and resource allocation in batch plants. Comput Chem Eng. 2011;35(12):2990–3001.

38. Tosto GD, Parunak VD. Multi-agent-based simulation X: international workshop. Budapest: MABS; 2009.

39. Venditti L. Production scheduling in pharmaceutical industry. PhD dissertation. Roma: Tre University; 2010.

40. Yu X, Li C, Shi Y, Yu M. Pharmaceutical supply chain in China: current issues and implications for health system reform. Health Policy. 2010;97(1):8–15.

24

Sustained-release methylphenidate in methamphetamine dependence treatment

Farzin Rezaei[1], Maryam Emami[1], Shakiba Zahed[2], Mohammad-Javad Morabbi[3], Mohammadhadi Farahzadi[3] and Shahin Akhondzadeh[4*]

Abstract

Background: The objective of this randomized, double-blind, placebo-controlled study was to evaluate the efficacy of sustained-release methylphenidate (MPH-SR) in treatment of methamphetamine dependence.

Methods: Fifty-six individuals who met DSM-IV-TR criteria for methamphetamine dependence participated in this 10-week trial. The participants were randomly allocated into two groups and received 18 to 54 mg/day sustained-released methylphenidate or placebo for 10 weeks. Craving was evaluated by a visual analogue craving scale every week. Urinary screening test for methamphetamine was carried out each week. The Beck Depression Inventory-II (BDI-II) was used to monitor participant depressive symptoms at baseline and bi-weekly during the treatment period.

Results: At the end of the trial, the MPH-SR group was less methamphetamine positive compared to the placebo group and the difference was significant ($p = 0.03$). By the end of the study, MPH-SR group showed significantly less craving scores compared to the placebo group [MD (95% CI) = -10.28(0.88-19.18), t(54) = 2.19, p = 0.03]. There was greater improvement in the depressive symptoms scores in the intervention group compared to the placebo group [MD (95% CI) =2.03(0.31-3.75), t (54) =2.37, p = 0.02].

Conclusion: Sustained-released methylphenidate was safe and well tolerated among active methamphetamine users and significantly reduced methamphetamine use, craving and depressive symptoms.

Trial registration: IRCT201202281556N38

Keywords: Clinical trial, Dependence, Methamphetamine, Methylphenidate

Background

Methamphetamine is a psychostimulant that is highly addictive and affects monoamine neurotransmitter systems [1]. Methamphetamine and related stimulants are the second most frequently used illicit drugs worldwide, second only to cannabis. It is estimated that more than 35 million people around the world use this class of substance [2-4]. Methamphetamine dependence is associated with a number of psychiatric disorders including depression and psychosis [5-7]. Furthermore, methamphetamine use is accompanied with various medical consequences such as myocardial infarction, renal failure, cerebral hemorrhage, muscle damage, nasal and sinus damage and sudden death [8-12]. Methamphetamine abuse and dependence have become a major health problem imposing a great burden on the society [13-15]. In recent years, a dramatic rise in methamphetamine use has occurred in many countries [16]. There is evidence for significantly increased prevalence of methamphetamine abuse in Iran in past years [17].

In the last decade, many medications have been used for treatment of methamphetamine dependence including modafinil, antidepressants, ondansetron, risperidone, aripiprazole, baclofen, topiramate, N-acetyl cysteine, naltrexone, and gabapentin, but none demonstrated consistent efficacy [2,10,13,18-25]. Some studies suggested sustained-release

* Correspondence: s.akhond@neda.net
[4]Psychiatric Research Center, Roozbeh Hospital, Tehran University of Medical Sciences, South Kargar Street, Tehran 13337, Iran
Full list of author information is available at the end of the article

dextroamphetamine and methylphenidate as effective pharmacotherapy for methamphetamine dependence [26-30]. Given that methylphenidate antagonizes the effects of methamphetamine *in vitro*, some researchers have tried it as a potential candidate for treatment of methamphetamine dependence [31,32]. The results of some preliminary studies have demonstrated that a maintenance pharmacotherapy program of daily sustained-release amphetamine could increase retention of patients and decrease relapse rate of methamphetamine dependence [33] although a study has findings to the contrary [34]. Some studies questioned the notion of replacement therapy for amphetamine dependence (a cochrane review) [35]. The objective of this randomized, double-blind, placebo-controlled study was to evaluate the efficacy of sustained-released methylphenidate in treatment of methamphetamine dependence.

Methods

Trial design and setting

This study was a double-blind, randomized, placebo-controlled trial. The participants (consecutive patients screened for the trial) were men and women with methamphetamine dependence attending outpatient clinics in Sanandaj and Tehran from June 2013 to August 2014.

Participants

Inclusion criteria were diagnosis of methamphetamine dependence based on DSM-IV-TR between 18 to 65 years of age, and positive methamphetamine urine test at the beginning of the study. Participants met none of the following exclusion criteria: (1) any other mental disorder on axis I except for depression, (2) any serious medical or neurological problem (3), IQ <70, (4) abuse of other substances except for nicotine and methadone over the last six months; (5) history of Attention Defecit-Hyperactivity Disorder (ADHD) during childhood, (6) pregnancy and breast feeding, (7) development of psychotic symptoms requiring pharmacotherapy and (8) serious suicidal ideations. The study protocol was approved by the Institutional Review Board of Tehran University of Medical Sciences (Grant No: 16507) and was performed in accordance with the Declaration of Helsinki and its subsequent revisions. Patients gave written informed consent before entry into the study. Patients were informed they are free to withdraw from the study at any time, without giving a reason. The trial was registered at the Iranian registry of clinical trials (www.irct.ir; registration number: IRCT201202281556N38) prior to conducting the study.

Interventions

Fifty-six individuals who met DSM-IV-TR criteria for methamphetamine dependence participated in this 10-week trial.

The participants were randomly allocated into two groups. Group 1 received 18 mg/day sustained-released methylphenidate during the first week and 36 mg/day during the second week and then received 54 mg/day sustained-released methylphenidate for the remaining 8 weeks. Group 2 received placebo for 10 weeks. The medication was given daily under staff supervision.

Outcome

Our primary outcome was Methamphetamine craving. Craving was evaluated by a visual analogue craving scale every week that ranges from 0 (no cravings) to 100 (most intense cravings possible) [22]. Data was gathered by a demographic questionnaire and severity of addiction was assessed by Addiction Severity Index (ASI) at the beginning of the study. Several studies have shown that ASI had acceptable reliability and validity [36-38]. It has been reported that the Persian version of this inventory has good reliability and validity [38,39]. Urinary screening test for methamphetamine was carried out each week Urine samples were analyzed using radioimmunoassay (Phamatech, Inc, San Diego, CA) for qualitative tests of MA metabolite. The Beck Depression Inventory II (BDI-II) rating scale was used to monitor participant depressive symptoms at baseline and bi-weekly during the treatment period [40]. Medication adherence was measured using weekly tablet counts justified against participant reports of medication taking to calculate the proportion of dispensed medication doses that were taken.

Sample size

Assuming a clinically significant difference of 4 on the visual analogue craving scale score between MPH-SR and placebo groups with a standard deviation (SD) of 4.5 (based on our pilot study), a power of 80%, and a two-sided significance level of 5%, a minimal sample size of 40 was estimated. Considering an attrition rate of 10%, a total sample size of 48 was planned.

Randomization, allocation, concealment and blinding

Generation of randomization codes was conducted by permuted randomization block using Excel software (blocks of four, allocation ratio 1:1). Randomization was performed by an independent party who was not involved elsewhere in the trial. Concealment of allocation was performed using sequentially numbered, sealed, opaque, and stapled envelopes. Separate persons were responsible for generation of randomization codes, treatment allocation and interviewing. The patients, research investigators, nurses and interviewers were all blinded to the treatment allocation. MPH-SR and placebo were completely identical in their size, color, shape, texture and odor.

Statistical analysis

Mean differences between the groups were reported as mean (95% confidence intervals (95% CI). All analyses were based on the intention-to-treat sample and were performed using the last observation carried forward (LOCF) procedure. To compare the score and the behavior of the two treatment groups over the course of the trial, two-factor repeated measure analysis of variance (ANOVA) was used. Greenhouse Geisser's correction was used whenever Mauchly's test of sphericity was significant. Comparison of score change from baseline to each time point between the two groups was done using the unpaired t-test. A p value of <0.05 was considered significant.

Results

Basic characteristics

Eighty-seven patients were screened to participate in this study and a total number of 56 patients were entered into the study. Ten patients from the MPH-SR group and 12 patients from the placebo group dropped out before week 6 and 34 patients completed the trial (Figure 1). Baseline psychiatric characteristics, demographic and drug use of both groups were compared yielding no significance between the two groups (Table 1).

Urine drug screen results

There was no significant difference between the two groups in baseline methamephetamine positive urine drug screen tests. Nevertheless, at week 10, the MPH-SR group was less methamphetamine positive compare to the placebo and the difference was significant (P = 0.03) (Figure 2).

Methamphetamine craving

Baseline Methamphetamine craving scores were not significantly different between the treatment groups [MD (95% CI) = 0.57(-3.97 to 5.12), t(54) = 0.25, p = 0.39]. At the study endpoint, the result of repeated measure analysis demonstrated a significant effect of time × treatment interaction [F = 4.06, p = 0.046] (Figure 3). By the end of the trial, MPH-SR group showed significantly less craving scores compared to the placebo group [MD (95% CI) = -10.28(0.88-19.18), t(54) = 2.19, p = 0.03] (Figure 3).

Depressive symptoms

Assessment of the baseline *Depressive symptoms* scores did not reveal a significant difference between the treatment groups [MD (95% CI) = -0.10(-1.18-0.97), t(54) = -0.19,

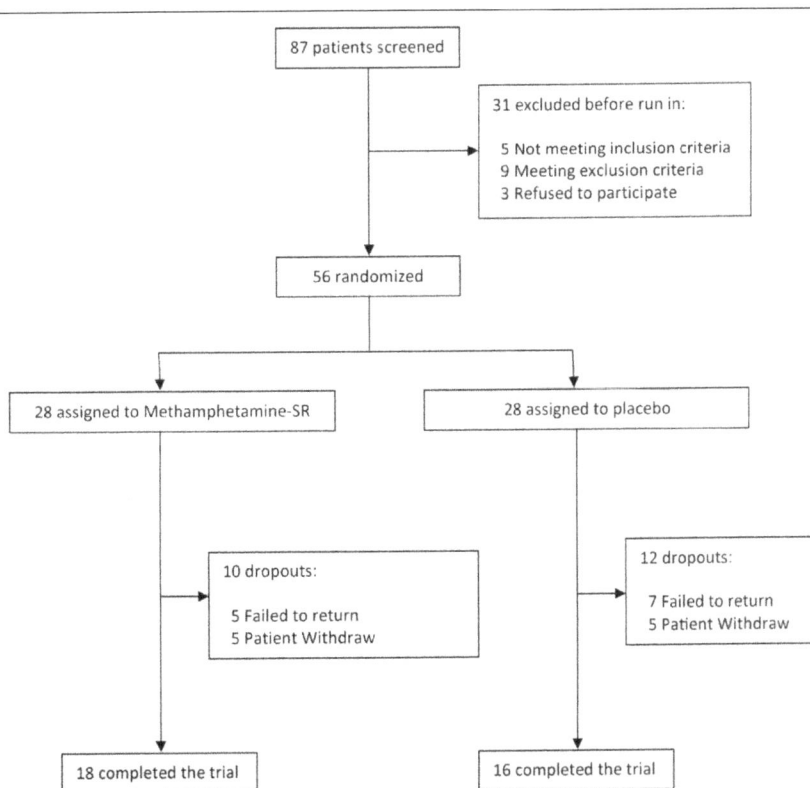

Figure 1 Flow diagram of the study.

Table 1 Baseline characteristics of the participants, drug use and psychiatric characteristics

	Mean (SD) or N Methylphenidate slow release (N = 28)	Mean (SD) or N Placebo (N = 28)	P value
Age (years)	35.6(10.8)	34.7(11.5)	ns
Gender, n	8	7	ns
· Female	20	21	
· Male			
Marital status, n			ns
· Single	18	19	
· Married	6	5	
· Divorced	4	4	
Level of education, n			ns
· Illiterate	2	1	
· Primary school	16	17	
· High school diploma	8	9	
· University degree	2	1	
Smoking, n	25	26	ns
Use of methadone	12	11	ns
Employed, n	5	7	ns
Years of methamphetamine use	13.3(8.5)	12.8(9.1)	ns
Days of methamphetamine use (past month)	10.2(8.7)	10.4(8.8)	ns
Route of methamphetamine use, n			ns
· Smoking	23	22	
· Nasal	3	2	
· Injection	1	1	
· Oral	1	3	
Addiction severity index composite score			ns
· Medical	0.25(0.31)	0.28(0.26)	
· Employment	0.22(017)	0.24(0.19)	
· Alcohol	0.15(0.10)	0.14(0.13)	
· Drug	0.28(0.1)	0.29(0.12)	
· Legal	0.08(0.17)	0.07(0.16)	
· Family/Social	0.22(0.23)	0.19(0.20)	
· Psychiatric	0.24(0.25)	0.22(0.23	

N: number; SD: Standard Deviation; ns: non-significant.

p = 0.84]. By the end of the trial, MPH-SR group showed significantly greater improvement in the depressive symptom scores compared to the placebo group [MD (95% CI) = 2.03(0.31-3.75), t(54) = 2.37, p = 0.02]. The effect of time × treatment interaction was also significant for the depressive symptom scores [F = 4.32, p = 0.02] (Figure 4).

Adverse events

No major adverse events or mortality occurred during the period of this trial. As summarized in Table 2, a total of 10 adverse events were recorded with no significant difference in their frequency between the two groups (Table 2).

Discussion

This preliminary study evaluated efficacy and safety of once-daily sustained-release methylphenidate using a double-blind, placebo-controlled design. Currently, there are no approved pharmacological treatments for methamphetamine dependence. This randomized placebo-controlled trial showed that slow-release methylphenidate can successfully be used in order to reduce drug craving.

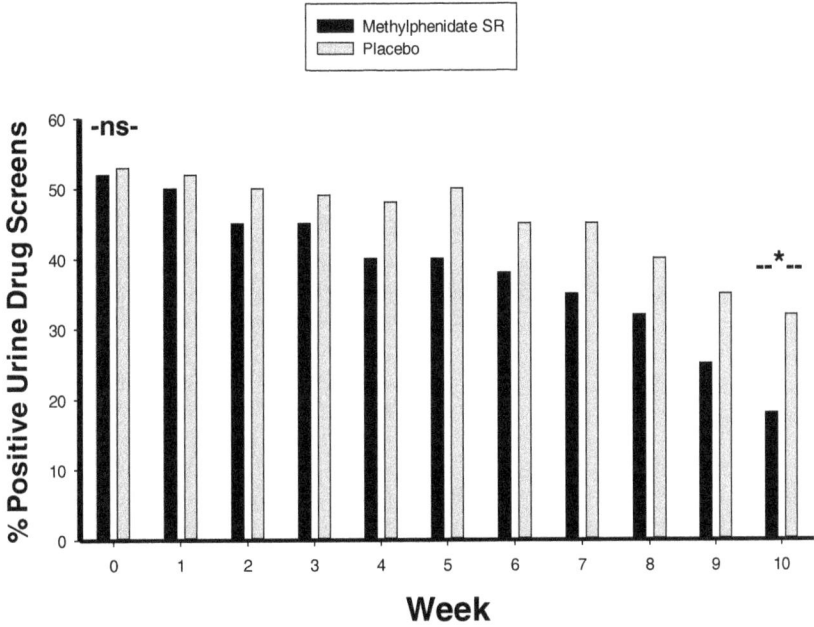

Figure 2 Positive urine drug screens in the two groups (%). NS indicates non-significant and * = p < 0.05.

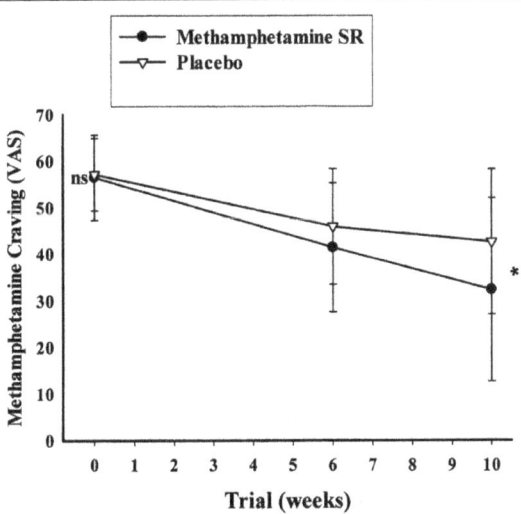

Figure 3 Repeated measure for comparison of the effects of two treatments on methamphetamine craving score. Values represent mean ± standard deviation of the mean. P-values demonstrate the result of the independent T-test for comparison of scores between two treatment groups at each time point. NS indicates non-significant; and * = p < 0.05.

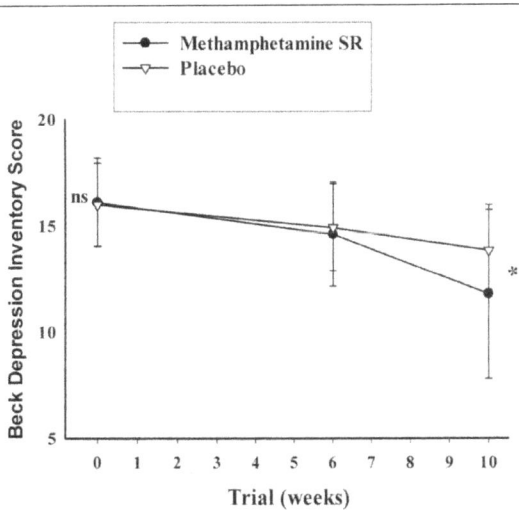

Figure 4 Repeated measure for comparison of the effects of two treatments on Beck Depression Inventory Score. Values represent mean ± standard deviation of the mean. P-values demonstrate the result of the independent T-test for comparison of scores between two treatment groups at each time point. NS indicates non-significant; and * = p < 0.05.

Table 2 Frequency of adverse events in the study groups

Averse events	Methylphenidate slow selease, n	Placebo n	P value
Anxiety	3	3	ns
Decreased appetite	3	2	ns
Depression	3	5	ns
Muscle aches	5	7	ns
Nausea	3	3	ns
Headache	10	5	ns
Irritability	5	8	ns
Stomachache	3	2	ns
Insomnia	8	9	ns
Dizzy	5	6	ns

ns: non-significant.

Furthermore, patients who received methylphenidate had less positive urine tests and it seemed that methylphenidate may decrease use of methamphetamine. The results of this study showed that depression decreased significantly more in the methylphenidate arm compared with the placebo arm.

Our results were in accordance with some previous studies [32,41,42]. Tiihonen and his colleagues have compared methylphenidate with aripiprazol for treatment of methamphetamine dependence, however, their study ended prematurely due to unexpected results of interim analysis and all of their patients were intravenous drug abuser; yet their results have been promising. Solhi et al. showed that both methylphenidate and risperidone were useful for decreasing drug craving in patients but the duration of this study was relatively short (3 weeks) and perhaps because of this the study failed to show the superiority of methylphenidate.

Methylphenidate blocks the methamphetamine-induced dopamine release and this effect may also antagonize the rewarding and reinforcing effects of methamphetamine and its use in dependent patients [31]. In addition, methylphenidate also increases dopamine levels and therefore may also act as substitution treatment for methamphetamine use [34,43]. Methamphetamine also releases norepinephrine and norepinephrine is thought to contribute to the acute effects of amphetamine-type drugs for the treatment of methamphetamine addiction [44]. Methylphenidate blocks the norepinephrine transporter and these drugs could also block methamphetamine-induced norepinephrine release [45].

Our results were inconsistent with the Miles study [34]. Miles et al. failed to confirm the usefulness of methylphenidate for amphetamine/methamphetamine dependence, but the retention rate in their study was low. In studies with long duration the Miles study was 22 weeks), the low retention rate is a major problem and one cannot necessarily conclude that all dropped out patients had experienced relapse. On the other hand, some studies show that amphetamine use began to decrease substantially as a function of time after 10 weeks of methylphenidate treatment reaching statistical significance at 18 weeks, which indicates that it may take an even longer period of time than 20 weeks to achieve full benefit from this treatment [32]. In these studies the participants were IV drug users which represented a more severe subtype of substance dependence. However, our participants used methamphetamine by smoking (the most common method of methamphetamine abuse in Iran) and perhaps because of this we could show the efficacy of methylphenidate in a shorter period of time. In the Konsteniusa study, sustained release methylphenidate could not affect craving for amphetamine or retention in treatment [46]. This study was carried out on abstinent persons, but in our study participants were active users. In terms of safety, the frequency of adverse events was not significantly different between the two study arms during this study. However, the present trial design was not particularly qualified for assessing the safety profile of MPH-SR, a point which merits further attention. This study has some limitations. The sample size was relatively small. Larger studies are required to replicate our findings. The effectiveness of methylphenidate beyond 10 weeks of treatment remains unknown.

Conclusion

Sustained-release methylphenidate was safe and well-tolerated among active methamphetamine users and significantly reduced methamphetamine use, craving and depressive symptoms. This randomized placebo-controlled trial showed that sustained-release methylphenidate can successfully be used for treatment of methamphetamine dependence.

Competing interests

No conflict of interest exists for any of the authors associated with the manuscript and there was no source of extra-institutional commercial funding. The funding organization had no role in the design and conduct of the study; in the collection, analysis, and interpretation of the data; or in the preparation, review, or approval of the manuscript and the decision to submit the paper for publication.

Authors' contributions

FR, ME, MJM and MF: Sample collection, SZ: Statistical Analysis, Article writing, SA and FR: Designer and project manager, Article writing. All authors read and approved the final manuscript.

Acknowledgments

This study was supported by a grant from Tehran University of Medical Sciences to Prof. Shahin Akhondzadeh (Grant No: 16507).

Author details

[1]Department of psychiatry, Kurdistan University of Medical Sciences, Sanandaj, Iran. [2]Department of Health Education and Health Promotion, Faculty of Health, Isfahan University of Medical Sciences, Isfahan, Iran. [3]Department of Neuroscience, School of Advanced Medical Technologies, Tehran University of Medical Sciences, Tehran, Iran. [4]Psychiatric Research

Center, Roozbeh Hospital, Tehran University of Medical Sciences, South Kargar Street, Tehran 13337, Iran.

References

1. Panenka WJ, Procyshyn RM, Lecomte T, MacEwan GW, Flynn SW, Honer WG, et al. Methamphetamine use: A comprehensive review of molecular, preclinical and clinical findings. Drug Alcohol Dep. 2013;129(3):167–79.

2. Degenhardt LHW. Extent of illicit drug use and dependence, and their contribution to the global burden of disease. Lancet. 2012;379:55–70.

3. Colfax G, Shoptaw S. The methamphetamine epidemic: implications for HIV prevention and treatment. Cur HIV/AIDS Rep. 2005;2(4):194–9.

4. Singleton J, Degenhardt L, Hall W, Zabransky T. Mortality among amphetamine users: A systematic review of cohort studies. Drug Alcohol Dep. 2009;105(1–2):1–8.

5. Plüddemann A, Dada S, Parry CDH, Kader R, Parker JS, Temmingh H, et al. Monitoring the prevalence of methamphetamine-related presentations at psychiatric hospitals in Cape Town, South Africa. Afr J Psychiatry (South Africa). 2013;16(1):45–9.

6. Salo R, Flower K, Kielstein A, Leamon MH, Nordahl TE, Galloway GP. Psychiatric comorbidity in methamphetamine dependence. Psychiatry Res. 2011;186(2–3):356–61.

7. Semple SJ, Patterson TL, Rant I. Methamphetamine use and depressive symptoms among heterosexual men and women. J Substance Use. 2005;10(1):31–47.

8. Akindipe T, Wilson D, Stein DJ. Psychiatric disorders in individuals with methamphetamine dependence: prevalence and risk factors. Metab Brain Dis. 2014;29(2):351–7.

9. Chen JP. Methamphetamine-associated acute myocardial infarction and cardiogenic shock with normal coronary arteries: Refractory global coronary microvascular spasm. J Invas Cardio. 2007;19(4):E89–92.

10. Ciccarone D. Stimulant Abuse: Pharmacology, Cocaine, Methamphetamine, Treatment, Attempts at Pharmacotherapy. Prim Care. 2011;38(1):41–58.

11. Gould MS, Walsh BT, Munfakh JL, Kleinman M, Duan N, Olfson M, et al. Sudden death and use of stimulant medications in youths. Am J Psychiatry. 2009;166(9):992–1001.

12. Kaye S, Darke S, Duflou J, McKetin R. Methamphetamine-related fatalities in Australia: Demographics, circumstances, toxicology and major organ pathology. Addiction. 2008;103(8):1353–60.

13. Brackins T, Brahm NC, Kissack JC. Treatments for methamphetamine abuse: A literature review for the clinician. J Pharm Pract. 2011;24(6):541–50.

14. Degenhardt L, Baxter AJ, Lee YY, Halle W, Grant E, Sara GE, et al. The global epidemiology and burden of psychostimulant dependence:Findings from the Global Burden of Disease Study 2010. Drug Alcohol Dep. 2014;137:36–47.

15. Hendrickson RG, Cloutier R, McConnell KJ. Methamphetamine-related emergency department utilization and cost. Acad EmerMed. 2008;15(1):23–31.

16. He J, Xie Y, Tao J, Su H, Wu W, Zou S, et al. Gender differences in socio-demographic and clinical characteristics of methamphetamine inpatients in a Chinese population. Drug Alcohol Dep. 2013;130(1–3):94–100.

17. Khajeamiri AR, Faizi M, Sohani F, Baheri T, Kobarfard F. Determination of impurities in illicit methamphetamine samples seized in Iran. Forensic Scie Int. 2012;217(1–3):204–6.

18. Coffin PO, Santos GM, Das M, Santos DM, Huffaker S, Matheson T, et al. Aripiprazole for the treatment of methamphetamine dependence: a randomized, double-blind, placebo-controlled trial. Addic. 2012;108:751–61.

19. Cruickshank CC, Montebello ME, Dyer KR, Quigley A, Blaszczyk J, Tomkins S, et al. Placebo-controlled trial of mirtazapine for the management of methamphetamine withdrawal. Drug Alcohol Rev. 2008;27(3):326–33.

20. Elkashef A, Kahn R, Yu E, Iturriaga E, Li SH, Anderson A, et al. Topiramate for the treatment of methamphetamine addiction: A multi-center placebo-controlled trial. Addic. 2012;107(7):1297–306.

21. Heinzerling KG, Shoptaw S, Peck JA, Yang X, Liu J, Roll J, et al. Randomized, placebo-controlled trial of baclofen and gabapentin for the treatment of methamphetamine dependence. Drug Alcohol Dep. 2006;85(3):177–84.

22. Heinzerling KG, Swanson AN, Kim S, Cederblom L, Moe A, Ling W, et al. Randomized, double-blind, placebo-controlled trial of modafinil for the treatment of methamphetamine dependence. Drug Alcohol Dep. 2010;109 (1–3):20–9.

23. Johnson BA, Ait-Daoud N, Elkashef AM, Smith EV, Kahn R, Vocci F, et al. A preliminary randomized, double-blind, placebo-controlled study of the safety and efficacy of ondansetron in the treatment of methamphetamine dependence. Int J Neuropsychopharmacol. 2008;11(1):1–14.

24. Ling W, Shoptaw S, Hillhouse M, Bholat MA, Charuvastra C, Heinzerling K, et al. Double-blind placebo-controlled evaluation of the PROMETA™ protocol for methamphetamine dependence. Addict. 2012;107(2):361–9.

25. Shoptaw S, Huber A, Peck J, Yang X, Liu J, Jeff D, et al. Randomized, placebo-controlled trial of sertraline and contingency management for the treatment of methamphetamine dependence. Drug Alcohol Dep. 2006;85(1):12–8.

26. Elkashef A, Vocci F, Hanson G, White J, Wickes W, Tiihonen J. Pharmacotherapy of methamphetamine addiction: an update. Subst Abus. 2008;29(3):31–49.

27. Galloway GP, Buscemi R, Coyle JR, Flower K, Siegrist JD, Fiske LA, et al. A randomized, placebo-controlled trial of sustained-release dextroamphetamine for treatment of methamphetamine addiction. Clin Pharmacol Therapeut. 2011;89(2):276–82.

28. Grant JE, Odlaug BL, Kim SW. A double-blind, placebo-controlled study of N-acetyl cysteine plus naltrexone for methamphetamine dependence. Eur Neuropsychopharmacol. 2010;20(11):823–8.

29. Herin DV, Rush CR, Grabowski J. Agonist-like pharmacotherapy for stimulant dependence:preclinical, human laboratory, and clinical studies. Ann New York Acad Scie. 2010;1187:76–100.

30. Laqueille X, Dervaux A, El Omari F, Kanit M, Baylé FJ. Methylphenidate effective in treating amphetamine abusers with no other psychiatric disorder. Eur Psychiatry. 2005;20:456–7.

31. Simmler LD, Wandeler R, Liechti ME. Bupropion, methylphenidate, and 3,4-methylenedioxypyrovalerone antagonize methamphetamine-induced efflux of dopamine according to their potencies as dopamine uptake inhibitors: implications for the treatment of methamphetamine dependence. BMC Res Notes. 2013;6:220.

32. Tiihonen J, Kuoppasalmi K, Föhr J, Tuomola P, Kuikanmäki O, Vorma H, et al. A Comparison of Aripiprazole, Methylphenidate, and Placebo for Amphetamine Dependence. Am J Psychiatry. 2007;164:160–2.

33. Longo M, Wickes W, Smout M, Harrison S, Cahill S, White JM. Randomized controlled trial of dexamphetamine maintenance for the treatment of methamphetamine dependence. Addiction. 2010;105(1):146–54.

34. Miles SW, Sheridan J, Russell B, Kydd R, Wheeler A, Walters C, et al. Extended-release methylphenidate for treatment of amphetamine/methamphetamine dependence: a randomized, double-blind, placebo-controlled trial. Addiction. 2013;108(7):1279–86.

35. Pérez-Mañá C, Castells X, Torrens M, Capellà D, Farre M. Efficacy of psychostimulant drugs for amphetamine abuse ordependence. Cochrane Database Syst Rev. 2013;9:CD009695.

36. Zanis DA, McLellan AT, Cnaan RA, Randall M. Reliability and validity of the Addiction Severity Index with a homeless sample. J Subst Abuse Treat. 1994;11(6):541–8.

37. Hendriks VM, Kaplan CD, van Limbeek J, Geerlings P. The Addiction Severity Index: reliability and validity in a Dutch addict population. J Subst Abuse Treat. 1989;6(2):133–41.

38. Mokri A, Ekhtiari H, Edalati H, Ganjgahi H. Relationship between Degree of Craving and different Dimensions of Addiction Severity in Heroin Intravenous Users. Iranian J Psychiatry Clin Psychol. 2008;14(3):298–306.

39. Ekhtiari H, Mokri A, Edalati H, Safaei H, Jannati A, Razzaghi ME. Designing and evaluation of reliability and validity of a visual cue – induced craving assessment task for intravenous heroin users. Eur Psychiatry. 2007;22 (Supplement 1(0)):S186–7.

40. Steer RA, Clark DA, Beck AT, Ranieri WF. Common and specific dimensions of self-reported anxiety and depression: the BDI-II versus the BDI-IA. Behav Res Ther. 1999;37:183–90.

41. Solhi H, Jamilian HR, Kazemifar AM, Javaheri J, Rasti Barzaki A. Methylphenidate vs. resperidone in treatment of methamphetamine dependence: A clinical trial. Saudi Pharmaceut J. 2014;22(3):191–4.

42. White R. Dexamphetamine substitution in the treatment of amphetamine abuse: an initial investigation. Addiction. 2000;95:229–38.

43. Sandoval V, Riddle EL, Hanson GR, Fleckenstein AE. Methylphenidate Alters Vesicular Monoamine Transport and Prevents Methamphetamine-Induced Dopaminergic Deficits. J Pharmacol Exp Ther. 2003;304(3):1181–7.

44. Rothman RB, Baumann MH, Dersch CM, Romero DV, Rice KC, Carroll FI, et al. Amphetamine-type central nervous system stimulants release

norepinephrine more potently than they release dopamine and serotonin. Synapse. 2001;39(1):32–41.

45. Hannestad J, Gallezot J, Planeta-Wilson B, Lin S, Williams W, van Dyck CH, et al. Clinically relevant doses of methylphenidate significantly occupy norepinephrine transporters in humans in vivo. Biol Psychiatry. 2010;68(9):854–60.

46. Konstenius M, Jayaram-Lindström N, Beck O, Franck J. Sustained release methylphenidate for the treatment of ADHD in amphetamine abusers: a pilot study. Drug Alcohol Depend. 2010;108(1-2):130–3.

25

Challenges of access to medicine and the responsibility of pharmaceutical companies

Saeed Ahmadiani and Shekoufeh Nikfar[*]

Abstract

The right to health as a basic human right- and access to medicine as a part of it- have been a matter of attention for several decades. Also the responsibilities of different parties- particularly pharmaceutical companies- in realization of this right has been emphasized by World Health Organization. This is while many companies find no incentive for research and development of medicines related to rare diseases. Also some legal structures such as "patent agreements" clearly cause huge difficulties for access to medicine in many countries. High prices of brand medicine and no legal production of generics can increase the catastrophic costs- as well as morbidity-mortality of medication in lower income countries. Here we evidently review the current challenges in access to medicine and critically assess its legal roots. How societies/governors can make the pharmaceutical companies responsible is also discussed to have a look on possible future and actions that policy makers- in local or global level- can take.

Keywords: Access to medicine, Pharmaceuticals, Pharmaceutical companies, Human rights

Background

Responsibilities of pharmaceutical companies with regard to human rights have been matter of debates for many years. In August 2008, the Secretary-General of United Nations published a report which mentioned that over 2 billion people all over the world do not have sufficient access to essential medicine [1]. The message was clear, two billion people (about one third of the world population at the time) were in danger of death or major harm to their health as a result of the lack of access to essential medicines, either because of not enough attention from pharmaceutical companies, or because the state parties could not fulfill their obligation in regards to essential medicines.

Now after a couple of years it might be still a question that, what the responsibilities of different parties (such as pharmaceutical companies, governments, NGOs, world organizations etc.) are for solving this problem, and how we can assure that the realization of access to essential medicines takes place? This paper will discuss these questions briefly from a human rights perspective, and we will try to find and summarize some legal solutions for controversies and complexities in this field.

What are the roots of the problem?

Huge part of barriers in access to medicine returns to patent law and its consequences. Although patent law generally has been used for centuries [2], the manifestation of TRIPS agreement in 1994 turned it to a new form of challenge. This agreement force the World Trade Organization (WTO) members to take action for protecting intellectual property rights, which entails that any patented product should be produced, imported, sold or used under permission of the patent owner [3]. This includes medicine, thus the production of each medicine is initiated with a period of monopoly in the market with the highest possible price. In this period there will be no low price generic drugs in the market after signing the agreement by one state (for those drugs which are still under patent), and hence, patients should provide the expensive branded medicine either out of pocket or by using their insurance.

* Correspondence: shekoufeh.nikfar@gmail.com
Department of Pharmacoeconomics and Pharmaceutical Administration, Faculty of Pharmacy, Tehran University of Medical Sciences, 16Azar St, Tehran, Iran

The problem will rise up when it comes to a developing country where population not only have lower economic status, but also lower health status and higher needs to medicine. According to WHO, life expectancy in developed countries was 1.7 fold higher than developing countries in 2002, showing a 32-years gap in life expectancy between these societies [4]. Also, data shows that infectious diseases such as TB have a negative relationship with GDP per capita of the country [5] (also see Fig 1). These health measures make it obvious that in developing countries there is a higher need to medical technologies which many of them are under patent. At the same time, health insurance coverage is usually poor in these countries and patients often have to pay for the branded medicine out of their own pockets. Evidence shows that the lower the national income is, the higher the out of pocket share of health spending will be [6]. With higher needs and lower economic ability, providing

branded medicine will result in a large load of expenditure for states, catastrophic expenditures for patients [7] and increase of mortality and/or morbidity because of low access to medicine (see Fig 2).

Moreover, if any TRIPS member produce or provide an under patent product, the company can sue the member state and ask for a fine compensating the market loss. This was the case for South Africa in late 90s, when giant pharmaceutical companies such as GlaxoSmithKline filed a lawsuit to the Pretoria High Court against the South African government because of importation of generic anti-retroviral medicine- for treating HIV/AIDS endemic situation [8]. The Pharmaceutical Association was using this law to save their presence in

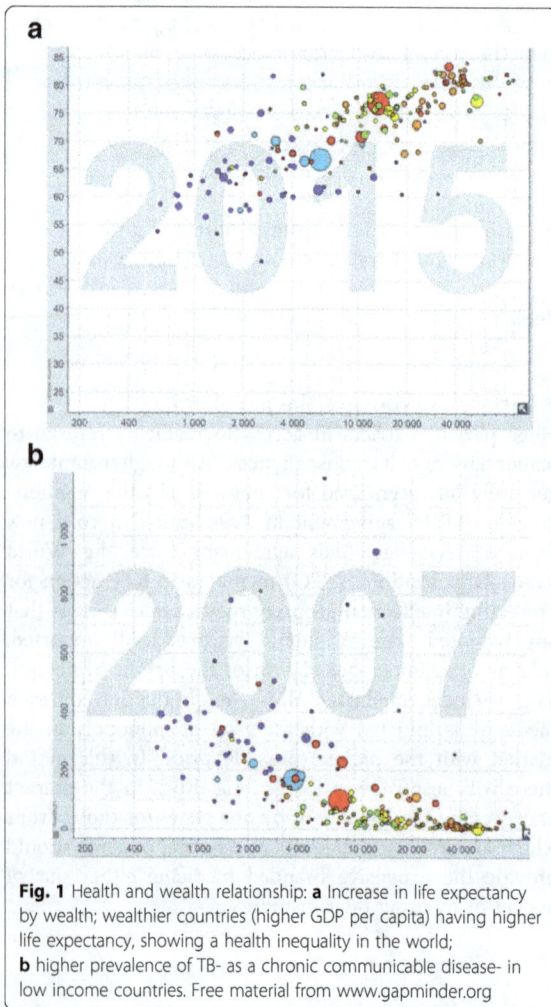

Fig. 1 Health and wealth relationship: **a** Increase in life expectancy by wealth; wealthier countries (higher GDP per capita) having higher life expectancy, showing a health inequality in the world; **b** higher prevalence of TB- as a chronic communicable disease- in low income countries. Free material from www.gapminder.org

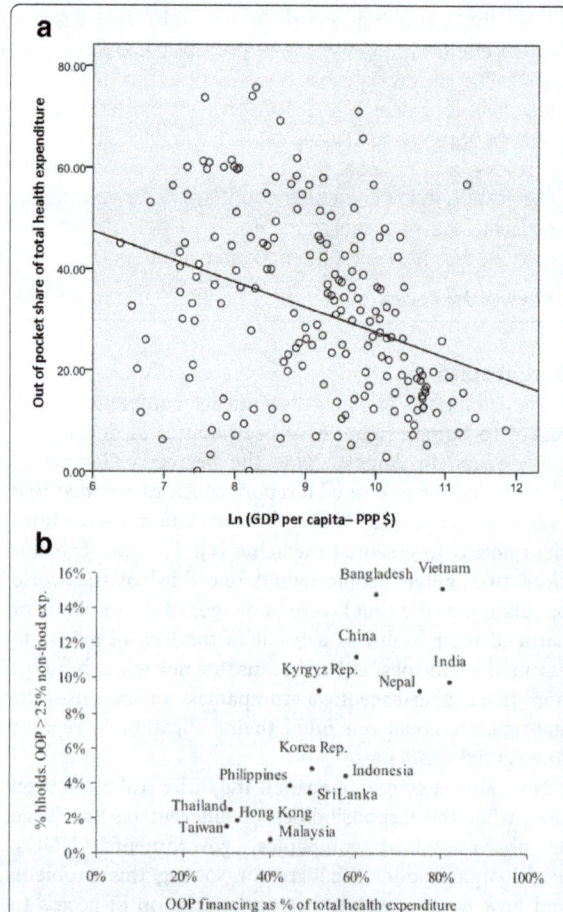

Fig. 2 Lower health insurance services in lower income countries: **a** decrease in out-of-pocket (OOP) share of health expenditures by increase in GDP per capita (Data from World Bank [21, 22]); **b** increase in catastrophic expenditures by increase of OOP share; plot from Van Doorslaer et al. [7] (with copy right permission from John Wiley and Sons). These figures depict that lower income can result in lower health insurance services (higher out-of-pocket expenditure for health) and hence higher incidence of catastrophic expenditures consequently, which can cause an inequality in health and social gaps between populations

the pharmaceutical market of South Africa. However, there were millions of people suffering from HIV/AIDS while could not afford the original brand medicine and the South African state was trying to find a way to guarantee their health. After three years of clashes, the court overruled the patent law in the case and recognized the right to health as a basic human right for the South African patients. Consequently big pharma companies withdrew the lawsuit and started negotiations for dropping the price of original brand to come into the South Africa market [9].

Although this was a happy-ending experience, no country can be sure that the court will give the right to the member state again and hence, in many cases the government prefer to import the branded medicine from the beginning, even if it is not affordable for a part of population.

The TRIPS agreement is not the end of story. Less than a decade after the first TRIPS agreement, United States started to make bilateral trade agreements with other TRIPS members to expand and deepen the TRIPS agreement. These agreements (generally known as TRIPS-plus) decrease the flexibilities which were anticipated for some exceptional situations- particularly for developing countries- and increase the duration of patents in some cases. Until now, there are 20 countries that accepted such an agreement with US [10], which surprisingly 80 % of them are developing countries. If we consider the economic power of United States and its role in pharmaceutical industry, then it is not hard to guess about the effect of these agreements on the access to medicine in the subjected developing countries.

Besides the patent law and TRIPS-plus agreements, there is always a bias towards maintenance medicine-the controlling medicine for chronic conditions. Pharmaceutical companies have a substantial desire in developing drugs which are focused on disease areas within the developed world, such as chronic diseases and cancer treatments, not only because of high prevalence, but also because these drugs are often used in long term, which means a long term costumer for the company, particularly if one can take the advantage of patent. As an instance, a new anti-hypertensive medicine not only has more costumers, also most of the costumers have to use the medicine until the end of their lives, let's say 10–15 years in average. On the other side, giant pharmaceutical companies are less interested in modern anti-parasites, antibiotics and other medicines related to acute conditions, while these medicines are more needed in developing countries and this bias cause a lower access to medicine- and a lower health in result-in these low income areas.

The mentioned bias also can be seen against "rare diseases" (i.e., diseases with prevalence less than 1/2000),

even if they might be chronic. This inattentiveness to some specific diseases forms when the disease is rare or restricted to some particular areas and population, hence pharmaceutical companies find no incentive to invest on research and development of new medicine specified for a limited population, specifically when there is a large possibility that the state does not have the ability to pay for the medicine and the company should provide it underprice.

To see it evidently, from over 1500 drugs which have been approved during 1975–2004, only about 1 % of them were related to the diseases which are known as neglected [11], while over 10 % of global burden of disease is caused by these diseases [12]. This is also reflected in 10/90 phenomena: only 10 % of R&D expenditures is related to problems of 90 % of world population [13]. These facts clearly show an insufficient attention from pharmaceutical companies to this field of health needs. According to WHO, already over one billion people are affected by neglected tropical diseases [14], which may considerably decrease both the life expectancy and quality of life. By considering the higher rate of these diseases in low income countries, it is to say that this situation can cause a huge discrimination between high and low income societies, not only in terms of health, but also economically as a consequence of low health level.

All these modern structures, from patents and TRIPS-plus agreements to bias in pharma industry, cause a decrease or imbalance in access to medicine, and hence an inequity in health between and within the communities, which can be considered as a breach of human rights as will be explained further.

Human rights and the role of pharmaceutical industry

Previously in 2000, United Nations established eight goals as Millennium Development Goals and 190 countries agreed to help to achieve these goals by 2015. At least three of these goals- reduction of child mortality, improve of maternal health, and combating HIV/AIDS, malaria, and other diseases- are extremely dependent on accessible and affordable medicine. Even the role of pharmaceuticals is clearly mentioned in the millennium declaration: "Develop a global partnership for development- In co-operation with pharmaceutical companies, provide access to affordable, essential drugs in developing countries; proportion of population with access to affordable essential drugs on a sustainable basis" [15].

The strong influence of pharmaceutical companies on accessibility and affordability of medicine is clear. But should they be responsible for the realization of access to medicines?

As first point, health is considered as a basic human right, as it is stated in article 12 of International Covenant on Economic, Social and Cultural Rights, "the States Parties to the present Covenant recognize the right of everyone to the enjoyment of the highest attainable standard of physical and mental health" [16]. And we should beware that, according to UN, the responsibilities which are stated in human rights declaration are not solely an obligation for the member states, but the private sector is equally subjected to human rights responsibilities [17].

Moreover, investing on modern chronic disease and neglecting other diseases such as tropical infections (e.g., leishmaniasis), is clearly inequitable and can increase the rich-poor gap. This socioeconomic gap is an issue to be noticed and should be prevented, which is not possible without serious contribution of pharmaceutical companies. One may mention the super costly research and development in the field of rare disease, but in response we should look at the both sides; costs and revenues. Although it is said that pharmaceutical companies spend around $60 billion for research and development, it should be also mentioned that the annual revenue of these companies exceeds 300 billion [18], which easily covers the cost of R&D. With such an income, it is just an insincere gesture to talk about the R&D costs as a reason of keeping high price for the products.

But even with accepting all these responsibilities, what or who can make the pharmaceutical companies responsible and to make commitment to human rights?

Making big pharma responsible: legal and social capacities

Since start of these debates, there have been several suggestions for achieving accountability of pharmaceutical companies. These suggestions are mainly classified in two groups of top-down (interventions from governments and international regulators) and bottom-up (pressure from NGOs and social organizations).

Top-down

As mentioned before, highest attainable standard of health, which includes access to essential medicines, is one of the human rights that states should ensure. Legally, governments that have signed the international treaties of human rights are expected to prevent violation of human rights even. Legislative bodies can play a major role in steering the activities of big pharma and prevent such violations. At first glance, governments might not be able to restrict the pricing directly and/or their trade activities since it is against WTO regulations and TRIPS agreement. Moreover, it is too complicated to define a definite crime in this field, in a way that no one can escape from the law, and at the same time not

making barriers for the enjoyment of the right of free trading. But in the wide field of pharmaceutical trading, there are still other ways to make appropriate restrictions, directly and indirectly.

Currently the most applicable way is antitrust or competition law, which protect the presence of competition in the market and fight against corruptions. Many patent owner may find it tempting to have the monopoly of market and be the only brand even after patent expiration. Hence these companies may form secret agreements with generic producers to postpone the entrance of low price generic medicine into the market. Antitrust law bans any act that big pharma companies can take to stop other companies from producing the generic products after patent expiration. By saving the competition, this law guarantee the decrease of price in a reasonable time and hence, increase of affordability of the medicine. This way can be very effective for medicines which their patent is already expired or is going to expire in near future.

Another important step to solve the patent problem was taken by WTO itself with Doha Declaration in 2001. After all debates and discussions on how TRIPS agreement can harm human population health, finally member states decided to make an escape way for emergency situations by waiving the strict TRIPS agreement: "the gravity of the public health problems afflicting many developing and least-developed countries, especially those resulting from HIV/AIDS, tuberculosis, malaria and other epidemic... the TRIPS Agreement does not and should not prevent Members from taking measures to protect public health" [19]. It also clearly mentions the assuming public health problems in paragraph 5 (c): "Each Member has the right to determine what constitutes a national emergency or other circumstances of extreme urgency, it being understood that public health crises, including those relating to HIV/AIDS, tuberculosis, malaria and other epidemics, can represent a national emergency or other circumstances of extreme urgency" [19]. Unfortunately these efforts were not much of success and major countries such as United States, Japan, Switzerland and Australia did not make any domestic legislative implementation for TRIPS Waiver while over 100 countries had accepted to do so [20].

There are also indirect ways for states to control big pharma and steer them to accept more responsibility for human rights. As an instance, it is suggested to mandate a certain level of transparency for pricing and its details, so that everyone will know if the price is logical in comparison to the costs. Although it seems to be an applicable effective approach, it has its own shortages. First of all, it can harm the market and competition since it reveals companies secrets and can be abused by other companies. Also, it can be misinterpreted by people and the media, since nobody knows which margin of interest is fair enough for the company, particularly by considering next projects and future investment programs. Similar suggestion may be made for disclosure of exact amount of donations and also the tax benefit resulted from this donation. In this way the company clearly shows their social contribution and the amount of effort they make to increase accessibility. This method might be more applicable; it is less problematic and makes more sense to public opinion.

All in all, while these top-down approaches might be helpful, the legal complexities have resulted in a long lasting pause in the current situation.

Bottom-up

The other group of actions are known as bottom-up, which means actions that are taken by society (as individuals or NGOs) to control and/or affect pharmaceutical companies.

The best known- and probably most effective- project in this area is "Access to Medicine Index". This index was innovated and introduced in 2008 by Bill & Melinda Gates Foundation and measures the amount of activities of biggest pharmaceutical manufacturers in means of increasing access to essential medicine all around the world [21]. In this index 7 fields of activities have been considered with different weights: "Pricing, manufacturing and distributing" with 25 %, "research and development" with 20 %, "Patent and licencing" with 15 % and "general access to medicine management", "market influence", "capacity building", "product donations" each with 10 % share of scores. Each of these fields are assessed based on 4 main criteria: commitment, transparency, performance and innovation. As an instance, Gilead Science Inc. had the highest score in the two fields of "pricing" and "patents" in recent years. This is probably because of increasing access to its new anti-viral medicine sofosbovir (Sovaldi) which has been provided 99 % off price for developing countries [22]. Although this medicine is provided with about $1200 per pill in US [23], Gilead allowed generic licencing in developing countries so that the medicine can be accessible in very low price and save lives of millions of people with hepatitis C, as well as its benefit from the market. Other examples also can be seen in the index report which clearly shows the improvements and lacks of the companies' policies.

At first glance it might be a simple index like thousands of other scientific measures. However, looking closer at the index one can notice that it is effectively encouraging big pharma to increase the access to their products in their own way and without any legislative obligation. Hogerzeil et al. showed that average score of these big pharmaceutical companies increased since 2010 to 2012 and we can be hopeful about continue of this increasing trend [24]. The reasons that may explain this positive effect, first is the attempts of companies to improve their image in the public opinion, which might be a promotion for their products and attract direct costumers. And second, the effect of improving public image on share values and convincing more shareholders to invest on the company. However, this encouraging effect is still a theory and not proven yet, particularly in long term. By looking at the index for 2014 we can see a decreasing trend for most of the companies since 2012. It seems that even if it is effective, it cannot be a guarantee for improvement of access to medicine overtime.

In addition, this measure potentially can be used as a precise definition for crimes, and to make legal actions for controlling pharmaceutical companies. As a broad example, we can imagine a law that mandates having a minimum score of Access to Medicine Index, and companies which get lower score will be penalized. In this way Access to Medicine Score is not just an honor which can be neglected by some companies or in some situations, but pharmaceutical companies have to try for it. This can be an answer to our question about "definition of crime" which mentioned before.

Other bottom-up approaches are also using the same trick. "Naming and shaming" by NGOs and world organizations can be an effective way, using "punishment" instead of encouragement. In this way, campaigns and movements can be used to openly blame the companies which explicitly avoid helping for improving access to medicine, so that the public opinion and media stream may make a pressure to these companies for accepting their responsibilities.

Current legal challenges and future efforts to make

Although it is 2015 and at least main parts of this problem were supposed to be solved by now, there is still a big capacity to change the situation. Having only some ethical guidelines and declarations after all these years shows a hanging situation and can be a clue that we need a break in the current framework to make a new paradigm. This new paradigm might be a different point of view in assumptions and philosophical theories that are being used as basis of world legal systems.

As an example, currently human rights are still interpreted from its conventional point of view. Human rights were initially established to protect mainly 'human' from the 'state', and majority of laws gave the originality to individuals and their freedom. But during these decades there has been a shift in the society to where the state does not have its previous major role in many areas, and non-state actors like pharmaceutical companies have started to play a more important role, which means there is a need to protect individuals from other 'individuals' who are free to make inequitable conditions- such as inequity in medicine production or pricing. Despite all these shortages and complications, there are no legal obligations for the private sector to obey human rights, i.e., the human rights are not 'legally binding' directly to pharmaceutical companies. The new legal framework is to find new ways to guarantee the proper contribution of these companies in human rights.

As a legal suggestion, an international effort can be made to oblige big pharma to sign the human rights treaties. By this mean, the enquiry of pharmaceutical companies and the assessment of their practice will be legally possible by international organizations. The first question will be if pharmaceutical companies are legally allowed to sign the treaty. One may refer to International Covenant on Economic Social and Cultural Rights (ICESR) article 8, where trade unions are known as legal persons in this law to have the right, and by definition, we may conclude that legal persons may be addressed to legal obligations as well as legal rights. Following this interpretation, even if pharmaceutical companies are not able to sign the covenants themselves, their professional union or association-either international or domestic- can be obliged to sign treaties and accept the commitments to provide affordable and accessible medicine for all disease categories.

Moreover, one of the major problems with current paradigm is the lack of incentives for states to make these new regulations, either because they do not see the access to medicine as their own problem, or because they are taking the advantage of the taxes coming from these pharmaceuticals, and restricting them is equal to losing part of this huge tax. Hence, governments might not be much interested in these types of regulations even though it is against their commitments to human rights covenant. Drawing on this point of view, world authorities may be able to establish new laws not only for controlling the trade and accountability of manufacturers, but also for more contribution of states. If member states be known as main responsible (instead of pharmaceutical companies) they will have enough incentives to find new ways to make pharmaceutical companies to co-operate or to compensate their share of contribution.

Legitimacy of TRIPS-plus agreements also can be criticized as a barrier for realization of human rights. According to Article 41 the Vienna Convention on the Law of Treaties, although having unilateral or multilateral agreements or modifications within members is allowed, it should be only in a way which does not affect the enjoyment of other members of treaty from the enjoyment of their rights as defined in the treaty. In our case of pharmaceutical companies, when United States- as one of the major owners of pharmaceutical companies- makes TRIPS-plus agreements and expand the patent duration in several countries- while some of them own big generic producers, and many of them are big generic consumers- it can be against the enjoyment of other member states, either those which want to buy generic products, or those that want to export generic products to subjected developing countries. Hence these agreements are not just restricting for the countries signing them, but also for many other TRIPS members.

In addition to these flaws of TRIPS-plus agreement, it can be also criticized in a human rights point of view that suggestion of such an agreement to developing countries- while it is predictable that the country will have big problems in purchase of medicine- is against human rights.

To sum up, the most important actions to take are making pharmaceutical unions or associations responsible by signing human right treaties, increasing the responsibility and contribution of member states and making TRIPS-plus agreements less effective.

Conclusion

Health is a basic human right and access to medicine is a basic tool to ensure health. This right and its tools are facing major issues in the world. Pharmaceutical companies play a substantial role in increasing the access to medicines in order to guarantee health.

Till now and despite all shortages and difficulties, remarkable efforts have been made. Major pharmaceutical companies are helping billions of dollars by donating medicine to poor population or patients with neglected disease. WHO and human rights committee of United Nations also make several heads-up every year and seek new ways to improve the situation of access to medicine in co-operation with NGOs and governmental organizations. Also states have tried to create a better circumstance for increasing the availability and affordability of medicine. However, there is still a substantial need for improvements, as well as the notable potential for making changes.

More realistic accountability of different parties- including both states and big pharmaceutical companies- is the main necessity in this way. Without this accountability, there will be no real and long term change in the situation and every step would work as a temporary painkiller, but not as a cure.

Also it should be considered that this accountability cannot be realized automatically or through ethical advice, but needs serious legal acts in terms of defining crimes, binding state and non-state parties to increase their co-operation and to make a safe way for access to generic medicine in developing countries by restricting TRIPS and TRIPS-plus agreements. With all these efforts we can be hopeful that delayed goals for increasing health and decreasing inequity will be achieved.

Competing interests
The study had no external funding source and any conflict of interest is disclaimed.

Authors' contributions
Both authors read and approved the final manuscript.

References
1. The right to health-Note by the Secretary-General. [http://www.who.int/medicines/areas/human_rights/A63_263.pdf]
2. Hulme E. History of the patent system under the prerogative and at common law. Law Q Rev. 1896;46:141–54.
3. A more detailed overview of the TRIPS agreement. [https://www.wto.org/english/tratop_e/trips_e/intel2_e.htm]
4. The world health report 2003- shaping the future [http://www.who.int/whr/2003/chapter1/en/index2.html]
5. Graph of TB against GDP per capita [http://www.gapminder.org/world]
6. Musgrove P, Zeramdini R, Carrin G. Basic patterns in national health expenditure. Bull World Health Organ. 2002;80(2):134–46.
7. van Doorslaer E, O'Donnell O, Rannan-Eliya RP, Somanathan A, Adhikari SR, Garg CC, Harbianto D, Herrin AN, Huq MN, Ibragimova S, et al. Catastrophic payments for health care in Asia. Health Econ. 2007;16(11):1159–84.
8. Ncayiyana D. Antiretroviral therapy cannot be South Africa's first priority. CMAJ. 2001;164(13):1857–8.
9. PLM E. Drug companies should be held more accountable for their human rights responsibilities. PLoS Med. 2010;7(9):e1000344.
10. Free Trade Agreements [https://ustr.gov/trade-agreements/free-trade-agreements]
11. A needs-based pharmaceutical R&D agenda for neglected diseases [http://www.who.int/intellectualproperty/topics/research/Needs%20based%20R&D%20for%20neglected%20diseases%20Els%20Pierre%20Martine.pdf]
12. Priority Medicines for Europe and the World "A Public Health Approach to Innovation" [http://www.who.int/medicines/areas/priority_medicines/BP6_9NTD.pdf]
13. The10/90 Report onHealth Research 2003–2004 [http://announcementsfiles.cohred.org/gfhr_pub/assoc/s14789e/s14789e.pdf]
14. Global Health Observatory (GHO) data: Neglected Tropical Disease [http://www.who.int/gho/neglected_diseases/en/]
15. GOAL 8: DEVELOP A GLOBAL PARTNERSHIP FOR DEVELOPMENT [http://www.un.org/millenniumgoals/global.shtml]
16. International Covenant on Economic, Social and Cultural Right. [http://www.ohchr.org/EN/ProfessionalInterest/Pages/CESCR.aspx]
17. Human rights guidelines for pharmaceutical companies in relation to access to medicines. [http://www.ohchr.org/Documents/Issues/Health/GuidelinesForPharmaceuticalCompanies.doc]
18. Pharmaceutical Industry. Trade, foreign policy, diplomacy and health [http://www.who.int/trade/glossary/story073/en/]
19. World Trade Organization. Declaration on the TRIPS agreement and public health. Doha: World Trade Organization; 2001.
20. Pogge T, Rimmer M, Rubenstein K. Access to essential medicines: public health and international law. In: Incentives for Global Public Health. edn. New York: Cambridge University Press; 2009:12.
21. What Is The Index? [http://www.accesstomedicineindex.org/what-index]
22. Gilead offers Egypt new hepatitis C drug at 99 % discount [http://www.reuters.com/article/us-hepatitis-egypt-gilead-sciences-idUSBREA2K1VF20140321]
23. Sofosbuvir. Drug information. In: UpToDate. Edited by Post TW. Waltham, MA: UpToDate; 2016.
24. Hogerzeil HV, Iyer JK, Urlings L, Prasad TSB. Is the pharmaceutical industry improving with regard to access to essential medicines? Lancet Glob Health. 2014;2(3):e139–40.

Permissions

The contributors of this book come from diverse backgrounds, making this book a truly international effort. This book will bring forth new frontiers with its revolutionizing research information and detailed analysis of the nascent developments around the world.

We would like to thank all the contributing authors for lending their expertise to make the book truly unique. They have played a crucial role in the development of this book. Without their invaluable contributions this book wouldn't have been possible. They have made vital efforts to compile up to date information on the varied aspects of this subject to make this book a valuable addition to the collection of many professionals and students.

This book was conceptualized with the vision of imparting up-to-date information and advanced data in this field. To ensure the same, a matchless editorial board was set up. Every individual on the board went through rigorous rounds of assessment to prove their worth. After which they invested a large part of their time researching and compiling the most relevant data for our readers.

The editorial board has been involved in producing this book since its inception. They have spent rigorous hours researching and exploring the diverse topics which have resulted in the successful publishing of this book. They have passed on their knowledge of decades through this book. To expedite this challenging task, the publisher supported the team at every step. A small team of assistant editors was also appointed to further simplify the editing procedure and attain best results for the readers.

Apart from the editorial board, the designing team has also invested a significant amount of their time in understanding the subject and creating the most relevant covers. They scrutinized every image to scout for the most suitable representation of the subject and create an appropriate cover for the book.

The publishing team has been an ardent support to the editorial, designing and production team. Their endless efforts to recruit the best for this project, has resulted in the accomplishment of this book. They are a veteran in the field of academics and their pool of knowledge is as vast as their experience in printing. Their expertise and guidance has proved useful at every step. Their uncompromising quality standards have made this book an exceptional effort. Their encouragement from time to time has been an inspiration for everyone.

The publisher and the editorial board hope that this book will prove to be a valuable piece of knowledge for researchers, students, practitioners and scholars across the globe.

List of Contributors

Anchal Sankhyan and Pravin K Pawar
Chitkara College of Pharmacy, Chitkara University, Chandigarh-Patiala Highway, Rajpura, Patiala, Punjab 140401, India

Nazila Gholipour
Department of Radiopharmacy, Faculty of Pharmacy, Tehran University of Medical Sciences, P.O. Box: 14155–6451, Tehran, Iran

Amir Reza Jalilian, Fariba Johari-Daha, Kamal Yavari and Ali Reza Khanchi
Radiation Application Research School, Nuclear Science and Technology Research Institute, P.O. Box: 14395–836, Tehran, Iran

Ali Khalaj
Department of Medicinal Chemistry, Faculty of Pharmacy, Tehran University of Medical Sciences, P.O. Box: 14155–6451, Tehran, Iran

Omid Sabzevari
Depatment of Toxicology and Pharmacology, School of Pharmacy, Tehran University of Medical Sciences, P.O. Box: 14176–14411, Tehran, Iran

Mehdi Akhlaghi
Research Center for Nuclear Medicine, Tehran University of Medical Sciences, P.O. Box: 14117–13137, Tehran, Iran

Mohammad Mahdi Rezaee, Mohammad Taghi Kazemi, Saeed Gharooee, Elham Yazdani and Hoda Gharooee
Department of Pharmacology, Babol University of Medical Sciences, Babol, Iran

Mohammad Reza Shiran
Department of Pharmacology, Mazandaran University of Medical Sciences, Sari, Iran

Ali Akbar Moghadamnia and Sohrab Kazemi
Department of Pharmacology, Babol University of Medical Sciences, Babol, Iran
Cellular and Molecular Biology Research Centre, Babol University of Medical Sciences, Babol, Iran

Fatemeh Yousefbeyk, Ahmad Reza Gohari, Fereshteh Golfakhrabadi and Gholamreza Amin
Department of Pharmacognosy, Faculty of Pharmacy and Medicinal Plants Research Centre, Tehran University of Medical Sciences, Tehran 14155-6451, Iran

Zeinabsadat Hashemighahderijani, Sayed Nasser Ostad and Mohamad Hossein Salehi Sourmaghi
Department of Toxicology, Pharmacology and Nanotechnology Research Centre, Tehran University of Medical Sciences, Tehran 14155-6451, Iran

Mohsen Amini
Department of Medicinal Chemistry, Faculty of Pharmacy, Tehran University of Medical Sciences, Tehran 14155-6451, Iran

Hossein Jamalifar
Department of Drug and Food Control, Faculty of Pharmacy and Pharmaceutical Quality Assurance Research Centre, Tehran University of Medical Sciences, Tehran 14155-6451, Iran

Faezeh Vahdati Hassani and Vahideh Naseri
School of Pharmacy, Mashhad University of Medical Sciences, Mashhad, Iran

Bibi Marjan Razavi
Targeted Drug Delivery Research Centre, Department of Pharmacodynamics and Toxicology, School of Pharmacy, Mashhad University of Medical Sciences, Mashhad, Iran

Soghra Mehri and Hossein Hosseinzadeh
Pharmaceutical Research Center, Department of Pharmacodynamics and Toxicology, School of Pharmacy, Mashhad University of Medical Sciences, Mashhad, Iran

Khalil Abnous
Pharmaceutical Research Center, Department of Medicinal Chemistry and Department of Biotechnology, Mashhad University of Medical Sciences, Mashhad, Iran

Hamid Nadri, Alireza Moradi and Amirhossein Sakhteman
Department of Medicinal Chemistry, Faculty of Pharmacy and Neurobiomedical Research Center, Shahid Sadoughi University of Medical Sciences, Yazd 8915173143, Iran

Morteza Pirali-Hamedani, Mohammad Abdollahi and Abbas Shafiee
Faculty of Pharmacy and Pharmaceutical Sciences Research Center, Tehran University of Medical Sciences, Tehran, Iran

Alireza Vahidi
Herbal Medicine Center, Shahid Sadoughi University of Medical Sciences, Yazd 8915173143, Iran

Vahid Sheibani and Ali Asadipour
Neuroscience Research Center, Kerman University of Medical Sciences, Kerman, Iran

Alireza Foroumadi
Neuroscience Research Center, Kerman University of Medical Sciences, Kerman, Iran
Drug design & Development Research Center, Tehran University of Medical Sciences, Tehran, Iran

Nouraddin Hosseinzadeh
Drug design & Development Research Center, Tehran University of Medical Sciences, Tehran, Iran

Renata Cavalcanti Carnevale, Caroline de Godoi Rezende Costa Molino, Marília Berlofa Visacri and Priscila Gava Mazzola
Department of Clinical Pathology, Faculty of Medical Sciences (FCM), University of Campinas (UNICAMP), Alexander Fleming, 105, 13083-881 Campinas, SP, Brazil

Patricia Moriel
Department of Clinical Pathology, Faculty of Medical Sciences (FCM), University of Campinas (UNICAMP), Alexander Fleming, 105, 13083-881 Campinas, SP, Brazil
Faculty of Pharmaceutical Sciences (FCF), University of Campinas (UNICAMP), Sérgio Buarque de Holanda, 25, 13083-859 Campinas, SP, Brazil

Zargham Sepehrizadeh and Neda Setayesh
Department of Pharmaceutical Biotechnology and Pharmaceutical Biotechnology Research Center, School of Pharmacy, Tehran University of Medical Sciences, Tehran 1417614411, Iran

Negar Mottaghi-Dastjerdi and Mohammad Soltany-Rezaee-Rad
Department of Pharmaceutical Biotechnology and Pharmaceutical Biotechnology Research Center, School of Pharmacy, Tehran University of Medical Sciences, Tehran 1417614411, Iran
Pharmaceutical Sciences Research Center, Sari School of Pharmacy, Mazandaran University of Medical Sciences, Sari, Iran

Gholamreza Roshandel
Golestan Research Center of Gastroenterology and Hepatology, Golestan University of Medical Sciences, Golestan, Iran

Farzaneh Ebrahimifard
Department of General Surgery, School of Medicine, Shahid Beheshti University of Medical Sciences, Tehran, Iran

Saad Ahmed Ali Jadoo
United Nations University-International Institute for Global Health (UNU-IIGH), Kuala Lumpur, Malaysia
International Centre for Case-Mix and Clinical Coding (ITCC), University Kebangsaan Malaysia Medical Centre, Jalan Yaacob Latiff, 56000 Cheras, Kuala Lumpur, Malaysia.

Syed Mohamed Aljunid, Amrizal Muhammad Nur and Zafar Ahmed
International Centre for Case-Mix and Clinical Coding (ITCC), University Kebangsaan Malaysia Medical Centre, Jalan Yaacob Latiff, 56000 Cheras, Kuala Lumpur, Malaysia

Dexter Van Dort
Pharmacy of Hospital University Kebangsaan Malaysia Medical Centre, Jalan Yaacob Latiff, 56000 Cheras, Kuala Lumpur, Malaysia

Masoumeh Alipour
School of Chemistry, University College of Science, University of Tehran, P.O.
Box 14155–6455, Tehran, Iran

Mehdi Khoobi, Saeed Fallah-Benakohal, Seyedeh Farnaz Ghasemi-Niri, Alireza Foroumadi and Abbas Shafiee
Department of Medicinal Chemistry, Faculty of Pharmacy and Pharmaceutical Sciences Research Center, Tehran University of Medical Sciences, Tehran 14176, Iran

Saeed Emami
Department of Medicinal Chemistry and Pharmaceutical Sciences Research Center, Faculty of Pharmacy, Mazandaran University of Medical Sciences, Sari, Iran

Mohammad Abdollahi
Department of Toxicology and Pharmacology, Pharmaceutical Sciences Research Center, Faculty of Pharmacy, Tehran University of Medical Sciences, Tehran 14176, Iran

Muhammad A Malana and Rubab Zohra
Chemistry Department, Bahauddin Zakarya University, Multan, Pakistan

Naga Raju Chamarthi, Kuruva Chandra Sekhar, Rasheed Syed and Madhava Golla
Department of Chemistry, Sri Venkateswara University, Tirupati 517 502, India

Jyothi Kumar MV
Department of Biotechnology, Sri Venkateswara University, Tirupati 517 502, India

Nanda Kumar Yellapu
Biomedical informatics Center, Vector Control Research Centre, Indian Council of Medical Research, Puducherry 605006, India

Appa Rao Chippada
Department of Biochemistry, Sri Venkateswara University, Tirupati 517 502, India

Niayesh Mohebbi, Mohammadreza Javadi, Mojtaba Mojtahedzadeh and Kheirollah Gholami
Department of Clinical Pharmacy, Faculty of Pharmacy, Tehran University of Medical Sciences, Tehran, Iran

Alireza Khoshnevisan, Soheil Naderi and Sina Abdollahzade
Department of Neurosurgery, Tehran University of Medical Sciences, Tehran, Iran

Jamshid Salamzadeh
Department of Clinical Pharmacy, Shahid Beheshti University of Medical Sciences, Tehran, Iran

Mehdi Farhoudi, Mahdi Najafi-Nesheli, Mazyar Hashemilar, Behzad Baradaran, Aliakbar Taheraghdam, Daryoush Savadi-Oskouei and Homayoun Sadeghi-Bazargani
Neuroscience Research Center (NSRC), Imam Reza Hospital, Tabriz University of Medical Sciences, Tabriz, Iran

Ata Mahmoodpoor
Department of Anesthesiology and critical care medicine, Imam Reza Hospital, Tabriz University of Medical Sciences, Tabriz, Iran

Elyar Sadeghi-hokmabadi, Hosein Akbari, Reza Rikhtegar and Ehsan Sharifipour
Student Research Committee, Tabriz University of Medical Sciences, Tabriz, Iran

Seyed Behzad Jazayeri
Students' Scientific Research Center, Tehran University of Medical Sciences, Tehran, Iran Department of Medicinal Chemistry, Faculty of Pharmacy and Medicinal Plants Research Center, Tehran University of Medical Sciences, Tehran, Iran

Arash Amanlou and Massoud Amanlou
Department of Medicinal Chemistry, Faculty of Pharmacy and Medicinal Plants Research Center, Tehran University of Medical Sciences, Tehran, Iran

Naghmeh Ghanadian and Parvin Pasalar
Department of Clinical Biochemistry, Faculty of Medicine, Tehran University of Medical Sciences, Tehran, Iran

Jinho Lee, Jina Kim and Victor Sukbong Hong
Department of Chemistry, Keimyung University, Daegu 704-701, Korea

Jong-Wook Park
Department of Immunology, Keimyung University School of Medicine, Daegu 704-701, Korea

Jason C Hsu
School of Pharmacy and Institute of Clinical Pharmacy and Pharmaceutical Sciences, College of Medicine, National Cheng Kung University, No.1, Daxue Rd., East Dist., Tainan City 70101, Taiwan R.O.C.

Christine Y Lu
Department of Population Medicine, Harvard Medical School and Harvard Pilgrim Health Care Institute, Boston, MA, USA

Mohammadreza Amirsadri and Abbas Hassani
Department of Clinical Pharmacy and Pharmacy Practice, Faculty of Pharmacy and Pharmaceutical Sciences, Isfahan University of Medical Sciences, Isfahan, Iran

Fatemeh Ramezani and Hashem Rafii-Tabar
Department of Medical Physics and Biomedical Engineering, Shahid Beheshti University of Medical Sciences, Tehran, Iran

Massoud Amanlou and Mostafa Habibi
Department of Medicinal Chemistry, Faculty of Pharmacy and Pharmaceutical Sciences Research Center, Tehran University of Medical Sciences, Tehran, Iran

Radhe Shyam Bahare and Swastika Ganguly
Department of Pharmaceutical Sciences, Birla Institute of Technology, Mesra, Ranchi 835215, Jharkhand, India

Kiattawee Choowongkomon and Supaporn Seetaha
Department of Biochemistry, Faculty of Science, Kasetsart University, Bangkean, Bangkok 10900, Thailand

Priyanga Ranasinghe, Shehani Pigera and Priyadarshani Galappatthy
Department of Pharmacology, Faculty of Medicine, University of Colombo, Colombo, Sri Lanka

Prasad Katulanda and Godwin R. Constantine
Diabetes Research Unit, Department of Clinical Medicine, Faculty of Medicine, University of Colombo, Colombo, Sri Lanka

Pilar Pérez Lozano, Encarna García Montoya, Montserrat Miñarro, Josep R Ticó and Josep M Suñe Negre
Pharmacy and Pharmaceutical Technology Department, Faculty of Pharmacy, University of Barcelona, Avda Joan XXIII s/n 08028, Barcelona, Spain

Paloma Flórez Borges
Pharmacy and Pharmaceutical Technology Department, Faculty of Pharmacy, University of Barcelona, Avda Joan XXIII s/n 08028, Barcelona, Spain
Reig Jofre Group, c. Gran Capitá 6 08970, Sant Joan Despi, Barcelona, Spain

Enric Jo
Reig Jofre Group, c. Gran Capitá 6 08970, Sant Joan Despi, Barcelona, Spain

Gökçe Candan and Harun Reşit Yazgan
Industrial Engineering Department, Sakarya University, 54187 Sakarya, Turkey

Farzin Rezaei and Maryam Emami
Department of psychiatry, Kurdistan University of Medical Sciences, Sanandaj, Iran

Shakiba Zahed
Department of Health Education and Health Promotion, Faculty of Health, Isfahan University of Medical Sciences, Isfahan, Iran

Mohammad-Javad Morabbi and Mohammadhadi Farahzadi
Department of Neuroscience, School of Advanced Medical Technologies, Tehran University of Medical Sciences, Tehran, Iran

Shahin Akhondzadeh
Psychiatric ResearchCenter, Roozbeh Hospital, Tehran University of Medical Sciences, South Kargar Street, Tehran 13337, Iran

Saeed Ahmadiani and Shekoufeh Nikfar
Department of Pharmacoeconomics and Pharmaceutical Administration, Faculty of Pharmacy, Tehran University of Medical Sciences, 16Azar St, Tehran, Iran

Index

9 781632 425102